Language-Related Learning Disabilities

Language-Related Learning Disabilities

Their Nature and Treatment

by

Adele Gerber, M.A., CCC-SLP

Professor Emeritus
Department of Speech, Language, and Hearing
Temple University
Philadelphia, Pennsylvania

with invited contributors

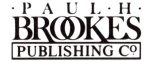

·P·A·U·L·H·
BROOKES
PUBLISHING CO

Baltimore • London • Toronto • Sydney

Paul H. Brookes Publishing Co.
P.O. Box 10624
Baltimore, Maryland 21285-0624

Typeset by Brushwood Graphics, Inc., Baltimore, Maryland.
Manufactured in the United States of America by
The Maple Press Company, York, Pennsylvania.

Library of Congress Cataloging-in-Publication Data
Gerber, Adele.
   Language-related learning disabilities : their nature and
treatment / by Adele Gerber, with invited contributors.
       p.   cm.
   Includes bibliographical references and index.
   ISBN 1-55766-053-0
   1. Language disorders in children.   2. Learning disabilities.
3. Neurolinguistics.   I. Title.
RJ496.L35G468   1992
618.92'85889071—dc20
                                                                                    92-17959
                                                                                    CIP

British Library Cataloguing-in-Publication data are available from the British Library.

Contents

About the Authors

Adele Gerber, M.A., CCC-SLP, Professor Emeritus, Department of Speech, Language, and Hearing, Temple University, Philadelphia, Pennsylvania 19118

Adele Gerber, M.A., CCC-SLP, is Professor Emeritus, Temple University, and Fellow, American Speech-Language-Hearing Association. She has had professional training, certification, and experience in the fields of education and speech-language pathology. She has taught in the elementary school classroom and has served as a speech-language pathologist in the public schools. She was a member of the faculty in the Department of Speech, Language, and Hearing at Temple University for 20 years, where she provided clinical supervision and instruction for graduate students in speech-language pathology and taught academic courses in language and learning disabilities. She has published books on preschool language intervention, language and learning disabilities, and articulation remediation. She has published journal articles and has presented numerous papers, short courses, and miniseminars at national, state, and local conferences.

Betty H. Bunce, Ph.D., LAP Educational Coordinator, Schiefelbusch Speech-Language Hearing Clinic, 2101 Haworth Hall, University of Kansas, Lawrence, Kansas 66045

Betty H. Bunce, Ph.D., has served as educational coordinator for the Language Acquisition Preschool at the University of Kansas and as courtesy assistant professor of speech-language-hearing at the University of Kansas from 1988 to the present. She holds certification in education in Colorado, Louisiana, and Kansas, and has taught in the kindergarten classroom. She also holds certification in speech-language pathology. She has conducted a preschool language program for 10 years and served as a speech-language pathologist in public schools for 2 years. She earned the first doctorate in child language at University of Kansas and has taught courses at the university in the areas of reading and language arts for prospective elementary school teachers. She has published book chapters and numerous journal articles, and has presented many papers and workshops at national, state, and local conferences.

Jack S. Damico, Ph.D., CCC-SLP, Department of Communicative Disorders, University of Southwestern Louisiana, P.O. Box 43170, Lafayette, Louisiana 70504-3170

Jack S. Damico, Ph.D., CCC-SLP, currently holds the Doris B. Hawthorne Chair in Special Education and Communicative Disorders at the University of Southwestern Louisiana. He has worked for 15 years in the area of speech-language pathology in numerous work sites including 6 years in the public schools. Dr. Damico received his M.S. in communication disorders from the University of Oklahoma Health Sciences Center and his Ph.D. in linguistics from the University of New Mexico. He has worked extensively in the areas of descriptive language assessment, naturalistic language intervention, and discourse analysis. Due to his interests with multicultural populations, Dr. Damico has worked with numerous school systems and boards of education on ways to best address language and cultural diversity issues. These consultations have included work for the Navajo Nation, the Jicarilla Apache Tribe, and six of the ten largest school districts in the United States. He has published extensively in the fields of speech-language pathology, special education, bilingualism, and applied linguistics, and has strived to make his research and writing directly relevant to the practicing school-based clinician.

Diana Kaufman, Ph.D., CCC, Department of Psychology, Temple University, Philadelphia, Pennsylvania 19122

Diana Kaufman, Ph.D., CCC, is visiting assistant professor in the Department of Psychology at Temple University, and consultant to the Infant Language Laboratory at Temple. She is also a consultant to the Temple site of the National Institute for Child Health and Human Development (NICHD) Study of Early Child Care. This national study is designed to assess the effects of early child care on children's social, emotional, and intellectual development in the first 3 years of life. Dr. Kaufman received her master's degree in speech and language pathology from Temple University in 1963. From 1963 to 1973 she worked as a speech-language pathologist in private practice. In her practice she dealt with children and adults with a variety of communication problems, including language, stuttering, and voice and articulation disorders. From 1972 to 1978 she worked at Wordsworth Academy, Fort Washington, Pennsylvania, a school for children with learning disability. While at Wordsworth Academy she served as a field supervisor for students from Temple University who were studying for their master's degrees in speech-language pathology. Dr. Kaufman received her Ph.D. from the Department of Speech, Language, and Hearing Science at Temple University in 1988. Her major area of study was psycholinguistics. Her doctoral and subsequent research have been in the area of language acquisition.

Charlann S. Simon, M.A., 5630 South Rocky Point Road, Tempe, Arizona 85283

Charlann S. Simon, M.A., began her career in education as a junior high school English and U.S. history teacher after her graduation from Northwestern University. After receiving her M.A. in speech-language pathology from the University of Kentucky in 1969, she worked in a child development center, on an educational research team, and in private and public schools. She has taught at the University of Kentucky and is an adjunct faculty member at Arizona State University. Simon is a member of ASHA's Task Force on Schools and the Publications Board. Currently she divides her time among writing, consulting with school systems in the United States and abroad, and working as an M.A. candidate in English as a Second Language at Arizona State. Her publications include journal articles, monographs, books, tests, and educational materials.

Preface

This volume is designed for the graduate student preparing to serve the needs of individuals with language-related learning disabilities as well as practitioners in such professions as regular education, special education, and speech-language pathology. It is also for reading specialists, resource room teachers, and school psychologists interested in acquiring current information relevant to the field of language-related learning disabilities. Those of us who are scholars or practitioners involved in the study and/or treatment of language-related learning disabilities require some measure of understanding of both phenomena—language and learning—each of which in its own right is daunting in its complexity. The interaction between these two areas of human function compounds the complexity.

The recent movement aimed at integrating students with special needs into the regular education system has required professionals from different disciplines to share responsibility and knowledge. As educators and as language specialists, it is incumbent on us to become conversant with key theoretical concepts and major lines of research in allied disciplines without necessarily laying claim to the depth and breadth of scholarship attained by those whose primary professional concerns lie in those domains. In the Introduction (Chapter 1) I have provided an overview of developments in the fields concerned with disabilities in learning and language, in the belief that some knowledge about their evolution would render current theory, practice, and issues more meaningful.

In writing this book, I have operated with the conviction that efforts to understand disabilities are facilitated by a foundation of at least basic knowledge about pertinent normal processes. Therefore, Part I consists of chapters devoted to those aspects of normal language and cognition considered relevant to areas of dysfunction identified and described in the literature on language/learning disabilities.

In writing such a book, the author is confronted with the challenge of meeting the needs of readers at different levels of scholarship, from varied disciplines, whose academic/professional preparation may not equally include certain bodies of information. Readers with different needs may choose to use the contents of this book with a certain degree of flexibility. For example, while we may be confident that the study of child language, its normal development, and its disorders is invariantly included in the preservice curriculum of the speech-language pathologist, we may not make such an assumption about the academic background of many classroom teachers. Therefore, to meet an assumed need, Chapter 2 presents a summary of information about the nature of language and aspects of its development that are regarded as a necessary prerequisite for further reading within this text. Although some of this material may be redundant for the language specialist, the chapter is likely to be valuable by virtue of the selection of its content as relevant to our present concerns. Furthermore, even the informed reader may find Kaufman's succinct expositions about extant theories of language acquisition illuminating, to the point of sharpening conceptualizations and focusing on outstanding issues in this area of scholarship.

Chapter 3 presents a review of research and theory about selected cognitive mechanisms, their functions in information processing, and their interaction with aspects of language, both oral and written. This material is viewed as indispensable to an understanding of the nature of information processing in education. Here, again, readers with extensive knowledge about cognitive psychology may want to skim this chapter. However, it should be considered that the material selected for inclusion here is particularly germane to aspects of disabilities discussed later in the book. In addition, all readers should benefit from the lists of questions at the conclusion of each section that highlight the pertinence of the information about normal cognitive processes to subsequent attempts to understand aspects of dysfunction.

Chapter 4 provides an overview of language processing at the level of discourse. Thus, its content represents a shift in focus from that of Chapter 2, which is essentially concerned with the phenomenon of language as an isolated entity, to the study of language use in context. That is, this chapter addresses the nature of more extended units of language, serving as a background for understanding the deficits in comprehension and expression that contribute to academic failure.

Chapter 5 is a natural extension of the foregoing material to the domain of our most immediate concern, the nature of educational discourse and the demands it places on the language-related learning abilities of the student. Bunce contrasts the contextualized language of social discourse with the decontextualized language of education in both the written and oral modalities. Patterns of classroom discourse are described from linguistic, cognitive, and pragmatic perspectives. This chapter also provides information about recent trends that view language skill development holistically and learning as a cooperative enterprise.

Part II is devoted to research and theory in the relevant fields of language-related learning disabilities. As is the case in all areas of normal processes addressed in Part I, investigations into the nature of the disabilities and the possible etiological or contributing factors have yielded a vast literature in each of the separate disciplines. Each of the chapters in this section provides information gleaned from these sources to the extent permitted by the constraints of the scope of the subject matter and space available in a multifaceted text.

Chapter 6 surveys the literature exploring possible neuropsychological factors underlying or contributing to language and learning dysfunction, in theories ranging from diversity in individual genetic predisposition to malfunction caused by maturational anomalies or brain pathology. In the last part of this chapter a report in condensed, tabulated form on recent technological research is presented. Those readers who are interested in securing more information about these investigations may consult the sources in the literature cited in the table.

Chapter 7 examines and reports on the extensive research describing various aspects of language deficits manifested by a substantial segment of the population having learning disabilities, with heavy emphasis on the relations between oral and written language, particularly reading disability. The length of this chapter is justified by the centrality of the subject matter to the topic of the book.

Chapter 8 presents an overview of deficits in those cognitive processes discussed in Chapter 3 that are reportedly characteristic of individuals with learning disabilities. It also includes information about the debilitating effects of learning disabilities on personal and social adjustment, describing some of the emotional overlays concomitant with a history of academic failure.

Part III contains material for the practitioner interested in methods of service delivery based on the foregoing research and theory. In Chapter 9, Damico and Simon address assessment of school-age children's language abilities from a functional-pragmatic perspective reflecting a synergistic view of language. Their philosophy and recommended procedures are at the leading edge of developments in the field and should provide the practitioner with valuable tools for securing educationally relevant information about the language status and needs of students as well as with the bases for decision making about intervention.

Chapter 10 focuses on the processes and products of interdisciplinary interaction among professionals engaged in providing services to students with language-related learning disabilities. The regular education initiative movement has provided impetus for increased classroom-based intervention, thereby necessitating a greater degree of collaboration between language specialists and teachers. This chapter describes a continuum of service delivery models and provides examples of a variety of approaches to such interdisciplinary intervention.

Chapter 11 offers a broad compendium of intervention procedures for children and adolescents throughout the various educational levels from preschool to secondary education. The overall approach underlying these procedures is designed to increase the probability of success in those areas that have all too frequently contributed to failure and frustration for those with language-related learning disabilities. The philosophy that has motivated the selection and/or development of many of these intervention procedures is similar, in certain aspects, to approaches just recently emerging in the literature and in the classroom—holistic language and cooperative learning. The procedures are regarded, to varying degrees, as suitable for use in the classroom and/or in small group/individual treatment of those children enrolled in a program for students with language impairment. Thus, the chapter is addressing an interdisciplinary readership.

Although, for the most part, professionals in the domains of education and language disorders have, until recently, approached language-related learning problems from different perspectives, developments in theory and research have resulted in greater current convergence among scholars and practitioners across disciplinary boundaries. The scope of information pertaining to our topic has imposed limitations on comprehensiveness and depth of scholarship in any single area. In certain chapters, content is provided essentially at the level of overview, with substantial but not exhaustive sampling of research. The criterion for selection of information for inclusion has been its relevance to the understanding of language-related learning disabilities. It is hoped that the style in which this review and analysis has been presented will be comprehensible and useful for readers of varying backgrounds but similar concerns.

Acknowledgments

I want to express my heartfelt gratitude to Betty Bunce, Jack Damico, Diana Kaufman, and Charlann Simon for their gracious and ready acceptance of my invitation to contribute their specialized scholarly expertise to this volume and for their dedication to fulfilling their commitments under extremely difficult circumstances. The content of their chapters is indispensable to the design and intent of the book, and the high caliber of their authorship adds immeasurably to its quality.

I am deeply indebted to the following people for their assistance in the preparation of this book: Katherine Butler, for her meticulous review of the manuscript and for her invaluable critique and recommendations; Melissa Behm, Sheila Fagan, and Megan Westerfeld for their extraordinary editorial competence and concern that brought to fruition the transition from manuscript to textbook format in accordance with their high professional standards; and Roslyn Udris and Ken Foye for their commendable commitment to accuracy and style of text production that have enhanced the book's quality and readability.

To my husband,
Irving Gerber,
with love and gratitude
for his patience and support
during the writing of this book

Language-Related Learning Disabilities

INTRODUCTION

Historical Trends in Learning Disabilities and Language Disabilities

1

PART I: HISTORICAL TRENDS AND
STATE OF THE ART IN LEARNING DISABILITIES

The opening sentence in a book coauthored by the present writer approximately a decade ago stated: "The field of learning disabilities has been characterized by rapid and extensive growth and by diversity of opinion about the nature of the problem, etiology, terminology, methods of assessment and treatment" (A. Gerber & Bryen, 1981, p. 1). This statement is an apt characterization of the current state of affairs at the time of writing the present volume. The number of children classified as learning disabled in almost every state in the United States exceeds those classified in other high-incidence categories (Algozzine & Ysseldyke, 1986) such as mental retardation; speech, hearing, and vision impairments; orthopedic problems; emotional disturbance; and so on (Education of the Handicapped Act Amendments of 1990, PL 101–476). The percentage of school children receiving services for learning disabilities has increased from 1.80% in 1976–1977 to 4.41% in 1987–1988. The percentage of special education students identified as having learning disabilities had risen from 21.5% in 1976–1977 to 47.0% in 1987–1988 (MacMillan, 1993). In actual numbers, enrollment of students with learning disabilities in public school special service programs increased from around 1 million to almost 2 million during that period (Doris, 1993; Will, 1986). Conversely, services to children identified as having mental retardation decreased over that time span (MacMillan, 1993). Many professionals have expressed their concern about the need to develop more valid procedures for defining, classifying, and identifying students with learning disabilities (Adelman & Taylor, 1985; Doris, 1993; Fletcher, Francis, Rourke, Shaywitz, & Shaywitz, 1993; Levine et al., 1993; MacMillan, 1993; Morris, 1993; Speece, 1993).

DEFINITION

In response to a 1984 survey of professionals' views about significant issues in the learning disabilities field, 59% noted lack of consensus about definition of the term *learning disabilities* as a fundamental concern (Adelman & Taylor, 1985). Different definitions have been formulated and advocated by various agencies and organizations over the years. The following definitions exemplify efforts to refine the characterization of "learning disabilities" during the period extending from the mid-1970s to the end of the 1980s and reflect some of the major shifts in the evolution of defining concepts and criteria.

Federal legislation passed in the 1970s included an early definition of learning disabilities:

> Individuals with specific learning disabilities are those who have a disorder in one or more of the basic psychological processes involved in understanding or in using language, spoken or written, which may manifest itself in an imperfect ability to listen, think, speak, read, write, spell, or do mathematical calculations. The term includes such conditions as perceptual handicaps, brain injury, minimal brain dysfunction, dyslexia, and developmental aphasia. The term does not include children who have learning problems which are primarily the result of visual, hearing, or motor handicaps, of mental retardation, or of environmental, cultural, or economic disadvantage. (PL 94-142, Education for All Handicapped Children Act of 1975)[1]

The National Joint Committee on Learning Disabilities (NJCLD) revised this definition in order to address several problems that were noted in it. Hammill, Leigh, McNutt, and Larsen (1981) presented an analysis of the reasons for the development of an early NJCLD version and gave their interpretation of the intention of the revised phrasing:

1. The term *children* was eliminated because of its overly restrictive characterization of a population that includes adolescents and adults.
2. The phrase "basic psychological processes" was eliminated because of the extensive debate generated within the field about the nature of these processes. Dispute centered largely around the application of the intended or misinterpreted theoretical concept to training programs whose results were called into question.
3. The list of "conditions" included within the learning disabilities classification was eliminated. These terms were considered ill-defined and had been the subject of much heated argument among members of the various professions serving the population with learning disabilities.
4. Emphasis was placed on the possible cooccurrence of learning disabilities with any of the handicapping conditions listed in the "exclusion" clause.

The positions of the NJCLD included such critical elements as the heterogeneous nature of learning disabilities and the presumed, although not always demonstrable, central nervous system dysfunction cause of the condition.

The most recent in a progression of revisions has been constructed by the NJCLD as follows:

> Learning disabilities is a general term that refers to a heterogeneous group of disorders manifested by significant difficulties in the acquisition and use of listening, speaking, reading, writing, reasoning, or mathematical abilities. These disorders are intrinsic to the individual, presumed to be due to central nervous system dysfunction, and may occur across the life span. Problems in self-regulatory behaviors, social perception, and social interaction may exist with learning disabilities but do not by themselves constitute a learning disability.
>
> Although learning disabilities may occur concomitantly with other handicapping conditions (for example, sensory impairment, mental retardation, serious emotional disturbance) or with extrinsic influences (such as cultural differences, insufficient or inappropriate instruction) they are not the result of those conditions or influences. (NJCLD, 1988, p. 1)

The changes included in this definition represent attempts made by the NJCLD to address problems inherent in existing definitions of learning disabilities. These problems and the ra-

---

[1]In 1990, the title of PL 94-142 was changed to the Individuals with Disabilities Education Act (IDEA). Now PL 101-476, the Education of the Handicapped Act Amendments of 1990 changed the name of EHA to the IDEA.

tionales for modifications of aspects of the definition reflect some of the historical developments that are described in greater detail in a subsequent section of this chapter.

Hammill (1990b) listed the critical characteristics included in moie than 70% of the definitions of learning disabilities formulated over more than 2 decades:

> Attribution of underachievement to intraindividual versus external factors
> Central nervous system dysfunction
> Persistence of learning disabilities across the life span
> Language-related academic deficits

Adelman and Taylor (1986c) reviewed aspects of the arguments about definition that have been
continuous since the inception of the field. Lack of agreement has existed among researchers
and practitioners about the nature and etiology of the phenomenon. Definitional ambiguity has
been exploited by special service delivery agencies operating under federal and state laws.
Failure to establish consensus about criteria has resulted in variability in standards and practices employed in identification of students with learning disabilities (Keogh, 1993; Zigmond,
1993).

CLASSIFICATION

Lack of consensus about definitions is inextricably related to the processes and methods of
classification aimed at differentiating individuals with learning disabilities from those without
learning problems and from those whose problems are attributable to other causes, such as
mental retardation or emotional/behavioral disorders (Fletcher et al., 1993; MacMillan, 1993).

Questions remain about the relative efficacy of approaches that attempt to classify a target
population on the basis of a list of attributes judged necessary and sufficient to qualify for
inclusion (monothetic model) or on the basis of subsets of attributes from longer lists, whereby
the presence of some is sufficient and all are not necessary for inclusion (polythetic model)
(Blashfield, 1993; Fletcher et al., 1993). It is considered likely that a monothetic approach to
classification is best suited to differentiating children with learning disabilities from those with
mental retardation (Fletcher et al., 1993). However, in view of the admitted heterogeneity of
learning disabilities, either a polythetic approach or some sort of prototype model is probably
preferable for discriminating between individuals with learning disabilities and those without
learning disabilities in the population at large (Fletcher et al., 1993; Morris, 1993; Speece,
1993).

IDENTIFICATION AND ASSESSMENT

Although classification processes are based on conceptual foundations, they are purported to
be free of the effects of measurement procedures. In contrast, identification is constrained by
the technical adequacy of measurement instruments and the expertise of their administration
and interpretation (Keogh, 1993).

A controversial issue related to both classification methods and identification procedures
is the use of a measured discrepancy between ability and achievement as one of the attributes
of a learning disability. The psychometric approach to documenting intellectual aptitude, both
clinically and in research studies, has come under attack for a variety of reasons:

1. Use of single-number scores from IQ tests is subject to measurement errors (Swanson,
   1993).

2. Computation of discrepancies between such IQ scores and achievement scores involves complex statistical procedures and diagnostic interpretation rather than merely straightforward comparison (Fletcher et al., 1993; Swanson, 1993).

3. IQ cutoff points for distinguishing between learning disabilities and mental retardation have varied in practice to the point of blurring boundaries between these groups (Zigmond, 1993). Recent redefinition of mental retardation has shifted the upper boundary to an IQ of 70, thereby excluding from that category borderline cases with IQs ranging from 70 to 85 (MacMillan, 1993).

4. Results on standardized tests may be negatively influenced by attentional disorder or reduced motivation, resulting in depressed scores that obscure actual ability (Swanson, 1993).

5. Use of global IQ scores, combining verbal and performance scores, may obscure the effects on estimated aptitude of relative weaknesses or strengths in either area (Morris, 1993).

6. Use of either a Verbal Scale IQ or a Performance Scale IQ from the Wechsler Intelligence Scale for Children–Revised (WISC–R) (Wechsler, 1974) as an index of aptitude may result in either over- or underestimation of those abilities particularly pertinent to academic achievement. With specific reference to reading disability, probably the most prevalent of all learning disabilities, even the widely used Verbal Scale of the WISC–R does not include assessment of phonological awareness, a specific area considered central to prominent theories about dyslexia (Morris, 1993; Stanovich, 1993; Torgeson, 1993).

Scholars agree on the need for a multifaceted test battery designed on the basis of a strong theoretical model (Levine et al., 1993; Swanson, 1993).

THEORETICAL FOUNDATIONS

An overriding concern expressed by many scholars is the need to improve theory and research as a key to maintaining the integrity of the field of learning disabilities (Adelman & Taylor, 1986b; Bauer, 1988; Kavale 1988, 1993; Levine et al., 1993; Poplin, 1988a; Swanson, 1988b; Torgeson, 1988a, 1993). Assumptions that have served historically as theoretical and practical foundations of the field have been called into question. The lack of consensus is attributed, in part, to the complexity of the phenomenon under study, demonstrated by the absence of any single variable identified as a primary source of learning disabilities in more than 1,000 studies reviewed (Kavale, 1993).

Beyond the complexity of the object of research, methods may vary widely according to disparate perspectives of scholars and practitioners whose conceptualizations may be unidimensional (Kavale, 1993; Morris, 1993). For example, research and theory formulation in the discipline have been faulted by some scholars for failure to remain current with and parallel to research in cognitive psychology (Swanson, 1993). There has also been an expressed need to delineate defensible theories about brain–behavior relationships adequate for explaining specific cognitive deficits identified through detailed analysis of learning difficulties (Torgeson, 1993). From another perspective, it has been reasoned that research in learning disabilities must take into account variations manifested across age and developmental levels as one aspect of theory formulation addressing the heterogeneity of the population (Levine et al., 1993).

In a broader sense, Kavale (1993) has argued for the construction of a larger theoretical framework that would encompass all relevant domains and establish relations among them by synthesizing available knowledge and extending its boundaries. The need for a metatheory about learning disabilities has been advanced by Swanson (1988b) and urged by Kavale (1993) "as the means through which a field is bound together and focuses on core ideas, assumptions, and procedures."

Current theoretical diversity and controversy may be understood by reviewing historical developments over the past half-century and by grouping theories into models or paradigms under which they are subsumed. A number of prominent authorities have organized influential theories into systems that are similar but not identical.

HISTORICAL THEORETICAL TRENDS

Torgeson (1986) characterized the paradigms determining theory and research in the field of learning disabilities as follows:

> The Neuropsychological Paradigm
> The Applied Behavior Analysis Paradigm
> The Information Processing Paradigm

Poplin's (1988a) organization of models includes dates of preeminent influence:

> The Medical Model (1940s and 1950s)
> The Psychological Process Model (1960s)
> The Behavioral Model (1970s)
> The Cognitive/Learning Strategy Model (1980s)

To differing degrees, these models have been oriented toward explanatory accounts of etiology *or* toward principles and practices in intervention.

The present historical overview describes developments in the field using a similar but slightly modified system of perspectives:

> The Neurological/Medical Perspective
> The Psychological Processes Perspective
> The Applied Behavior Analysis Perspective
> The Cognitive/Information Processing Perspective

Accounts of historical developments reflecting the different trends are followed by critiques of each perspective and, subsequently, by an overall analysis of the state of the art (or science) of the field.

The Neurological/Medical Perspective

Early in the history of the learning disabilities field, a medical model placed strong emphasis on diagnosis in terms of organic etiology. A major focus was the attempt to explain certain types of academic failure in terms of damage to specific brain functions by disease or accident (Torgeson, 1986).

Alfred Strauss and Heinz Werner were involved in the study of mental retardation during the 1940s. Their early theoretical formulations were strongly influenced by K. Goldstein's (1942) work on effects of brain damage in adults, with resultant attempts to determine whether the symptoms observed in adults with central nervous system damage could be observed in children with mental retardation.

In their comparison of *exogenous retardation* (resulting from neurological impairment) and *endogenous retardation* (resulting from familial factors), they noted different behavioral patterns (Werner & Strauss, 1941). In visual-perceptual motor studies, the performance of subjects with exogenous retardation was disorganized and characterized by poor figure-ground discrimination (i.e., they had greater difficulty than control subjects in perceiving an object embedded in a background—e.g., a pictured bird in a leafy tree). The performance in this regard of subjects with endogenous retardation was similar to that of people who were not retarded. This same difference between the performance of the two populations was noted on auditory-vocal tasks in the form of melody-pattern imitation (i.e., the ability to hear and re-produce a group of tones).

From these studies emerged the theory that children with neurological impairment are deficient in the ability to direct attention to the task at hand because of the interference of nonessential stimuli in pattern perception and resultant concept formation. That is, in a figure-ground task the experimental subjects demonstrated an inability to inhibit responses to extra-neous stimuli and to focus solely on critical information. Thus, from these observations it was hypothesized that problems existed in the related areas of perception, visual-motor perfor-mance, and selective attention.

The exogenous retardation (neurologically impaired) population was characterized as dis-tractible, hyperactive, impulsive, and disinhibited. Since the behavior patterns observed were similar to those manifested by adults with brain injury, they were regarded as evidence of brain injury in such children. These behavior patterns were viewed as the result of subcortical im-pulses discharging neural energy directly and intensely, and Strauss believed that increased cortical control and reduction of driven behavior could be achieved by training (Myers & Ham-mill, 1976). The educational environment was designed to reduce or eliminate all distracting visual stimuli, and extraneous stimuli were removed from teaching material to ensure focus of attention on essential aspects of the task (Strauss & Lehtenin, 1947).

From his examination of a body of literature reporting on investigations of minimal brain dysfunction in children, Clements (1973) abstracted 10 characteristics most often cited, listed in order of frequency:

1. Hyperactivity
2. Perceptual-motor impairments
3. Emotional lability
4. General coordination deficits
5. Disorders of attention (short attention span, distractibility, perseveration)
6. Impulsivity
7. Disorders of memory and thinking
8. Specific learning disabilities:
   a. Reading
   b. Arithmetic
   c. Writing
   d. Spelling
9. Disorders of speech and hearing
10. Equivocal neurological signs and electroencephalographic irregularities (p. 172)

To varying degrees, most of these symptoms of the syndrome identified as minimal brain dys-function by Clements (1973) have continued to receive the attention of scholars and practi-tioners in the field of learning disabilities. However, theories about causality and interrelations among symptoms remain topics of ongoing research.

Hyperactivity/Attention Deficit Disorder Theories   From one perspective, motor problems and perceptual problems were viewed as necessarily linked, because the lack of a stable motor response can alter the original perceptual input (Kephart, 1960). Hyperactivity, or excessive, non–goal-directed motor activity, was believed to interfere with perception and learning (Ayers, 1974). Early accounts of learning disabilities were likely to include descriptions of hyperactivity, along with distractibility and impulsivity. These characteristics are included in the definition of attention-deficit disorder (ADD) described in the *Diagnostic and Statistical Manual of Mental Disorders* (third edition) (*DSM–III*) of the American Psychiatric Association (1980) as a syndrome of generally maladaptive behaviors.

The *DSM–III* included the labels ADD with hyperactivity and ADD without hyperactivity as clinical entities. In the revision of the *DSM–III (DSM–III–R)* (American Psychiatric Association, 1987), this dual category was replaced with a single category, attention-deficit hyperactivity disorder (ADHD), and another category, undifferentiated attention-deficit disorder, was added. Confusion in the use of these terms has resulted, with some authors using ADD to signify both ADHD and undifferentiated ADD and other authors using ADD synonymously with hyperactivity.

Whereas learning problems may coexist with hyperactivity and other attentional disorders, current views do not equate them (Shaywitz & Shaywitz, 1988). There is a recognized need to resolve classification problems stemming from the lack of a clear distinction between the two disorders (Epstein, Shaywitz, Shaywitz, & Woolston, 1991). It has been estimated that approximately 20% of children with learning disabilities manifest hyperactivity and/or distractibility (Silver, 1987).

Among neurologists, ADD is generally attributed to some central nervous system dysfunction (Denckla, 1972; Silver, 1981). However, from a psychological perspective, research across the past decade has provided support for the hypothesis that "basic information-processing skills are intact, and observed deficits are attributable to self-regulatory processes" (Henker & Whalen, 1989, p. 217).

Medical treatment has consisted of administration of psychostimulant drugs, predominantly methylphenidate (Ritalin), dextroamphetamine (Dexedrine), and pemoline (Cylert) (Silver, 1987), to strengthen feeble inhibitory function and increase control of attention and motor activity (Denckla, 1972). A current medical view is that, while psychostimulants may lessen hyperactivity and/or decrease distractibility, they do not directly treat the learning disability. "They can, however, make the student more available for learning" (Silver, 1987, p. 498).

A fine-grained analytical review of studies published from the mid-1970s to the mid-1980s provides evidence supporting the beneficial effects of psychostimulant drugs on laboratory learning tasks and aspects of classroom achievement by at least a subset of children with ADD and learning disabilities (Pelham, 1988). Other reviews over the past decade have led to the conclusion that medication with stimulant drugs *by itself* does not appear to produce gains in achievement over the long term (Doris, 1993; Henker & Whalen, 1989). This issue remains the subject of controversy. It will receive further attention in subsequent chapters.

Theories About Minimal Brain Damage   A number of perceptual-motor theorists were influenced by the theoretical formulations of Werner and Strauss. One notable example is Cruikshank, who studied a population whose brain damage was clearly evident: children with normal or near-normal intelligence who had cerebral palsy. Cruikshank (1955) found striking similarities between many of the characteristics of children with cerebral palsy and those who had exogenous retardation. Numerous studies demonstrated these performance patterns on different learning tasks, including the task of learning to read. Ultimately, the findings of studies of children with normal or near-normal IQ who had cerebral palsy were extended to children with normal IQ scores who did not have cerebral palsy but exhibited similar disabilities of learning. In contrast to *severely* brain-injured children with cerebral palsy, these children who did not have cerebral palsy were classified as *minimally* brain damaged. Thus, one of the early characterizations of children with learning disabilities was: normal or near-normal intelligence coupled with perceptual and attentional deficits. This characterization of minimal brain damage with its concomitant perceptual and attentional deficits led to the emergence of perceptual-motor accounts of learning disabilities.

Perceptual-Motor Theories   Perceptual-motor theorists have maintained that early development in visual-spatial and motor abilities is prerequisite to later, higher levels of learning (Ayers, 1974; Barsch, 1968; Frostig, LeFever, & Whittlesey, 1964; Kephart, 1960), and that deficits in perceptual and motor development may account for problems in learning, including difficulties in learning to read. Within this conceptualization, Frostig et al.'s primary focus was on the visual-perceptual, rather than the motor, base of academic learning. They analyzed various types of perceptual difficulties observed in children with learning problems, including eye-motor coordination, figure–ground relationships, form constancy, position in space (rotation), and spatial relationships. From Frostig et al.'s theoretical viewpoint, reading was regarded as essentially a visual-perceptual act, and difficulties in learning to read were attributed to visual-perceptual and related motor problems resulting from neurological impairment. As noted above, minimal brain damage was inferred based on comparison with characteristics of other populations of adults and children with brain injury. However, insufficient knowledge about brain–behavior relationships prevented accurate prognosis of educational performance (Torgesen, 1986).

A multitude of training programs was designed to remediate or ameliorate these perceptual-motor deficiencies and thus to foster improvements in academic learning, particularly in reading. Reviews of research on the efficacy of such programs have called into question the purported relationship between visual-perceptual skills as measured and academic achievement. Larsen, Rogers, and Sowell (1976) found that many children who do poorly on these tests exhibit no difficulty in mastering academic subjects, with the reverse also being found to be the case in numerous instances. These authors found no general agreement on what constitutes the perceptual disorders characteristic of learning disabilities. Others have challenged the adequacy of visual-perceptual and motor theories for characterizing learning disorders involving language and thought (P.I. Myers & Hammill, 1976). Extensive research on the nature of dyslexia has refuted the notion of a perceptual deficiency as a major cause (Vellutino, 1979). This research and the related theory is presented in Chapters 7 and 8.

Language-Based Theories   Parallel in time to the perceptual-motor movement, an alternate view of reading and learning disabilities as part of a language disability exerted a marked influence on the conceptual evolution of the field. Orton (1937) proposed the concept of specific dyslexia or specific reading disability to describe those children whose language problem was the result of neurological involvement. He attributed reading and writing disabilities to disruptions in the establishment of cerebral dominance, maintaining that this cerebral ambilaterality was responsible for the letter reversals and mirror writing observed in children with reading problems. He argued that mirror images were represented in the right visual cortex because of poorly established hemispheric specialization and the resulting inability to suppress such mirror images. However, Bryden (1982) maintained: "Orton's specific arguments have not stood the test of time very well. . . . There is little evidence that poor readers actually perceive visual stimuli in mirror image orientation" (p. 242).

More recent theory maintains that orientation reversals are a developmental phenomenon. The young child, for whom orientation is less salient than shape, must eventually learn that object constancy, while crucial to other perceptual operations, is not relevant for letters (Kinsbourne & Caplan, 1979). For example, a chair is perceived as a chair regardless of its position or rotation in space. On the other hand, the position of the vertical line to the left of the curve in a "b" distinguishes it from a "d," which has the vertical line to the right of the curve. The work of Shankweiler and Liberman (1972) also questioned Orton's neurological explanation of letter reversals by demonstrating that these problems may be attributable more to deficits in linguistic processing than to defective processing of optical characteristics.

Theories About Abnormal Cerebral Structure and Function   Despite the challenges to Orton's theory, the more general notion of *some* disruption of the process of optimal cerebral dominance is still considered one possible causal factor of learning/reading disability. The idea that lateralization of specialized functions to the two hemispheres occurs over time as the result of maturation (Lenneberg, 1964) has been largely disputed by evidence that marked asymmetries are present in infancy; the magnitude of this asymmetry does not appear to increase with age in the normally developing individual (Hiscock, 1983).

According to prevailing theory about cerebral abnormality, the following conditions may contribute to learning impairment related to deviant brain function (Hiscock, 1983; Kinsbourne, 1983a):

1. *Structural abnormality*: At the present time there is no compelling evidence from standard neurological evaluations of such abnormalities in children with learning disabilities.
2. *Neurodevelopmental lag*: Such a delay may be attributed to some early covert damage that interferes with normal maturation. Or, some physiologic abnormality, such as excessively high or low levels of neurotransmitters, may disrupt the function of a structurally normal brain.
3. *Deviant lateralization of function*: Lateralization is the establishment of dominance of specific functions in the left or right hemisphere of the brain. Some abnormality in hemispheric dominance might produce interference between two functions coexisting in a single hemisphere. For example, overlap of linguistic and visual-spatial functions might interfere with normal linguistic and sequential functioning within the left hemisphere.
4. *Abnormality in the corpus callosum*: Either structural or functional deviance in the nerve fibers connecting the two hemispheres (corpus callosum) could result in:
    a. diminished flow of information between the hemispheres, distortion of information transmitted between hemispheres, or transmission of information to the wrong region of the opposite hemisphere; or
    b. excessive interconnection between hemispheres, thereby causing interference between verbal-visual-spatial functions in the same hemisphere.

A detailed account of current neuropsychological theory and research relevant to learning disabilities forms the content of Chapter 6; therefore further discussion of this topic is reserved for that chapter.

Neurological Evaluations: Early Results and Recent Advances   Apart from studies of the pathological brain through postmortem or invasive medical techniques, information about brain function is usually secured from interpretation of behavioral patterns, from the administration of a clinical neurological examination, and from a variety of measures of behavioral laterality. It is acknowledged that the standard clinical neurological examination is too crude a tool for detecting brain injury, since there is evidence that such examinations do not consistently reveal abnormalities in children with documented, indisputable brain damage (Rutter, Chadwick, & Shaffer, 1983). Attempts to study cerebral lateralization by means of behavioral laterality techniques are fraught with difficulties because of possible confounding variables, such as attention, prior experience, or strategies used (Bryden, 1982; Hiscock, 1983).

In contrast, an extensive review of the literature on results of standardized neurological examinations revealed that detection of *soft signs* provides a valid and reliable index to existent abnormality of function. Soft signs are single aberrations (e.g., language delay, motoric clumsiness) that, existing in a constellation of such signs, are regarded as syndromes or symptom complexes suggestive of brain dysfunction (Denckla, 1972). Soft signs are significant predictors of cognitive and behavioral function. However, "in general the base rate of neurological 'soft signs' in children who do not show problems is so high as to make these phenomena of only limited value for such exercises as screening, prediction and so forth" (Shaffer, O'Connor, Shafer, & Prupis, 1984, p. 159).

Rutter (1984) concluded that correlations between cognitive syndromes and neurophysiology are not known at the present time. While soft signs do appear from empirical evidence to be related to cognitive/learning dysfunction, they have not as yet been linked to the type of malfunction in a diagnostically useful way.

Some of the assumptions of the neurological/medical perspective of learning disabilities theory and practice have been subjected to challenge. Because of the limitations of traditional procedures and their interpretation, and because there has been a broader application of the concept of learning disabilities, recent developments have diminished adherence to the neurological dysfunction account of learning disabilities (Adelman & Taylor, 1986c). Inadequate knowledge about brain–behavior relationships caused early theories about the neurological basis for academic failure to have limited practical value (Torgeson, 1986).

Despite shifts away from the traditional neurological/medical position on etiology and treatment, recent technological advances have spurred resurgent interest in exploration of brain–behavior relationships. Capabilities have been expanded for studying neurophysiology and for observation of function during the performance of selected tasks by the use of technology such as computerized tomography (CT scan), magnetic resonance imaging (MRI), event-related cortical potentials (ERP), regional cerebral blood flow (rCBF), brain electrical activity mapping (BEAM), and others (Bigler, 1987; Hynd, Hynd, Sullivan, & Kingsbury, 1987; Languis & Wittrock, 1986; Obrzut & Hynd, 1983; Pelham, 1988).

Much of the current emphasis represents another shift from traditional neurology, which during the recent past had dissociated itself from the "mentalistic" functions that had been the concerns of psychology and psychiatry. Denckla (1972) was a pioneering proponent and practitioner of the use of a more extended neurological examination (beyond the classical neurological motor and sensory examination), exploring performance in the following areas: language; gross and fine motor (including eyes, mouth, and fingers); visuospatial; perceptual; memory (visual, verbal, and combinations); and "observation of specifics of behavior, strategy, and control" (p. 404).

Recent development of the subspecialty of neuropsychology has stimulated research and theory to expand the conceptualizations of learning and learning disabilities by integrating aspects of neurological and cognitive sciences. Torgesen (1986) expressed optimism tempered by caution about the current trend:

> The recent development of a more complete scientific paradigm in the area of child neuropsychology provides a firmer base from which to develop useful theories about brain–behavior relationships in children with learning disabilities than has been available in the past. . . . [However,] we must regard the practical value of these assumptions as essentially untested and should await with interest the outcome of further research and theorizing in this area. (p. 402)

Recent neurological perspectives differ in significant ways from the early medical model of the 1940s and 1950s. Special education services for children with learning disabilities have largely shifted from highly structured, sterile environments in private institutions to public schools that have tended to place less reliance on the medical model (Poplin, 1988a). A general disenchantment within the educational community through the late 1960s and the 1970s about the effectiveness of neurological procedures in identifying students with learning disabilities or in providing bases for appropriate intervention led to the development and adoption of a new perspective.

The Psychological Processes Perspective

Frustration over the unfulfilled expectations of neurological/medical theory and its application to special education resulted in a shift in emphasis from diagnostic/etiological concerns to a focus on identifying underlying processes and training specific abilities believed prerequisite to academic learning. In addition to the prior emphasis on perception, other processes, such as memory, attention, sequencing, and closure, in the visual, auditory, motoric, and tactile modalities, were selected as areas of focus for remedial training. This shift from a medical to a psychological/educational perspective began in a period during which behavioral learning theory was dominant in American psychology. From this perspective, mentalistic concepts and covert phenomena were not considered appropriate subjects for scientific study. Therefore, "Those who wanted to develop theories of [learning disabilities] that used psychological processing concepts as explanatory variables were forced to do so in a relative conceptual and scientific vacuum" (Torgesen, 1986, p. 402).

Thus, the pioneering efforts of early psychological process theorists and practitioners were largely based on assumptions that were adopted with widespread enthusiasm but lacked the undergirding of an appropriate established scholarly discipline. The early proliferation of programs designed to train specific perceptual and motor abilities viewed as prerequisite processes for learning fell far short of the expected effects on academic achievement. However, they continued to exert an influence within the prevailing psychological processes paradigm. Reviews of research reporting on the results of such training led Myers and Hammill (1976) to assert that, in the absence of a firm data base, assumptions about the benefits of these kinds of activities were no longer warranted. To secure such a data base, Kavale and Mattson (1983) analyzed reports of 180 experiments assessing the efficacy of perceptual-motor training. The results, reported in Kavale and Forness (1985), led to the conclusion that: "In no instance were perceptual-motor interventions effective. In fact, among the lowest ESs (mean effect sizes) were those found for learning/reading disabled children for whom perceptual-motor training is a favored approach" (p. 19).

Other approaches to assessment and training emerged during the late 1960s and the 1970s. One of those viewed as promising was *differential diagnosis–prescriptive teaching* (DDPT). It involved assessment of those psycholinguistic and perceptual motor abilities presumed necessary for acquiring basic academic skills. Profiles of individual abilities were derived from such assessment, with major emphasis placed on determining relative modality strengths and weaknesses. Teaching methods were then prescribed that were congruent with these modality strengths. For example, children with strengths in the visual modality and weaknesses in the auditory modality received reading instruction by sight word rather than phonics methods (Arter & Jenkins, 1977, 1979).

Research on the efficacy of DDPT led Arter and Jenkins (1977) to the conclusion that "children were not differentially helped by instruction which was congruent with their modality strengths" (p. 295). Their findings raised questions about the validity of the DDPT model and its practical applicability. Furthermore, it was argued that modality purity itself is difficult to demonstrate: "Even seemingly modality-pure instruction would not prevent a child from using other stimuli than those intended" (p. 295).

Most prominent among the instruments for process assessment and related training programs was the Illinois Test of Psycholinguistic Abilities (ITPA), designed by Samuel Kirk and his colleagues (Kirk & Kirk, 1975; Kirk, McCarthy, & Kirk, 1968). This approach assigned higher priority to analysis of each learner's relative strengths and weaknesses in specific abilities/disabilities than to the use of classificatory labels, such as *minimal brain damage* or *minimal brain dysfunction*. The ITPA was designed to assess and provide profiles of specific abilities and disabilities, which could then serve as the basis for prescriptive remedial education. That is, the psycholinguistic processes examined by the test were assumed to underlie academic achievement, and deficiencies in *specific* processes were viewed as characteristic of learning disability as opposed to a generalized deficiency that is characteristic of mental retardation.

The ITPA was constructed on the basis of an adaptation of Osgood and Sebeok's (1954) model of communication, which was, in essence, a behaviorally based account of semantics. The term *psycholinguistic* within that behavioral context is sharply at variance with more recent theoretical concepts in the contemporary field of psycholinguistics.

The ITPA purportedly assesses the 12 discrete underlying mental functions judged most crucial for learning through the auditory and visual modalities, including:

> Auditory and visual reception
> Auditory and visual association
> Verbal and motoric expression
> Auditory and visual sequential memory
> Grammatical and visual closure

Its widespread use in special education stemmed from the assumption that deficits in these psycholinguistic abilities are related in some causal or contributory way to problems in academic achievement. It simultaneously enjoyed popularity in the field of language disorders. However, the ITPA—indeed, the entire theoretical framework and related training programs of the processes approach—came under attack during the mid-1970s and became the focus of intensive research and controversy.

Research on the Diagnostic Validity of the ITPA   Because of the extensive use of the ITPA, it has been subjected to a great deal of research on its concurrent validity (Arter & Jenkins, 1979) and its diagnostic and predictive validity (Larsen et al., 1976; Newcomer & Hammill, 1976), and on the effectiveness of training programs based on its theoretical constructs. Reviews of the literature by the above scholars led to the conclusion that available research failed to support the assumption that the ITPA can be used to validly identify deficits that underlie academic failure in particular areas such as reading, spelling, and arithmetic. Its value in identifying young children at risk for school failure was challenged. Doubt was cast upon the utility of the subtests as a basis for the development of individualized remedial education programs designed to match a child's psycholinguistic characteristics. The extensive work in this area by Hammill and his colleagues is summarized in Hammill (1990a).

Interpretations of research formed the basis of lively debate between opponents and proponents of the ITPA. Relationships between certain academic skills and automatic versus representational processes were reported by Kirk and Kirk (1975), McLeod (1965), and M. Sanders (1979). McLeod (1976) called into question the quality of Newcomer and Hammill's (1976) research and their "simplistic notions of diagnosis" (p. 131). Kauffman and Hallahan (1976) stressed the diagnostic value of the ITPA in assessing relatively neglected psycholinguistic functions of students with learning disabilities. With reference to this last point, Newcomer and Hammill acknowledged that their findings pertained only to the relationship between the ITPA and academic learning: "The conclusions regarding its lack of practical value should not be generalized to the area for which it was developed—psycholinguistics" (p. 63). (For evaluation of the ITPA from a language perspective, see Part II of this chapter.)

Evaluation of Specific Abilities/Psycholinguistic Training   Process training research has produced equivocal results. On the one hand, positive effects were reported from extensive reviews of the literature by Kavale (1981), Kavale and Forness (1985), and Lund, Foster, and McCall-Perez (1978). On the other hand, from their review of over 100 studies, Arter and Jenkins (1979) found "little evidence to support the trainability of underlying psycholinguistic abilities" (p. 540).

Debate ensued about these conflicting findings. Some authors suggested that lack of consensus about training effectiveness might be attributed to the different meanings assigned to the term *psycholinguistic training* by different practitioners and investigators (Lund et al., 1978), and that each psycholinguistic area selected for evaluation and training by the ITPA is actually a complex aggregation of many subareas (Minskoff, 1976). However, L. Bloom and Lahey (1978) have made the point that apparent benefits evidenced in improved subtest scores may be the result of training that duplicates the type of material tested, but may not, in fact, reflect gains "within the entire domain of the ability supposedly measured" (p. 544).

Beyond the controversy about ITPA assessment and training, a more generalized view in the field found the processes approach lacking in theoretical and/or empirical support (Poplin, 1988a; Reid & Hresko, 1981; Wong, 1985a). Extending the concept of psychological processes beyond those identified as psycholinguistic, Kavale and Forness (1985) concluded from their own research and reviews of other investigations that selected disabilities had little if any demonstrated relationship to academic achievement.

This admittedly brief account reflects the controversial history of process theory and practice. The very concept of the isolated existence of specific abilities (a virtually synonymous term for psychological processes) has been the subject of ongoing debate in special education, with particular relevance to the field of learning disabilities. A dramatic example illustrating such continued controversy is the expression of differing views by two prominent authorities on the issue in their coauthored book. In L. Mann and Sabatino (1985), L. Mann acknowledged that the idea of identifying and retraining specific abilities is appealing and should not be completely discarded. However, he cogently argued that *general* abilities are likely to be involved in most cognitive activities, making it difficult to single out the *specific* ability responsible for a particular cognitive activity. He therefore discounted the degree to which such evaluation practices may be predictive of academic achievement or may translate into effective remediation. He argued that, in view of the failure of specific ability (process) approaches to remediation, the burden of demonstrating their effectiveness rests on their proponents. In contrast, Sabatino's view, cited from an earlier publication (Sabatino, Miller, & Schmidt, 1981), continued to advocate renewed efforts to train specific cognitive abilities. Wong (1986) commended as worthy of further study and theoretical reformulations those concepts that can more satisfactorily explore the covert processes underlying learning disabilities (Wong, 1986).

The Applied Behavior Analysis Perspective

Powerful currents shifted the direction of the field of learning disabilities away from the exploration of inferred cognitive processes and toward the analysis and control of overt behavior. The influence of behavioral learning theory on special education, including the field of learning disabilities, was pervasive from the late 1960s into the early 1980s. Behavior analysis has been characterized by its proponents as "a systematic, empirical methodology for accomplishing academic and social behavior change and for conducting applied research" (C.M. Nelson & Polsgrove, 1984, p. 6). From this perspective, the primary concern of the scholar or practitioner is the identification and analysis of abnormal behavior rather than the application of classification labels derived from hypothesized etiologies (Lovitt, 1975a), since research using applied behavior analysis has demonstrated that labels are less predictive of behavior than are specific environmental variables (C.M. Nelson & Polsgrove, 1984). Indispensable to claims of scientific status is the ability to predict and control events, the ultimate test of how well a phenomenon is understood (Perkins, 1971).

Applied behavior analysis has promoted close inspection of the antecedent and consequent events that influence learning and performance within the social and educational domains. It has also developed a technology capable of programming procedures for effecting desired changes according to individual needs and level of entry (Koorland, 1986).

In the application of applied behavior analysis to learning disabilities, levels and instructional targets are generally determined by documenting significant discrepancies between measured ability and achievement (Poplin, 1988a). Recommended procedures in the classroom then consist of the following steps (Koorland, 1986; Lerner, 1985; Lovitt, 1975b):

> Identification of the behavior to be taught
> Establishment of the appropriate criteria level for mastery
> Arrangement of the situation in which the identified behavior will occur
> Direct and repeated measurement of the behavior at baseline and over an initial observation period

Analysis of students' performance

Selection of appropriate intervention technique involving control of antecedent and/or
    consequent events

Evaluation of results and repetition of the procedures if goals are not attained

Termination of the teaching technique upon achievement of criterion

Generalization of newly acquired behavior

Direct teaching of academic skills through the use of applied behavior analysis has been
considered by some to be more effective for remediating learning disabilities than training
underlying processes. Central to behavioral technology is the analysis of complex behaviors
into discrete constituent components and the sequencing of those component behaviors along a
gradation of steps designed to facilitate mastery at criterion level, ultimately resulting in the
acquisition of the final targeted behavior (Staats & Staats, 1966). Until recently, operant conditioning in conjunction with systematic programming has been the most prevalent model for
instruction in special education (C.M. Nelson & Polsgrove, 1984).

Advocates of the applied behavior analysis approach to instructing students with learning
disabilities maintain that such procedures are applicable to the academic tasks of oral reading,
reading comprehension, spelling, handwriting, and arithmetic. Hallahan and Kauffman
(1976) have attested to the effectiveness of direct instruction, programmed to meet each student's level and needs in these areas. For example, significant gains were reportedly made in
training visual discrimination first for pictures, then for letters and words, as an approach to
reading instruction. Successful outcome of oral paragraph reading instruction was reported
from the combination of the following techniques: 1) reinforcement of correct production of
new words, 2) prompts for correction of misread words, and 3) repeated oral reading until the
paragraph was error free.

In reading comprehension training, reinforcement is seen as serving primarily a motivational function; however, for remedial instruction, systematic programming through such steps
as factual, sequential, and interpretive comprehension has been considered necessary. Thus,
the more covert phenomenon of comprehension may not be viewed as readily amenable to
some of the operant procedures, as are overt behaviors. However, objectives tend to be stated
in behavioral terms and evaluated on the basis of quantified results.

The practice of operationalizing objectives and establishing quantitative criteria for
achievement of behavioral objectives has dominated educational legislation and implementation (Poplin, 1988a). For example, since the mid-1970s compliance with PL 94-142 has required that an individualized education program (IEP) must include:

1. A statement of the child's present levels of educational performance
2. A statement of annual goals, including short term instructional objectives
3. Appropriate objective criteria and evaluation procedures and schedules for determining, at
   least on an annual basis, whether short term objectives are being achieved. (Implementation
   of Part B of the Education of the Handicapped Act, 1977, Section 121a.346)

Koorland (1986) reviewed 19 research reports on the use of the applied behavior analysis
model for the achievement of academic objectives for subjects with learning disabilities, dating
from 1979 through 1984. The overwhelming majority of these treatment studies utilized, singly or in combination, the following behavior modification techniques: cues and prompts,
modeling, various types and schedules of reinforcement, and verbal intervention and feed-

back. Koorland noted that "Generally, conclusions about the effectiveness of behavioral procedures have been favorable. On a short term basis, academic deficits have been alleviated" (p. 312). However, proponents and critics alike have noted serious problems with generalization and maintenance of changes in academic skills and disruptive behaviors resulting from the use of operant procedures (Baer, Wolf, & Risley, 1987; Koorland, 1986; Lovitt, 1975a; Meichenbaum, 1980).

More than a decade ago, while the literature was replete with evidence of effectiveness of behavior modification, review of the reported success acknowledged that evidence of long-term generalization was conspicuous by its absence (Keeley, Shemberg, & Carbonell, 1976). Ten years later, Baer and his colleagues (Baer et al., 1987), in a retrospective review of the previous 20 years of applied behavior analysis, continued to address these issues: "In the past 20 years, we have changed behavior as specified *and* shown experimental control of its appropriate generalization just often enough to make clear that the discipline is capable of such outcomes" (p. 321). Yet, they proceeded to acknowledge that the problem is still not solved and that there is no certainty that a system exists that is capable of effecting generalization in the breadth and complexity of social context. These proponents of applied behavioral analysis envision future progress involving system-wide interventions and maintain:

> But it should be current theory that is built on—not some replacement of it—current theory has worked far too well to be abandoned in the face of what are far more parsimoniously seen as technological rather than theoretical failures. (p. 325)

Some models of behavior modification have diverged from exclusive adherence to observable phenomena and have incorporated cognitive components. The observational learning model (Bandura, 1969) accorded to the individual the ability to learn without direct training, depending on the cognitive equipment of the observer, characteristics of the model and opportunities for perceived reinforcement of the model, and the observer (C.M. Nelson & Polsgrove, 1984). Cognitive behavior modification, employing self-instructional training and/or social problem solving training, was developed in response to the perceived inadequacies of operant procedures in achieving generalization and maintenance of training effects (Meichenbaum, 1980). Yet all extant models operate upon the principle that applied behavior analysis is a science, and that rigorous adherence to the scientific method can increasingly lead to "more profound discoveries of the basis of human behavior and learning" (C.M. Nelson & Polsgrove, 1984, p. 14).

With particular reference to the efficacy of the behavioral model in the field of learning disabilities, Poplin (1988a) stated that earlier hopes were not fulfilled. "Proponents as well as critics noted that students were not making the kind of pervasive and lasting progress necessary for school success" (p. 392). Others (Adelman & Taylor, 1982) have criticized the behavioral perspective for the superficiality of assumptions underlying its skills-oriented approach to learning disabilities. Questions have been raised about the validity and appropriateness of focusing on a restricted set of selected behavioral outcomes that are associated with predetermined hierarchies of knowledge and skills. Increased pressure to state short-term objectives in behavioral terms has resulted in a trend among special educators to resort to commercially prepared materials for assessment and programmed instruction. Adelman and Taylor (1982) expressed the concern that such a mechanistic model tends "to ignore the affective dimensions that may be crucial in unblocking learning and performance and expanding interests" (p. 159).

From a similar perspective, Torgesen (1986) cautioned against accepting the behavioral model as the dominant approach to learning disabilities because of its failure to provide a framework for considering the usefulness of information about organismic variables that may be important contributors to learning problems. While acknowledging the advances in accountability made by the behavioral movement in treatment conditions, he regarded an exclusively behaviorist approach as regressive since movement in psychology during the last 20 years has been away from behavioral learning theory and toward the investigation of internal processing mechanisms hypothesized to explain intellectual functions.

The Cognitive/Information Processing Perspective

In contrast to the behavioral view of learning as the reaction of a passive organism to an external reality, cognitive psychology regards learning as the result of the human being's active operation on environmental input. Instead of a stored one-to-one correspondence to external reality, input information is believed to be transformed, constructed, and reconstructed by the individual through cognitive processes.

The mainstream of American cognitive psychology has directed its research to the study of processes and mechanisms presumed to be involved in thinking, knowing, and learning, focusing at the outset predominantly on adults. The Geneva (Piagetian) school of psychology was concerned with investigation of the stages of intellectual development in children. Both American and Genevan cognitive psychologists have been engaged in the search for understanding *how* human beings process information. Within the recent past, attempts have been made to employ information processing theory and research methodology to operationalize Piagetian developmental stage constructs (Klahr & Wallace, 1976; Pascual-Leone & J. Smith, 1969) and/or to examine aspects of information processing in children from a Piagetian perspective (Flavell, 1977).

A powerful impetus to the development of current cognitive theory also emerged from computer technology, whereby the components and operations of computer information processing served as a metaphorical model of human information processing. "The problem for the theorist is to chart this flow of information—from input to output" (Rumelhart, 1977a, p. 2). Increasingly, cognitive/information processing conceptualizations have had an effect on education and on efforts to explain the problems children with learning disabilities experience in mastery of crucial academic tasks.

A recent series of articles was devoted to examining the application of information processing theory and research to various aspects of learning disabilities (M.M. Gerber & Hall, 1987; Pellegrino & Goldman, 1987; Samuels, 1987; Swanson, 1987). Considerable research has compared children with and without learning disabilities in experiments on perception, attention, memory, organization, and so on that contribute to an increased understanding of the areas of cognitive/linguistic deficit that impede academic success. Unlike the earlier processes approach, the cognitive/information processing approach has attempted to develop facilitative learning strategies and an enhanced knowledge base *in conjunction with direct instruction in academic skills*. Modifications in direct instruction are designed to take into account the identified areas of deficit, providing the necessary supports and/or compensatory adjustments to minimize the probability of failure and frustration.

Because Chapters 3 and 8 are devoted to extensive discussions of normal information processing and the information processing deficits of individuals with learning disabilities, respectively, further consideration of these topics is not provided here. Suffice it to state at this point that much of the literature reflects optimism about the identification and training of information processing strategies in such areas as selective attending, on-task behavior, comprehension and memory of academic material (Loper & Hallahan, 1982; Reid & Hresko, 1981; Ryan, Short, & Weed, 1986; Schumaker, Deshler, & Hills, 1986; P.L. Seidenberg, 1988; R.J. Sternberg & Wagner, 1982; Torgesen & Greenstein, 1982). However, the optimism is tempered by recognition of the fact that this science is in an incipient stage of its maturation. Proponents are aware of the current absence of comprehensive theories to explain relationships between processing deficits, school failure, and the outcome of various treatments (Swanson, 1987; Torgesen, 1986).

It should be noted that endorsement of an information processing approach is not unanimous among learning disabilities scholars. Some remain skeptical about advocacy of instructional procedures based on hypothetical models, which, without adequate proof, remain "a useless mental construction" (P.I. Myers & Hammill, 1990, p. 12).

The present author, in conjunction with those cited above, recognizes that the processes underlying learning and cognition are covert, and therefore not amenable to direct observation. Inevitably, scholarship in cognitive psychology is engaged in formulating and testing hypothetical constructs about such unobservable mechanisms and operations. The vast body of recent and current research into normal cognitive processes is here regarded as a rich source of support for those theoretical constructs of interest to scholars studying aberrant cognitive processes. Admittedly, as mentioned above, proponents of an information processing approach to learning disabilities bear the burden of proof in translating promising theory into effective educational intervention practices. A substantial part of the material in Chapters 10 and 11 reflects such an effort.

Another challenge to information processing theory as a basis for understanding learning disabilities asserts that such an approach takes inadequate account of complex psychosocial forces and task-related variables that shape cognitive style (Gavelek & Palinscar, 1988). From this author's perspective, consideration of psychosocial factors is indispensable to theory and practice in the field of learning disabilities. However, it is here viewed as supplementary to information processing theory instead of as a substitute for it. In Chapter 8, psychosocial correlates of learning disabilities are discussed, in addition to descriptions of cognitive information processing deficits.

CURRENT ISSUES AND DIRECTIONS

The history of diverse perspectives and current lack of consensus has provoked extensive critical analysis and self-evaluation by leaders in the field of learning disabilities, to the point of voicing doubts about its scientific legitimacy. Journals have published results of questionnaires about professional concerns (Adelman & Taylor, 1985) and conducted forums consisting of position papers and responsive commentaries.

Theory and Research

Concern has been expressed about the lack of a comprehensive theoretical structure to serve as the underpinning for research and practical application (Kavale, 1988; Swanson, 1988b). The history and current state of affairs in research is described as fragmented into isolated areas without full specification of the components approximating the actual phenomenon of learning disabilities (Kavale, 1988). Therefore, the field is viewed as an immature science, continuing to operate on such assumptions as underlying neurological abnormality in the absence of direct evidence after 40 years of research (Bauer, 1988; Carnine & Woodward, 1988).

Furthermore, classification on the basis of established descriptions, definitions, and diagnostic procedures is considered flawed in view of the excessive overlap of populations with various types of learning problems (Adelman & Taylor, 1986c; Algozzine & Ysseldyke, 1986). Indeed, there has been a strong movement in the direction of including many students with learning disabilities in regular education classes.

The Regular Education Initiative

The movement to counter the segregation of students with special problems received impetus from a report to the Secretary of Education by Madeleine Will (1986) making a commitment by the federal Office of Special Education and Rehabilitative Services (OSERS) to search for ways to encourage a partnership between regular and special education. "The objective of the partnership for special education and other special programs is to use their knowledge and expertise to support regular education in educating children with learning problems" (Will, 1986, p. 20). The regular education initiative (REI) emerged as an effort to clarify the mandate of PL 94-142 to provide services for special students in the least restrictive environment (Sailor et al., 1989). The literature reflects two major options advocated by those supporting REI. One option is to aim for the education of children with disabilities of all types and degrees of severity in a regular education school (Sailor et al., 1989; Will, 1989). The other is to educate students with mild to moderately handicapping conditions in the regular classroom (Stainback & Stainback, 1989) or to find ways of integrating students having disabilities at all levels of severity in the regular classroom (Lipsky & Gartner, 1989). Wang (1989) has advocated a partnership between regular and special education for better serving the needs of students with a variety of mild disabilities in the regular classroom.

Some advocates of REI have cited evidence of the failure of special education to benefit students with learning problems. Lipsky and Gartner (1989) reported on a review of 50 studies that compared academic achievement of children with mildly handicapping problems in mainstreamed and segregated programs. Analysis revealed a mean performance at the 80th percentile for the integrated group in contrast to a mean performance at the 50th percentile for segregated students. These authors have also sharply questioned the diagnostic validity of the classification of present concern. In concurrence with Algozzine and Ysseldyke (1986), they have asserted: "There is little in school practice to justify labeling nearly 2 million students as learning disabled; similarly, an analysis of the professional literature suggests it is unwarranted" (p. 13). Lipsky and Gartner (1989) cited one study that reported that 40%–50% of students classified as having learning disabilities failed to achieve expected benefits from a special education program.

In addition to assertions of a flawed special education system in terms of academic outcome, advocacy of REI is based on philosophical positions. For example, Will (1989) stressed the need to educate students for integration into society. "Education in an integrated environment is the best way to prepare students to live in integrated communities as adults" (p. vii). It is further assumed that placement in regular versus special education classes would remove the stigma of "handicap" labels: "when special education is made available by both regular and specialized staff to both exceptional and non-exceptional students, students are less likely to develop perceptions of themselves as 'exceptions' or 'failures'" (Wang & Birch, 1984, p. 393).

To accomplish this goal, a need has been recognized for "broadening the knowledge base and understanding of how to provide effective special education services within the context of the regular classroom" (Wang & Baker, 1985–1986, p. 504). Proponents of REI have called for a restructuring of both regular and special education to reduce the need for costly special education programs for mildly and moderately handicapped students and to provide more effective education for all students.

One prominent approach to regular education for diverse populations with learning problems is the Adaptive Learning Environments Model (ALEM) (Wang & Reynolds, 1985). This model contains a built-in diagnostic component and a highly structured prescriptive learning component adapted to individuals' optimal pace for skill acquisition (Wang & Birch, 1984). It is thus designed to be responsive to needs of students with marginal handicaps by virtue of:

Effective teaching methods drawing upon practices from regular, special, and compensatory education
Team teaching
Consultation
Cooperative learning techniques

Implementation of such programs is believed to require retraining of regular education teachers to prepare them to assume primary professional roles in teaching all mildly and moderately handicapped students together with regular education students, and to require that special educators function in supportive roles along with paraprofessionals (Reynolds & Wang, 1983; Sailor et al., 1989). It has also been urged that preservice teacher training include both regular and special education coursework and field experience (Sailor et al., 1989).

Review of research on mainstream programs (i.e., full- or part-time placement in regular education settings) during the period 1975–1984 yielded data supportive of the overall positive effects of mainstreaming on improved academic performance, attitudes, and classroom processes (Wang & Baker, 1985–1986). However, data from some studies suggested that "mainstreaming is effective only for students with certain special education classifications" (p. 517).

The REI has not met with universal approval. A number of prominent special educators and scholars in the field of learning disabilities have expressed reservations about how the REI would meet the needs of students with different types and degrees of disability (Hammill, 1990b). E.W. Martin (1993) has called into question its applicability to providing services for students with learning disabilities. He has contested the practice of attempting to meet their needs by regular education in conjunction with brief special education supplements, and he has challenged the view of learning disabilities as similar to other mild handicapping conditions. With regard to the "myth" of mildness, E.W. Martin (1993) cited the statistic that "almost 50% of all disabled children who drop out are children with learning disabilities." He further characterized the severity of the problem in terms of the difficulty experienced by many individuals with learning disabilities in securing and maintaining employment, thus attesting to the persistence of the disability beyond education into adulthood.

E.W. Martin (1993) stated that a second "myth" is the assumption that integrated placement per se guarantees successful outcome for these students. He maintained that there is insufficient evidence of the long-term efficacy of regular education for students with learning disabilities. Research on the ALEM has been subject to criticism for a number of methodological limitations, including inadequate data on effectiveness with all types of mildly handicapped students (Hallahan, Keller, McKinney, Lloyd, & Bryan, 1988). Information available has shown mixed results across categories. However, of particular interest in the present context, students with learning disabilities were shown to benefit more from special than regular education placement (Carlberg & Kavale, 1980; Wang & Baker, 1985–1986).

Other concerns expressed include the following:

Possible reduction in funding needed services for special students (J.D. McKinney & Hocutt, 1988).

Unrealistic expectations of regular education teachers' ability to meet the widely varying needs of the heterogeneous group of students with learning disabilities (Bryan, Bay, & Donahue, 1988).

In the context of the educational reform movement, doubts about the feasibility of simultaneously aiming at higher mean achievement scores and meeting the needs of low-achieving students (Kauffman, Gerber, & Semmel, 1988; Keogh, 1988).

Inadequate research on attitudes of regular education teachers toward incorporating difficult-to-teach students in their classrooms (Kauffman et al., 1988) and those of special educators toward being assigned a secondary role in this process (J.D. McKinney & Hocutt, 1988).

Possible negative effects of poor performance by special students in competition with nonhandicapped students in regular education classes (Kauffman et al., 1988).

The NJCLD (1991) stated its position on this issue as follows:

The regular education classroom is regarded as an appropriate setting for educating some, but not all, students with learning disabilities. When provided with adequate support services many students with learning disabilities are able to meet academic requirements in the regular education classroom while maintaining self-esteem and developing social skills. However, there are problems that may result from attempts to mainstream such students, some of which are:

the regular education teacher's lack of adequate preparation for providing services beneficial to a wide variety of learning problems

lack of curricular flexibility to permit adaptation to individual students' needs

inadequate support services, time, and technology for the teacher and the student with learning disabilities

inadequate evaluation of program effectiveness for meeting student needs

A number of recommendations were made for successful implementation of regular classroom placement of students with learning disabilities, some of which are:

collaboration among various professionals, parents and students in planning, implementing, and evaluating regular classroom programs

establishment of instructional conditions that permit capitalization on individual strengths and compensation for areas of weakness

availability of support services by qualified professionals

modification of programs as needed, based on systematic evaluation of regular education effectiveness

inservice programs to provide teachers with knowledge and skills needed for effective education of students with learning disabilities

Subtyping

The thrust of recent developments in the neuropsychological research on learning disabilities has been toward identifying groups of individuals with different patterns of learning disabilities. The use of a number of statistical classification techniques in the search for subtypes of learning disabilities has been found productive in demonstrating the existence of more homogeneous groups (J.M. McKinney, 1985). These advances are regarded as promising in providing "descriptions of subtypes on a number of neuropsychological domains" (Bryan et al., 1988, p. 25). The topic of subtyping and research findings in this area are addressed in Chapters 6 and 8. Of particular relevance to our present concerns is the recognition of the prevalence of language deficits in a large subset of children with learning disabilities. "Because literacy is the ultimate value of the school system, it is not surprising that Vellutino (1979) finds that those students called learning disabled in the school primarily have language problems" (Poplin, 1988a, p. 396).

The widespread recognition of the coexistence of language problems and learning problems in the population labeled learning disabled serves as justification for the contents of this book. Although some striking differences have existed between the theoretical issues in the fields of learning disabilities and language disabilities, as well as in their philosophies and methods of service delivery, substantial parallels have marked shifting trends in neurological, psychological, and behavioral emphases.

PART II: HISTORICAL DEVELOPMENTS IN THEORY AND PRACTICE IN LANGUAGE DISABILITIES

The professional primarily concerned with the nature, assessment, and treatment of disordered, delayed, or deficient language is most frequently the speech-language pathologist. The profession of speech-language pathology has a relatively brief history, starting as speech pathology approximately half a century ago. It has been regarded as an offspring of "mixed parentage" (psychology and speech arts education) (LaPointe, 1983; McLean, 1983) as well as a foster child of medicine.

PRECURSOR TO THE FIELD OF LANGUAGE DISABILITIES: SPEECH PATHOLOGY

The early literature of the field contains infrequent mention of child language disorders. However, all widely used texts of that period do include *delayed speech* among the categories of communication problems requiring evaluation and treatment (Backus & Beasley, 1951; Berry & Eisenson, 1956; Van Riper, 1954). The exclusive focus on speech behavior is not surprising considering the roots of the profession. Another influence determining the imposed limitations was the medical orientation of quite a few members of the profession during its formative years. Disorders were classified as organic or functional. Individuals with such organic disorders as cerebral palsy, cleft palate, and hearing impairment were deemed appropriate candidates for speech therapy. However, conditions severe enough to militate against speech development (language acquisition) were attributed to biological constraints not accessible to existing functional remedial approaches and were therefore excluded from the province of speech pathology and assigned to the domain of medicine. Thus, speech correction was considered feasible in the presence of developed but defective speech (McLean, 1983).

However, descriptions of delayed speech patterns in the earlier literature are recognizable from our current vantage point as delayed language development. The clinical approach to diagnosis and treatment of delayed speech was strikingly holistic in its philosophy, in all likelihood reflecting the psychodynamic school of clinical psychology that was prevalent during the 1930s, 1940s, and 1950s. Certain communication disorders, including delayed speech, were viewed organismically as manifestations of not only possible neurological or structural impairment, but also psychosocial problems such as disrupted interpersonal relations, low self-esteem, noxious environmental conditions, intrinsic emotional disturbance, and so forth. Some of the possible causes for delayed speech listed in the diagnostic literature (Berry & Eisenson, 1956; Van Riper, 1954) were:

Mental deficiency
Short auditory memory span
Neuromotor disorders
Hearing loss
Emotional disturbance
Inadequate environmental stimulation

Since verbal communication was viewed as a pervasive aspect of personality and adjustment, diagnosis and treatment took into account, in addition to prenatal, perinatal, and postnatal history, the family constellation and interaction, educational experiences, and the general social milieu of the client. Remedial training procedures were admittedly atomistic, for the most part focusing on speech sound perception and production; combinations of trained sounds in words, phrases, and sentences; and ultimately connected units of communication. However, other nonreductionist approaches were employed that took into account the child's level of emotional maturity and psychological state. The practice of using games to motivate young children's participation was widespread. A more holistic approach consisted of parallel play accompanied by self-talk, thus coupling meaningful context with verbal input in a non-pressuring clinician–client relationship.

Early on, Backus and Beasley (1951) conceptualized remediation of delayed speech in pragmatic terms, emphasizing the communicative functions of speech. They utilized a group setting, in which interpersonal relationships were optimized, with the provision of a corrective emotional experience as the major aim. Children who were diagnosed as too immature or emotionally disturbed to benefit from direct remedial procedures were recommended for non-direct play therapy to work through barriers to communication (Hahn, 1961).

The above account of the early state of the art describes the model generally prevalent in clinical practice with children. In school settings the use of such an in-depth model was not widespread. Excessively large caseloads, composed mainly of children with defective articulation (at times developmental in nature), restricted practice to a more superficial level of training perceptual-motor aspects of speech behavior.

PIONEERS IN CHILD LANGUAGE DISORDERS: EARLY NEUROLOGICAL PERSPECTIVES

The subsequent course of development within the field of language disabilities may be viewed metaphorically as a complex river system, starting with the "headwaters" of the early years and growing in scope and power as the result of numerous "tributary" contributions. One such surge was propelled by developments in the treatment of adult language disorders during and after World War II. Improvements in medical science kept alive soldiers with brain injury who later required treatment for aphasia, providing impetus to research the relationship between neuropathology and language disorders and to develop rehabilitative methods (LaPointe, 1983).

Theories postulated neurological impairment as one cause of "delayed speech." For example, Berry and Eisenson (1956) mentioned slow myelinization of cranial motor nerves, absence or delayed development of various elaboration areas in different brain systems, lack of sufficient power at the synapses as a result of low electrochemical potential, or failure to establish cerebral dominance as possible causes of delayed speech. Furthermore, they commented on the apparent relationship between speech retardation, reading disability, and ambilaterality.

Eisenson (1968) advanced the theory that developmental childhood aphasia is caused by central nervous system dysfunction, presumably via either a maturational lag or cerebral damage. His research and clinical observations led to speculations about deficits in the perception and storage of speech signals and difficulty in processing and sequencing auditory signals at the normal rate.

Another tributary branching in a different direction was the contribution of Helmar Myklebust, whose background of professional specialization was education of the deaf. His book, *Auditory Disorders in Children* (1954), provided a significant advance in the description and differential diagnosis of childhood developmental language disorders. He subsequently focused on the study and treatment of language-related learning disabilities and is generally regarded (along with his colleague and collaborator, Doris Johnson) as a leading figure in the formative period of this field.

The work of D.J. Johnson and Myklebust (1967) represents a confluence of the fields of language pathology and special education. These authors described the processes of learning (verbal and nonverbal) in hierarchical terms that include sensation, perception, imagery (memory), symbolization, and conceptualization, with the possibility of disability at any level. They advanced a psychoneurological theory of language-related learning disabilities, hypothesizing semiautonomous neurological systems subject to overloading under certain circumstances. In some instances, difficulties were attributable to impaired function in a single system (*intraneurosensory*), such as the auditory system (reduced ability to comprehend the spoken word). In other instances (e.g., reading) involving cross-modal learning, the disability was characterized as *interneurosensory*, or deficient integration of functions in more than one system.

Katrina de Hirsch, an adherent of Orton's theory of maturational lag, worked intensively with young children whose language problems, both oral and written, were attributed to delay in lateralization of the language function to one cerebral hemisphere. She described many of these children as manifesting a pervasive immaturity, emotionally as well as linguistically. Her research documented the relationship between early language processing problems, both receptive and expressive, and later reading failure. Publication of this investigation (de Hirsch, Jansky, & Langsford, 1965) served as a landmark in the development of a vast body of research and publication in the area of language-related learning disabilities. de Hirsch maintained that linguistic and cognitive competencies, rather than perception, were most essential to reading and academic performance (1981).

CONVERGENCE OF PSYCHOLINGUISTIC AND BEHAVIORAL PERSPECTIVES

In retrospect, the impact of the specific psycholinguistic abilities approach represented in the ITPA (Kirk et al., 1968) was widespread but not enduring. During the period from the mid-1960s to the mid-1970s, when increasing demands for services to children with language impairments were being placed on practitioners whose backgrounds of training and experience in this area were limited, a structured approach to assessment and training was welcomed.

The challenge to the construct validity of the test from the educational point of view was discussed earlier in this chapter. From a psycholinguistic perspective, the theory has been sharply questioned in light of subsequent developments in the field. The assumption that certain designated specific abilities are necessary and sufficient to account for the development and use of language does not accord with contemporary views of language or its disorders (Rees, 1973). It has been argued that attempts to identify specific language-related abilities are confounded by difficulties in isolating such abilities from the effects of generalized language knowledge (L. Bloom & Lahey, 1978). These authors have challenged both the diagnostic and remedial value of the specific abilities approach inherent in the ITPA. Within the framework of advances in the study of the phenomenon of language, the special abilities perspective has been displaced by other conceptualizations and concomitant remedial practices.

NORMAL LANGUAGE THEORIES: THE GREAT DEBATE

The behaviorist position conceived of language as verbal behavior, subject to the laws of learning, with "no unique emergent properties that require either a separate causal system, an augmented general system, or recourse to mental way-stations" (MacCorquodale, 1969, p. 832). Thus, language from this perspective has been regarded as learned behavior that is amenable to functional analysis of how the environment impinges on the organism and how the behavior of the organism acts upon the environment (Bricker & Bricker, 1974).

Emphasis on Linguistic Structure

Movement toward the contemporary view of language (in contrast to speech or verbal behavior) received powerful impetus from the dynamic revolution in linguistics and the subsequent surge of research in developmental psycholinguistics. Chomsky's (1957, 1965, 1968) generative-transformational grammar model of linguistic structure altered and expanded understanding of aspects of language, particularly in the area of syntax and morphology.

Nativist theories of acquisition (Chomsky, 1965; Lenneberg, 1964; McNeill, 1970) minimized the impact of environmental experience beyond the function of triggering innate biological capacities whose development was determined by the maturation of the organism. Across cultural variations and even in the presence of retardation (Lenneberg, 1964), order of emergence of linguistic patterns has been found to be remarkably invariant (R. Brown, 1973), attesting to the existence of a discrete linguistic module of cognition, separate from general learning capacities and relatively impervious to environmental influence.

The initial focus on structure blind to meaning, established by the abstract theory of syntax, was eventually recognized as unduly restrictive to research and theory. Dissatisfaction with the adequacy of orthodox transformational grammar on the part of a new generation of linguists and psychologists interested in the various factors involved in and accounting for language development resulted in a shift from exclusive focus on syntax to the development of generative semantics and to a semantically based account of child language acquisition.

Emphasis on Content

In developmental psycholinguistics, research was directed at the semantic relations underlying the structure of early child language (L. Bloom, 1970; L. Bloom, Lightbown, & Hood, 1975; Bowerman, 1973; R. Brown, 1973; Schlesinger, 1971), revealing a relatively invariant order of emergence across subjects studied. In the field of linguistics, contributions such as Fillmore's (1968) Case Grammar formulated understanding of the system of meaningful relations among structural components.

In the domains of both research and theory, it became increasingly evident that semantics was inextricably bound to context, whether in the interpretation of early child utterances or in the types of information required to provide an account of sentence meaning in conversational exchanges. Thus, "within both linguistics and psycholinguistics, the effort to formalize semantics led inevitably to an effort to formalize contextual information, or pragmatics" (Bates, 1976, p. 420).

Emphasis on Function

The pragmatics revolution radically changed theory about language acquisition and use. Hymes (1971) broadened the notion of linguistic competence from syntactic to communicative, or competence for use. From the pragmatics perspective, "Language is a shared social system with rules for correct use in given contexts" (Rees, 1978b, p. 194). From studies on the acquisition of pragmatics, it has been concluded that, during the earliest stages, "semantics emerges developmentally from pragmatics, in much the same way that syntax has been shown to emerge from semantic knowledge" (Bates, 1976, p. 420).

Interest in semantic and pragmatic development led scholars to the investigation of possible relationships between cognition and language (Bowerman, 1974; Leonard, 1976, 1978). In addition, the pragmatics revolution, attributing an important role to environment context, stimulated a great deal of research on the effects of social interaction on child language development (Bruner, 1975; Cross, 1978, 1981; Halliday, 1975; Snow, 1981), an issue that had been relegated earlier to a peripheral status. In a sense, some of the intuitive notions about the significance of interpersonal relations, characteristic of the more holistic views of an earlier period, were reinstated at a more sophisticated level in the state of the art.

IMPLICATIONS OF THEORY ABOUT NORMAL LANGUAGE FOR PRACTICE IN THE FIELD OF LANGUAGE DISABILITIES

Impact of Behavioral Theory and Technology

Behavioral theory and technology had a marked effect on intervention with individuals with speech and language disorders. Even prior to the impact of generative grammar theory on language training, operant conditioning programs had been designed to institute communication in the nonverbal child and to shape limited or deviant language toward a functional level (Kent, Klein, Falk, & Guenthe, 1972; Lovaas, 1968; Risley & Wolf, 1968). In these programs for autistic or severely retarded subjects, behaviors regarded as interfering with learning were extinguished, and useful behaviors present in the repertoire were shaped toward vocalization and verbalization.

Impact of Generative-Transformational Grammar

The broadened perspective of language resulting from the theory of a generative-transformational grammar spurred research on disordered child language structure (J.R. Johnston & Schery, 1976; Menyuk, 1969; Morehead & Ingram, 1973). Although the generative grammar theories expanded the practitioner's model of language and motivated increased efforts to serve the needs of students with language disabilities, the accompanying innatist hypothesis provided little if any help or hope for intervention. In the face of this void, the speech-language pathologist resorted to behavioral technology to train language structure (McLean, 1983), either indifferent or oblivious to the incompatibility of psycholinguistic and behavioral perspectives.

Synthesis of Psycholinguistic and Behavioral Models

Some designers of operant conditioning language training programs, taking cognizance of the futility of trying to train all language forms, have adopted the principle of training a rule-based mini-language that has the potential for developing into a generative system (Gray & Ryan, 1973, 1975). A multitude of other programs have, to varying degrees, attempted to synthesize psycholinguistic and behavioral models, in which the content is psycholinguistically determined and behavior management is judged the most effective instructional method (Bricker & Bricker, 1974; J.F. Miller & Yoder, 1972, 1974). Some programs used a developmental logic to train syntax based on semantic relations (J.F. Miller & Yoder, 1972). Others selected classes of content and form most readily trainable and most functional for the children (Guess, Sailor, & Baer, 1974).

A number of such programs for training speech and language in populations with severe impairments were reviewed to evaluate generalization of trained behaviors, but data were not yet provided to demonstrate the extent to which spontaneous use could be taught (Guess, Keogh, & Sailor, 1978): "It appears to be easier to *establish* a rudimentary language repertoire in language deficient children than to teach the *spontaneous* use of the skills in nontraining situations" (p. 375).

BASES OF LANGUAGE INTERVENTION APPROACHES

Meaning-Based Intervention

The semantic revolution, emphasizing the relationship between meaning and structure, had its impact on intervention approaches. One example of this shift from abstract form to contextually based meaning was the Environmental Language Intervention Strategy (MacDonald & Blott, 1974). This program's major objective was to teach functional language to children already using single words by training the use of semantic relations that underlie eight grammatical rules characteristic of early language development. Training procedures included structured play and conversation as accompaniments to presentation and elicitation of targeted utterances. The semantic encoding of children with language impairment is believed to be enhanced through adult mediation "by framing, focusing and feeding back salient features of environmental experience" (Nelson, 1986b, p. 7).

Approaches similar to the above reflect a marked shift from the operant conditioning paradigm of modeling, imitation, and reinforcement of elicited responses. Focused stimulation has been employed as a technique for facilitating the acquisition and use of new lexical items, action words as well as object labels (K.L. Chapman & Terrell, 1988; Fey, 1986). In this approach, training consisted of intensified verbal input in conjunction with play activity, requiring *no* child production of the words (in contrast to the emphasis in operant approaches, wherein response elicitation was indispensable to behavioral reinforcement).

Cognitive-Based Intervention

Other perspectives viewed cognitive development as the necessary precursor to early language development and adopted procedures for fostering the child's cognitive and conceptual growth prior to or concurrent with language intervention efforts. Efforts to link Piagetian stages of sensorimotor development to language development were found to be provocative but inconclusive in their application to intervention (Leonard, 1978). In a somewhat similar vein, Rees (1983) raised questions about whether the relationship between cognition and language is a one-way or bidirectional interaction.

Communication-Based Intervention

As noted in the section describing developments in the study of various aspects of normal language, semantics and pragmatics are not clearly separable. Reports on research on various aspects of communicative competence in children with language impairments have appeared with increasing frequency in the literature (Rees, 1978b). Examples of topics under study are: 1) request-response sequences (Brinton & Fujiki, 1982); 2) conversational aspects of language-disordered speech in children (Brinton, Fujiki, & Sonnenberg, 1988; Gallagher & Darnton, 1978); 3) pragmatic analysis of the communicative behavior of an autistic child (Bernard-Opitz, 1982); and 4) requests for clarification (Brinton, Fujiki, Winkler, & Loeb, 1986; Fey, Warr-Leeper, Webber, & Disher, 1988). Increasing emphasis has been placed on procedures for assessing pragmatic abilities as part of the clinical evaluation process, such as assessment of attention-gaining skills, initiation of play routines by child and/or caregiver, patterns of turn taking, conversational skills and access to peer play (Corsaro, 1981; Damico, 1980; Prutting, 1982; Roth & Spekman, 1984).

Summary of Approaches

It has been observed that, in the specialty of disordered language, there seems to be a regrettable propensity for considering the syntactic, semantic, and pragmatic perspectives as mutually exclusive (Carrow-Woolfolk & Lynch, 1982). There is a recognized need to integrate clinical approaches to various aspects of language and to reexamine the validity of certain widespread practices, such as imitation (Snow, Midkiff-Borunda, Small, & Proctor, 1984). The following features of behavioral, psycholinguistic and sociolinguistic approaches have been extracted from Snow et al.'s overview of clinical procedures represented in the literature:

Behavioral: elicited imitation in response to clinician-controlled stimuli; drill that is product oriented; elaborate extrinsic reinforcement; a single communication partner.
Psycholinguistic: tasks at the child's cognitive level; meaning-based elicitation reinforced by linguistic feedback; control of stimuli by child as well as clinician; a process versus product orientation in the presence of one or more communication partners.

Sociolinguistic: functionally based meaningful language models in tasks at the child's social and cognitive level; turn taking in control of stimuli; reinforcement intrinsic to conversational interaction; one or more communication partners engaging in receptive-expressive role exchanges.

Generalization

In the field of language disabilities intervention, accommodation of practice to theoretical shifts has been motivated, to no small degree, by the search for solutions to the problem of generalization. Similar to the reported effects of behavioral training in special education, generalization of trained language responses to functional use has failed to meet expectations (Costello, 1983; Warren & Kaiser, 1986). The very concept of generalization in the domain of language has been called into question or redefined in a recent series of papers addressing this issue. From a psycholinguistic perspective, increased linguistic competence is attributable to growth in linguistic knowledge (Connell, 1988), increased capacity for the extension and application of that knowledge (Kamhi, 1988), and, in addition, other developmental changes "that are fundamentally different from generalization" (J.R. Johnston, 1988, p. 320).

From a "soft behavioral" perspective, which takes into account cognitive processes and linguistic knowledge but adheres essentially to operant conditions for learning, it is recognized that stimuli do not occur in isolation in the natural environment but, rather, occur as stimulus complexes in situational contexts (Warren, 1988). This view has led Warren (1988), along with other contemporary behaviorists, to adopt a "systems approach" in contrast to former efforts designed to have specific localized effects on the modification of complex behaviors.

Therefore, although the debate about the nature of language and the processes involved in its acquisition continues, there has been a shared recognition across theoretical boundaries that past intervention models are in need of revision.

FROM THE CLINIC TO THE WORLD

Naturalistic and Child-Oriented Approaches

Reflecting the impact of accumulated understanding of the various aspects of language and the need for greater ecological validity in intervention, innovations in remedial approaches have proliferated from the late 1970s through the 1980s and into the 1990s. Some have rejected the sterility of the clinic environment in favor of settings that provide a genuine social-educational environment, in which language serves *actual* versus *simulated* communicative needs (Berry, 1980). In other cases, combinations of structured and unstructured procedures and settings have been used to integrate systematic training of form with meaning and function (Waryas & Stremel-Campbell, 1978), thus imposing trainer-controlled structure on a naturalistic environment.

Incidental language teaching, or milieu language teaching (Hart & Rogers-Warren, 1978), has continued to apply a behavioral model of language learning, but in a naturalistic setting wherein the language elicited and reinforced serves real-world functions. Results of numerous studies of incidental language teaching have provided evidence of its effectiveness in fostering generalization of both form and function across time, settings, and persons (Warren & Kaiser, 1986).

In contrast to trainer-controlled approaches, child-oriented approaches have reemerged, based on the assumption that growth in child language may be best fostered by effecting optimal adjustments between the child and significant others. Procedures used in this approach include facilitative play, following the child's lead, self-talk and parallel-talk, expansions, recasts, and so forth (Fey, 1986). It is noteworthy that these procedures characterize approaches employed during an earlier period of the field's development (described above).

Most recently, Norris and Hoffman (1990) have designed procedures for imposing on language intervention for young children within naturalistic contexts the organization necessary for effectively promoting growth in verbal communication. While maintaining a child-oriented approach, they have developed means of setting goals and implementation strategies that combine systematic control with spontaneously occurring events.

School-Based Approaches

Beyond the clinic, the concerns of an increasing number of practitioners have extended to more advanced levels of communicative competence in older school-age children and adolescents. Prominent in early efforts in this area is C.S. Simon's (1979, 1980, 1987) work in the development of a functional-pragmatic approach to communication skills for primary and secondary school students.

For the past decade, there has been increased emphasis on integrating students with disabilities with students without disabilities and on providing services in the least restrictive environment. This has created a major trend toward classroom-based intervention. The literature contains a growing number of reports of speech-language pathologists functioning in schools who have been including in their services the assessment and treatment of language problems that have an impact on academic performance. This type of intervention has necessitated consultation and collaboration between speech-language pathologists and educators for the sharing of information about curricular demands and student needs. Extensive documentation of this interdisciplinary development is provided in Chapter 10.

> The impact of service delivery within the regular education milieu will continue to determine the functions of the speech-language pathologist in the schools. Some state and local education agencies are considering policies that would require speech-language pathologists to play more of a consultative role. By team teaching with classroom teachers and providing in-service instruction to train teachers to accommodate students' needs within classroom settings, speech-language pathologists would reduce direct service delivery to students with mild communication problems and restrict service delivery to students with more severe communication disorders. This trend in service delivery is seen as a response by state and local education agencies to fiscal shortfalls and increased federal mandates to provide services to younger populations. (C. Lynch, Director of State Policy Division, American Speech-Language-Hearing Association, 1992, personal communication)

LANGUAGE DISABILITIES AND LEARNING DISABILITIES

Inevitably, with developments in the field of learning disabilities implicating language deficits in a sizable proportion of those classified as having learning disabilities, the field of language disabilities has become inextricably involved with this allied discipline in research, theory formulation, and service delivery. Indeed, for more than a decade, the American Speech-Language-Hearing Association (ASHA) has been a member of the NJCLD and has issued position papers attesting to the relationship between language disabilities and academic failure, asserting the role of speech-language pathologists and audiologists in the assessment and treatment of language-related learning disabilities (ASHA, 1976, 1979, 1989).

Prominent in the journal *Topics in Language Disorders*, edited by Katherine Butler, former president of ASHA, have been issues devoted to the language of education and language-related learning disabilities. A growing number of speech-language pathologists have specialized in the language of literacy and language-related learning disabilities (e.g., L. Miller, 1990; Moran, 1988; Nelson, 1986b; Roth & Spekman, 1989a; Van Kleeck, 1990; Wallach, 1990). Kamhi and Catts (1989) have made important contributions to the understanding of dyslexia. From the results of their own research and their review of the literature, they have argued that dyslexia is not restricted to reading disability, but is a manifestation of a more general developmental language deficit. This view is in accord with that of Ceci (1987), a learning disabilities scholar, who has stated his preference for the term *language-related learning disability* instead of *reading disability* (Ceci & Baker, 1987). This convergence between the disciplines of learning disabilities and language disabilities is also evident in the interdisciplinary perspective of the present book.

Appendix:
Major Organizations and Publications
in the Field of Learning Disabilities

For descriptions of the composition and professional functions of the organizations, the reader is referred to Hammill (1990a).

The Council for Learning Disabilities (CLD)
P.O. Box 40303
Overland Park, KS 66204
> Publishes *The Learning Disabilities Quarterly*

Division for Learning Disabilities of the Council for Exceptional Children (DLD)
1920 Association Drive
Reston, VA 22091
> Publishes *Learning Disabilities Focus* and *Learning Disabilities Research,* currently a single journal titled *Learning Disabilities Research and Practice*

Learning Disabilities Association of America (LDA)
4156 Library Road
Pittsburgh, PA 15234
> Publishes *Learning Disabilities*

The Orton Dyslexia Society Inc.
724 York Road
Baltimore, MD 21204
> Publishes *Annals of Dyslexia* and *Perspectives on Dyslexia*

National Joint Committee on Learning Disabilities
c/o The Orton Dyslexia Society
724 York Road
Baltimore, MD 21204

Journal of Learning Disabilities (published by PRO-ED, 8700 Shoal Creek Boulevard, Austin TX 78758-6897)

NORMAL PROCESSES RELATED TO LANGUAGE AND LEARNING

I

2 / The Nature of Language and Its Acquisition

Diana Kaufman

In the normal course of development, all children acquire a human language. This miraculous achievement has apparently been viewed as the natural state of affairs given that adults in general, and parents in particular, make no special arrangements for the explicit teaching or learning of language. For most laymen uninitiated into the complexities of the systems of human language and communication, this acquisition is nothing more than a part of growing up. During the preschool period, ranging from birth to 5 years of age, children are expected to pass easily, uneventfully, and uniformly through the stages of uttering and understanding sounds, single words, simple two- or three-word combinations, and, finally, complex sentences. Remarkably, all children except those with the most severe disabilities do just that. They grow up speaking and understanding the language of their parents and peers and, for the most part, becoming proficient in using this language in social and educational contexts such as those described in this text.

In this chapter, the goal is to initiate the reader into the complexities of the systems of human language and communication, to briefly discuss and evaluate some of the theories of how children acquire these systems, and to give an overview of the course of acquisition. The purpose of this presentation is to familiarize the reader with the various aspects of language and communication that are described as delayed or deficient in the succeeding chapters on language and learning disabilities.

In order to understand what human language is, it might be useful to begin with a definition: Language is a finite system of principles and rules that allows a speaker to encode meaning into sounds and a hearer to decode sounds into meaning. The relationship of the sounds to their meanings is not stimulus-bound and is essentially arbitrary. This rule-governed system of language is by necessity finite since it must be capable of being stored in the brain. However, this finite system has the property of being infinitely creative in that it allows the speaker/hearer to create and understand an infinite set of novel grammatical sentences.

Knowledge of this structured system of principles and rules, characterized as an unconscious mental grammar, constitutes a speaker/hearer's language competence. This language competence underlies the use of language in performance. However, language performance is not synonymous with language competence, since the former includes and is affected by other competencies such as conceptual, social, and pragmatic knowledge. In addition, performance is affected by factors such as memory, attention, and fatigue.

LANGUAGE COMPETENCE

Phonological Rules

Knowledge of a language includes knowing the phonological system of that language—the inventory of sounds that occur in the language and the rules for combining the sounds into meaningful units. Speech sounds constitute a subset of all of the possible sounds human beings are capable of producing, and each particular language uses a subset of these.

Speech sounds, or *phones,* can be described by their phonetic properties (their manner or place of articulation) and their acoustic properties (their pattern of sound waves). Phones sharing the same phonetic properties (or features) are grouped into classes of consonants or vowel sounds, voiced or voiceless sounds, oral or nasal sounds, and so on. All of the phones thus classified make up the inventory of possible sounds of the languages of the world.

When particular phones occur in the same word environment and signal a difference in meaning (i.e., produce two different words in a language), they are by definition distinct *phonemes.* For example, the words *boy* and *toy* in English differ only in terms of their initial phones. Since the difference produces two different words, the *b* and the *t* are two distinct phonemes of English. These contrasts are language specific since the sounds that are distinctive in one language, and therefore are phonemes of that language, may not be distinctive in another. Knowing which sounds are distinctive in one's language is part of one's phonological knowledge.

Phonological knowledge of a particular language also includes knowing the rules for combining the phonemes of that language. For instance, the speaker/hearer of English knows that English, unlike Japanese, allows many consonant clusters. This includes, for example, the clustering of three consonant sounds in the word-initial position of a syllable, but only if the first consonant sound is an *s,* the second a voiceless stop, and the third a liquid or glide, as in the word *splash.* In addition, the speaker/hearer of English knows that certain sound combinations are not permissible in English, such as the *dv* in the word *Dvorak,* and that certain phonemes cannot occur in the word-initial position, such as the final sound in the word *ring*.

Finally, in addition to these segmental rules, there are phonological rules governing the use of suprasegmental features such as pitch, stress, and vowel and consonant length. Various combinations of these features are contrastive and therefore phonemic in some languages and not in others. For example, Mandarin Chinese is a tone language in which differences in word meaning are signaled by differences in pitch. English is not a tone language since word meaning is unaffected by pitch changes. English is an intonational language in which pitch variations across phrases and sentences create differences in meaning.

Morphological Rules

A second system of rules that characterizes the speaker/hearer's linguistic competence is the system that deals with the internal structure and formation of words. Although for the layman the word is usually regarded as the smallest meaningful unit of language, it is often possible to break words down into smaller units each of which can be assigned a meaning. These minimal meaningful units of language are called *morphemes*.

Words can consist of one or more morphemes. Consider, for example, the words *brother* and *hunter.* The word *brother* consists of one morpheme since neither of its two syllables can stand alone and the meaning of the word is determined for the word as a whole. The word *hunter,* on the other hand, consists of two morphemes, the free morpheme *hunt* and the bound morpheme *-er.* Free morphemes can stand alone but bound morphemes must always be affixed to a free morpheme.

Bound morphemes, such as the *-er* in *hunter,* are called derivational morphemes since their affixation to a free morpheme results in the creation of a new word. As in the case of *hunter,* in which the verb *hunt* has been changed to a noun, there is often a change in syntactic category as well. Bound morphemes that do not create new words by changing their meaning or syntactic category but instead modify or add meaning are called inflectional morphemes. Examples of inflectional morphemes in English include the progressive of the verb *-ing,* the possessive *'s* (e.g., *Dad's*), the plural *-s,* and the past tense *-ed.* The pronunciation of these inflections varies depending on the last sound of the morpheme being inflected. Speaker/hearers of English know the complex set of rules that enable them to add the inflectional morphemes to words they have never heard before.

Semantic Rules

Semantic knowledge, or knowledge about meaning in human language, includes information about the meaning of individual morphemes, words, phrases, and sentences. Information about morphemes and words is contained in the speaker/hearer's mental dictionary or lexicon. Competent speaker/hearers can make judgments about word and sentence meaning. They can recognize instances of ambiguous words and sentences, anomalous (nonsense) words and sentences, synonymous words and sentences (paraphrases), referential and coreferential words and relations, truth and falsity of utterances, and so on.

Although it has been possible for theorists to agree on some of the aspects of the meanings of words and sentences for which semantic knowledge must account, it has been difficult for anyone to arrive at an adequate theory to explain the nature of meaning. One theory of word meaning distinguishes the *intension,* or inherent sense of a word, from the *extension,* or the set of entities in the real world to which the word refers. Thus the intension of the word *baby* would include such properties as "human" and "young" and its extension would be the set of entities (babies) that it picks out in the real world. Both the notions of sense and reference have been important in characterizing the meanings of words even though there have been many problems equating a word's meaning with either its sense or its reference.

Another important theory about the meanings of words has been developed in terms of the semantic features that words share (J. Katz, 1972). Thus, *girl, woman, mother,* and *sister* share the features of being [+human, +female] as opposed to *boy, man, father,* and *brother,* which are [+human, +male]. By decomposing words into features such as these it is possible to group words into different semantic categories that share similar features. By specifying more features, one can attempt to arrive at the particular feature composition that characterizes the meaning of a particular word. However, establishing which features are both necessary and sufficient to define a word or a particular class of words has been very difficult (Armstrong, Gleitman, & Gleitman, 1983).

Despite the fact that semantic features, unlike phonological features, have not been reducible to a small, well-defined set, semantic feature theory has been useful in defining certain meaning relations among words. One of these is the relationship of antonymy. Words that are antonyms (i.e., opposites) share all features but one (*boy* and *girl*). Other types of semantic relations among words include synonymy, polysemy, and homophony. Words that are synonyms (or near-synonyms) are defined as sharing the same features (*sofa* and *couch*). Polysemous words are those that have two or more meanings that are related. An example is the word *diamond,* which can mean a baseball field or a precious stone (the relation being the shape). Homophonous or homonymous words are two different words that have a single phonetic form and the same (the three meanings of *bank*) or different (*bear* and *bare*) spelling.

Polysemy and homophony can create lexical ambiguity, as in the case of the sentence, "I walked by the *bank.*" Usually the discourse context will make the intended meaning of the sentence clear. However, lexical ambiguity is often the source of many jokes, riddles, and puns. Awareness of the ambiguity of the word meanings is required to appreciate the source of the humor. In addition, many sentences have both a literal and a nonliteral (idiomatic or metaphorical) interpretation. Understanding idioms requires knowledge of the meanings of the expressions as a whole, and interpreting metaphors requires knowing both the literal meanings of the expressions and the facts about the real world that allow for their novel application.

Semantic knowledge is evident in the recognition of sentences that have the same meaning. These sentences are called paraphrases. Paraphrase can be created by the use of synonymous words or expressions, as in "Show me the way to go home" and "Indicate the way to my habitual abode" (lexical paraphrase), or it can be the result of a difference in syntactic structure, as in the active/passive sentence pairs "The man caught the fish" and "The fish was caught by the man." In this latter case, the sentences are recognized as meaning the same thing (except for the difference in focus or topic) because the noun phrases (*the man* and *the fish*) play the same semantic roles in the two sentences. The man is the *agent* and the fish is the *recipient* of the action of the verb *caught.* These semantic or thematic roles, and others such as goal, source, instrument, and location, are assigned to the noun phrases by the verb.

Both semantic and syntactic knowledge are involved in the determination of coreference relations among noun phrases in sentences. For example, pronouns, reflexives and other types of "proforms" can replace full noun phrases in sentences, as in "*John* said *he* is going," "*Bill* told Peter to call *him*," "Dan has *a ball* and Andy has *one* too," and "Jenny said *Sharon* gave her a picture of *herself*." In all of these sentences the proform must be related to another noun phrase (its antecedent) in order to get its reference. Principles of syntactic structure constrain the possibilities for the coreference relations of these noun phrases and proforms within a sentence. Other factors involving pragmatic knowledge determine the coreference relations of noun phrases and proforms across sentences within the discourse or in the nonlinguistic context.

Syntactic Rules

Knowledge of a language means knowing the rule system that governs the way in which words are combined to form phrases and sentences. First, words share properties that allow them to be grouped into major syntactic or lexical categories (nouns, verbs, adjectives, and adverbs) and minor lexical categories (pronouns, auxiliary verbs, determiners, conjunctions, and prepositions). Major lexical categories are often referred to as the open-class words and minor lexical categories as the closed-class words. The entry for each word in the speaker/hearer's lexicon or mental dictionary contains information about syntactic category membership, as well as phonological, morphological, and semantic (or meaning) features.

Second, lexical categories can be grouped in certain ways to form phrasal categories, such as noun phrase (NP), verb phrase (VP), prepositional phrase (PP), and so on. A phrasal category consists of a lexical category, which is its *head*, and modifiers, which can be other lexical categories or other phrasal categories. So a noun heads a noun phrase, a verb heads a verb phrase, and so on. Phrasal categories can be represented as trees, as in the examples in Figure 1.

Syntactic knowledge includes an understanding of the relationships among the lexical elements in the phrasal categories; thus knowledge of English includes knowing that noun phrases may contain determiners (Det) followed by nouns (N), but not nouns followed by determiners. In addition to knowing about the internal organization of phrases, speaker/hearers are able to combine phrases into sentences, as in Figure 2.

Competent speakers of a particular language know the canonical word order of basic sentences in that language, such as the sentence in Figure 2. Also, they know the rules for transforming basic sentences into sentences such as: "Did the little boy throw the ball?", "What did

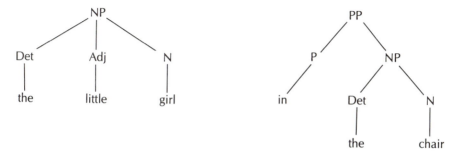

Figure 1. Examples of phrasal categories represented as trees. *Left,* Noun phrase (NP). (Det, determiner; Adj, Adjective, N, noun.) *Right,* Prepositional phrase (PP). (P, preposition; NP, noun phrase; Det, determiner; N, noun.)

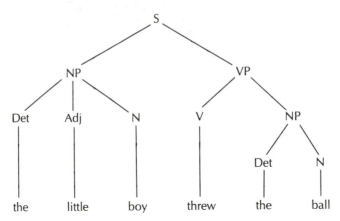

Figure 2. Combination of phrases into a sentence (S) requires grammatical knowledge, including canonical word order of basic sentences and the function of constituents. (NP, noun phrase; VP, verb phrase; Det, determiner; Adj, adjective; N, noun; V, verb.)

the little boy throw?", "The ball was thrown by the little boy", and "The little boy did not throw the ball." In addition to these single-clause sentences, speaker/hearers know the rules for formulating and comprehending compound sentences and sentences with embedded clauses.

Grammatical knowledge includes knowledge of the function of the constituents in phrases and sentences. Thus in the sentence in Figure 2, the noun phrase *the little boy* is the immediate noun phrase under S (sentence) and therefore the structural subject of the sentence. The noun phrase *the ball* is the immediate noun phrase under VP and therefore the structural object of the sentence. These relationships are called grammatical relations.

Syntactic knowledge accounts for the competent speaker/hearer's ability to create and understand an unlimited number of novel sentences, to create sentences of indefinite length, and to judge sentences as grammatical or ungrammatical. Finally, syntactic knowledge is reflected in the speaker/hearer's ability to recognize sentences that are structurally ambiguous and sentences that are paraphrases.

LANGUAGE PERFORMANCE

For expository purposes, the component rule systems of language have been discussed separately. However, it should be apparent from a number of the examples given above that these systems interact in the determination of linguistic competence. Equipped with this lingusitic competence, the speaker/hearer is free to use language in thought and communication. However, effective communication involves more than just grammatical competence. It also involves pragmatic knowledge, or awareness of the rules that govern the use of language in social contexts. This latter knowledge has been called communicative competence (Hymes, 1971).

In the discussion of syntactic rules, the competent speaker/hearer is characterized as being able to produce and comprehend a variety of sentence types, each of which expresses a different meaning. These include declaratives (statements), imperatives (commands), and interrogatives (questions). However, there is no one-to-one correspondence between a particular sentence type and the speech act it is used to perform (Austin, 1962). Various sentence types can be uttered by a speaker with a variety of intents in order to produce different responses on the part of the hearer. For example, in order to get something to eat, a speaker might say:

"I love your cooking." (statement)
"Would you please give me something to eat?" (request)
"Feed me or I'll pass out." (command)
"Isn't it 12 o'clock yet?" (question)

While the choice of any particular sentence is infinitely variable, the speaker with communicative competence knows which sentence type might be more appropriate to the context of the utterance, more expressive of her or his intent (to flatter, praise, threaten, etc.), and more likely to produce the desired response. Some of the factors that she or he might consider in making these choices include: the age, relationship, and status of the speaker and hearer; the formality of the situation; and rules of politeness. While there is no guarantee that any particular utterance will be followed by any particular type of response, since the hearer is free to choose how to respond, if at all, the hearer with communicative competence knows something about how to interpret the communicative intent of the speaker.

Another aspect of communicative competence involves having knowledge of the kinds and amount of information that are required to get intended messages across. People differ in their knowledge, attitudes, and beliefs about the world. An effective speaker is capable of assessing the status of her or his listener and of providing the background information necessary for that listener to understand the message. Many utterances are indirect and/or involve presuppositions about earlier events or states. For example, in uttering the sentence, "Are you free to tell me why she stopped writing to you each week?", the speaker presupposes that the person being referred to was writing each week and that the listener knows why that person stopped writing. In addition, the use of the proform *she* indicates that the speaker and hearer must already know who is being referred to. Such knowledge must have been provided by an earlier utterance in the discourse or perhaps by the physical presence of the person to whom the sentence refers. The use of pronouns and other referring expressions that require contextual knowledge such as time, place, and identity of the speaker for identification is called *deixis*.

Grice (1975) pointed out that utterances in discourse, such as those given in the examples above, do not usually occur as a succession of disconnected remarks. Instead they are usually part of "talk exchanges" in which speakers are attempting to carrying out suitable, coherent, communicative conversations. Such conversational exchanges are characterized as cooperative endeavors in which the participants try to be informative, truthful, relevant, unambiguous, brief, and so on. Speaker/hearers with communicative competence are aware of these cooperative principles or maxims of conversation. Of course, as Grice acknowledged, having this type of communicative competence does not assure that the speaker will not violate these principles of cooperation or maxims of conversation for a variety of reasons. Violating maxims, for example, is one way of attempting to assure metaphorical rather than literal interpretation of a message (Kempson, 1977).

THEORIES OF LANGUAGE ACQUISITION

Linguistic Theory of Acquisition

Implicit in the discussion of language competence and language performance presented above is the view that language is an autonomous system, one aspect of human cognitive capacity (Chomsky, 1975). This system of grammatical principles and rules, while extremely complex, is constructed and acquired by children during the preschool years. During these years children also construct and acquire conceptual categories of objects and events in the world, develop an awareness of social relationships, and begin to learn the complex rules governing the use of language in academic and social interactions.

This description of language competence as an autonomous system developing alongside but separate from conceptual and social competence is most consistent with a linguistic approach to language acquisition (see Bohannon & Warren-Leubecker, 1989, for a detailed discussion of this approach and the others to follow). Researchers in this approach view language (as characterized by Chomsky, 1957, 1965, 1975, 1981, and other writings) as arising out of an innately specified cognitive structure. This cognitive structure is viewed as uniquely human and responsible for the universal aspects of human language.

In Chomsky's earliest writings the term Language Acquisition Device (LAD) was used to describe the cognitive structure that determined the child's initial hypotheses about the nature of language and the mechanisms for arriving at an adult grammar. In more recent work, the child's prelinguistic initial state has been characterized as a universal grammar (UG). A universal grammar consists of interacting subsystems of principles and rules that are common to language in general. Particular languages are characterized as varying along certain parameters in terms of the ways in which the principles are instantiated. The child's task is to construct a grammar by using the input data from the language to which she/he is exposed to set the parameters for the principles of universal grammar. For example, the child exposed to English gets evidence that English is a configurational language in which semantic relations are encoded primarily by word order and that *wh-* question formation in English involves movement of the *wh-* word to the sentence-initial position.

Proponents of the linguistic approach to language acquisition (of which this author is one) point to several sources of evidence that can be interpreted as supportive. First, all children appear to follow a similar course of acquisition (at least in regard to the core properties of language), thus supporting the existence of an innately specified universal grammar. This is true regardless of race, social class, intelligence, or cultural background. Second, acquisition is relatively rapid. Third, it takes place with no formal instruction and little or no correction (Braine, 1971; R. Brown & Hanlon, 1970). Even if present, the correction is considered to be of questionable usefulness to the child (Grimshaw, 1986; Hirsh-Pasek, Golinkoff, Braidi, & McNally, 1986; Maratsos, 1986). Fourth, the input data are in many ways degenerate and deficient and do not provide the kind of evidence that would allow children to induce the structural principles that characterize linguistic competence (see C.L. Baker, 1970, and Hornstein & Lightfoot, 1981, for discussion). Fifth, in the many attempts to teach language to nonhuman primates, no one has succeeded in teaching anything resembling a human language. (This latter point is controversial and the subject of much debate; for example, see Limber [1976], Savage-Rumbaugh [1987], Savage-Rumbaugh, MacDonald, Sevcik, Hopkins, and Rupert [1986], and Seidenberg and Petitto [1979, 1987].)

Critics of the linguistic approach (see Bohannon & Warren-Leubecker, 1989, for further discussion and some specific citations) have used data from acquisition studies to suggest that language acquisition is not as rapid as this approach would predict, that individual differences in acquisition must be accounted for, that child-directed language is especially suited for language learning, and that, at the very least, the input from the environment must be responsible for the particular language learned. However, linguistic theory has provided a rich framework within which to study the ways in which universal grammar constrains children's early hypotheses about many aspects of language. These include knowledge in such areas as question-formation (Crain & Nakayama, 1987), intrasentential pronominal coreference (Crain & McKee, 1985, 1987; D.K. Kaufman, 1987, 1988; Lust, 1986, 1987; Wexler & Chien, 1985), and optionality of pronominal subjects (Hyams, 1983, 1986), to mention a few of the growing number of studies within this paradigm.

Behavioral Theory of Acquisition

The linguistic approach to language acquisition contrasts sharply with the behaviorist approach, such as that advocated by Skinner (1957) in *Verbal Behavior.* Strict behaviorists do not view language as a mental grammar with a rich deductive structure, but rather as verbal behavior similar to all other learned behaviors. This verbal behavior is the result of stimulus-response learning that takes place through imitation, practice, and selective reinforcement. Behaviorists emphasize the role of the caregiver in modeling the correct adult forms and in selectively reinforcing (punishing and rewarding) the child's imitative productions. Through this process the child eventually becomes a mature communicator.

Chomsky (1959) criticized Skinner's account of both language and language learning as too impoverished to account for either the complexity of the system or the facts of acquisition cited above. In addition, some of the mechanisms on which verbal learning is supposedly dependent have not been found to be crucial or even operant in the acquisition of language. First, in regard to the role of imitation, children are found to be unable to imitate structures that they have not yet learned. Also, children produce many sentences that they could never have heard adults produce. Examples taken from productions of the author's daughter (at 4;6 years) include:

> What you was doing downstairs Mommy?
> I just only kidding.
> That what we did.
> I taked it off.

Notice that in the last example the child's use of the verb *taked* is evidence that she is attempting to apply the grammatical rule for the formation of the weak form of the past tense rather than imitating the irregular strong form *took,* which is found in the adult speech.

Second, in terms of the role of practice, children who cannot imitate because of neurological or physical impairment still learn to understand language and to communicate. Third, in regard to reinforcement, it has already been pointed out that children do not appear to receive correction very often. Even when they do, it does not appear to be very effective in changing the child's utterance if the correct form is in advance of the child's grammatical knowledge.

It should be pointed out that, although few people would consider language as being as structurally impoverished as Skinner's theory would suggest, many treatment programs designed to remediate the speech and language problems of the child with language/learning disability appear to have effectively utilized techniques growing out of the behavioral tradition. These include the language specialist's modeling, cueing, and prompting of stimulus targets, the child's imitation of these targets, and the specialist's reinforcement of correct responses. However, while these special techniques may be necessary and effective in remediation, it does not follow that they are operative in the normal course of language development.

Cognitive Theory of Acquisition

A third approach to language acquisition views language as dependent on and emerging from cognition. Many proponents of this approach embrace Piaget's theory of cognitive development. According to Piaget (1962, 1980), there is no need to posit an innate language acquisition device to explain the development of language. Rather, language emerges as a result of the child's construction of cognitive operations and structures through his/her early sensorimotor interactions with the world.

At first (from birth to approximately 18 months) the child is characterized as being presymbolic and prelinguistic. During this stage the child relates to and develops an understanding of the world through his or her actions upon it. Important in this development is the child's active imitation of his or her own actions and the actions of others both for exploration of the environment and for purposes of sensorimotor play. Initially this sensorimotor imitation and play is tied to the child's immediate perception of people and objects in the environment. However, at about 18 months of age the child gives evidence of an awareness of the existence of objects, actions, and relations outside of his or her immediate environment (object permanence). This awareness is demonstrated in the child's ability to represent these objects, actions, and relations through "deferred imitation" and symbolic play. Through the development and integration of deferred imitation and symbolic play, the child becomes capable of representational intelligence and language.

Influenced by the work of Piaget, many developmental psychologists and psycholinguists have argued that the cognitive concepts arising out of sensorimotor intelligence are the precursors for language. Representing this position, Sinclair-deZwart (1973) suggested that the child's "first direct-action differentiations—i.e. between the subject's own action and the object acted upon on the one hand, and the child himself as an agent and some other person or object as agent—give rise to the first grammatical functions of subject-predicate and object-action" (p. 23).

Slobin (1982) discussed two ways in which early cognitive development has been claimed to be related to early language. First, the child's early semantic categories have been claimed to be a direct reflection of his or her cognitive categories. In this regard, R. Brown (1973) stated: "In sum, I think that the [child's] first sentences express the construction of reality which is the terminal achievement of sensori-motor intelligence (the permanence of form and substance of immediate objects) and the structure of immediate space and time does not have to be formed all over again on the plane of representation" (p. 200). Second, Slobin (1982) reported that many cognitive theorists have viewed the word order of child language as a natural reflection of the order of thought or of the child's perception of the environment.

However, while himself a proponent of the position that social and cognitive development prepare the child for the acquisition of language, Slobin (1982) presented data from a number of cross-linguistic studies that do not support either of the above claims. Citing the differences among languages in the ways in which they encode various semantic relations, Slobin concluded "that language, in itself, constitutes a complex body of knowledge which must be discovered and structured in its own terms" (p. 129). Notwithstanding his statement about meaning relations quoted above, R. Brown (1973) appeared to agree, stating, "I do not mean to say that such grammatical relations as subject of the sentence, object of the predicate, and so on, defined as Chomsky (1965) defines them, are a part of sensorimotor intelligence. . . . The formal relations which express semantic relations are peculiarly linguistic, and I see nothing like them in sensori-motor intelligence" (p. 201).

Aside from the work related to the early representation of semantic categories and word order, a number of researchers have looked for evidence that the emergence of particular linguistic forms (e.g., morphological markers) is dependent on acquisitions in the cognitive domain. This dependence has been argued for on the basis of studies that show either that conceptual understanding seems to precede linguistic expression or that there is a correlational relationship between the two domains (see Bohannon & Warren-Leubecker, 1989, for specific citations). However, as many researchers (e.g., Chomsky, 1980; Curtiss, 1981; Newport, Gleitman, & Gleitman, 1977) have pointed out, the demonstration of precedence, co-occurrence, or correlation does not prove causation.

Also, although it seems trivially true that children will have to have some knowledge of a concept before they will be able to express that concept in language, it has not been unequivocally demonstrated that the attainment of any particular cognitive skill is necessary for or directly related to the attainment of any particular language form. (For example, see Moore and Harris [1978], in which they demonstrate that, contrary to what would be predicted by Piagetians, the concept of "reversibility" is not necessary for children's understanding of passive sentences in English.)

Finally, studies of children with varying sensorimotor and cognitive deficiencies and deprivations, including retardation, deafness, blindness, and cerebral palsy (see, e.g., Feldman, Goldin-Meadow, & Gleitman, 1978; Fowler, Gelman, & Gleitman, 1980; Landau & Gleitman, 1985), argue further for the separation of language and cognition, since in these cases language does emerge and often is quite advanced relative to cognitive development.

Competition Model of Acquisition

The linguistic and cognitive theories of acquisition share the goal of accounting principally for what is universal in language development (although they do attempt to find explanations for aspects of cross-linguistic diversity as well). They are "theories" of the mental structures that putatively constrain the nature and course of language acquisition. A much different approach to acquisition is presented by a model arising out of the information processing paradigm—the competition model of Bates and MacWhinney (1987; MacWhinney, 1987).

First, according to Bates and MacWhinney (1987), the competition model does not have the status of a theory. (As a matter of fact, Bates and MacWhinney claimed that, in areas such as psychology, one must be satisfied with models, not with theories, the latter being possible only in areas such as physics and genetics.) Thus, they characterize their model as having "much less internal coherence [than a theory], insofar as it reflects an open-ended or 'bottom up' attempt to describe or simulate aspects of the world" (p. 174). Second, the competition model is a performance, not a competence, model. Third, the competition model is proposed to account principally for what is variable (not universal) in language acquisition across languages and possibly within individual learners of the same language.

Bates and MacWhinney (1987) posited the existence of a general processing mechanism that is able to take advantage of cues in the environment in order to map the forms of the language to the functions they serve. The cues vary in terms of their validity or information value depending on their statistical properties—how available the forms are and how reliable they are in leading to correct conclusions about the functions they serve. The learner possesses the psychological mechanism necessary to bring him/her in tune with the differing values of the cues. Although this processing mechanism is essentially data driven, the learner is not seen as passive (as in the behavioral theory presented above) since the learner's goals, expectations, and functional readiness play a role in determining what is learned.

Bates and MacWhinney (1987) claimed that "the major developmental prediction of the Competition Model is that cue validity will determine the order in which grammatical devices are acquired" (p. 171). Presenting evidence from studies of the acquisition of many languages (Hungarian, Polish, French, Italian, English, Russian, Serbo-Croatian, and Turkish), they concluded that "the relative timing of semantic, syntactic and morphological development is at least a partial function of cue validity. There is no universal schedule [as predicted by other theories] that determines the order in which children will acquire these surface forms" (p. 174).

Despite the evidence presented by Bates and MacWhinney for the adequacy of the competition model in predicting the course of acquisition, there seem to be some potential problems with the model. First, although Bohannon and Warren-Leubecker (1989) criticized the model as endowing the child with a too-powerful learning mechanism, it is difficult to imagine how this general, unconstrained learning mechanism could be "powerful enough" to guide learning in just those ways that are necessary for learning the complex rule systems that appear to underlie language comprehension and production. Second, Bates and MacWhinney (1987) reported that a number of constraints have had to be added to the model in order to account for cross-linguistic variations that have proved to be exceptions to their predictions. Although the researchers claim that these *ex post facto* constraints and principles have independent justification, there seems to be no theoretical limit on the number or kinds of principles that could be added to the model to handle recalcitrant data.

Social Theory of Acquisition

This final approach to acquisition views language as emerging primarily out of the social interactions of the child with his or her caregivers (see D. Bernstein & Tiegerman, 1989, for a discussion of this approach). These social interactions are the settings within which the child actively participates with the mature language user in learning the communicative function of language. The child learns that language can be used to express his or her intentions and to direct the behaviors of others. Many nonlinguistic aspects of these early interactions, particularly between mothers and infants, such as mutual gaze, joint attention, and turn taking, have been claimed to be the precursors and facilitators of language development and communicative competence (Bruner, 1975).

The speech of mothers (and other caregivers) to their young children, called "motherese" (Newport et al., 1977), "baby talk" (Ferguson, 1977), and "child-directed speech" (Bohannon & Warren-Leubecker, 1989), has been described as particularly well adapted to the task of assisting the child in language acquisition. A number of researchers have investigated the properties of this speech (for reviews see Bohannon & Hirsh-Pasek, 1984; Bohannon & Warren-Leubecker, 1989; Snow & Ferguson, 1977; Wanner & Gleitman, 1982). On the basis of their findings, researchers have characterized child-directed speech as high in pitch, syntactically and propositionally simple, clearly enunciated, limited in vocabulary, contextually based, repetitive and redundant, and matched to the child's developing linguistic sophistication. (Actually, this speech style has been observed in a diversity of settings by a variety of speakers to a variety of listeners perceived as immature or inadequate communicators.)

Interestingly, although there is general agreement that child-directed speech is special in ways such as those listed above, there is disagreement about whether or how these special properties could facilitate the language development process. At one extreme are those who argue for a direct causal relationship between what the caregiver says and does (in speech and gesture) and the actual language forms that the child learns. Believing that these external factors are the primary determinants of the course of acquisition, these researchers often see no need for hypothesizing an innate component.

Shatz (1982) reviewed and discussed two sorts of dependency relations that are proposed by researchers of this persuasion—the direct mapping of grammatical structures onto already known nonlinguistic action patterns and gestures, and the learning of structural constituents and variations (substitutions, deletions, movements) on the basis of conversational devices such as reformulations, expansions, and recasts. Shatz (1982) presented arguments and evidence against this strong form of the "motherese hypothesis," concluding that "the environment does not seem sufficiently or appropriately structured to control the course of language acquisition as we know it" (p. 125).

At the opposite extreme are those who argue for an innate component, noting that child-directed speech, if characterized as simple or "finely tuned" (i.e., that the mother's speech changes in response to the child's language growth), could not in principle aid the child in inducing the structural principles that characterize the adult grammar (see Wexler, 1982; Wexler & Culicover, 1980). As a matter of fact, these researchers argue that simplified input might actually make it more difficult for the learner to converge on an adult grammar since there will be fewer data available to the child from which to induce the structural principles of the language. In addition, certain aspects of the grammar, such as the structure-dependent movement transformations that take place across clauses, are only revealed in complex sentences. Therefore, the latter must be available to the child at some stage in acquisition, and preferably early if the child is not to form incorrect rules from which he or she will not be able to retreat (L.R. Gleitman & Wanner, 1982; L.R. Gleitman, Newport, & Gleitman, 1984).

There are also researchers who appear to take a more moderate position, attributing to motherese varying degrees of importance in aiding the acquisition process (see Bohannon & Warren-Leubecker, 1989, for an extensive review). One important correlational study that highlights the differential effects of motherese on language learning is by L.R. Gleitman and colleagues (1984). (This study is a reanalysis and replication of a study by Newport et al. [1977], made in response to conflicting results obtained by Furrow, Nelson, and Benedict, [1979].) While urging some caution in interpreting the results of correlational studies, L.R. Gleitman et al. found that two properties of the maternal corpus appeared to be most important in the learning process. The first was related to the finding of a significant positive correlation between maternal usage of more syntactically complex speech (as measured by sentence [S] nodes per utterance and mean length of utterance [MLU]) and child language growth. As L.R. Gleitman et al. pointed out, if this finding holds up, it is in direct opposition to the usual motherese hypothesis that simple input is best. These researchers discuss the ways in which this particular type of complexity might aid the child in the learning of structure-dependent rules.

The second important property of the maternal corpus was related to the finding of a significant positive correlation between the mothers' use of the subject/auxiliary inverted yes/no questions and the children's learning of the English auxiliary. L.R. Gleitman et al. (1984)

discussed this second finding as evidence for the importance of environmental input in the learning of closed-class items (determiners, pronominals, prepositions, inflectional markings, etc.) as opposed to open-class items (nouns, verbs, etc.), which appear regardless of input. They relate this finding to the learners' bias to pay attention to material in the input that is sentence initial and, more generally, stressed (see L.R. Gleitman, Landau, & Wanner, 1988, for further discussion). Finally, L.R. Gleitman et al. concluded that, "while language is learned through experience with the environment, its ultimate character is materially an effect of the learner's own dispositions as to how to organize and exploit linguistic stimulation" (1984, p. 76).

LANGUAGE ACQUISITION

The above presentation of these many theoretical approaches to language acquisition should make it clear that there is considerable disagreement as how best to account for the facts of acquisition. In truth, theorists of different orientations often have difficulty in agreeing on what the facts really are. In the rest of this chapter an overview of some of the current findings about acquisition in the preschool and school-age years is given. As with the earlier discussion of the grammar, the acquisition of the component rule systems of language is discussed separately. However, again it should be apparent that these systems develop in parallel and interact in acquisition as they do in the determination of linguistic competence.

Phonological Acquisition

Speech Perception   Research on infant speech perception has shown that shortly after birth infants demonstrate an impressive ability to discriminate between acoustic parameters that signal speech differences. (For an extensive review of this literature see Aslin, Pisoni, and Jusczyk [1983], on which the following discussion is based.) In a ground-breaking study by Eimas, Siqueland, Jusczyk, and Vigorito (1971), infants as young as 1 month were able to discriminate syllables differing solely in voice onset time (VOT)—for example, /pa/ and /ba/. These researchers concluded that the perceptual mechanisms underlying this capacity to discriminate were probably innate, that infant perception appeared to be similar to categorical perception in adults, and that infant perception was probably linguistic in nature. Subsequent research has upheld the first two conclusions in nearly all of the phonetic contrasts that have been presented to infants. However, there is considerable controversy over whether this perceptual ability is unique to humans and whether it is derived from properties related specifically to speech perception or more generally to auditory perception.

Cross-linguistic research has demonstrated that, in the early months, infants are able to discriminate among many speech sound contrasts (phonetic differences) that are not phonemic in their native language, rendering them able to learn any language to which they are exposed. However, with continual exposure to the particular language of their community, infants become less able to discriminate among sounds not in their native language and more sensitive to those aspects of the acoustic signal that are phonologically meaningful in the specific language to which they are being exposed (Aslin et al., 1983).

In terms of the role of speech perception in phonological development, Menyuk and Menn (1979) reported that by 9–13 months of age children begin to understand the meaning of phonological sequences as they relate to specific contexts. At this age children prefer to listen to word-length utterances as opposed to connected speech. Phonological analysis appears to be limited to word-level units, which are identified and contrasted as a whole. During the second year of life children become able to recognize phonological contrasts in syllables. Most studies suggest that by 3 years of age children give evidence of being able to discriminate the adult phonological contrasts based on distinctive feature contrasts between segments. However, Grunwell (1986) cited several studies that suggest that children continue to mature in their perceptual skills during their school years.

Speech Production   In the early period of speech production infants again demonstrate the ability to produce sounds that go beyond those that are present in their linguistic environment. (See Locke [1983] for a discussion from which much of the following is derived.) Cross-linguistic studies indicate that initially babbling (which starts around 6 months of age) is similar among infants all over the world. Also, deaf children and hearing children of deaf parents babble, suggesting that babbling is not dependent on acoustic, auditory input. As children continue to babble, their speech sound patterns (pitch and intonational contours) begin to resemble those of the language they are acquiring. Finally, while babbling is a stage that all normal children appear to go through, it does not seem to be necessary for language acquisition. Infants who because of physical motor problems are unable to babble have been claimed to develop normal articulation once their disability has been corrected.

Menyuk and Menn (1979) described the transition from babbling to speech as a gradual one. They described the child's speech during this transitional time as containing made-up words (proto-words that do not appear to be modeled on any adult word), stretches of jargon, and real words that more closely resemble the adult models. While there is some variation, most children begin to produce their first real understandable words at about 1 year of age. During this early stage of word acquisition, children often appear to avoid words they cannot say and to have a bias for words they can say (Menyuk & Menn, 1979).

Ingram (1976, 1979) characterized children's first words as being phonologically simpler than adult speech in a number of ways. First, the syllable structure of the child's first words usually consists of single consonant-and-vowel combinations (*da, at*) or consonant-vowel (CV) reduplications (*dada, baba*). Reduplications are found most commonly in the child's first 50 words. Within a few months consonant-vowel-consonant (CVC) combinations appear. Second, the inventory of sounds produced in words is initially more limited than that found in adult speech, or even in the child's earlier babbling.

There is some variability in the order of sound emergence, apparently related to both cross-linguistic differences and variations among children learning the same language (see Macken, 1980). However, the following features have been found to be characteristic of early sound production in many children (see Ingram, 1976):

Vowels emerge earlier than consonants.

Generally, among the consonants nasals and glides appear early, followed by stops.

Among the stops, voiceless are acquired before voiced and front before back.

Fricatives (*s, z*), affricates (*ch, zh*), and liquids tend to be late-emerging sounds for most children.

Ingram (1976, 1979) described the early speech patterns of children (from approximately age 1;6 to 4;0) as reflecting general simplifying phonological processes that affect entire classes of sounds. First, reduction of syllable structure to the basic CV syllable is accomplished through deletion of final consonants, reduction of consonant clusters, and deletion of unstressed syllables. Second, certain sounds are commonly substituted for other sounds. Thus, there are the processes of *stopping*, in which fricatives (*s*, *z*) and affricates (*sh*) are replaced by a corresponding stop (*t*, *d*); *fronting*, in which sounds made in the back of the mouth (velars such as [k]) are replaced by sounds made in the front (alveolars, such as [t]); *gliding*, in which liquids (*l*, *r*) are replaced by glides (*w*); and *denazalization*, in which nasals (*n*, *m*) are replaced by a corresponding nonnasal stop (*d*, *b*). Third, there are processes in which one segment is assimilated to a neighboring segment as a result of *voicing* of a consonant in anticipation of a vowel, *devoicing* of final consonants, *consonant harmony*, and *progressive vowel assimilation*.

While believing the above processes to be useful in describing the speech of children between ages 1;6 and 4;0, Ingram (1979) pointed out other factors that must be considered in an adequate characterization of phonological development. He reported that some children demonstrate much variability in their pronunciation of words. This variability is related to the children's simultaneous production of old words and new words (learned in a more advanced form), their idiosyncratic styles of organizing the adult models, and their demonstration of phonological preferences. Mastery of the phonetic inventory in production appears to take a number of years, being completed by most children by the age of 7 or 8.

Finally, Grunwell (1986) stated that both phonemic awareness (as mentioned in the discussion of speech perception above) and pronunciation continue to develop in the school years. Development of phonemic awareness is demonstrated in the appreciation and use of rhyming, the understanding of riddles (based on homophones), and the appreciation of phonological jokes and puns. The development of pronunciation is seen in the achievement of mature articulatory control, complex sound pattern production, and full use of allophonic variants. Grunwell (1986) reported that many authorities believe certain metaphonological skills (e.g., knowledge of word-size units, word boundaries, and word constituent structure) must be acquired in order for children to learn to read. Conversely, other authorities suggest that reading provides the experience that leads to the development of these metaphonological skills.

Morphological Acquisition

Children's first words consist of a single free or root morpheme. L.R. Gleitman and Wanner (1982) argued that these morphemes, which are the phonologically *open-class* elements (nouns, verbs, etc.), are the most salient for the child because they are stressed in the speech signal. Morphological development involves the acquisition of more complex open-class words and the phonologically *closed-class* elements. These include bound morphemes, such as inflectional and derivational affixes, and free morphemes, such as determiners, prepositions, and uncontracted auxiliaries and copulas. Morphological development also includes the learning of morphophonemic and word formation rules.

In a pioneering study of the acquisition of grammatical morphemes in English by three children (ages 1;6–4;0), R. Brown (1973) found the developmental sequence shown in Table 1. Although there is some variation in the exact ages at which these morphemes are acquired, subsequent studies have generally replicated this order. One question that has been of interest is the role of environmental input in the acquisition of closed-class elements. This has been studied rather extensively for the English auxiliary system (see Newport et al., 1977; L.R. Gleitman et al., 1984; Shatz, Hoff-Ginsberg, & Maciver, 1989; and the references therein).

Table 1.   Mean order of acquisition of 14 morphemes across three children

1.	Present progressive *-ing*
2–3.	*in, on*
4.	Plural *-s*
5.	Past irregular
6.	Possessive *'s*
7.	Uncontracted copula—main verb forms of *be*
8.	Articles (*the, a*)
9.	Past regular *-ed*
10.	Third person singular regular (*-s*)
11.	Third person singular irregular (*does, has*)
12.	Uncontractible auxiliary (*is, are, am*)
13.	Contractible copula
14.	Contractible auxiliary

Source: Based on R. Brown (1973).

Much of this research has supported the positive effect of the presence of fronted auxiliaries (e.g., in yes/no questions) in the speech of the mother on the child's auxiliary acquisition.

In accounting for cross-linguistic variations in the acquisition of the closed-class elements, Slobin (1982) listed a number of factors that appear to result in earlier acquisition. These include:

1. The occurrence of the morpheme in the *postposed* or word-final position (children pay attention to word endings)
2. The *syllabic* and/or *stressed* status of the morpheme (uncontracted or free is more salient than contracted or bound)
3. The *obligatoriness* of the morpheme (optionality presents the child with more problems)
4. A *clear relationship between form and function*
5. *Regular* (i.e., exceptionless), *consistently applied*, *distinct* (nonhomonymous) morpheme paradigms

In addition to learning the individual morphemes listed in Table 1, English-speaking children must acquire the morphophonemic rules that account for the allophonic variations in the English plural (/s/ in cats, /z/ in bugs, /iz/ in churches) and the English past tense (/t/ in clapped, /d/ in wagged, /id/ in wanted). Jean Berko (1958) invented the basic method used in the study of children's morphophonemic rules. She presented children ages 4;0 to 7;0 with nonsense syllables to which they had to add the plural or past tense form. This test was possible because there are obligatory contexts for the application of these endings signaled, for instance, by a word like *two* for plural and a word like *yesterday* for past. Nonsense words were chosen in order to test the productivity of the children's rules and to avoid responses made on the basis of memorized forms.

In Berko's study the children were shown a picture of a strange animal and then told, for example:

This is a wug. Now there is another one. There are two of them. There are two _____.

The results of this study indicated that the easiest inflections for the children were those that followed the general rule of voicing assimilation—/s/ and /t/ added to nonsense words ending in voiceless consonants (*heafs, ricked*) and /z/ and /d/ added to nonsense words ending in voiced consonants (*wugz, zibbed*). With these inflections the preschooler's scores ranged from 63% to 76% correct and the first grader's ranged from 73% to 97% correct. More difficult for the children was the inflecting of words ending in vowels, nasals, or liquids, to which a voiced ending /z/ or /d/ must be added (*luns, spowed*). On these the preschoolers scored from 36% to 68% correct and the first-graders from 59% to 92% correct. Finally, most difficult for the children was application of the allomorphs /iz/ or /id/ to words ending with fricatives and affricates (*gutches, motted*). Preschoolers scores ranged from 28% to 57% correct and first graders' scores from 33% to 56% correct on these.

In addition to these inflectional rules, English-speaking children must master the rules of English derivational morphology. These, too, appear to be learned in a relatively fixed order. Derwing and Baker (1979) studied the development of the following four patterns of derivational morphemes:

1. *-er* nominalizations (agentive—*teach + er = teacher*; instrumental—*erase + er = eraser*)
2. *-y* adjective formation (*dirt + y = dirty*)
3. *-ly* adverb formation (*slow + ly = slowly*)
4. Compound noun formation (*bird + house = birdhouse*)

Presentation frames were constructed to elicit each of these forms (e.g., "A man who teaches is called a . . . .") and the subjects were given sentences with both real words and nonsense syllables.

As should be apparent in Table 2, there is considerable variability in the time taken to master these word formation rules, related to the productivity of the rule (how freely it can be applied to root morphemes yielding grammatical forms). Thus, compounding and the application of agentive *-er*, which are very productive in English, are learned early, whereas adverbial formation, which is restricted to a small set of adjectives, is learned much later.

Semantic Acquisition

According to Carey (1982), "learning a word includes the pairing of a phonological representation of its sound with a representation of its meaning" (p. 348). As discussed above in the section on phonological acquisition, by 1 year of age most children give evidence of being able

Table 2. Percentage correct for nonsense root morphemes

Construction	Preschool	Elementary	Junior high	High school	Adult
Agentive *-er*	7	63	80	86	96
Instrumental *-er*	7	35	45	64	59
Adjective *-y*	0	30	55	86	100
Adverb *-ly*	0	13	20	79	81
Compounds	47	50	65	79	70

Adapted from Derwing and Baker (1979, pp. 214–215).

to do this mapping of phonological representation to meaning representation in the comprehension and utterance of their first words. How children develop these representations of meaning and how these representations come to be lexicalized is at the core of semantic acquisition.

Carey (1982) pointed out that most accounts of the mapping of phonological representations to meaning representations assume that meanings are concepts. Therefore, hypotheses about the development of word meaning in children and interpretations of the descriptive facts of acquisition vary with the theory of conceptual representation and development that the researcher holds. Thus, researchers holding a feature theory view of meaning and concepts have looked for evidence that children's word meanings are incomplete when compared with adults' meanings. Also, they have assumed that the development of word meaning consists of acquiring more and more of the features until the word meaning is complete.

While there have been a number of challenges to the feature theory view of concepts (see Carey, 1982, for discussion), much work in the acquisition of word meaning in children has been carried out in this framework. In critically reviewing these studies, Carey concluded that, "there is simply no evidence that a word's meaning is composed, component by component, in the course of its acquisition" (p. 369). If meaning is not acquired in this way, Carey believes that, given the inadequacy of the other theories that have been tendered, "we are left with no theory of lexical development to replace the semantic feature hypothesis."

Despite this rather pessimistic assessment of the state of the art in semantic theorizing, meanings do get lexicalized, as evidenced by the fact that children begin learning words. The initial words, mapped onto "simple" concepts that the child has somehow represented, are predominantly names for people or objects that move by themselves (*mama, dada, dog, baby, car*) or that the child can manipulate (*juice, milk, sock, ball*). Action words (*give, up, see*) and adjectives (*hot, mine, dirty*) are the next most common. There are also personal-social words (*no, yes, please*) and words for social routines (*bye-bye*).

By 18 months most children have developed a vocabulary of 50 words or more. This is followed by a period of rapid expansion during which children may acquire on average as many as 9 or 10 words a day. This rapid rate of acquisition suggests that children must be able to enter words into their mental lexicon on the basis of just one or a few exposures to a word. Carey (1978) presented evidence that what she calls "fast mapping" can take place in the initial representation of a word. This representation may be narrower and more context specific than the adult representation. Once a word has been entered into the lexicon, the child can continue to expand its representation through additional encounters with the word, on the basis of his or her growing conceptual knowledge in general and lexical, semantic, and syntactic knowledge in particular.

There are a number of experiments that have demonstrated that children can use certain aspects of syntactic context in order to learn the meaning of a word. Carey (1978, 1982) discussed two of these. The first is a study by B. Katz, Baker, and Macnamara (1974) in which 18-month-old girls were able to use the presence or absence of a determiner to distinguish between common and proper nouns (a *dax* versus *Dax*). When told that a new doll was a *dax*, they identified a second as another one. When told that a new doll was *Dax* they restricted that name to that doll alone.

In the second study discussed by Carey, R. Brown (1957) demonstrated that 4-year-old children who had already acquired the conceptual distinctions between actions, things, and stuff and the syntactic distinctions between verb, count noun, and mass noun were able to use this knowledge in learning the meaning of a new word, *seb*. They correctly acted out the requests to show *sebbing,* to show *a seb,* and to show *some seb.*

By age 6 most children have mastered as many as 14,000 words, or 8,000 root morphemes (Carey, 1978). From the early primary school years to the midsecondary years, the size of total vocabulary at least doubles (Durkin, 1986). In addition to this growth in the number of words, the child's vocabulary development involves the "enrichment of the child's knowledge of the organizational structures relating items in the lexicon, and the refinement of knowledge of the meanings of individual words" (Durkin, Crowther, & Shire, 1986). With this development comes appreciation of synonymous, homonymous and polysemous terms. (For an interesting study of the acquisition of polysemous vocabulary in the school years, see Durkin et al. [1986].)

In addition to the acquisition of the meaning of individual words, semantic development includes the development of an understanding of both the literal and figurative meaning of sentences. This is discussed below in relation to the acquisition of syntax.

Syntactic Acquisition

There is considerable debate in the acquisition literature as to when syntactic knowledge is first exemplified. Children begin to produce one-word utterances at about 1 year of age. However, even at this *holophrastic* stage children give evidence of understanding more than they can say. For example, they can obey two-word commands (Sachs & Truswell, 1978) and they give evidence of preferring to look at a representation of a scene that matches a sentence, such as "She's kissing the keys," as opposed to one that does not match (Golinkoff, Hirsh-Pasek, Cauley, & Gordon, 1987).

A few months after children begin uttering their first words they begin to produce two-word utterances. These utterances are characterized as expressing semantic relations that are universal in the speech of children at this stage. L. Bloom (1970) gave the following examples:

Child's utterance	Semantic relation
Mommy slipper	possessor-possessed
girl write	agent-action
Kathryn raisin	agent-object
touch milk	action-object
baby chair	agent-location

During this stage there are no syntactic or morphological markers (plurals, past tense, prepositions, etc.), so it is difficult to know whether children have knowledge of these closed-class elements.

As the children begin to string more words together, their speech begins to resemble the sentences used in telegrams, in which the "content" words are present and the small "function" words are missing. Therefore, this speech has been characterized as being *telegraphic.* Some examples from L. Bloom (1970) are:

Kathryn want raisin
cat more meat
Gia more read book

no want that
make all gone
make this sit down

Development during this stage is characterized by the gradual emergence of the grammatical morphemes discussed in the section on morphological acquisition above. The interesting thing about the sentences produced during this stage is that, although they often lack bound morphemes and minor lexical items, they almost always reflect the canonical word order of the language being learned (i.e., all of the word categories are in the expected order).

Children's first use of negative and interrogative sentences is characterized by a maintenance of canonical structure as well. Thus, in their early production of negative sentences (from approximately 18 to 25 months) the negative element is at the beginning of the sentence (e.g., "No Daddy hungry", "No car going there"). Next (from approximately 26 to 42 months), negative elements occur sentence internally but the auxiliary verbs are usually missing ("Man no go in there", "I don't want play"). At this stage *can't* and *don't* appear, but not *can* and *do*, so it seems that the former are learned as unanalyzed lexical items. Finally (after 42 months), the forms *not* and *-n't* appear sentence-internally with auxiliary verbs.

Question formation follows a similar pattern, with yes/no questions and *wh-* questions being produced first without auxiliary inversion. The presence of a rising intonation and/or the occurrence of a *wh-* word in the sentence initial position signals a question (e.g., "Why Daddy go?", "I play ball?"). In the next stage the auxiliary appears and is inverted in yes/no questions, but not in *wh-* questions. Finally, *wh-* questions appear with auxiliary inversion.

The first complex sentences begin to appear in spontaneous speech after simple sentences of approximately 4 words long become common in the child's speech (see Bowerman, 1979, for a review and citations, on which the following is based). The first complex sentences are embedded sentences in which the embedded clause functions as a direct object of the matrix verb (e.g., "I wanna read book"). Shortly after the appearance of object complement sentences, simple coordinations without the coordinating conjunctions appear (e.g., "You lookit that book, I lookit this book"). Parts of sentences are also conjoined (e.g., "He has book and paper"). Next, *wh-* constructions appear, first adverbially (e.g., "Can I take it when we go?"), and then with verbs that take complement questions (e.g., "I show you how to do it"). Next come relative clauses modifying abstract nouns of place and manner (e.g., "I show you the place I went", "That's the way Mommy talks"), and then relative clauses attached to "empty" head nouns (" . . . ones Mommy get"). Finally, relative clauses begin to appear on common nouns in the object position (e.g., "Where's a book I can read?").

Generally, object complementation appears before subject complementation in child language. Limber (1976) suggested that this is based on pragmatic factors rather than on linguistic or information processing factors, since the subject noun phrases are mostly proper names, demonstratives, and pronouns that do not lend themselves to modification. Object nouns, in contrast, are mostly common nouns or empty nouns like *one* that do allow modification. Object complementation continues to be more prevalent than subject complementation in adult speech as well, since subjects (particularly in spoken language) are almost always pronouns (Scott, 1988b).

The order or age of occurrence of the production data cited above is generally uncontroversial, with most researchers agreeing that complex sentences emerge in spontaneous speech between the ages of 2 and 4. However, there is considerable controversy over the ages at which these more complex structures are understood. For years researchers have engaged children in act-out tasks to determine the age of comprehension for the above sentence types as well as for sentences that violate canonical order (passives) or reverse the temporal order of events (*before* and *after*). Most of the earliest research indicated that children were having difficulty understanding complex or passive sentences even up to age 9 or 10 (see Bowerman, 1979, for a review).

However, in more recent years, a number of researchers have focused on uncovering and controlling possible pragmatic, cognitive, or methodological factors that have interfered with children's demonstration of their knowledge of syntactically complex sentences in experimental situations. While the findings are still controversial, many of these researchers have demonstrated comprehension of complex sentences—for example, sentences with relative clauses (Hamburger & Crain, 1982), passives (Naigles, Golinkoff, & Hirsh-Pasek, 1989), and clauses embedded under verbs like *promise* and *tell* (Sherman & Lust, 1988)—at much earlier ages than previously demonstrated.

While the studies cited above have focused mainly on children's understanding of the literal meaning of sentences, many researchers have been interested in children's understanding of the figurative use of language. As with lexical knowledge, where children have been found to know more about words than they can reflect in their definitions (Nippold, 1988b), children's understanding of figurative language in sentences (idioms, proverbs, metaphors, and similes) as demonstrated in multiple-choice and picture identification tasks exceeds their ability to actively explain what they know (Nippold, 1988a).

There have been a number of studies demonstrating that with the use of age-appropriate materials and testing procedures even preschool children are able to comprehend figurative language (see Nippold, 1988a, for citations and discussion). However, despite this early understanding of some aspects of figurative language, it seems clear that there is further development with age. Nippold (1988a) related this development to the growth in lexical knowledge, syntactic complexity, world knowledge, and analytical reasoning.

Finally, while development of language in the early years is characterized as rapid and salient in all areas, Nippold and Martin (1989) stated:

> it is now a well-documented phenomenon that language development during adolescence—especially in the areas of semantics, syntax, pragmatics, reading, and writing—unfolds in a slow and protracted manner and that growth becomes obvious only when sophisticated linguistic phenomena are analyzed and nonadjacent groups are compared. (p. 65)

More research in later language development is needed to determine the nature and extent of this growth.

SUMMARY

In this chapter, human language was defined as a structured system of principles and rules for relating sound and meaning. Within the language system four subsystems of rules were described: phonological rules for classifying and combining the sounds of language; morphological rules for determining the internal structure and formation of words; semantic rules for defining the meanings of individual morphemes, words, phrases, and sentences; and syntactic rules for combining words and phrases to form sentences. Knowledge of these rule systems of human language characterizes linguistic competence. The latter accounts for the speaker/ hearer's ability to produce and comprehend the sounds and meanings of language and to make judgments about sentence grammaticality, ambiguity, and paraphrase.

Linguistic competence was described as being a part of communicative competence, the latter being defined as knowledge of the ways in which language is used in social contexts. Communicative competence includes: knowledge of the sentence types that are most appropriate for eliciting the desired response; awareness of the background information required to convey the intended message; and understanding of the cooperative principles that underlie conversational exchanges.

Five approaches to acquisition were described:

The linguistic theory approach, which views language as arising out of innately specified cognitive structure and resulting from the setting of parameters for principles of a universal grammar (UG)

The behavioral theory approach, which sees language as similar to all other learned behaviors and as the result of stimulus-response learning

The cognitive theory approach, which perceives language as dependent on and emerging from general principles and concepts of cognition

The competition model approach, which arises out of the information processing paradigm and attempts to account for the individual variations in language learning

The social theory approach, which focuses on the effects of caregiver language input on child language output in the social contexts of early childhood

While proponents of each of these competing accounts of acquisition give evidence supporting their positions, this author views the linguistic account as being most consistent with the earlier description of language competence.

Much of linguistic competence is seen to emerge during the preschool years. Shortly after birth children give evidence of being able to discriminate speech sound contrasts. By 9 months to 1 year of age children are doing phonological analysis of word-level units, and during the second and third years of life they become able to recognize and discriminate phonological contrasts in syllables and feature segments. Speech production is characterized as going from babbling to word production in the first year of life. While there is some variation in the order of sound emergence, the early speech patterns of all children appear to reflect general simplifying of phonological patterns. Mastery of the phonetic inventory continues into the school years, and is attained by most children by the age of 7 or 8.

Morphological acquisition follows a similar course of acquisition for most children. Simple open-class root morphemes are learned first, followed by more complex morphemes and closed-class elements. Cross-linguistic variations in the acquisition of closed-class morphemes are said to arise from differences in the regularity, obligatoriness, and consistency of application of the morpheme paradigms in individual languages. In addition to learning the individual morphemes, morphological development involves the acquisition of word-level inflectional and derivational rules.

Semantic acquisition is seen to begin with the mapping of words onto "simple" concepts that the child has represented in the first year of life. By 1 year of age most children have uttered their first word. Around 18 months of age children experience a growth spurt in their vocabulary development, going on to acquire as many as 9 or 10 words a day. Vocabulary development continues during the school years and into adulthood. Not only are new words acquired, but the meanings of old words are refined and expanded.

Syntactic development is characterized by an increase in the length of children's utterances. Children begin to produce one-word utterances by 1 year of age. They begin combining two words by about 18 months of age and produce sentences of three or more words by around 2 years of age. Early two-word utterances are made up of "content" words that are combined to express universal semantic relations. "Function" words appear later as sentences become longer and more complex. The development of negative and interrogative sentences is marked by the maintenance of the canonical or lawful word order of the target language in the early stages, followed by the introduction of sentence permutations and contracted word forms.

Another aspect of syntactic development is the emergence of complex sentences in the speech of children between 2 and 4 years of age. Object complementation precedes subject complementation and continues to be more prevalent in the speech of adults as well. While there is considerable agreement on the order and age of emergence of complex sentences in production, there is considerable controversy regarding the age at which complex sentences are understood. In recent years, researchers have demonstrated understanding of complex sentences in children at younger and younger ages. Finally, the development of more complex knowledge of figurative language is seen to continue into the adolescent years.

3 / Cognition and Information Processing

In efforts to understand the nature of language-related learning disabilities, it is necessary to become informed, to some degree, about theories of normal cognition and its interaction with language. Cognitive psychology has been concerned with the study of how we think, learn, and know. *Thinking* is regarded as a conscious, intentional mental act, generally directed at achieving a desired outcome, such as the solution of a problem, a plan of action, or simply satisfaction of the need to understand. *Learning* involves memory and selective attention in the acquisition of new knowledge structures. *Knowing* has been described as the transformation and reduction of complex information to a simpler state, in which patterns have been abstracted out of a multiplicity of stimuli. The process of knowing is not necessarily conscious or volitional.

MAJOR COGNITIVE THEORIES

Cognitive psychology has been dominated by two major theoretical movements: traditional cognitive theory and behavioral learning theory. Traditional cognitive theory has been exemplified by Gestalt psychology and Piagetian theory, both largely European in origin, whereas behavioral learning theory has been dominant in America. Andre and Phye (1986) have compared these movements along a number of dimensions, a few of which are as follows:

Behavioral learning theory	Traditional cognitive theory
The learner is passive but reactive to environmental input.	The learner is active, operating on and transforming input.
Learning consists of associations among stimuli and responses and through the transfer of responses across situational similarities.	Learning consists of construction and reorganization of mental structures as a result of the interaction between prior knowledge and new information.
Theory verification consists solely of empirical research directed at observable phenomena.	Theories about mental functions are derived largely from observational research and logical analysis.

COGNITIVE INFORMATION PROCESSING

The cognitive information processing (CIP) model now in the mainstream may be characterized as an integration of some aspects of both of the earlier movements. As in behavioral psychology, the formation of associations is accorded a role in learning. However, current views regard associations as complex networks connecting mental structures called schemata. In the cognitive information processing model, the mind possesses structural components and processes for receiving, transforming, storing, and retrieving information. Figure 1 represents a model of the cognitive system as conceptualized by Andre and Phye (1986). The five basic components in this model are:

1. *Input* or *sensory registers*—for example, auditory and visual sensation as data for operations performed in perception (receives information)
2. *Short-term memory*—that is, limited capacity for current information processing (briefly stores and transforms information)
3. *Long-term memory*—that is, virtually unlimited capacity for storage of episodic and semantic information
4. *Executive component*, in control of information flow and allocation of processing resources (selects and performs operations on information)
5. *Output buffer* (speculative)—that is, the operation of well-learned skills at the automatic level requiring minimal allocation of attentional resources

In summary, external information is registered by the senses. Sensory information to which the individual attends is passed on to short-term memory, where a perceptual representation is briefly held until processed. The transformed information is either acted on or trans-

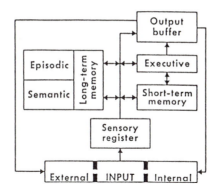

Figure 1. A model of the cognitive system. (From Andre, T., & Phye, G.D. [1986]. Cognition, learning and education. In G.D. Phye & T. Andre [Eds.], *Cognitive classroom learning: Understanding, thinking, and problem solving* [p. 4]. San Diego: Academic Press; reprinted with permission.)

ferred to long-term memory for storage. The executive component controls the selection, processing, and transfer of information and initiates retrieval of stored information. Varying degrees of attentional resources are brought to bear on the system, as modified by a hypothetical output buffer that engages automatic cognitive skills (i.e., those requiring low levels of attention). Thus, in the cognitive information processing model, heavy emphasis has been placed on such mechanisms as perception, attention, and memory, and the interrelations among these mechanisms in knowing, thinking, and learning. Research in cognitive information processing has been aimed at describing, to the degree that such descriptions are possible, the mechanisms, sequences, and interactions of human mental operations.

One segment of cognitive psychology has been involved in formulating computer simulation models that require explicit delineation of the information that must be represented and of the operations that must be performed in order to account for the internal thought processes leading to desired outcomes. In these models, cognitive psychologists have attempted to describe such processes and/or structures as:

Data input, including feature detection (bottom-up processing)

Encoding of input data into patterns matched to stored information (top-down and bottom-up processing)

The internal organization of memory, in terms of information stored in a network of interconnected nodes (structural knowledge of concepts and the relations among them)

Operations of spreading activation within a network of nodes in long-term memory (in higher level processes of comprehension and inference)

Although still in the experimental stages, this line of scholarship has had a significant impact on concepts and terminology employed in information processing theory and research. With particular application to the processing of language and discourse, oral and written, cognitive information processing provides a useful framework for investigating possible deficits in individuals with learning disabilities in the areas of perceptual input, attentional allocation, short-term memory capacity, and/or strategies for storing, integrating, and retrieving verbally coded information. These topics are explored in Chapters 7 and 8.

In the opinion of this author and others (Swanson, 1987; Torgeson, 1987), cognitive information processing theory and research findings are rich with promise for increased understanding of problems in learning, since the types of deficits reportedly manifested by individuals with learning disabilities lie in the very areas that are the subject of extensive investigation in this field.

This chapter is limited to considerations of those aspects of cognition that can serve as a foundation for conceptualizing the nature of these deficiencies: perception, attention, and memory. For each of these three topics, material selected for inclusion in this chapter is that deemed relevant to understanding problems manifested by individuals with language-related learning disabilities. A series of questions are posed at the end of the discussion of each of these aspects of cognition that anticipate the content of later chapters on disabilities, inviting the reader to reflect on the information presented here as it relates to such disabilities.

PERCEPTION

The following discussion of perception focuses on the manner in which information is taken in from the environment, predominantly through the auditory and visual modalities, which are central to educational learning. A grasp of some of the fundamental characteristics and processes of perception is necessary to understand the possible problems experienced by some individuals with language-related learning disabilities. Present concerns focus on the following key areas:

1. Input of information from the environment through the senses
2. Feature detection and pattern recognition
3. The relative roles of data-driven bottom-up processing and concept-driven top-down processing
4. Interactions between perception and other cognitive functions

One issue that has been debated is the degree to which the human being internalizes a *copy* of external stimuli or creates a *transformed representation* of the input. Although different schools of thought in cognitive science attribute varying degrees of importance to the extraction of stimulus information from the external environment through the senses, most are in agreement that the individual is an active processor on, rather than a passive receiver of, sensory information.

Sensory Storage

Numerous studies have demonstrated that, in the absence of further processing, visual and auditory impressions from sensation have brief duration (Matlin, 1989). In the visual modality, the duration of the icon (visual impression) is approximately 200–400 milliseconds. In the auditory modality, there is evidence of two types of echoic (auditory impression) storage reported under different experimental conditions: short echoic store (approximately 1/4th second) and long echoic store (approximately 2–3 seconds) (Cowan, 1984). Visual information in the environment is likely to be static or enduring, permitting reinspection during input. Auditory information is usually fleeting, existing temporally and therefore not accessible to reinspection. Therefore, the more persistent trace in echoic storage is viewed as a necessary precondition for processing. This brief stage has been labeled *preperceptual storage*.

Distinctive Features

There is fairly general acceptance of the assumption that sensory information is received in the form of *distinctive features* (Rumelhart, 1977a) picked up by certain physiological receptors (Matlin, 1989). Distinctive features are those aspects of sensory information that distinguish one set of items from other sets contrastively (Gibson & Levin, 1975). Feature detection represents data-driven, bottom-up processing, in which the individual actively searches the environment with the aim of discovering invariant, distinctive features and the systematic patterning of such features in a world of change (Gibson, 1969).

With regard to language, two types of distinctive features are important: visual and auditory. An example of visual distinctive features is letter configurations. Gibson (1969) developed a system of distinctive features for discriminating letters, regardless of their representation in print, type, or handwriting. This model continues to receive support through ongoing research. It is generally accepted that relatively few features serve as the basis for discrimination among and identification of letters. The main classes of features are:

Straight (including horizontal, vertical, and diagonal features)
Curve (including open and closed features)
Intersection
Redundancy (including symmetry and cyclic change)
Discontinuity (including vertical and horizontal features)

Examples of the application of distinctive feature analysis to some letters are:

Letter	Distinctive features
A	Straight (horizontal and diagonal)
	Intersection
	Discontinuity (vertical)
G	Straight (horizontal and vertical)
	Curve (open)
P	Straight (vertical)
	Curve (closed)
	Intersection
	Discontinuity (vertical)

In the auditory modality, a limited number of distinctive features serve to contrast phonemes along a number of dimensions. For example:

Stopping contrasts /t/ and /s/, both being voiceless consonants produced in the same place of articulation.
Voicing contrasts /t/ and /d/, both being stop consonants produced in the same place of articulation.

Distinctive features are not absolute; they are relational and contrastive. While members of a set of objects may share features, each object is characterized by its own unique pattern (Gibson & Levin, 1975). Models of perception tend to place feature detection at an earlier stage or a lower level of processing, whereas pattern recognition is regarded as a higher level of cognition.

Pattern Recognition

The process of perception involves recognizing patterns that correspond to information stored in memory. The crux of perception is believed to reside in the synthesis of features into a unitary code. Coding reduces the amount of information the system must process into more economical entities—for example, coding features of shapes into a face, or coding features of lines, curves, and angles, into a letter. It is speculated that, in early stages of perceptual learning, a considerable amount of attention is required to actively scan features and integrate them into a coded pattern. At subsequent stages this coded information is used as a filter, screening out irrelevant features from the processing operations. For example, in perceiving a face, the presence of eyes may not be differentially coded because all faces have eyes; thus a "face" (including eyes) is a recognized coded pattern. However, the color of the eyes may be discriminated, and thus "color of eyes" functions as a distinctive feature. With continued exposure to a pattern, a reduced amount of processing resources is believed to be allocated, with resultant perception at the automatic level (LaBerge, 1976); this idea may exemplify the hypothesis of an output buffer in the CIP model.

Bottom-Up and Top-Down Processing

The foregoing simplified account of feature detection and pattern recognition represents, to at least some degree, *bottom-up processing*, which is generally regarded as inadequate in characterizing perceptual learning and other cognitive functions from contemporary cognitive information processing viewpoints. There is widespread agreement that perception operates on nonsensory as well as sensory information. A considerable amount of information processing research has provided support for the assumption that pattern recognition involves more than identification of features in the face of substantial variation of actual physical stimuli (Rumelhart, 1977a). A *top-down processing* model assigns importance to the nonsensory information brought to bear both from context and from expectancies based on prior knowledge.

Cognitive psychologists have focused intensively on the interaction between bottom-up feature detection and top-down context-based expectancies, as presented in Figure 2. In this model,

1. Features from the sensory image are input to a pattern synthesizer.
2. Expectations are input to the pattern synthesizer simultaneously with sensory feature input.
3. A reconstructed representation of the target input is produced by the pattern synthesizer.
4. The representation is transferred into memory.
5. The memory system uses both stored knowledge and the current reconstructed representation to form a new set of expectancies.

The operation of this model can be seen in both speech perception and visual-verbal pattern recognition.

In the auditory domain, speech perception models have taken into account the relationship between stored linguistic knowledge, feature detection, and pattern recognition.

Speech Perception   Over the past two decades research has supported the theory of categorical perception, that is, the lack of a one-to-one correspondence between acoustic information and phoneme identification and discrimination (A.M. Liberman, Cooper, Shankweiler, &

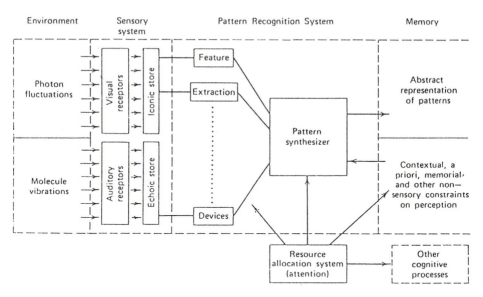

Figure 2. Diagram illustrating the interaction among environment, sensory system, pattern recognition system, and memory system. (From Rumelhart, D. [1977]. *Introduction to human information processing* [p. 100]. New York: John Wiley & Sons; reprinted with permission.)

Studdert-Kennedy, 1967; Studdert-Kennedy, Liberman, Harris, & Cooper, 1970). Speech sound perception has been observed to be related to the way the speaker/listener's language categorizes segments of the acoustic information and contrastively identifies such segments by label. "This means that, in speech, equal stimulus differences do not produce equal perceptual experiences" (Massaro, 1976, p. 305). Categorical perception has been demonstrated, for example, by studies showing that speakers of different languages differ in their perceptions of phoneme boundaries on the same acoustic continuum (Borden, Gerber, & Milsark, 1983). Korean speaker/listeners differed from English speaker/listeners in their identification of and discrimination between English-language phonemes. A substantial body of such evidence attests to the top-down influence of the individual's linguistic knowledge and the perception of acoustic input.

Figure 3 presents a model of speech perception from an information processing perspective. Massaro (1976) described some of the components of this model as follows:

Feature detection—the preperceptual reception and storage of raw auditory information at the sensory level.

Primary recognition—the perceptual discrimination of acoustic information and recognition of patterns that match representations of such patterns held in long-term memory. Perception may utilize knowledge of stored phonological rules of the listener's language through which the input is processed. Meaning is not a component at this level.

Secondary recognition—the transformation of perceptual information into meaningful units, involving access to the lexicon stored in long-term memory and the possible utilization of syntactic, contextual, and abstract semantic knowledge. Secondary

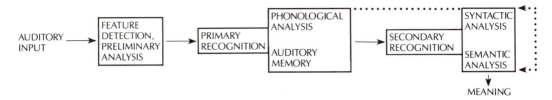

Figure 3. A model of speech perception. (Based on Massaro [1976] and Pisoni & Sawusch [1975].)

recognition might facilitate primary recognition in a top-down processing manner; for example, semantic-syntactic closure in conjunction with phonological closure may facilitate the processing of acoustic information.

The effects of stored knowledge on perception are illustrated by the well known phenomenon of "foreign accent." The sound patterns of a second language are perceived through the phonological system of the hearer's first language in a top-down processing fashion. This leads to misperceptions reflected in linguistic productions by the second-language speaker that represent the phonology of the first language. Thus, the speech output of a second-language speaker is usually marked by discernible differences from the output produced by a native speaker of the language.

In summary, in auditory verbal perception, sensory information being processed in a bottom-up fashion interacts with varying nonsensory information being processed in a top-down fashion. This nonsensory information may include:

1. Phonological knowledge about feature combinations, permissible sounds, and sequences of sounds in the language
2. Knowledge of word configurations
3. Sentence context (syntactic and semantic knowledge)
4. Thematic knowledge in discourse processing

Similar principles apply in the visual-verbal domain.

Visual-Verbal Pattern Recognition   The literature on perceptual processes involved in reading is vast. Psycholinguists generally accord a predominant role to top-down processing in the perception and interpretation of printed language. One example is the view of reading advanced by Smith (1973), in which the process was described as a trade-off between the amount of stored information behind the eyeball and the amount of visual information in front of the eyeball that required processing. That is, the burden placed on visual perception during the act of reading (bottom-up processing) is substantially reduced because of the knowledge (linguistic and general) that is stored in the reader's brain and invoked during the process of decoding the printed information (top-down processing).

Also, the greater the expectation of a particular stimulus, the greater the probability that it will be perceived. Knowledge of familiar words has been found to be more advantageous to perception of letters within a presented word than perception of letters in a nonword string. For example, letters tend to be more readily or rapidly perceived in *c h a i r* than in *i r h a c*. These effects have been demonstrated repeatedly in laboratory experiments (Rumelhart, 1977a; Rumelhart & McClelland, 1982; Whittlesea & Brooks, 1988).

Furthermore, sentence context has been found to facilitate perception more than individual word context. In an early study of this effect, Tulving, Mandler, and Baumel (1964) reported that subjects exposed to 8, 4, 2, or 0 words from stimulus sentences perceived target words more rapidly in response to a larger amount of contextual information. Results demonstrated a trade-off between the amount of contextual information available and the amount of time required to perceive the word. That is, the more words presented in the context sentence, the faster was perception of the target word.

Interaction of Bottom-Up and Top-Down Processing in Reading During the 1980s, cognitive psychologists increasingly turned their attention to further delineation of the role of bottom-up feature detection in interaction with the contextual influences of top-down processing. A series of studies by Rumelhart and McClelland (1982) provided support for the following proposed interactive model during the reading process. Seeing a string of letters in words or word-like configurations causes activation of features from which compatible letter units are activated. Knowledge of words (and pseudowords composed of pronounceable sequences of letters, such as *worl* or *owdr*) tends to activate perception of candidate letters. As one or more letters are activated, they serve to facilitate perception of other letters. For example, in processing the word "slant," the curved, straight, and vertical features of "a" are likely to be activated in the context of *sl_nt*, because other feature configurations in letters such as *i* or *o* would not satisfy the contextual constraints of a familiar English word. This effect has been termed "contextual enhancement on the perception of letters in words" (Rumelhart & McClelland, 1982, p. 72). Thus letter identification in words is facilitated through the interaction of both top-down and bottom-up processing.

In a study by Rueckl and Oden (1986), subjects presented with letter strings such as *b e a _ s* selected stimuli for word completion from an array of letters and letter-like characters ranging from *n* to *r* (bottom-up, data-driven processing):

ɒ ɒ ɾ ɾ

In addition, different contexts were presented for word choice (top-down processing):

The [dairy farmer/zookeeper] raised bea_s to supplement his income.

If the sentence context was about a zookeeper, subjects were more likely to choose the "bears" response when the letter-like character they were shown had a shortened rather than a lengthened right side. They were also more likely to choose the "bears" response in the context of the zookeeper than in that of the dairy farmer. Thus, *both* bottom-up features and top-down contextual knowledge were influential in pattern recognition.

In a recent study, Whittlesea and Brooks (1988) attempted to determine the relative influence of stored general knowledge about word structure and specific experimental training on perceptual recognition of letters, letter strings, pseudowords, and natural words. They found, as anticipated, that letters presented in words or pseudowords were more readily perceived than letters in nonword strings. However, they also found that prior training in orientation toward altered features produced some bottom-up advantage in the relative and absolute perceptibility of the letters alone as well as in their occurrence in words, pseudowords, and phrases.

Recent opinion in visual cognition has called into question the unduly heavy reliance on top-down processing accounts of perception. Pinker (1985) voiced some of the concern in terms of failure of the research and theory to clarify what kind of knowledge is brought to bear on recognition and how it is brought to bear. He, along with some other contemporary scholars, has reaffirmed some of the earlier claims made by Gibson (1969):

> Given the enormous selection advantage that would be conferred on an organism that could respond to what was really in the world as opposed to what is expected to be in the world whenever these two descriptions were in conflict, we should seriously consider the possibility that human pattern recognition has the most sophisticated bottom-up pattern analyses that the light array and the properties of our receptors allow. (Pinker, 1985, p. 32)

In other words, in recent theory a greater role is being assigned to bottom-up processing than was heretofore the case. A contemporary position accords important functions to both bottom-up and top-down processing in a collaborative interaction.

Perceptual Development

There is reason to believe that, as a result of both maturation of the sensory receptors in terms of their increased ability to differentiate critical features and the accumulation of knowledge from experience, perceptual development progresses through the interaction of bottom-up and top-down processing. From an information processing perspective, it is suggested that, developmentally, there is progress from the considerable allocation of resources to such processes as figure–ground discrimination (detecting a target pattern against a background), feature detection, and coding to the automatization of such rudimentary processes. Thus, as a result of automatization of lower level processes, resources are freed up for the higher level cognitive processing related to the ability to combine present input information with stored information (Collins & Hagen, 1979; LaBerge, 1976).

The abilities to volitionally focus perception and attention may be viewed as complementary developmental processes. The young child's relative inability to focus attention is believed to result in scattered perception, and the failure to develop automatized focal processing is likely to place excessive demands on the system, with perception and attention dispersed (Collins & Hagen, 1979). Therefore, gains in automatized focus of perception may represent the liberation of resources from demands of effortful processing at earlier levels of maturation for use in higher levels of processing at subsequent levels of development.

Summary

Perception involves detection of stimulus features and the recognition of pattern synthesizing features on the basis of information stored in memory. Both bottom-up data and top-down knowledge and expectations are believed to interact in perception of information from the external environment. Perceptual development appears to reflect increasing automaticity of feature detection and growth in the knowledge brought to bear in pattern recognition.

Questions To Be Considered About
Perception and Language-Related Learning Disabilities

1. Does perception figure largely in the reading process?
2. Is there evidence of perceptual impairment or delayed development in the visual and/or auditory domains of individuals with learning and reading disabilities?

3. In the auditory domain, to what extent may sensory or nonsensory factors contribute to language processing problems?
4. In reading disability, to what extent may problems reside in perception versus other cognitive mechanisms such as attention and/or memory?

ATTENTION

Attention is a multifaceted phenomenon that defies simplistic, unitary definition. Over the years, various definitions have attempted to account for some of the major components encompassed in the concept of attention, including, among others, mental concentration, informational search, and selection (Stankov, 1983). A definition of attention eloquently expressed a century ago by William James (1890) is cited in contemporary literature with surprising frequency:

> Everyone knows what attention is. It is the taking possession by the mind, in clear and vivid form, of one out of what seems several simultaneously possible objects or trains of thought. Focalization, concentration, of consciousness are of its essence. It implies withdrawal from some things in order to deal effectively with others. (p. 403)

Some more recent efforts at definition relate attention to perception in a rather straightforward manner. For example, Gibson and Rader (1979) described attention as "the perceptual pickup of information that has optimal utility for the task at hand" (p. 3). They added that this perceptual attending may be internally or externally motivated. The attending process is generally believed to consist of both a perceptual component and a decision-making component. Stankov (1983) favored a definition of attention as related to intelligence: "the ability of the organism to deal with increasing amount of information" (p. 472). In succinct fashion, Matlin (1989) stated: "Attention is a concentration of mental activity" (p. 47).

The overlap between attention and perception is aptly illustrated by Neisser's (1979) investigation of information pickup in selective looking, using the umbrella woman experiment. Two groups of subjects were presented with a tape of a ball game. One group of subjects was instructed to press a key when a dark-shirted team member passed the ball (the focused attention group). The other group of subjects simply watched the tape without instructions to focus on the passing of the ball (nonattending group). About halfway through the 1-minute tape of the ball game, a woman carrying an open umbrella walked across the playing field. Subjects in the focused attention group never saw the umbrella woman. When the tape was replayed, they expressed surprise at her presence. The subjects in the nonattending group always noticed the umbrella woman immediately.

The conclusion drawn from a series of studies using this technique (with some variations) was that people fail to notice *unexpected* events, particularly when they are keenly focusing on a task perceived as difficult. In the absence of a task focus requiring concentrated effort, pickup of information is less constrained. Central to these findings are the effects of directed attention on information processing.

Characteristics of Attention

In an earlier paper, Posner and Boies (1971) suggested three characteristics of attention:

1. *Alertness*, or the ability to maintain optimal sensitivity to external stimuli
2. *Selection*, or the ability to concentrate awareness on one source of information rather than another

3. *Limited processing capacity*, a term that reflects the difficulty people have in processing two tasks simultaneously

The concept of attention as a limited-capacity system was heavily influenced by Broadbent's (1958) pioneering filter model that described the processing of information held in brief sensory storage until selected by the attention mechanism for conscious awareness and perception. This model posits a limited-capacity channel with a filter that blocks out all messages except the one selected for attention and for subsequent processing. More recent research has led to theories attributing greater flexibility to the attentional mechanism, as illustrated by the umbrella woman studies described above. Neisser (1975) pointed out that, in real life, people simultaneously perform tasks requiring different degrees and kinds of attention. Examples provided by Matlin (1989) include:

Listening to a lecture and taking notes at the same time

From two radio stations tuned in simultaneously, making a decision about which to attend to and which to tune out

It is acknowledged, however, that under many real life circumstances, people become inefficient if they try to attend to too many things at the same time. Thus, there is reason to continue to regard attention as a relatively fixed fund of resources that may be reallocated but not immeasurably increased. Therefore, a key assumption in many information processing accounts of attention is that, from the overwhelming number of stimuli impinging on the organism at any moment, only a small amount can be processed accurately and meaningfully. A contrast has been drawn between parallel processing of a multitude of information concurrently and serial processing, which can accommodate only one type of information at a time (Hirst, 1986). This contrast may have a rough correspondence to controlled (conscious) versus automatic (unconscious) processing (see discussion below).

Areas of Theoretical Consensus

Because there are different facets of attention and varying techniques are employed to study them, conflicting research findings and their attendant theories abound. Therefore, material included in this section of the chapter is confined to areas of relative consensus that most directly contribute to understanding interactions among aspects of attention and learning.

One assumption on which consensus has been achieved is that both semantic and sensory cues influence certain aspects of attention (Hirst 1986). This attests to the complementary roles of data-driven bottom-up and meaning-driven top-down processing. Furthermore, goals, motivation, and emotional states are considered to have a significant influence on the allocation of attentional resources (Eysenck, 1982). The positive impact of this mix of meaning and motivation on attention was asserted a century ago by James (1890):

The only pedagogic maxim bearing on attention is that the more interest the child has in advance in the subject, the better he will attend. Induct him therefore in such a way as to knit each new thing on to some acquisition already there. (p. 424)

Another well-researched and generally accepted aspect of attention is the existence of two modes of information processing: automatic and controlled. A.D. Fisk and Schneider (1984) described the two types of processing as follows:

Automatic Processing	Controlled Processing
Fast	Slow
Parallel	Serial
Effortless	Effortful
Not limited by short-term memory	Capacity limited
Not under direct control	Regulated by direct control
Reflects well-developed skills	Deals with novel or inconsistent information
Result of consistent processing over many trials	Easily modified, suppressed, or ignored
Once learned, difficult to suppress, modify, or ignore	

Shiffrin and Schneider (1984) believed that all tasks are carried out by combinations of automatic and controlled processing in parallel fashion without cost to either type of processing. However, an essential component of this theory is that two or more controlled processes cannot occur simultaneously without cost in the sharing of resources. That is, for the most part, only one controlled process may be effectively performed at any time, because controlled processing is believed to be more time consuming and effortful, utilizing substantially more of available resources in a limited-capacity system and placing heavier demands on short-term memory. One prominent model of a limited-capacity system proposes that short-term memory limitations may constrain attention (Shiffrin, 1976). In certain attentional processes, a search of features and decision making about their task relevance is required before this information is lost from short-term memory.

The development of automaticity has been empirically demonstrated as an effect of consistency in training during laboratory experiments. It is believed to result from well-practiced perceptions and decisions, probably as a result of the activation of sequences of maximally developed links between nodes (i.e., hypothesized clusters of stored information about features, words, or concepts) (A.D. Fisk & Schneider, 1984). Acquisition of a new skill starts out as controlled processing, "but as learning progresses, automatic detection begins to operate in parallel with controlled search and eventually provides the dominant response basis" (Shiffrin & Schneider, 1984, p. 273). This operation is judged to be crucial to the acquisition of critical academic skills, and disturbances in the balance between automatic and controlled processing may be one of the dimensions of attention that contribute to certain learning disabilities.

Dimensions of Attention

Attention has a number of dimensions that have been extensively studied in laboratory experimentation. Different bodies of research have investigated the following aspects of attention:

Arousal or alertness: the degree to which an organism is in an attentional state

Selective attention: the choice of one message of concern out of many that may be present simultaneously

Divided attention: processing information from two or more simultaneously present messages or stimuli

Focused attention: concentration on task-relevant stimuli in the presence of incidental or distracting stimuli

Vigilance: the ability to sustain attention to a task over extended time periods

Preparatory set: the influence of advance cueing or priming on attentional performance

A necessarily limited number of the key concepts current in the theoretical and research literature on each of these dimensions is presented.

Arousal and Vigilance   Arousal refers to a number of physiological and behavioral states associated with heightened excitation or increased mobilization of energy. Shifts from a state of low arousal to a higher level of arousal are accompanied by a variety of changes in the autonomic and central nervous systems. For example, in response to different conditions or task demands, alterations may occur in heart rate, blood pressure, electrical activity in the brain, and/or muscle tone (Parasuraman, 1984). The level of arousal tends to decline during tasks requiring attentional vigilance under conditions of prolonged and monotonous activity.

It has been reported from studies of repetitive, prolonged responding that subjects have failed to detect stimuli on some of their presentations, made incorrect decisions, or slowed their response rate. Apparently they "switched off" for brief periods of time, particularly when input stemmed from the same sensory source (e.g., visual). This decline in performance, indicating decreases in vigilance or sustained attention, was systematically reduced in reaction to frequent shifts to new signals (Posner, 1973).

In contrast to effects of lowered arousal, evidence exists that, in states of high arousal, there is a reduction in the ability to resist distraction from the environment (Eysenck, 1982). There are implications here for later considerations of attentional factors related to some learning disabilities.

Selectivity   "Selective attention refers to the differential processing of simultaneous sources of information" (W.A. Johnston & Dark, 1986, p. 44). In other words, out of all current input from external and internal stimuli, the individual selects particular information for further processing. Among the frequently used techniques for studying selective attention are *message shadowing* (speaking aloud words as soon as they are heard) and *dichotic listening* (hearing two messages simultaneously presented to different ears). Early pioneering studies by C. Cherry (1953) and Treisman (1960) found that subjects shadowing a message presented in one ear, to which they were attending, were frequently unaware of a message presented in the unattending ear. They were best able to ignore the competing message in the unattending ear when voices were of a different gender, were spatially separated, or spoke a different language.

These studies led to the conclusion that selection was based on some stimulus characteristic. However, subsequent modification of the experimental procedures and materials provided evidence of the influence of semantic content on message selection. For example, from the well-known "cocktail party effect," it is evident that some meaningful features of unattended messages are processed. That is, despite the ability to focus attention on a particular conversation in the context of competing messages, hearing one's own name mentioned elsewhere tends to capture one's attention. This phenomenon suggests that irrelevant information is not completely blocked out. If it has some particular significance, the attention filter "only attenuates it, like a volume control that is turned down but not off" (H. Gleitman, 1986).

Levels of Analysis   It is considered quite possible by some scholars that there are two levels of analysis of sensory information (signals). Treisman and her colleagues (Treisman, 1986; Treisman & Gelade, 1980; Treisman & Souther, 1985) presented evidence of a *preattentional processing* stage and a *focused attention* stage. In a preliminary stage (preattentive), information features are processed in an automatic, parallel fashion. For instance, the presence of a red object among many objects that are not red is rapidly, effortlessly noted. This effect is likely to occur when single or simple features are processed. However, when a number of features must be integrated into some entity, such as finding a red X among a number of red and blue letters, attention becomes focused and operates in slower, serial fashion.

From a slightly different viewpoint, two signal analyzing mechanisms, one passive and the other active, have been proposed. The passive system is believed to be capable of only rough preliminary analysis of many events. At this level there is only passing awareness without retention for processing at the more active level that permits understanding and later retrieval. Such incoming sensory information is believed to be held very briefly in a temporary storage buffer. At the level of preliminary analysis, only enough information is extracted to restrict the input that may be deserving of attention to a small, manageable number of signals. The active device uses meaning, context, and situational expectations from previously analyzed material to further reduce the number of signals that may require additional consideration to a still smaller, workable set. Thus, both top-down and bottom-up processing function in the selection processes.

W.A. Johnston and Dark (1986) reviewed a number of prominent theories about the relative effects of bottom-up sensory processing and top-down semantic processing on selective detection of relevant and irrelevant information. The absence of complete agreement on this issue may be the result of variations in processing conditions that are too intricately detailed to be comprehensively reviewed here. Under some conditions, in early stages of processing information that is the object of focus (particularly visual), selection is guided by sensory cues. This bottom-up selection tends to be less effortful and more accurate than semantic selection (p. 48).

However, under certain conditions, top-down semantic processing in the form of previously learned and currently activated knowledge may influence attention to irrelevant as well as relevant information (p. 48). This effect has been recognized in the well-known "cocktail party" phenomenon. In selective attention studies, listening to an unfamiliar relevant passage required greater effort in the presence of a familiar irrelevant passage. "One way to interpret this finding is that selective processing of relevant information is difficult when the irrelevant information conforms to active schemata" (W.A. Johnston & Dark, 1986, p. 64).

Voluntary and Involuntary Selection   Selective attention may operate at either a conscious/voluntary level or a passive/involuntary level believed to be relatively automatic. James (1890) provided examples of automatic (involuntary) attention to salient sensory cues, such as a sudden loud noise, and subtle semantic cues, such as a soft signal from a lover. Examples of voluntary selective attention include the ability to follow a particular conversation at a noisy party while ignoring other conversations, or selecting one radio program out of two that may have been picked up simultaneously: "If you listen closely to one program, you notice only the superficial characteristics of the other" (Matlin, 1989, p. 49).

Knowledge and Selective Attention   W.A. Johnston and Dark (1986) emphasized the role of schematic knowledge in selective attention. That is, selective attention is primed by knowledge possessed by the message receiver and the effects of prior processing of information. Put succinctly by James (1890), "Attention *creates* no idea; an idea must already be there before we can attend to it" (p. 450). As expressed in contemporary terms, "Most students of attention now conclude that the psychological event we think of as attention must occur after sensory information has contacted our base of knowledge in long-term memory" (Tomblin, 1984, p. 33).

Some early findings have supported the assumption that even information that is ostensibly ignored has been meaningfully processed. For example, in one such study, when a sentence such as "He threw stones at the bank" was presented to the attending ear while a single disambiguating word such as "river" or "savings" was presented simultaneously to the other ear, subjects tended to report the sentence in light of the meaning of the word heard in the unattending ear, even though they had no conscious recollection of its having been presented (MacKay, 1973). Thus, even though subjects were not able to remember or report on the information presented to the unattending ear, these results were interpreted as evidence that the unattended message had been processed sufficiently to have accessed the semantic structures related to the attended message (Posner, 1973). More recently the interpretation of such results has been questioned because of the failure of other investigators to replicate this effect (Matlin, 1989).

Which information is selected for attention in natural conditions is generally believed to be determined by both the meaningfulness of the information and its relevance to present context-sensitive, goal-oriented processes. The extraction and analysis of information appears to be aided, to a nontrivial degree, by prior contextual information stored in long-term memory and expectations related to the situation. Therefore, selective attention is viewed as a highly active process. In the opinion of some researchers, attention itself is considered to be the result rather than the cause of perception and cognition (Neisser, 1979; Tomblin, 1984).

Focused Attention   Focused attention may be regarded as an artifact of selective attention. That is, what has been selected for attention among competing stimuli is the object or event on which focus will be placed. Carver and Scheier (1981) pointed out one possible distinction in focus that could be made selectively by a relatively fixed-capacity attentional mechanism: focus on the environment versus focus on the self. "As attention outward increases, attention to the self will decrease, and vice versa" (p. 35). They considered the possibilities of rapidly shifting focus or divided attention as equally plausible means of coordinating these two types of focus.

Internal Versus External Focus   Much, but not all, self-focus involves awareness of internal states such as cues indicating embarrassment, fear, pain, and so forth. Research has demonstrated that external focus of attention tends to occur in response to events that are novel or that occur with increasing speed or complexity. Under such conditions, focus on the self tends to diminish, accounting for such phenomena as reduced awareness of pain in the face of external distractors. Conversely, excessive self-focus would tend to reduce attentional focus on external information (Carver & Scheier, 1981).

Senf (1972) took account of such internal cues as distractors in his information processing model of attention. Within this model, he postulated an information array of limited capacity and suggested that cues from internal states, such as anxiety, may occupy a relatively large amount of space in such an array, thereby reducing attentional focus on external stimuli relevant to successful performance on learning tasks.

Active Versus Passive Attention   Two attentional modes are contrasted to describe different degrees of attentional focus:

> *Active, analytical attention*, believed to result in the fuller occupation of available space in the information array, leaving less space for the intrusion of distracting information
> *Passive, global attention*, believed to result in reduced entry of information into the array, thus leaving more space available for irrelevant, distracting entries

From this perspective, active attention contributes to the maintenance of focus, whereas passive attention is subject to disruption of focus as a result of either the intrusion of irrelevant external input or internal subjective distraction.

Divided Attention   According to much of prevailing theory, divided attention must allocate some portion of available resources to different functions performed simultaneously. Most people are familiar with the phenomenon of divided attention in everyday situations, such as the ability to walk and think at the same time. Walking is so automatic it requires a minimal allotment of attentional capacity, freeing up processing resources for the more demanding task of concentrated thought. However, walking on a tightrope would compel one to make a drastic shift of attentional capacity to the act of walking, severely limiting capacity to think about anything else at that time.

Studies of divided attention using dual process or time-sharing tasks have yielded evidence of demands on separate resource pools, that is, different modalities such as vision, audition, speech, and motor function (J. E. Hoffman, Houck, MacMillan, Simons, & Oatman, 1985; Kinsbourne & McMurray, 1975). These results "suggest that automated tasks may well use limited capacity resources that are highly specific to particular information processing functions" (Hoffman et al., 1985, p. 51). It has been found that, when automated attentional responses are required under conditions demanding increased allocation of resources to another task in the *same* modality, such as listening to two messages simultaneously and making a response to one of them, accuracy and speed of response tend to be reduced.

Hoffman and his colleagues, using a physiological measure (event-related evoked brain potentials), secured objective evidence of the relative amount of attention allocated to competing components in a dual-task performance. Reductions in the physiological measurement of attentional activity correlated positively with reductions in task performance accuracy on automatic targets.

In studies that experimentally manipulated the relative allocation of attention to controlled processing (i.e., effortful, serial, slow) and automatic processing (i.e., effortless, parallel, fast) in divided attention tasks, it has been found that accurate automatic processing can occur while leaving no record in long-term memory. A commonplace example of such a phenomenon may be locking the extra security lock on the door when leaving for work in the morning and later worrying that the house may be burglarized because by midafternoon there is no recollection of having performed this highly automatic act. Conversely, other divided attention experiments have found that even very brief controlled processing produced changes in long-term memory: "The close parallel between attention and memory literature suggests when we process information, we can perform serial controlled processing in a stage and remember, or parallel processing in a stage and forget" (Fisk & Schneider, 1984, p. 196).

Divided Attention and Intelligence   Stankov (1983) argued that dual task performance, requiring greater processing effort and the deployment of more processing resources, may be relevant to measures of intelligence. He noted that such tasks as dichotic listening appear to assess memory span and to serve as indicators of intelligence. The existence of individual differences in strategies selected for task performance may be interpreted as one example of the relationship between attention and intelligence. In a dual task situation, greater effectiveness may be related to a choice to work first on the easier task of the two, freeing up capacity for further work on the remaining task. Furthermore, Stankov concluded that speed of perceptual search and speed of attention switching are indications of the general speed of information processing, assumed to be an important characteristic of intelligence. This mental quickness, related to efficiency of working memory, may be related to the ability to allocate attentional resources.

Flexibility Versus Fixed Capacity   The notion of limited resources as an explanation for the effects of divided attention in time-sharing tasks is challenged by Hirst (1986). Some dramatic results of experimental training in simultaneous reading of demanding prose and writing from dictation lent support for the contention that the capacity of the cognitive system may grow with experience and intensive practice. Hirst (1986) argued that the subjects in this study "were learning to do two meaningful tasks at the same time, neither of which are simple enough to permit automaticity" (p. 129). From Hirst's (1986) point of view, the fixed resource capacity theory is viewed as less appealing in its explanation of dual task performance than one positing a more flexible concept of *skill*, which takes into account such variables as individual differences and practice.

While debate continues on this and previously mentioned issues, the various theories do serve to provide fresh perspectives in our attempts to understand attentional factors contributing to academic success or failure.

Preparatory Set or Cued/Primed Attention   External cues given in advance of subsequently presented information appear to induce expectations regarding what is to be perceived. This expectation is represented as "attentional activation of the particular pattern code to a level of excitation above the code's base rate of activity" (LaBerge, Petersen, & Norden, 1977, p. 287). Such a selective increase in prior attentional activation has been found to facilitate response to displayed patterns, in terms of more rapid reaction times, in laboratory experiments (LaBerge et al., 1977). Under more natural instructional conditions in reading comprehension tasks, questions presented to students before they read a text led to a significant increase in memory for information related to the questions. These adjunct questions are thought "to provide a task schema which controls the allocation of processing attention during study" (Kulhavy, Schwartz, & Peterson, 1986).

Attentional Development

At the conclusion of the section on perceptual development, it was observed that the immature child's relative inability to focus attention results in scattered perception. Until the young child develops automatized focal processing, it is likely that both perception and attention will tend to be diffused. Kinsbourne and Caplan (1979) reported on the inefficient attentional strategies used by young children:

> The way young children inspect things is *incomplete*: Their gaze is arrested by eye-catching features so they ignore other parts of the display. It is also *redundant*: Certain features are repeatedly inspected although they were understood at first glance. And it is *unsystematic*: Attention flits from salient feature to salient feature without consistent direction or any other organization . . . (p. 56)

The young child's attention is readily trapped by features described as high in the perceptual hierarchy. For example, in visual information, dimensions of form and color are more salient than dimensions of size, location, orientation, sequence, and texture. With increased development, the child's attention is detached from the more salient but possibly irrelevant aspects and becomes more focused on critical features that may be less perceptually salient. According to Kinsbourne and Caplan (1979): "Thus the ability to detach and redirect attention accompanies brain maturation. What exactly is attended to is determined by experience" (p. 56).

This growing ability to regulate response to relevant stimuli is believed to be related to cognitive development that engages higher level internal processes in the control of reactions to external percepts (H.A. Simon, 1972). Evidence exists of a developmental trend in the ability to focus critical amounts of attention on central versus incidental stimuli (P.H. Miller & Weiss, 1981).

Hale (1979), who had earlier reported similar results from a series of studies, has questioned such findings as experimental artifacts, since his observation of spontaneous performance yielded evidence of a developmental trend toward *broader* attentional deployment. With maturation, heightened awareness of specific, independent dimensions such as size, shape, hue, and brightness have been observed. Furthermore, with increased age, children have reportedly demonstrated greater flexibility in using either selective attention or broader attentional deployment to meet specific task demands. Younger children were observed to continue to employ the same attentional deployment pattern regardless of the nature of the task. In this respect, they remained relatively unaffected by instruction to alter their strategy (Hale, 1979).

A series of studies by Miller and her colleagues (DeMarie-Dreblow & Miller, 1988; P.H. Miller & Weiss, 1981; Woody-Ramsey & Miller, 1988) has demonstrated a complex relationship between developing ability to employ selective attention strategies, memory, and processing capacity. Preschool children and children in grades 2, 5, and 8 were shown an array of small doors that concealed pictures of classes of objects, such as household items or animals. Pictures on the doors symbolized the class of concealed pictures (e.g., a house for household objects). Subjects were instructed to inspect the items pictured behind the doors and to try to remember as many of them as possible. Clear developmental patterns were observed in the selective strategies employed and the resultant performance on the recall task:

1. Preschool children were not observed to use an organized strategy for selective attention spontaneously or to restrict their attention to stimuli that were task relevant (Woody-Ramsey & Miller, 1988).
2. Second-grade children tended to open doors in no perceivable selective pattern relevant to the task. They generally opened doors that were adjacent in a row, rather than selecting those whose characteristics met task requirements (e.g., opening all doors on which a house was pictured).
3. Between grades 2 and 5 there was a marked gain in the use of efficient selective attention strategies.
4. Between grades 5 and 8, further progress in selective attention strategy use was only moderate (P.H. Miller & Weiss, 1981).

The use of recall as an instrument for measuring selective attention does provoke some questions about the information processing dynamics involved in relation to age. Young children, apparently less able to use their own selective strategies to enhance recall, have performed as well as older subjects when adults have demonstrated and guided application of the strategy (DeMarie-Dreblow & Miller, 1988). It is suggested that, without external support, the degree of effort needed for second-grade children to try to use a self-generated selective atten-tion strategy reduced their capacity for efficient retrieval. However, with external support, reduction of effort by young children facilitated recall, suggesting that when strategy effort was low "even young children had capacity to devote to further mnemonic processes" (DeMarie-Dreblow & Miller, 1988, p. 1511). This complex interaction among available resources (includ-ing knowledge base), degree of effortfulness, and strategy use is discussed in greater detail in the section on memory.

Summary

Attention consists of the following dimensions: arousal or alertness, selectivity, dual process-ing, focus on central versus incidental information, and heightened response in reaction to preparatory set. Attentional resources, although limited in capacity, may be differentially allo-cated in automatic and controlled processing tasks. Selection and subsequent processing of some but not all available information is largely determined by the significance of the informa-tion and the relevant knowledge possessed by the individual. It is possible to attend to two or more tasks simultaneously if certain skills have been well practiced to the point of relative automaticity. The active analytical focus of attention on central, task-relevant information tends to reduce the intrusion of distractors. All of these aspects of attention reflect develop-mental trends.

Questions To Be Considered About
Attention and Language-Related Learning Disabilities

1.   May delay in attentional development negatively affect educational performance?
2.   Do all individuals with learning disabilities manifest attentional impairment?
3.   Are there subgroups of people with learning disabilities who have specific deficits in sus-taining attention or selective attention?
4.   May attentional deficits be a result rather than a cause of learning failure?
5.   May differences in verbal ability affect selective attending to linguistically coded infor-mation?

MEMORY

Memory is widely believed to be central to cognition. The rich body of literature in this area provides information that contributes to an understanding of the interaction of memory with attention, perception, language, and learning. Certain central concepts relevant to the role of memory in learning have been selected for consideration here.

The "Stores" Model of Memory

Traditionally in cognitive psychology, the mechanisms for memory processing have been con-ceptualized as a system of information storage stages: sensory registers, short-term stores, working memory, and long-term stores. The model formulated by Atkinson and Shiffrin (1971) is presented in Figure 4.

Sensory Registers   Sensory input from the environment is held for a very brief period. Traces of visual input are believed to endure for less than 1 second and traces of auditory input for possibly 2 seconds (Craik & Levy, 1976). Because of the rapid decay of sensory informa-tion, it tends to be lost unless it is quickly transferred to short-term storage. During transfer

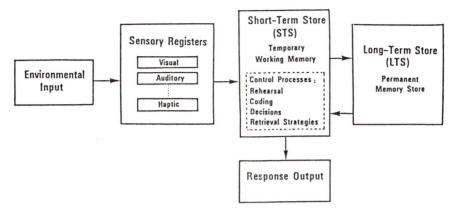

Figure 4. The Atkinson-Shiffrin model of memory. (From Atkinson, R.C., & Shiffrin, R.M. [1971]. The control of short-term memory. *Scientific American, 225,* p. 82; reprinted with permission.)

from sensory registers to short-term storage, information may be recoded in different modalities. For example, visual information may be verbally coded or verbal input may be recoded into a visual image.

Memory codes are related to the different modalities of input and the different formats for storage of information in the memory systems. The *iconic code* consists of images in the visual modality. The *echoic code* consists of patterns in the auditory modality, both verbal and non-verbal. The *enactive code* consists of images in the motoric modality.

Sensory information is recognized and becomes meaningful through perceptual processes discussed above, in which patterns stored in long-term memory are thought to play a role. Attention is believed to determine which sensory information is to be retained for further processing and which is to be ignored and forgotten.

Short-Term Stores Short-term memory is characterized by limited capacity (five to nine chunks of information) and by limited duration (approximately 15 seconds) unless it is subjected to some form of active processing such as rehearsal. Maintenance rehearsal consists of the repetition of items of information in short-term storage prior to transfer to long-term storage. There is strong evidence that phonemic coding is more effective than semantic or visual coding for retaining information in short-term memory. That is, representing information in some acoustic/articulatory form enhances its retention over short intervals (Craik & Levy, 1976).

The longer information is retained in short-term storage, as in maintenance rehearsal, the more information will be transferred to long-term storage. In addition, the quantitative limitations of short-term memory may be substantially increased through the imposition of higher levels of organization. Such elaborative rehearsal involves the use of more active strategies such as the formation of associations among items and the recoding of many low-information chunks into fewer high-information chunks (Loftus & Loftus, 1976). For example, the digits in Example 2 are easier to retain than those in Example 1:

1. 6 0 1 9 5 3 6 8 4 7 1 2
2. 601   953   368   712

The letters in Example 4 are easier to retain than those in Example 3:

3.   D H M A O T X I F
4.   HOT   MAD   FIX

The words in Example 6 are easier to retain than those in Example 5:

5.   rapid keep is to in hard with up world changes the it
6.   It is hard to keep up with rapid changes in the world

Thus, structure from the grouping of digits into hundreds, the morphology of words, and the syntax of sentences all have an enhancing effect on the amount of information that can be retained in short-term storage.

Working Memory   Working memory is considered more robust than short-term memory and more ephemeral than long term storage. Its primary function is to transfer information from short-term to long-term storage and to facilitate verbal reasoning and comprehension. During task performance, "Working memory refers to the role of temporary storage in information processing" (Baddeley, 1981). The information in working memory is believed to consist of currently encoded input and the declarative and procedural knowledge retrieved from long-term memory relevant to immediate processing functions in task performance (J.R. Anderson, 1983). According to Anderson, *declarative knowledge* refers to what is known and *procedural knowledge* is information about how cognitive activities are performed. A substantial part of declarative knowledge is believed to be stored in propositional form. A *proposition* is an abstract representation of the relationship between concepts (Matlin, 1989) in the smallest unit of knowledge that can be judged true or false (J.R. Anderson, 1976). Each term abstractly represented within a proposition itself represents a network of associations, as illustrated in Figure 5.

The function of working memory is considered to be goal oriented. For example:

1.   Goal: setting the time on a new watch
2.   Retrieval of procedural knowledge: look at instruction book
3.   Declarative knowledge held in working memory: propositions (e.g., the watch has three buttons), and visual images (e.g., location of the buttons) (Black, 1984)

Baddeley (1981, 1986) provided a tentative model of working memory consisting of three components:

> Two peripheral systems:
>> An *articulatory loop* serving to maintain information through subvocal verbal rehearsal
>> A *visuospatial "scratch pad"* serving to maintain visualization of spatial information
> A central *executive* that selects and controls the operation of various higher level processes (e.g., organization of information, retrieval of relevant information from long-term memory, reasoning)

An earlier premise that increases in the current memory load, in excess of the capacity of the peripheral systems, would detrimentally reduce resources of the executive control system has not been fully substantiated by later research. More recent evidence supports the notion of

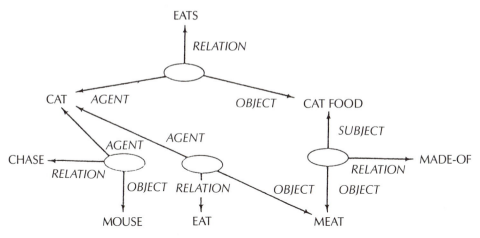

Figure 5. A partial representation of the proposition representing *cat* in memory. (From Matlin, M.R. [1989]. *Cognition*. Orlando, FL: Holt, Rinehart, and Winston, Inc. ; reprinted with permission.)

a separate verbal memory component (for maintenance rehearsal) that does not necessarily compete for resources in such high-level processes as reasoning. To illustrate this point, it was found that, in a study of the effects of length of digit span on reasoning, "some subjects were able to hold seven or eight digits while performing a complex verbal reasoning task with no apparent decrement in speed or accuracy" (Baddeley, 1981, p. 22). This finding and its interpretation within the theoretical model is relative rather than absolute, because all subjects did demonstrate reductions in performance on the reasoning task if the digit load was large enough.

Baddeley (1981) is inclined toward viewing the central executive as separate from the memory system, assigning it to the mechanism of attention. While arguing that the above results are inconsistent with the notion of a single pool of general processing capacity for the peripheral and control systems, he acknowledged that:

> Once the memory system becomes overloaded, however, it requires the controller to bring in further resources in an attempt to avoid breakdown and consequent loss of the stored material. The more attention that is devoted to supporting the memory component, the less is available for reasoning, and the slower and more error prone is the reasoning performance. (p. 22)

From the above perspective, it may be inferred that individual differences in efficacy of encoding incoming information in verbal and/or visual short-term memory and in effectiveness of interfacing current input with information from long-term memory affect the transfer of new information to long-term storage. This may be regarded as a major facet of learning, a point of central interest in this book.

Primacy and Recency Effects   Craik and Levy (1976) provided an extensive review of theory and research on primary (short-term) memory and its interaction with secondary (long-term) memory. One of the many aspects examined is the primacy and recency effect noted in numerous studies. When a list of items is presented for subjects to recall, different experimental conditions have been found to determine whether initial items are more effectively remembered (the *primacy* effect) or terminal items are better remembered (the *recency* effect). Many studies have reported a higher proportion correct for the most recent items under conditions of immediate free recall, in which terminal items of a single list are permitted to remain in the rehearsal buffer of primary memory. Other studies, requiring subjects to memorize multiple lists and then engage in final free recall of all lists, reported that items in the terminal position of all the lists are recalled less well.

However, under certain conditions, the first item is recalled better than words in the middle or end of the list, as in initial free recall of the first few lists in a series of lists. This primacy effect has been attributed to the allocation of full attention to the first item, in contrast to the shared attention available for subsequent items. In general, because of both the primacy and recency effects, middle items fare more poorly than either initial or final items in lists of material freely recalled. Such results are interpreted as support for the limited capacity theory of primary or short-term memory. Attentional allocation and rehearsal are viewed as two of the mechanisms operating in the transfer of information from short-term to long-term storage.

Long-Term Stores   Long-term memory functions include the acquisition of information, an enduring trace of which is believed to be left in the nervous system in some form whose nature continues to be debated. Storage of information is facilitated by integrating new information into current knowledge structures and by the retrieval of information from long-term storage. In contrast to a behaviorist view, cognitive psychology conceives of memory as a constructive process rather than a faithful record of input. That is, internal processes transform input into representations that are reconstructed upon retrieval (Schacter & Graf, 1986).

Information stored in long-term memory is generally envisioned as a "loosely structured network . . . in which associative relationships exist within a network and possibly between structures" (Solso, 1974, p. 200). The basic elements of memory structures are believed to be conceptual storage nodes, each of which is characterized as the combination of a concept and the array of perceptual codes linked to it (Atkinson, Herrmann, & Wescourt, 1974). The following example from Atkinson and his colleagues serves as an illustration: "the sight of an actual dog, the auditory perception of the spoken word, the display of the printed word, etc." (Atkinson et al., 1974, p. 104), linked together with the concept of "dog," would form a conceptual storage node. It is proposed that the activation of the network has a neurophysiological base: "At some level of abstraction it is reasonable to identify activation with rate of neural firing (although nodes probably do not correspond to simple neurons)" (J.R. Anderson, 1983, p. 27).

Some argue against the notion that information is stored in memory in any special place, suggesting that the term "memory store" is used by many psychologists as a convenient shorthand rather than a strict definition (Weisberg, 1980). Indeed, the actual nature of the representation of information in memory is open to different interpretations according to the type of information stored and the model for conceptualizing memory systems. J.R. Anderson (1983) postulated three types of memory representations:

> Temporal strings to record the sequential structure of events
> Spatial images that preserve configural information
> Abstract propositions that preserve semantic relations

Such a conceptualization of the contents of long-term memory is in accord with Tulving's (1972, 1986) classification of stored information into episodic and semantic memory.

Episodic and Semantic Memory   Tulving (1986) contrasted the two types of memory, episodic and semantic, as follows:

> Episodic memory refers to "unique, concrete, personal, temporally dated events" (p. 307). Semantic memory refers to "general, abstract, timeless knowledge that a person shares with others" (p. 307).

Episodic memory is described as the storage of perceptual events that are temporally dated and consist of temporal-spatial relations among experienced events, that is, event knowledge (J.R. Anderson, 1983). Episodic memories of actual events may be autobiographical in nature, containing perceptible attributes and properties. For example, a thunderstorm may be remembered as the experience of having seen a streak of lightning followed by a loud clap of thunder.

Semantic memory refers to information integrated within the knowledge structures as concepts, lexical meanings, relational systems, rules, and so forth, independent of the original autobiographical source of their perceptual or episodic input. Thus, the semantic memory of a thunderstorm is likely to include the generalization that sound takes longer to travel than light, all of which may influence episodic recall of the time interval between the lightning and the thunder. Semantic memory involves linguistic encoding of experience and, reciprocally, serves as the basis for the use of language. The linguistic translation of experiences into abstract concepts and their relationships in the form of semantic memory is apparently protected from loss by virtue of rich, multidimensional structure. Semantically encoded information is described as knowledge that is essentially permanent "because it is part of so inclusive and unified an organization that it is never disrupted" (Restle, 1974, p. 208).

Recently, some psychologists have had reservations about efforts to identify subcomponents of memory. M.K. Johnson and Hasher (1987) expressed doubts about the conceptualization of semantic (versus episodic) memory and its attendant research methodology. A hypothesis that these two types of memory may represent different brain functions or structures has been challenged on the basis of insufficient evidence. The critics do, however, acknowledge that the episodic-semantic distinction has served to generate many interesting data. In his conceptualization of the memory system, Tulving (1985, 1986) proposed that episodic memory is a subsystem of semantic memory. While the two systems are viewed as hierarchically related, each is believed to possess unique capabilities. Continuing to adhere to the distinction between the two memory types as a valuable classification device, Tulving concurred with the need for further validation through research.

The very term *semantic memory* as used by many psychologists has been called into question because of the lack of distinction between language-based information and real-world knowledge abstracted out of experience (A.L. Brown, 1979; K. Nelson, 1977). However, while G.A. Miller (1978) concurred that semantic knowledge should be divided into a lexical component, referring to knowledge of word meanings, and a practical component, referring to general world knowledge, he argued that lexical knowledge must include some nonlexical, practical knowledge in order to satisfy conditions of truth and possibility. For example, in the sentence "The Smiths saw the Rocky Mountains while they were flying to California," general world knowledge that mountains do not fly is brought to bear in interpreting the verbal information supplied (G.A. Miller, 1978, p. 314).

Organization and Recall

"Semantic memory is organized knowledge of the world" (Matlin, 1989, p. 192). Viewed from the more restricted perspective of symbolic information, semantic memory is organized knowledge about words and other symbols, their meanings, their referents, and the relations among these items (Tulving, 1972). In cognitive psychology, decades of research have supported the claim that "long-term recall depends importantly upon the encoding and organization of newly presented material in relation to the organized network of associations already existing in memory" (Estes, 1976, p. 14). One such aspect of semantic memory that has had a long history of investigation has been associations among words.

Word Associations   Word associations analyzed from patterns of list recall have been observed to be based on a variety of relationships, such as attributes, networks, serial ordering, and taxonomic categories (Friendly, 1979). Extensive experimentation has demonstrated that certain words tend to elicit associated words, but the underlying connections for word classes may differ (Deese, 1965). Associations among nouns tend to be made on the basis of common characteristics (e.g., *carpenter-apprentice*; *apprentice-trade*). Associations among frequently occurring adjectives are based on contrastive structure characterized by the polar opposite dimension (e.g., *big-little*; *hot-cold*). Less frequently occurring adjectives, however, tend to evoke not their opposite, but a syntagmatic association (e.g., *strenuous-exercise* rather than *strenuous-effortless*). *Syntagmatic associations* consist of words that may be adjacent in grammatical structure (e.g., *dog-bark*). In contrast, *paradigmatic associations* tend to reflect a similar grammatical class (e.g., *dog-cat*) (McNeill, 1966). Developmental shifts from syntagmatic to paradigmatic associations are viewed as evidence of a refinement in the organization of semantic features.

Categorization and Memory   The way information is organized affects how it is entered into the storehouse and how it is retrieved during recall (H. Gleitman, 1986). In many psychological experiments, it has been shown that people impose organization upon information even when they have not been instructed to do so, and when the material itself may be unrelated (Matlin, 1989). One form of organization observed to be widely prevalent in storage and recall is *categorization*.

One account of the way that knowledge is stored in semantic memory is the grouping of items that, despite their differences, are treated as equivalents (Matlin, 1989). For example, apples, oranges, peaches, and pears, while clearly distinguishable, possess a commonality that allows them to be included in the category of *fruit*. In other words, they are similar in some essential features and different in their properties from items excluded from that category. The formation of categories as proposed by Rosch (1978) serves the function of providing "maximum information with the least cognitive effort" (p. 28).

It is acknowledged that categories are, in part, *constructed* on the basis of culturally determined classification of entities and their linguistic coding within a particular culture. Nevertheless, it is also maintained that there are naturally occurring attributes that do coexist. For instance, whereas the concept of *bird* may be culturally distinguished from concepts of other creatures, in the objective world such attributes as *feathers* and *wings* do go together. In other words, categorization about the world is determined in part by organization imposed by the perceiver and in part by the structure inherent in what is perceived (Rosch, 1978).

In the work of Rosch, categorized information is analyzed into three levels:

Level of categorization	Examples	
Superordinate (highest level)	vehicle	animal
Basic (specific instance)	car	dog
Subordinate (lower level of specificity)	Ford	collie

Furthermore, recent theory has inclined toward the notion of *prototypes* as exemplars of categories in semantic memory that share the most attributes with other members of the class. For example, a *robin* has been found to be prototypical of the category *bird; apple* is a prototype of the category *fruit*. These instances of category membership are produced more frequently and recognized more rapidly in experiments than less typical instances. Research on prototypes within the larger domain of categorization has yielded insights into the nature of certain aspects of semantic knowledge organization. Another line of research has explored a different dimension of semantic knowledge: schematic structures.

Schema Theory   Schemas (or schemata) are knowledge structures that are broader than the organization of knowledge into word meanings or concepts. They consist of generalized knowledge about the world, such as familiar situations and events. For example, an individual would know from schemas about houses that, in general, cooking utensils would not be found in the bedroom.

Recent schema theory has been, in part, derived from the early work of Bartlett (1932) that established the premise that recall consists of a reconstruction of the past from partial knowledge. This notion of the constructive nature of memory was also espoused by Piaget. From these perspectives, it was maintained that original events are altered by the effects of stored knowledge on what is recalled from objective reality.

Debate is ongoing regarding the role of schemas on what is stored, recalled, or recognized. Alba and Hasher (1983) analyzed the theories that postulate ways in which information is selected and interpreted in its storage and retrieval. At issue are questions about the assumed effects of schematic knowledge on memory in terms of:

Abstraction of only some information from all of available original input
Alteration of input information according to which schemas are activated
Alteration of existing schematic knowledge by integration with new information

Support for these effects of processing information through existing schemas has been secured from numerous studies demonstrating the restructuring or reconstruction of stored information during recall.

However, evidence inconsistent with these notions has been provided by some studies of *recognition*, in contrast to studies of *recall*. Whereas recall has been found to vary substantially with the amount of prior knowledge activated, recognition has been found to vary minimally. Such results are considered as evidence that more is encoded than is consistent with the operation of a schema-based selection theory, and doubts have been cast on the abstraction principle in light of the degree of accurate detail observed in some well-learned material. It is suggested that schemas may, in fact, influence retrieval rather than selection for storage.

This point of view is not universally held. For example, it has been contended that underlying schemata guide both encoding and retrieval of story content (Mandler, 1984; Mandler & Johnson, 1977). However, it has been noted that reorganization of content occurs over time and that what is retrieved is dependent on the schemata operative at the time of recall. Various research paradigms have been used to show that subjects restructure input in accord with semantic, conceptual, or idiosyncratic categories. This assumption is compatible with Piaget's theories of active construction of stored knowledge structures and his premise that memory improves with increases in operativity. From such a perspective, memory is regarded as a constantly changing accumulation of knowledge, and what is recalled is not simply some fraction of what has been stored (Liben, 1977). Rather, it is assumed that what has been stored undergoes changes in the light of our own attitudes, expectations, or evolving schemas. Paris (1978) maintained that remembering transforms experience repeatedly over time

> according to social and cognitive rules available to the individual. Distortions in memory are often directed towards filling in gaps, reorganizing events and adding supplementary information, such that the resulting representation is internally consistent with the structural knowledge and social disposition of the person. (p. 131)

While the power of schema theory to explain aspects of comprehension and memory has been accepted by some psychologists, others have questioned the adequacy of a theory of fixed knowledge structures to account for the detail and flexibility of what is remembered (Alba & Hasher, 1983; Kintsch, 1988). To meet the demands of changing contexts, Kintsch (1988) proposed an alternate view: "Instead, a minimally organized knowledge system is assumed here in which structure is not prestored, but generated in the context of the task for which it is needed" (p. 164).

Retrieval   Retrieval is the process by which material stored in long-term memory is activated to recognize new input, perform a task, or solve a problem. "Retrieving stored information is preeminently a strategic process" (Wingfield & Byrnes, 1981, p. 8), requiring search activity that may take two forms: effortless or effortful.

Under experimental conditions, it has been demonstrated that the degree to which the cue provided at retrieval time resembles cues encoded during original storage influences the readiness of access. Furthermore, as a generalization, "success is most likely if the context at the time of retrieval approximates that during the original coding" (H. Gleitman, 1986, p. 237). Numerous studies have attested to the fact that information learned in one environment is recalled more easily either when tested in the same setting (e.g., a particular room) or when the same physical environment is recreated mentally. This phenomenon has been called the principle of *encoding specificity* (Tulving & Thomson, 1973).

Effortless retrieval occurs when there is a close match between organization of information at input and at recall. Material that has been classified into particular categories at the time of learning is more easily retrieved if such category labels are used as cues at time of retrieval. Effortful retrieval is believed to occur in two stages. In stage one, similar in nature to effortless retrieval, attention is directed to that part of memory in which the pertinent information is stored. For example, a face may be recognized as familiar before the name is recovered. The second, more effortful stage consists of slower search of information activated by effortless retrieval. Information stored in long-term memory is not always readily accessible.

While much retrieval is rapid and effortless (e.g., where a person was born), other information must be sought with more effort and varying degrees of successful outcome. The tip-of-the-tongue phenomenon is an instance of access to some relevant information about a word, such as beginning sound, number of syllables, or words of similar meaning, but not to the actual target word. This slow, effortful process may be likened to a search of the location in which the information sought is "filed." The act of thinking generally consists of this more difficult, highly conscious process of retrieval.

Recognition and Recall   Recognition is easier than recall. The dual-process theory of memory describes recall in terms of, first, retrieval of "candidate" items from long-term memory and, second, testing the candidates for an appropriate match to present task requirements (Weisberg, 1980). Thus, in recall, individuals must generate their own information. Recognition, in contrast, bypasses retrieval, since items are already retrieved in the presented material. Therefore, only a match to present requirements is needed.

Numerous studies have demonstrated that different types of processing are apparently involved in recognition and recall. A familiar situation demonstrating such a difference is the way students prepare for and react to objective examinations (multiple choice or true/false) and to essay tests. Studying for the former apparently requires strategies for recognition, in contrast to strategies for recall required in the latter instance (Weisberg, 1980).

However, recognition may involve different degrees of active operations in various types and levels of task difficulty. "Recognition decisions may be made quickly on the basis of partial information (familiarity) or they may be made more slowly, and more accurately, on the basis of an extended memory search" (Atkinson et al., 1974, p. 140). It would appear from numerous studies of recognition that the information needed for remarkably good recognition is acquired relatively effortlessly. However, closer inspection reveals that, even in these relatively effortless recognition tasks, active encoding must be done during the input stage (Weisberg, 1980). This issue of active encoding during the storage of information has been studied from a depth-of-processing perspective.

Depth of Processing

During the 1970s, Craik and his colleagues (Craik & Levy, 1976; Craik & Lockhart, 1972; Craik & Tulving, 1975; Jacoby & Craik, 1979) proposed a model of memory based on the levels at which information was processed. Rather than conceptualizing memory processes as "a series of discrete stages with transfer of information between the stages" (Craik & Levy, 1976, p. 166), this model viewed memory as a continuum of processing from shallow structural analysis to deep semantic analysis.

Experimental tasks designed within this conceptual framework have tended to contrast subjects' memory for verbal stimuli when oriented toward selected physical characteristics (e.g., word length or upper/lower case letters) with their memory for verbal stimuli when oriented toward meaning (e.g., sentence completion or categorization). The findings of superior results of deep versus shallow analysis led to the conclusion that "stimuli which do not receive full attention and are analyzed only to a shallow sensory level give rise to a very transient memory trace," whereas "stimuli that are attended to, fully analyzed and enriched by associations or images yield a deeper encoding of the event, and a longer lasting trace" (Craik & Tulving, 1975, p. 270).

The levels-of-processing paradigm was extended to encompass not only depth but breadth of processing in terms of degrees of elaboration of input. Jacoby and Craik (1979) claimed that distinctiveness of stimuli, resulting from the quality and quantity of discriminative analysis of incoming information, is an important determinant of retention. Breadth and depth of processing are, then, regarded as aspects of information elaboration during input encoding, influencing both storage and retrieval.

As an account of the structure of memory, the levels-of-processing model has been found wanting and no longer enjoys wide acceptance. Nevertheless, a substantial body of research employing the levels-of-processing paradigm has produced impressive evidence that processing information at deeper levels of meaning has led to more effective encoding and better memory with materials ranging from words to sentences to lengthy passages of expository text (Kulhavy et al., 1986). This beneficial effect of semantic encoding on recall has been attributed by a number of investigators to increased cognitive effort and the degree to which processing capacity is expended in the promotion of associations and elaborations of meaning (Horton & Mills, 1984; Koriat & Melkman, 1987). The implications of voluntary depth of processing in strategies for enhanced memory are examined in the section on memory and language.

Memory and Language

Language and memory are recognized as intimately related, both in development and in use. The relation between memory and language appears to be reciprocal in that memory is acknowledged to play a critical role in the acquisition of language, and language has been demonstrated to be a potential facilitator of memory. Thus, it has been suggested that syntactic structure minimizes the load on the limited capacity of short-term memory (Norman, 1972), and semantic structure plays a major role in the enduring nature of long-term memory. Some of these knowledge structures are believed to be stored in permanent form, readily available for rapid automatic use, as in the retrieval of words to label objects or actions. Others are thought to remain free elements subject to specific organizational structure to meet particular situational needs. An example of the latter condition would be tests of free recall of lists of items, requiring the construction of particular organizational structures from collections of possible structures, in contrast to the permanently stored organization of semantic structures that render function in real-life situations meaningful (Naus & Halasz, 1979).

These hypothesized aspects of semantic memory may represent the contrast between involuntary and voluntary memory. Automatic semantic processing, including such functions as integration and inferencing, is found to show few age-related changes during the processing of highly meaningful material (Naus & Halasz, 1979). For instance, no deliberate mnemonic strategies are required for a preschool child to recall a sentence such as, "When Nanny comes, take her to your room and show her the new dress we bought for your party." In contrast, lists of items are low in meaningfulness, so their memorization requires deliberate strategic planning and an imposed organizational structure. Many academic tasks share this characteristic and, therefore, involve voluntary memory processes in learning.

Language-Related Memory Strategies   The use of strategies for the encoding and recall of information frequently involves interaction between aspects of semantic knowledge and acts of voluntary memory.

Verbal Rehearsal   Verbal rehearsal serves as a time-binding, goal-directed strategy wherein the past is kept alive by carrying information that has been coded for future use into the recall period. Maintenance rehearsal consists of the repetition of items in the transfer of information from short-term store to long-term memory. Elaborative rehearsal involves the use of more active strategies such as the formation of associations among items and the organization of items into higher level categories (Loftus & Loftus, 1976). Developmental patterns have been observed in children's tendency to use both rehearsal and organization. These are discussed in the section on memory development.

Organization   For over 2 decades, memory research has been replete with studies of the effects of categorization at input and output, with results demonstrating that "clustering by category occurs during the recall of categorized lists" (Weisberg, 1980, p. 16). In addition, it has been found that subjects tend to construct subjective organizations during free recall and that recall is apparently causally related to such organization.

> To summarize, there is support for the assumption that organization must occur whenever large amounts of material are to be recalled. If such organization is not built in by the experimenter, it will be manufactured by the subject. Once again, this organization comes about because of the match between the person's knowledge and the to-be-remembered material. (Weisberg, p. 17)

The research on verbal recall alluded to above was largely conducted with adult subjects. Results of studies of children's use of organization via clustering or categorization on verbal memory tasks show age-related effects and are discussed in the section on memory development. Organization by theme is discussed in Chapter 4, on discourse processing.

Elaboration   The last aspect of verbal-memory interaction to be briefly considered here is the effect on recall of meaning elaboration as an aspect of depth and breadth of information encoding. J.R. Anderson and Reder (1979) provided a theoretical account of the relationship between greater elaboration during input and superior recall. From their view of memory as a network of interconnected propositions, they reasoned that, during any memory episode, a set of propositions is encoded. If multiple propositions that were partially redundant were encoded at input, the chance of recall at time of test would be increased because of the richness of the original encoding.

> Memory for any particular proposition will depend on the subject's ability to reconstruct it from those propositions that are active. This ability will in turn depend on the richness of the original set and hence on the amount of elaboration made at study. (p. 388)

Research methods for investigating the effects of elaboration on memory have included the use of questions about the material to be remembered. Two examples, one with children and one with adults, are summarized here.

Pressley and associates (Pressley, McDaniel, Turnure, Wood, & Ahmad, 1987) studied the effects of different kinds of elaborations of sentence meaning on both intentional and incidental learning of those sentences. Larger gains in recall followed adult subjects' precise elaborations of meaning in responses to *Why* questions than resulted from experimenters' precise elaborations. It is possible that attempts to generate an answer to such questions may heighten arousal and/or cognitive effort; force a deeper, more distinctive encoding; activate more links in the associative network, which would provide more retrieval routes; and so forth.

An earlier study of the performance of young nondisabled children and children with mental retardation on a paired association task examined the effects of labeling, sentence generation, sentence repetition, and *What* and *Why* questions on picture recall (Turnure, Buium, & Thurlow, 1976). The results demonstrated an overwhelming superiority of recall of the paired words as an effect of the *Why* questioning condition. It must be acknowledged that this study did not apparently tap voluntary memory strategy use. Rather, it invoked tacit semantic knowledge through elaboration procedures using the verbal modality as an enhancer of memory. In contrast, voluntary memory strategy use is more likely to invoke a heightened awareness of the value and appropriateness of selected strategies. This stored knowledge about strategies and their benefits is viewed as a component of metamemory.

Metamemory

Metamemory consists of knowledge or cognition about memory. In tasks involving voluntary memory, there is an apparent awareness of the need for deliberate storage for later recall and of the fact "that certain kinds of information are harder to learn and remember than others" (Flavell, 1985, p. 209). Flavell (1985) drew a distinction between metamemory knowledge and metamemory experience. He subdivided metamemory knowledge into three components: person knowledge, task knowledge, and strategy knowledge.

Person knowledge is what is known about one's own mnemonic abilities (e.g., the limits of short-term span, the occasional difficulty with retrieval of stored items). Such knowledge is exemplified in people's tendency to abandon efforts at retrieval of information never stored, in contrast to greater optimism about eventual retrieval of tip-of-the-tongue information.

Task knowledge refers to what is known about the memory demands of various tasks—the amount of effort required in studying certain kinds of material. For adults, experience gained over the years leads to reliable knowledge about what is easy or difficult to remember, reflected in a sensitivity to the need for varying amounts of effort at storage or retrieval in different situations. Research has investigated metamemory abilities in diverse experimental tasks such as prediction of ability to recall serial material, judgments of most efficacious strategies for sort and recall, estimates of study time and effort required for a learning task, and feeling of knowing in retrieval tasks (Schneider, 1985).

Strategy knowledge refers to what is known about the benefits of strategies in enhancing memory. Metamemory about strategies (MAS) is believed to constitute part of metamemory knowledge (Pressley, Borkowski, & O'Sullivan, 1985). According to these authors, metamemory about strategies includes both declarative knowledge (i.e., factual knowledge about the nature of strategies) and procedural knowledge (i.e., knowledge about how to use strategies). The components of metamemory knowledge of strategies have been hypothesized to emerge in the following order (Borkowski, Milstead, & Hale, 1988; Pressley, Forrest-Pressley, & Elliot-Faust, 1988):

1. *Specific strategy knowledge*—that is, knowledge about specific strategies (e.g., rehearsal or categorization) and their appropriate application to specific tasks
2. *Relational strategy knowledge*—that is, understanding of the comparative benefits associated with a number of strategies and the ability to contrast strengths and weakness of specific strategies for particular tasks
3. *General strategy knowledge*—growth in understanding that the use of strategies requires effort and that such effortful use of strategies may contribute to more successful outcome than nonstrategic approaches
4. *Metamemory acquisition procedures*—gaining assistance in learning about the use of strategies for specific tasks and in making decisions about how and when to use or switch strategies

Research on the relationship between metamemory and memory behavior has generally used the following types of measures to assess metamemory (Schneider, 1985):

Verbalized accounts of subjects' knowledge and use of strategies through interviews or questionnaires (e.g., "What did you do to help yourself to remember the pictures?")

Memory monitoring in terms of prediction, feeling of knowing (e.g., tip-of-the-tongue), judgment of readiness for recall

Nonverbal behavior such as reaction time for memory search, underlining textual material

One body of research has investigated the effects of training on the metamemory–memory behavior relationship, on the assumption that the connection would be more apparent in the transfer of newly acquired strategies to similar but modified tasks. One approach has studied the effects of training in self-testing for the purpose of evaluating the efficacy of new strategies (Pressley et al., 1985). Subjects monitored memory performance by asking themselves questions about the relative effectiveness of particular strategies. The evidence appeared to support the effectiveness of training in metamemory acquisition procedures (MAP) and was interpreted as having a profound bearing on "the theoretical position that metamemory is a general regulator of mnemonic behavior" (p. 145). Subsequently, Borkowski and his colleagues (Borkowski, Milstead, & Hale, 1988) reported on the long-term benefits of metamemory training and its spread of effect in terms of improved memory performance, heightened motivation, and increased self-esteem.

From his review of intervention studies, Schneider (1985) reported that "most of the studies . . . confirmed the assumption that the level of metamemory predicts strategy use and memory performance in maintenance and generalization tasks when organizational strategies are under investigation" (p. 95). Furthermore, analysis of results of almost 50 studies that used a variety of procedures for investigation of the metamemory–memory behavior relationship yielded a mean correlation of .41 between measures of metamemory and memory behavior (i.e., strategy use). These findings were viewed as support for the hypothesized metamemory–memory behavior relationship. This interpretation was incongruent with a view expressed by Flavell and Wellman (1977) that demonstration of a strong connection between memory knowledge and memory performance is unlikely in light of possible confounding effects of motivational or developmental variables.

Lack of consistency among results of certain bodies of research may be attributed not only to variations in motivation and subjects' age differences, but possibly to differences in measurement procedures as well. With regard to the latter variable, Flavell (1985) commented: "the emphasis is on verbalizable knowledge about strategies as distinguished from actual 'online' strategy use in memory situations" (p. 233). Schneider (1985) observed a closer relationship between behavioral versus verbalized measures of metamemory and memory performance in the research reviewed and concluded that such a finding "seems to shed some doubts on the validity of the interview data, especially for younger children" (p. 82). Discussion of research and theory about metamemory development is included in the section on memory development.

Memory Development

Within the past 2 decades, the attention of cognitive psychologists has been directed at changes occurring in memory with increased maturation. Some of the earlier work by Bruner (1964) postulated a developmental change in the way information was encoded by young children, progressing from enactive to iconic to symbolic representations. This view was in accord with Piaget's theory of sensorimotor schemas preceding symbolic thought.

Other later approaches have examined aspects of short-term and long-term memory and the development of strategies for enhancing the storage and recall of information. The interaction of increases in knowledge, both general and linguistic, has been studied from a developmental perspective. These issues are considered here.

Short-Term Memory   Short-term memory capacity appears to remain relatively constant over a wide age range (Ornstein, 1978). For example, young children's memory for pictures has been found to be similar to that of adults (G.M. Olson, 1973). Recognition of previously presented objects by 2- to 5-year-old children ranged from 81% to 92% (N.A. Myers & Perlmutter, 1978). However, one seemingly paradoxical finding is the often-reported developmental increase in digit span, a measure of short-term memory that has been found to correlate with chronological age (30 months, 2 digits; 36 months, 3 digits; 54 months, 4 digits; adulthood, 5–7 digits) and IQ.

G.M. Olson (1973) pointed out, however, that this ostensible measure of actual span capacity consists of verbal material. He interpreted these findings as support for Bruner's theory of children's progression from the iconic to the symbolic encoding mode, thereby judging it logical to expect that developments in memory would reflect a developmental trend in language acquisition. He explained the apparent increases in short-term memory span across age as reflection of a developmental trend in language acquisition and its use. However, the use of language in strategies for voluntary memory clearly develops with age.

Memory Strategy Development   Young children have been observed to engage inconsistently in such primitive strategies for remembering as pointing to the location of an item, ordering items, and looking attentively at material to be remembered. Recall in preschool children has shown a marked recency effect. That is, overwhelmingly, these young children's recall has been limited to the last items presented, attesting to their failure to engage in the use of those strategies that have been found to foster the primacy effect and transfer of information to long-term storage (N.A. Myers & Perlmutter, 1978; Wellman, 1988).

Entrance into the school situation creates task-related demands that necessitate the use of voluntary memory involving knowledge and control of the deliberate means of learning (A.L. Brown, 1979). The transition from preschool to school-age function appears to reflect, among other developmental factors, a shift from more passive, automatic processing to the use of more active techniques for memorization (Ornstein, Baker-Ward, & Naus, 1988).

A framework has been advanced for viewing development of memory strategies and their use (Ornstein et al., 1988, p. 38):

1. At early points along this continuum, the young child does not utilize strategies in the context of deliberate memory tasks.
2. Somewhat later, in the preschool years, a child may behave strategically in some situations that require remembering, but the effects of these mnemonic efforts may not be realized in actual memory "dividends."
3. Further along, in the early elementary years, the child's mnemonic efforts may be somewhat

effective, but the deployment of strategies may be in part determined by the salience of the stimulus materials.

4. Later still, strategies may be used in a variety of settings, with stimuli of varying degrees of saliency, and these strategies are effective.

5. Finally, strategy implementation becomes increasingly effective, reflecting the routinization and automatization that comes from both practice and the development of certain underlying information handling skills (such as retrieval and the ability to make interconnections in the knowledge base).

Developmental Trends in Rehearsal   A developmental pattern has been revealed in the ability to use verbal rehearsal to improve memory performance on a visual memorization task (Flavell, Beach, & Chinsky, 1966). Observable age-related differences between kindergarten, second-grade, and fifth-grade children's tendency to use verbal rehearsal as a mnemonic aid led to the conclusion that the development of linguistic competence in its broadest sense may include children's growing awareness of the benefits of "linguification" in certain situations. Young children do appear to benefit from instruction in the use of such memory strategies as rehearsal, but in subsequent spontaneous performance the strategy tends to be abandoned (Flavell, 1977).

Older children not only tend to use rehearsal more consistently, but have also been observed to use more varied and effective patterns of rehearsal than younger children (Ornstein & Naus, 1978; Ornstein et al., 1988; Ornstein, Naus, & Stone, 1977). For example, sixth-grade children tended to include a variety of items in a rehearsal set, sometimes drawing on previous items from the word pool, whereas third-grade children tended to combine each presented word with the same two other items from the list. For example (Ornstein & Naus, 1978, p. 80), the two age groups were presented with the following words separately, to be rehearsed cumulatively on successive trials:

apple   hat   story   dog   flag   dish

By the time the fifth word (flag) was presented, the rehearsal protocols of the two age groups differed as follows:

Third graders: flag, hat, apple, flag, flag, hat,
Sixth graders: flag, dog, story, flag, dog, story

On presentation of the sixth word, (dish), the two groups' rehearsal protocols differed as follows:

Third graders: dish, hat, apple, dish, dish, dish
Sixth graders: dish, flag, hat, dish, flag, hat, dish

Active rehearsal of unrelated or randomly presented related items appeared to lead to the development of an organizational plan at the time of input. It may be that this organization during rehearsal is the factor that renders the material more memorable. For example, when list material was preorganized according to taxonomic categories, rehearsal activity decreased in amount (Ornstein & Naus, 1978). Although the primary goal of this research was the study of developmental patterns of verbal rehearsal, these findings intersect with an extensive body of research on the relationship between organizational strategies and memory.

Developmental Patterns in Semantic Knowledge and Structure   Even in the absence of spontaneous use of strategies, memory does improve throughout the preschool years. Such improvement in young children's recall has been attributed to growth in world knowledge. This enriched knowledge base is believed to enhance the comprehension of first-hand experience at the involuntary level through the automatic spread of activation. Over the course of development, advances in the content and structure of the semantic or conceptual systems make input more familiar, meaningful, and conceptually related. The greater degree of meaningfulness is thought to result in increased depth of processing, contributing to improved storage and recall (Naus, Ornstein, & Hoving, 1978). Therefore, in both automatic, involuntary retrieval and conscious, deliberate retrieval, information is more readily reconstructed by virtue of the invocation of stored knowledge (Flavell, 1977).

Development of Organization and Recall

Preschool Children's Organization and Recall   Examination of the research on young children's abilities to sort objects for recall has revealed that even 2- to 5-year-olds are capable of clustering objects at unexpectedly high levels (Lange, 1978). On such tasks, preschool children have demonstrated the ability, when instructed, to impose organization on the material at hand, even though the strategy was applied only in approximately half the responses and was not used spontaneously. It is maintained that this ability to perceive some level of organization is more likely to occur in young children when the organization inherent in the material is readily recognizable and the demands for retrieval are minimal. "Highly associated items are likely to be recognized by the memorizer as preorganized, or intact, units, quite independent of any conscious attempt to interrelate the items" (Lange, 1978, p. 107). That is, age-related improvements in clustering may reflect changes in the permanent knowledge structure allowing for automatic storage and retrieval.

While some of these knowledge structures are believed to be stored in permanent form, readily available for rapid, automatic use, others are thought to remain relatively free elements, subject to specific organization to meet particular situational needs, perhaps reflecting availability for voluntary versus involuntary memory. Not until late childhood and early adolescences are children likely to deliberately search for underlying structures to organize material for memorization.

School-Age Children's Organization and Recall   School-age children as a group employ organization more readily and consistently than preschoolers, but age differences have been noted in the ability to sort material that has high or low semantic relatedness (Best & Ornstein, 1986). On highly related material sharing common attributes or functions (e.g., food, vehicles), third- and sixth-grade children were similar in their sorting patterns. Both groups' organization performance was less effective on material of lower semantic relatedness. Older children, however, appeared more capable of imposing their own subjective organization on items having relatively low associational value. (For example, presented with pictured items including, among others, a refrigerator, a light bulb, and an iron, older children may group them on the basis of their common use of electricity, a feature not observable in the perceptually present material.) During recall, both groups performed similarly on highly categorized material. However, on low-association items, sixth graders performed better than third graders. Sixth graders performed equally well on low- and high-association material.

Developmental Shifts in Organization   In another study, younger children instructed in the use of organization did not manifest the use of categorical organization in recall. That is, they appeared unaware that the strategy of organization had beneficial effects during recall

(Corsale & Ornstein, 1980). Regarding children's relatively less effective use of categorization for recall, "one might speculate that categorizing is not a spontaneous way of organizing the world but comes about only as a deliberate memorizing strategy" (Mandler, 1979, p. 290). Children seem to be more inclined to group items on a schematic than a taxonomic basis, and the differences in patterns of recall for story structure and list structure may indicate that semantic memory is episodic in nature. "Our taxonomic knowledge appears to be a secondary kind of organization that has been built onto a basically schematically organized memory system" (Mandler, 1979, p. 294). It is conceivable that the aforementioned developmental shift from syntagmatic associations (*dog-bark*) to paradigmatic associations (*dog-cat*) reflects such changes in the organization of semantic memory over age levels.

This effect was apparent in a study of retrieval cues for different age groups (B.P. Ackerman, 1985). Comparing responses of second- and fourth-grade children with those of college students, it was found that, for the younger subjects, cues that represented specific episodic context were more effective in retrieval than were generalized categorical cues signaling abstract relationships. In contrast, for the college-age subjects cues signaling taxonomic organization were more effective in stimulating recall. The following descriptions and examples drawn from the experimental materials and procedures will help to clarify interpretation of the results.

During the acquisition stage, subjects were presented with lists of word triplets, each of which was composed of an adjective (distinctive or general) + a noun + a noun (e.g., rotten/round + apple + *peach* [target word for retrieval is in italics]). For each triplet, questions were asked that oriented subjects toward either specific, episodic processing (e.g., "Would a grocer examine these carefully?") or relational processing (e.g., "Do these grow on trees?"). During the retrieval stage, either specific episodic cues (e.g., rotten, or rotten apple, or apple) or category name cues (e.g., fruit) were presented.

Results demonstrated that older subjects had significantly higher recall scores than younger subjects in response to relational orientation and category cues at retrieval. There was no significant difference among age groups in response to specific orientation questions and distinctive adjective cuing at retrieval.

> An appropriate conclusion here, then, is that young children may lack an associative infrastructure that can mediate the elaborative spread of taxonomic information, but do seem to possess a structure that will support such a spread for more singular or specific relations among concepts. (B.P. Ackerman, 1985, p. 436)

Thus, organization of knowledge in semantic memory may not be uniform in its character across age levels. From a Piagetian perspective, these changes in organization and recall are tied to stages in general intellectual development (Piaget & Inhelder, 1973). That is, memory transformations are revealed in the course of the child's advance to concrete operations, with retention of certain combinatorial structures not attained until the level of formal operations (approximately 11 or 12 years of age). The quality of recall changes with increasing age as a function of the level of knowledge structures, or schemata, achieved developmentally. Translated into information processing terms, the nature of the representations in memory are reorganized with maturation, permitting the storage of more data at higher levels of organization.

The tendency of older children to use memory strategies with greater flexibility and greater ease may be related to this growth in the knowledge base. "Thus, what a child knows about the materials to be remembered may dramatically determine just what can be done strategically with those materials" (Ornstein et al., 1988, p. 34). Therefore, it may be assumed that at later stages of development, along with increased declarative knowledge, individuals make gains in procedural knowledge, part of which is awareness of processes facilitative to memory, or metamemory.

Development of Metamemory Although earlier accounts describe preschoolers as lacking in metamemory abilities, more recent findings indicate that they do possess rudimentary knowledge in their understanding of such terms as *remember, forget, know*, and *guess* (Kail & Strauss, 1984). Children across all ages evidenced awareness of the greater ease of recognition than recall tasks (Flavell, 1985).

It has been demonstrated that older children have a more accurate notion than young children about how much effort is required to master a memory task. Younger children have been found to overestimate their ability to remember such experimental task material as a series of pictures. Only children of 7 years of age or older were found to be capable of accurately assessing their memory span (Flavell, Friederichs, & Hoyt, 1970). However, young children's prediction becomes more accurate when the task is reality based (e.g., a simulated shopping list) (Flavell, 1985) and when they are asked to predict memory for content rather than quantity (Schneider, 1985).

With regard to strategy awareness, older children have been observed to be capable of thinking of more things they could do to enhance recall, but even some kindergarten and first-grade children have demonstrated the ability to think of things they could do to help them remember. However, they tended to rely more on external strategies, such as putting something in a particular place or asking a parent to remind them, rather than on such internal strategies as rehearsal. Developmental trends have also been observed in children's awareness of the benefits of clustering or forming associations among materials during retrieval and in their recognition of the need for further study of material missed in recall tests (Flavell, 1985).

Despite the demonstrated metamemory *ability* in young children, it has been found that *use* of metamemory is not a necessary condition for their memory performance. That is, research has provided evidence of low metamemory use and high strategy use in kindergarten- and early elementary school–age subjects. This finding emerged from some studies that employed the interview as a metamemory measure; that is, subjects were required to verbalize their knowledge of the strategies used to remember.

For example, Bjorklund and Zeman (1982) asked first-, third-, and fifth-grade children to recall familiar material (e.g., names of their classmates) and less familiar material (e.g., categories of objects, such as furniture or body parts). No developmental differences were found across grade levels for recall of classmates' names, but age-related differences were observed on recall of categorically grouped object names. The major focus of the study was to determine the children's ability to verbalize the strategies they used for organization and recall.

Although examination of their output revealed that subjects tended to use organizational strategies, their verbal descriptions of memory strategies were, in many cases, unrelated to anything observed in their memory behavior. Younger children (i.e., first and third graders) were more likely to profess no strategy. That is, when asked what they did to help them remember, many first-grade children replied that they had used no strategy at all; they just knew their classmates.

In an effort to circumvent the possible invalidity of verbalization as a measure of metamemory, the experimenters used a recognition multiple choice technique. Subjects were presented with four possible strategies and asked which ones they had used to help them remember. Whereas older children were more likely to select a strategy that was consistent with observed memory behavior, approximately half of all children across grade levels selected a strategy that was inconsistent with the observed memory behavior.

Bjorklund and Zeman (1982) posited four stages in children's development of knowledge of their memory strategies:

1. No awareness of any special mnemonic technique
2. Lack of awareness until after being asked, albeit, at times, giving responses that are unrelated to actual performance
3. Entrance into task without predetermined strategy, but discovery of the benefits of strategy during task performance
4. Initiation of a retrieval plan at time of input

As Flavell (1977) had reported, awareness of the need for deliberate storage of information for later recall appears to develop later than acts of retrieval. Very young children may be induced to engage in memory-facilitating behavior and to use it deliberately to improve recall, but may not continue to employ the strategies "unless the link between their improved retention and their use of the strategy is made explicit" (Kail & Strauss, 1984, p. 8).

Metacognition

Metamemory may be regarded as a specific instance of the broader phenomenon of metacognition. Since the early 1970s there has been an upsurge of scholarly interest in research and theory in this area. Metacognition has been conceptualized as consisting of two major components: knowledge about cognition and regulation of one's cognition (A.L. Brown & Palinscar, 1982). Knowledge about cognition includes knowledge about oneself and one's abilities, knowledge about task variables, and strategies for monitoring progress in task performance (Wong, 1985a). Regulation of cognition includes planning activities before beginning a task, monitoring learning activity in terms of need to revise or reschedule particular strategies, and checking the outcomes in terms of effectiveness and efficiency of the strategies employed (A.L. Brown & Palinscar, 1982).

Study of the phenomenon of "thinking about thinking" (Yussen, 1985, p. 253) has considered the relationship of metacognition to memory, attention, reading, and social interaction, with growing interest in the role of metacognition in academic failure (Yussen, 1985). Synthesizing material from the literature (A.L. Brown, 1980; Flavell, 1978), Wiens (1983) derived a list of metacognitive skills needed for effective student learning:

Recognizing problem difficulty
Using inferential reasoning to check validity of information
Predicting outcome of strategy use
Planning study-time needs
Monitoring success of selected strategy
Checking outcome for internal validity
Checking outcome against common sense criteria

Narrowing the focus of metacognition and academic functions to a more particular area, L. Baker and Brown (1980) identified some of the metacognitive activities involved in successful reading comprehension:

Clarifying the purposes of reading
Identifying the important aspects of a message
Focusing attention on major content rather than trivia
Monitoring effectiveness of comprehension
Engaging in self-questioning to determine whether goals are being achieved
Taking corrective action when failures in comprehension are detected (Gordon & Braun, 1985, pp. 4–5)

A study of the effects of metacognitive training in terms of heightened reading awareness and informed strategy use by third- and fifth-grade students produced data supporting "the often hypothesized importance of metacognition for reading and studying" (Paris &Jacobs, 1984, p. 2092). These authors did, however, temper their enthusiasm about the effects of their experimental procedures by acknowledging that heightened reading awareness may develop from factors other than those employed in their study and that reading awareness (metacognition) may not be a significant factor in all reading tasks at all times. That is, certain measures (e.g., error detection) may be more sensitive to the effects of metacognitive instruction than others (e.g., standardized comprehension tests).

Subsequent developments in metacognitive research and theory with particular reference to learning and reading disabilities are discussed in greater detail in Chapter 8.

Summary

Memory involves the transfer of information from short-term storage to long-term storage and from long-term storage to working memory. Whereas information processed in short-term and working memory is relatively limited in quantity and duration, the capacity of long-term memory is relatively unlimited. The duration and retrievability of information in long-term storage, while more robust than that of information in short-term storage, are variable. Transfer of information to and from long-term memory is facilitated by the use of such strategies as organization and the integration of new input with old knowledge. Developmental factors influence the extent and structure of the knowledge base and how effectively it is applied to voluntary or involuntary memory performance.

Questions To Be Considered About
Memory and Language-Related Learning Disabilities

1. Is there evidence of a relationship between memory deficits and language-related learning disabilities?
2. In what aspects of memory may deficits be correlates of language-related learning disabilities: Sensory register? Memory span? The executive control component of working memory? Long-term store?
3. What are the prevailing theories about the nature of presumed memory deficits and learning disabilities: capacity limitations or maladaptive strategies for storing and retrieving information?

4. How may knowledge about memory and metamemory development in normal children contribute to an understanding of the problems of children with learning disabilities?
5. In what ways may the extent and structure of knowledge stored in semantic memory determine abilities or disabilities in the processing of oral and/or written discourse?

4 / Language and Discourse Processing

This chapter is concerned with those factors involved in the normal processing of oral and written discourse serving educational purposes. The primary goal is a measure of understanding about those cognitive-linguistic processes involved in comprehension and recall of educational discourse and the expressive skills needed to meet the communicative demands of the classroom. This information about normal processes is intended to serve as a foundation for understanding those deficiencies that interfere with language-related academic success in the population with learning disabilities. The material included in this overview chapter, far from being representative of psycholinguistic theory and research, reflects interest in selected areas pertinent to possible sources of cognitive-linguistic deficit in the student with language/learning disabilities. Thus, at the level of sentence processing, hypothesized interactions among the cognitive systems of perception, attention, and memory and the linguistic systems of phonology, syntax, and semantics are issues of legitimate concern.

Much of the research and theory about language in the fields of linguistics and psycholinguistics has been devoted to the sentence as a unit of study and analysis. The field of discourse has shifted from the earlier traditional linguistic focus on grammatical analysis of context-independent sentences to the study of context-dependent language (van Dijk & Kintsch, 1983). While it is acknowledged that phrases, clauses, and sentences are legitimate objects of study, it is maintained that, within the coherence of discourse, they are determined or shaped in important ways by the communicative intentions of the language users (de Beaugrande, 1985) and in a dynamic interaction, with previous utterances setting the scene for the interpretation of subsequent utterances (J.M. Sinclair, 1985).

In contrast to the preoccupation of traditional linguistics with the invention of abstract classifications in the narrower, uniform domains of syntax and phonology, text linguistics deals with the way language functions in the broader, more variegated areas of semantics and pragmatics (de Beaugrande, 1985). That is, discourse analysis examines the way language transmits meaning in actual communicative interactions.

This chapter considers both the processing of the sentence as a component of discourse and the larger phenomenon of discourse into which sentences are integrated. From this latter perspective, concerns focus on the overall structure of discourse and some of the theories about the influence of this structure on the processing of informational content. Subsequently, the chapter examines the devices of coherence and cohesion that bind the elements of discourse into a unified whole.

Of major interest in the context of this book is the comprehension of narrative and expository discourse, both of which loom large in academic learning. Therefore, a section of this chapter briefly addresses the nature of these two types of discourse and presents some research and theory about how they are processed. A final segment addresses a limited selection of pragmatic aspects of discourse. More extensive consideration of this topic is reserved for Chapter 5.

THE SENTENCE

Language processing occurs at different levels, singly or interactively. From the perspective of the sentence as a component of discourse, Perfetti (1979) advanced a multilevel model in which sentential information is processed in a top-down–bottom-up interaction. In this model, information is processed at varying levels:

1. Prelinguistic—acoustic properties of stress and pitch in the speech stream
2. Phonological—segmental (consonant and vowel) sequences
3. Syntactic—surface structure (phrasal and clausal units and relationships)
4. Propositional—relations among predicates and their arguments at the deep structure level
5. Referential—semantic descriptions of the content words accessed from the lexicon
6. Thematic—discourse value added to semantic interpretation, such as given versus new information or foregrounding (i.e., activation of memory structures necessary for sentence interpretation, in terms of topic constraints imposed by the theme)
7. Functional—deletion of text propositions determined by the speaker/writer's communicative intentions and assumptions about the listener/reader's assumed nontextual knowledge and motivation

Figure 1 presents a model of multilevel sentence processing within the context of discourse based on the above formulation by Perfetti (1979) and the work of Kintsch (1977).

Aspects of Sentence Processing

Top-Down Processing   Focusing for the moment on the sentence separate from its discourse context, it may be useful to recall Massaro's (1976) information processing account of speech perception, described in Chapter 3. Even at this relatively low level of processing, stored phonological and syntactic knowledge is believed to interact with reception and recognition of patterns from input, and semantic knowledge is invoked to render the patterns meaningful, thus involving multilevel processing within this more limited range. According to Fillmore (1985), the language user's linguistic knowledge is invoked at all levels; for example, phonemic

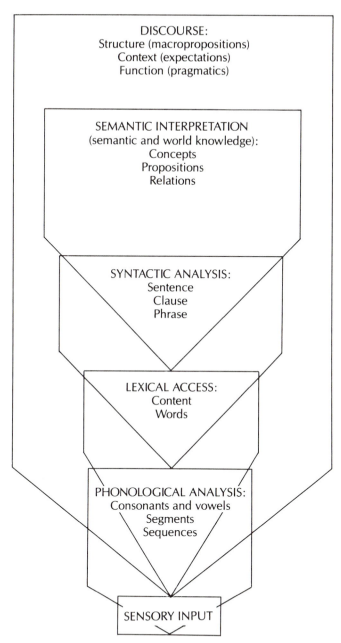

Figure 1. Multilevel processing of sentences within the context of discourse. (Based on Kintsch [1977] and Perfetti [1979].)

contrasts (e.g., *live/love*), inflectional contrasts (e.g., *dances/danced*), morphologically related words (e.g., *medicine/medical*), semantic contrasts (e.g., *thrifty/wasteful*), grammatical requirements of individual items within phrases and sentences, and knowledge of distant dependencies among sentences.

Attentional Allocation   Perfetti (1979) characterized processing at the level of form as transparent and generally automatic. Stated differently, under normal conditions of language processing, there is apparently a differential allocation of attention to the various levels, with phonological information making little demand on the limited capacity for attention (i.e., individuals are not consciously aware of this level of processing), thereby freeing up resources for processing at higher levels. While syntax is judged less automatic than phonology in its processing demands, as a linguistic form it is judged transparent relative to meaning, which is characterized as opaque, in that maximum attention is allocated to the propositional, referential, thematic, and functional levels.

Memory and Sentence Processing   Working memory is critically involved in the interactional processing of form and meaning. Extensive evidence attests to the fact that the limited capacity for verbatim information retention is one major determinant of the clause-by-clause processing of sentences. For the past two decades, it has been demonstrated that, once a syntactic unit has been processed (i.e., its meaning extracted), its superficial structure is no longer retained in memory (Jarvella & Herman, 1972). However, in sentences composed of more than one clause, the nonimmediate clause is "held in a still largely superficial form in the larger sentence representation until the sentence [is] complete" (Jarvella & Herman, 1972, p. 413). After the underlying propositions have been abstracted from the surface constituents, the verbatim information is allowed to decay, freeing up limited capacity for subsequent processing while retaining the semantic gist of prior clauses/sentences.

Sentence Processing Strategies

Various hypothetical accounts of sentence parsing (i.e., analysis of syntactic structure) into constituents have been suggested in terms of strategies employed by the language user. G.H. Bower and Cirilo (1985) listed some of these strategies drawn from the psycholinguistic literature:

Syntactic Strategies

1. A function word indicates the beginning of a new constituent (e.g., **the** boy)
2. Use affixes to help decide whether a content word is a noun, verb, adjective, or adverb (e.g., rain, raining, rainy)
3. Use the first word (or major constituent) of a clause to identify the function of that clause in the sentence (e.g., **after** the storm was over—adverbial)

Semantic Strategies

1. Using content words alone, build propositions that make sense and parse the sentence into constituents accordingly (e.g., Frightened and exhausted, his sick **wife** steadfastly **waited**.)
2. Identify the verb and look for noun phrases that fit its semantic requirements (e.g., The *chef* **baked** a fruit tart.)
3. Replace known definite noun phrases by their referents as soon as possible (e.g., The conference . . . /the annual convention of the association)
4. Expect "given" information to precede new information unless the sentence is marked otherwise (e.g., The conference was in New York.) (pp. 81–82)

It should be stressed that the use of the term *strategy* is not intended to imply consciousness or intentionality. In fact, comprehension strategies are believed to be unconscious (van Dijk & Kintsch, 1983).

A number of computational models have been constructed in the effort to describe the syntactic/semantic parsing process. Since these exceed the scope of technical detail judged appropriate for this overview, the interested reader is referred to other sources for further explication (e.g., J.R. Anderson, 1976; G.H. Bower & Cirilo, 1985; Rumelhart, 1977b).

Complex Sentences One aspect of sentence processing addressed by such models, and of particular concern to readers, is the processing of complex sentences such as *center-embedded* versus *right-branching* structures. Examples of each type, provided by G.H. Bower and Cirilo (1985), demonstrate that right-branching relative clause sentences like that in Example 1 are easier to process than center-embedded sentences like that in Example 2:

1. The cat chased the mouse that lived in the house that Jack built.
2. The house the mouse the cat chased lived in was built by Jack. (p.85)

In Example 2, the noun phrase parsing subroutine must be repeatedly interrupted and then be appropriately paired off with "a stack of verb phrases" (G.H. Bower & Cirilo, 1985, p. 85). Thus, certain types of center-embedded sentences appear to place heavy demands on short-term memory during the construction of underlying structure from the surface information, which serves as a data base for such syntactic operations.

Other factors beyond the location of the subordinate clause have been found to affect the level of processing difficulty in relative clause sentences. Object-focused relative clauses, as in Example 3, have been reported to be more difficult than subject-focused relative clauses, as in Example 4 (H.D. Brown, 1971; Hakes, Evans, & Brannon, 1976):

3. The boy whom the dog was chasing tripped and fell.
4. The boy who was chasing the dog tripped and fell.

In these examples, linguistic rather than cognitive demands are apparently the major source of increased processing difficulty. In particular constructions, ambiguity apparently increases the possibility of misinterpreting the object of an embedded clause as the subject of the main clause verb, particularly by preschool children:

5. The ball that is rolling toward *the sandbox is red.*

Processing Surface Structure Within the mainstream of American psycholinguistics throughout the past 25 years or so, it has been rather widely but not uniformly hypothesized that, in the processing of a sentence, clausal boundaries are constructed with relative independence of the surface structure manifested in the perceptual input. Foss and Hakes (1978) have reviewed the research and the controversies related to this issue, beginning with the well-known work by Bever and his associates on the "click" studies.

Early claims were made that listeners segment an input utterance into surface structure components of phrases and clauses and that extraneous stimuli, such as inserted clicks, were more likely to be perceived if they occurred *between* the perceptually structured units than if they occurred *within* those units. Research findings supported this hypothesis by providing evidence that subjects perceived the inserted clicks best when they occurred at major syntactic breaks. "Furthermore, Fodor and Bever reported that the clicks which had actually occurred in places other than the major boundary were perceived as located closer to the boundary" (Foss & Hakes, 1978, p. 118).

Later work by Bever and his colleagues (Bever, Lackner, & Kirk, 1969) led to a revision of the earlier conclusion. Observing that the click location is reported with greatest accuracy when it occurs at major clausal boundaries reflecting two underlying sentences, Bever more recently hypothesized that perception of click location was determined not by surface structure, "but rather by the underlying structure the listener extracts from the utterance" (Foss & Hakes, 1978, p. 119). This conclusion has not gone unchallenged, with further research by other investigators calling this assumption into question. Summarizing their review of the research in this controversial area, Foss and Hakes (1978) asserted: "Consequently, we cannot be sure whether the click location results are affected by surface structure alone, underlying structure alone or by a mixture of surface and underlying structure" (p. 119). In fact, Fodor, Bever, and Garrett (1974), in their analysis of processing strategies for different types of complement sentences (e.g., "John expected that Mary would leave," "John expected Mary to leave," "John expected Mary's leaving"), recognized the role of surface structure in providing clues to deep structure:

> Thus, it is self-evident that the analysis of "John expected Mary to leave" as an example of *for-to* complementation must be facilitated by the presence of "to" in the surface structure of that sentence. Similarly, the *poss-ing* interpretation of "John expected Mary's leaving" must be facilitated by recognition of the surface *s*, *ing*, etc. (p. 354)

From their research, van Dijk and Kintsch (1983) observed that the view of syntactically based strategies inherent in the above sentence recognition device, although distant from the earlier transformational grammar model, continues to ignore the importance of semantic and pragmatic information. "Yet it is precisely that information that yields powerful expectations about the meaning of a sentence and therefore also about the correct surface analysis of a sentence" (p. 75).

This latter alternative would appear to be reflected in the parallel processing, multilevel model posited by Perfetti (1979), in which information from all levels contributes, to differing degrees, to what is held in memory during the comprehension of a sentence. Studdert-Kennedy (1989) assigned higher priority to phonological input than is generally acknowledged in prevailing psycholinguistic theory, which is heavily oriented toward the primacy of syntax. He maintained that no syntactic analysis can be performed without phonological input. Thus, he judges phonology and syntax to be inextricably related.

Role of Phonological Representation   Since information in short-term memory is reportedly enhanced when phonetically encoded (see Chapter 3), and since syntactic structure is imposed, at least in part, on the phonological input, retention of that input in working memory during the derivation of a syntactic representation is highly plausible. This theory that a phonological representation of the raw speech signal is held in working memory during the derivation of a syntactic representation has been advanced by H.H. Clark and E.V. Clark (1977). R.C. Martin, Jerger, and Breedin (1987) agreed that such a phonological representation would be useful in preserving not only exact word order, but also the morphological information of inflectional endings and functor words that are important cues to syntactic analysis. However, they offer an alternate account of the role of phonological storage to that proposed by H.H. Clark and E.V. Clark (1977):

> In the Clark and Clark theory, phonological storage is used to maintain information downstream from the point at which syntactic analysis is taking place. Under our hypothesis, phonological storage only becomes critical for comprehension when sentence processing cannot keep pace with the incoming speech stream. When sentence processing is easy because the sequence of words

conforms to expected syntactic structure, each word may be immediately integrated into the developing interpretation of the sentence as it is perceived. However, when an unusual construction is encountered that causes sentence processing to lag behind the input, the retention of subsequent information in a phonological form would become necessary. (R.C. Martin et al., 1987, p. 147)

Although discussion of research on individuals with language impairment is reserved for Chapter 7, R.C. Martin et al.'s (1987) interpretation of the performance of a child with language/learning disabilities affords some provocative insights into possible interactions among components in normal language processing. Their subject manifested a severe deficit in short-term auditory memory in the presence of normal intelligence. Analysis of the findings of this study suggest that phonological short-term memory may be implicated, to a nontrivial degree, in auditory language comprehension, particularly in the processing of complex linguistic structures. Experimental tasks consisted of selecting pictures matching presented sentences in the oral and written modality or answering questions about an aspect of a test sentence. The subject demonstrated normal syntactic proficiency in written language when the input material was static versus transient. He also performed adequately with auditorially presented sentences containing subject-relative clause constructions, but exhibited difficulty with object-relative clauses and passive constructions in the relative clause, and with certain complement constructions. This difficulty did not occur when processing sentences in the written modality.

From the perspective of some current theories about divided attention, it is considered possible (although not as yet demonstrated) that the perception of speech (as input to the phonological representation stored in short-term memory) and syntactic processing may share the same (left hemisphere) attentional resources. It is speculated that "at a point in the sentence where syntactic analysis becomes difficult, less capacity is available for perception of subsequent words" (R.C. Martin et al., 1987, p. 147). After exploring possible reciprocal influences of a speech perception deficit, a phonological memory deficit, and auditory syntactic problems, R.C. Martin et al. conceded that, at the present time, the relationships remain unclear. Study of this particular case, exhibiting syntactic proficiency under visual conditions making minimal demands on auditory memory but reduced proficiency under conditions that taxed auditory memory, led to the following assertion:

> The dissociation between syntactic comprehension with auditory and visual presentation provides the first strong data linking a phonological short-term memory deficit and a syntactic processing deficit in a child for whom a deficit or delay in syntactic competence can be ruled out. (R.C. Martin et al., 1987, p. 148)

It is pointed out that, although auditory syntactic comprehension difficulty may stem from a memory deficit, the findings of this study do not suggest that memory plays as important a role in reading or that a memory deficit is implicated in reading comprehension difficulties involving syntactic information processing. Although the foregoing speculations address possible interactions among deficits in perception, attention, and memory in persons with language disabilities, they may also be pertinent to language processing under demanding conditions by the normal language user.

Individual Differences in Sentence Processing   Extending the above notions to the normal reading population, individual differences in the relative strength of verbal memory may not be ruled out as a facilitative or disruptive factor in optimal syntactic/semantic processing. A study by Daneman and Carpenter (1983) examined the relationship between memory span and the ability to detect and resolve ambiguities within and across clausal/sentence boundaries. They chose as a measure of short-term memory "reading span," that is, the number of words accurately recalled following the reading of a designated passage segment.

The experimental material consisted of sentences containing words with alternate meanings, such as *bat* (baseball implement or flying mammal), the ambiguity of which was subsequently resolved by information within or across the sentence boundary. Results revealed, not unexpectedly, that normally achieving college students varied in length of reading span and that short-term verbal memory so measured correlated positively with speed and accuracy of ambiguity resolution.

This process (detection of ambiguity and revision of interpretation) may be regarded as a more active metalinguistic function in reading comprehension than the primary linguistic processing involved in matching sentences (read or heard) to their appropriate pictured representations (as in the R.C. Martin et al., 1987 study). Thus, once again, increased task demands would appear to reveal, even in the normally functioning population, observable cost to a system with relatively lesser capacity.

Integration of Meaning Across Sentence Boundaries

Another task in the comprehension of discourse is the integration of meaning across sentence boundaries. As pointed out by de Beaugrande (1985), discourse consists of more than a sequence of sentences, in that semantic relations evolve and are constituted on a larger scale textually than sententially. Each utterance sets the scene for the next, and the way a subsequent utterance will be interpreted is dependent on interpretations of the previous ones (J.M. Sinclair, 1985).

Furthermore, it has been known for more than two decades that what is abstracted from individual sentences and integrated across sentence boundaries is the underlying gist or holistic ideas intersententially expressed (Bransford & Franks, 1971). In this well-known study, subjects recognized novel sentences composed of parts of originally presented items in relationships not previously expressed as "old" sentences.

Individual differences have been demonstrated in the efficiency with which prior sentence meanings are integrated with subsequent sentence meanings. Using a high-memory-load experimental task, Benninck (1982) studied the ability of college students classified as "global processors" and/or "analytical processors" to recognize sentences integrating information from prior presentation items and to answer inference questions about the integrated information. Further information on the study and its results is presented in Chapter 7. For present purposes, comments are limited to the finding that normally functioning subjects manifesting *both* global and analytical cognitive styles were equally capable of integrating old with new information across sentence boundaries, but that subjects who were global processors *only* were apparently less efficient in encoding and retaining sequences of sentences that taxed the limits of working memory. Thus, they required more processing time for the performance of the sentence integration task.

Discourse consists of more than sequential interaction among individual sentences. Rather, discourse is characterized by hierarchical interrelations among its elements that have as an ultimate goal the transmission of the purpose of the entire text (J.M. Sinclair, 1985). In other words, the linkage of individual sentence meanings adds up to a more complex whole with an overarching coherence. The language user must perform the cognitive task of establishing spatial, temporal, and/or causal relations among the propositions represented linearly by the component sentences (van Dijk, 1985). In this regard, de Beaugrande (1985) maintained that factors such as attention, memory capacity, and situational goals are more crucially involved in discourse processing than in sentence processing. Figure 2 presents Kintsch's (1977) model of comprehension as an interaction among linguistic knowledge, cognitive processes, and pragmatics within the structure of discourse.

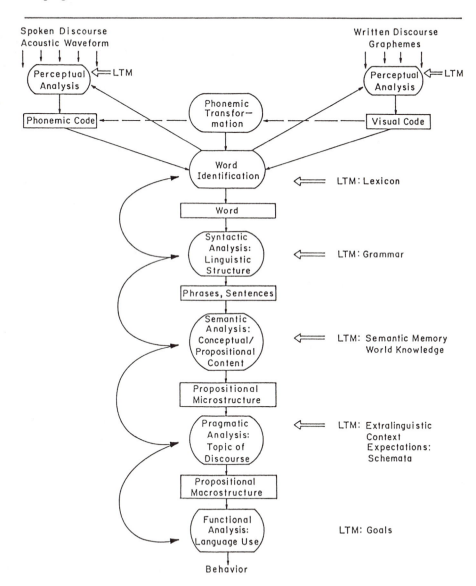

Figure 2. Processing stages in comprehension. (LTM, long-term memory.) (From Kintsch, W. [1977]. On comprehending stories. In M.A. Just & P.A. Carpenter [Eds.], *Cognitive processes in comprehension* [p. 34]. Hillsdale, NJ: Lawrence Erlbaum Associates; reprinted by permission.)

DISCOURSE STRUCTURE AND PROCESSING

Models of discourse structure and processing presented in Kintsch (1977), Kintsch and van Dijk (1978), and van Dijk and Kintsch (1983) have been prominent in theory and research within the field. The earlier models were predominantly structural, conceptualizing the relationships between macrostructure and microstructure in hierarchical organizations.

Structural Model

Macrostructure   The macrostructure of a discourse text consists of a synthesis of main ideas at the highest level of thematic organization. This higher level of organization tends to overcome limitations on storage and retrieval of information by summarizing information abstracted from micropropositions. Thus, at this level, macrostructures are assumed to include or reflect the meanings of the individual micropropositions and the relations among them, both explicitly stated and implied, even when those micropropositions are no longer accessible.

At the level of macrointerpretation, semantic detail is reduced; that is, the essence of a passage is retained while much of the specific information is lost. This abstraction of higher level organization from lower level detail is presumed to be a function of a number of "macro" rules that operate in text construction:

1. *Generalization*—selection of the smallest superordinate concept to preserve the incorporation of as much specific information as possible (e.g., "Education in the United States has failed to achieve universal literacy.")
2. *Deletion*—pruning away irrelevant propositions (e.g., in an anecdote of a car repair, omitting such details as time of arrival, name of the mechanic)
3. *Integration*—reduction through deletion of information already expressed or implied (expected facts or presuppositions) (e.g., "Henry was smoking his pipe" [Does not require statement that Henry lit his pipe].)
4. *Construction*—combination of a sequence of propositions into one unit, reducing without deleting information (e.g., "On the train to Paris, John showed his ticket to the conductor" [entailment of the propositions that John was traveling to Paris and that he had bought a ticket].)

Microstructure   The microstructure consists of the underlying network of ideas or propositions in the deep structure, which is mapped onto a sequence of sentences. The semantics of discourse involves the interpretation of these sentences relative to the interpretation of other, mostly previous, sentences. A critical function of the microstructure is the achievement of coherence, or connection between propositions. Each proposition contains a predicate and a number of arguments serving various case roles. The surface structure expression of those propositions must signal coherence through its employment of appropriate word and sentence ordering and by its effective use of cohesive devices (van Dijk, 1985).

Strategic Model

In their more recent model of discourse comprehension, van Dijk and Kintsch (1983) expanded the original model by placing greater emphasis on dynamic strategies of information processing rather than on structure. Undergirding this strategic model are a set of cognitive and contextual assumptions.

Cognitive Assumptions   Processing of events or verbal accounts of events (as in discourse) requires:

1. Construction of a mental representation, based on available visual and linguistic input data
2. Interpretation of the meaning of this mental representation
3. Understanding in on-line fashion (i.e., meaning is assigned gradually in an ongoing process rather than post hoc after all input data are processed)
4. Activation and use of stored knowledge leading to presuppositions

It is not assumed in this model that construction, interpretation, on-line processing, and presuppositions occur in discrete or linear fashion. Rather, language users are believed to have the ability to employ processing strategies flexibly; that is, "There is no fixed order, at each point, between input data and their interpretation. Interpretations may be constructed and only later matched with input data. . . . information that is interpreted may be incomplete" (van Dijk & Kintsch, 1983, p. 6).

Comprehension Strategies   The role of processing strategies is regarded as central to all levels of comprehension. Strategies are analogous to working hypotheses about the structure and meaning of a segment of text that may be disconfirmed in the light of subsequent processing. They are influenced by the language user's knowledge and goals and are acquired and automatized through practice and overlearning. New strategies are likely to be developed to meet the demands of new types of discourse (e.g., research literature versus narrative). The overall goal of strategies for discourse processing is the construction of a *text base* or semantic representation of the input data in episodic memory.

While comprehension continues to be viewed as an interaction between top-down and bottom-up processing in constructing meanings of words, clauses, sentences, and sequences of sentences, recently greater importance has been assigned to strictly bottom-up processes assumed to occur in initial stages (Kintsch, 1988). In this model, the attempt is made to delineate how word meanings and propositions are activated and elaborated independently of top-down contextual influence. Employing the metaphor of the spreading activation process derived from computer simulation models of cognition, Kintsch (1988) provided accounts of how different meanings may be activated. A simplified summary includes the following premises central to the model:

1. Knowledge is represented in an associated network consisting of interconnected conceptual or propositional nodes.
2. Meanings of concepts are *constructed* on the basis of their position in the network. That is, core concepts consist of the most immediate associations or "semantic neighbors" (p. 165). Full meaning is obtained by exploring other, more distant nodes in the network. The early stage of activation is probably automatic and context independent.
3. The constructed network in this early stage contains components that are not necessarily coherent, consistent, or appropriate to the discourse content.

For example, the occurrence of the word *bank* may activate associations with *money* and with *river*. Both meanings may be retained until further discourse information (*First National*) determines the retention of one meaning and the exclusion of another that is incompatible.

It is postulated, then, that text comprehension is cyclic. The meanings constructed from the activated network by bottom-up processes are believed to be integrated into the text through subsequent top-down processes that exclude unwanted elements and retain or reconstruct meanings consistent with coherent text. "The highly activated nodes constitute the discourse representation formed on each processing cycle. In principle, it includes information at many levels: lexical nodes, text propositions, knowledge-based elaborations (i.e., various types of inference), as well as macropropositions" (Kintsch, 1988, p. 168).

Propositional Strategies   Compelling evidence of the psychological reality of the proposition has been amassed from a large body of research demonstrating the holistic nature of propositions as semantic units in recall. The number of propositions in sentences has been directly related to processing time. It has been generally assumed that one clause expresses one proposition; however, the structural relationship may be complex. For example, a semantic role of *agent* and a grammatical role of *subject* might be assigned to the first noun occurring in the surface structure during the formation of propositional schemas. Thus, a semantic strategy is thought to be invoked prior to full analysis of the clause and ultimately the sentence.

> Surface ordering and heirarchy of clauses will be strategical indications for the ultimate organization of these complex propositional schemata, although other semantic information, for example, from previous sentences or the overall macrostructure, may assign a different structure to the semantic representation of the sentence. (van Dijk & Kintsch, 1983, p. 14)

Contextual Assumptions   In conjunction with the cognitive-linguistic factors, it is hypothesized that situational, social-interpersonal and cultural factors are important contributors to discourse comprehension. More specifically, these contextual assumptions would include: 1) the function of the communication in a particular social context; and 2) the pragmatics of the discourse in terms of the speech acts and the purposes and goals of the interactional communication along with the situational contexts (e.g., formal or informal) that shape style.

In the larger process of constructing a text base, then, relations among propositions are augmented by information external to the immediate sentence/clause/proposition. In addition, from a *situation model* perspective, such information may be derived from the activation and updating of previous experiential knowledge and/or text bases related to similar situations in episodic memory and, possibly, from the instantiation of relevant knowledge from semantic memory (van Dijk, 1987). Situational models invoked in the understanding of discourse may be constructed from:

1. Specific episodic memories of personal experiences, such as job interviews
2. Specific episodic memories of experiences related by others, such as admission to a hospital
3. Specific events experienced vicariously through the media, such as the political situation in Central America

All of these specific situational models contribute also to the formulation of more generalized situational models, such as housekeeping, working, food shopping, attending school, and so forth. Each unique event need not be kept available for retrieval, except for relating anecdotes. "Rather, we combine information from the particular models into more general (but still personal) models of such situations" (van Dijk, 1987, p. 178).

Coherence Strategies

Discourse coherence involves the linkage of propositions into a more complex meaning (van Dijk, 1985). It is necessary to explore the ways in which the ordering or organization of items affects the referential dimensions of discourse, and to examine the devices that are used in surface structure of propositional sequences to signal the underlying coherence connecting them. The following principles and examples serve as a partial listing of the information derived from studies of strategies that facilitate coherence:

1. A more global statement about time, place, or state of affairs should precede a more specific state or action:
   a. Next month we will be staying at Berkeley.
   b. We will be staying with friends.
2. Spatial ordering may require a linear ordering of the propositions, with objects introduced before properties:
   a. They have a big house on the hill.
   b. It has at least 10 rooms.
3. Temporal or conditional relations require that possible, probable, or necessary conditions should be mentioned prior to the statement of their consequences:
   a. This morning I had a toothache.
   b. I went to the dentist.
4. Coreference in consecutive sentences, earlier regarded as a primary contributor to coherence (Kintsch & van Dijk, 1978), is currently regarded as but one among a number of conditions fostering local coherence:
   a. George got some *beer* out of the car.
   b. The *beer* was warm.
5. More recently (van Dijk, 1985), coreference in consecutive sentences has been regarded as neither a necessary nor a sufficient condition for discourse coherence:
   a. We went to an expensive restaurant.
   b. John ordered trout with almonds.
   The inference made is that *John* in Example b was a member of the group denoted by *we* in Example a. It is generally agreed that such bridging inferences between discourse elements play an important role in establishing relations among propositions, thus contributing to both local coherence and comprehension.

Pragmatic Aspects of Coherence   The flow of discourse establishes local coherence in part by taking into account the informativeness, relevance, clarity, and quantitative appropriateness of sequences of propositions (Grice, 1975). It is expected that, at each point in the discourse, there should be some new information appropriately linked to old information assumed to be in the possession of the message receiver (van Dijk, 1985). That is, there is an assumed contract between speaker and listener (and writer and reader) that syntactically marked *Given* information resides in memory, and that *New* information, also syntactically marked, will be provided, extracted, and integrated with other information in memory (Haviland & Clark, 1974). New information may be signaled prosodically (i.e., by intonation and/or stress) as well as syntactically (Halliday, 1985).

This aspect of discourse is frequently manifested in the distinction between topic and comment. The *topic* function is generally assumed to be old information, that is, information introduced by prior text or known by the receiver. It therefore functions as given or presupposed information. The *comment* provides further information about the previously introduced topic entity.

Other terminology used in the literature to express this relationship between topic and comment refers to the *theme* and *rheme* components of discourse sentences; theme is the topic and rheme is the contribution of new information (predication) relevant to the development of the theme in a unit of discourse. Scinto (1986) provided examples of sentence sequences containing theme-rheme relations that are manifestations of local connectivity or coherence:

1. The book was published by Oxford University Press.
2. It appeared in the autumn.
3. Oxford University Press is second only to Cambridge University Press. (p. 114)

Scinto analyzes *the book* in Example 1 as the theme (T) and *was published by Oxford University Press* as the rheme (R). "Applying this procedure in turn for each sentence in the text we obtain the following pattern of theme and rheme (T–R)" (p. 115):

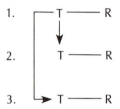

Thus, the theme of Example 1 is repeated in Example 2 marked by a pronominalized form *it*, and the rheme of Example 1 (*Oxford University Press*) appears as the theme of Example 3, as represented in the following notation:

1. T_1 ——— R_1

3. $T_3 (= R_1)$ ——— R_3

Cohesion

While coherence is the property of propositional connectivity that makes discourse more than just a collection of sentences, cohesion consists of the linguistic devices that signal connectivity and maximize the efficient management of textual information. Halliday and Hasan (1976) have classified types and subtypes of cohesion.

Devices Signaling Cohesion   The following classifications and illustrations constitute a compressed account of major cohesive devices.

Referents   There are three main categories of referents: pronouns, pro-verbs, and comparatives.

Pronouns may be grouped into two general types: *anaphoric*, referring to prior noun phrases in the text;

1. The cat purred. *It* rubbed against my leg.

and *cataphoric*, referring to subsequent information in the text:

2. Al heard *it* before he saw *it*. The cat was hissing in its hiding place.

Pronouns may also be grouped into the following grammatical types:

> Personal pronouns: *he, she, they*, etc.
> Possessive pronouns: *her, his, mine, theirs*, etc.
> Indefinite or neuter pronoun: *it*
> Determiners or demonstrative pronouns: *this, that, these*, etc.

Antecedent referents may consist of a single noun or elaborated noun phrase or an extended clause:

3. Amy and Bill enjoyed themselves. *They* went to the theater last night. *That* was their first outing in months.
4. Emigration from Eastern Europe reached record proportions at the end of the 19th and beginning of the 20th centuries. *This* was attributed to economic misery and religious persecution.

   Pro-verbs refer to prior verb phrases in the text:

5. Do—A flower dies. When it *does*, the petals fall off.

   Comparatives, which are adjectives and adverbs, can be grouped into two types: *general comparatives*, such as *same, similar, other, different, else,* and *likewise:*

6. Mort thought the government was too conservative. Harold held a *similar* view.
7. There were many kinds of flowers. Jenny took the roses and I took the *other* ones.
8. Harry became very angry. I never knew he had *such* a temper.

and *particular comparatives*, such as *better, more,* and *less:*

9. They were very proud of their house, but I thought ours was *better*.
10. He needs a lot of money to support his life-style. I can get along with *less*.

    Substitution   Substitution involves the use of different terminology for a coreferent:

11. A *bear* had wandered into the campsite while Joe and Henry were fishing. When they returned, they were amazed at the destruction the *animal* had caused.
12. They had a long, hard *climb* up the mountain. None of them had expected the *ascent* to be so difficult.

    Ellipsis   Ellipsis is substitution by zero; that is, information that is understood is deleted rather than reiterated:

13. Elsie tried to get there on time but found she couldn't [*get there on time*].
14. The Democrats were working hard to get out the vote, but the Republicans were [*working hard*] too.

Definiteness   Definiteness is usually expressed in the form of articles. In general (but not universally), definiteness activates known information and indefiniteness signals new information:

15.   In front of the house was *a* tree and some shrubs. *The* tree was half dead.
16.   *A* conference was held in Washington devoted to the topic of single versus dual certification, *an* issue that had been the subject of debate for more than a decade. *The* conference failed to resolve *the* issue.

Conjunctions   In contrast to all the above cohesive devices, which presuppose other components in the preceding or following text, conjunctions *specify* the type of relationship existing among textual elements. There are five main types of conjunctions.

Additive conjunctions, such as *and* or *furthermore*, link a series of points all related to one argument:

17.   The drought will probably produce a shortage in certain food products, *and* it may be anticipated that prices will rise.
18.   A learning disability generally causes difficulty in academic achievement. *Furthermore*, emotional problems are frequent as a result of a sensed inadequacy.

Temporal conjunctions are represented by prepositions and adverbials:

19.   *After* the battle they counted their losses. (preposition)
20.   They fought a battle. *Afterward*, they counted their losses. (adverb)
21.   The votes were counted. *Subsequently*, there was a recount.

Adversative conjunctions include *although* and *nevertheless*:

22.   *Although* he was uncomfortable, he fell asleep.
23.   He was uncomfortable. *Nevertheless*, he fell asleep.

Cause-effect conjunctions include *therefore*, *accordingly*, and *as a result*:

24.   She had studied diligently. *Therefore*, she felt confident.
25.   He had read the instructions carefully. *Accordingly*, he built a fine model.

Disjunctives include *but*, *instead*, and *on the contrary*:

26.   The program was no longer federally funded. *Instead*, state money was allocated.
27.   They never took a penny for their services. *On the contrary*, they contributed their own money as well as their time.

Processing Requirements   Although all of the foregoing cohesive devices increase the efficiency of discourse processing, they also add to the processing burden in terms of comprehension. Unless the import of the relations signaled by the various connectives is fully and precisely grasped, subtle but important shades of meaning may not be apprehended. During the processing of reference antecedents, ellipsis, substitution, and definiteness, there is the need for prior items to be held in mind or searched for, thus imposing, under varying conditions, different demands upon memory for the construction of a coherent interpretation. These demands are present in expressive formulations as well as receptive interpretations.

Linguistic Signals for Given and New Information   In addition to coreference and connective devices signaling cohesion, certain structures operate to signal Given and New Information. Several examples were provided by Haviland and Clark (1974). Given Information, for example, can be signaled by:

1. Restrictive relative clauses in the initial part of a sentence: "The house that Alice bought is expensive." (It is already known that Alice bought a house.)
2. Use of the adverbial *too*: "Evelyn's house was expensive, too." (It is already known that Evelyn bought a house.)

New Information can be signaled by structures such as the cleft construction. For example, in the sentence "It was Franklin who founded the University of Pennsylvania," the fact that the University of Pennsylvania had been founded was known or Given; New Information about the identity of its founder is signaled by the cleft construction *It was*.

In general, Given information must have an antecedent in memory. In the absence of an antecedent for New information in the text, one must be constructed either by elaboration of possessed information or from scratch. In the process of comprehension (discussed in greater detail below) difficulty and speed of processing reflect the accessibility of Given information in memory. That is, accessing readily available information in memory will take less time than will constructing a new antecedent or engaging in the inferential processes needed to establish meaning. Studies have demonstrated that this facilitation of comprehension attributable to given information is independent of the actual repetition of the critical antecedent noun (Haviland & Clark, 1974).

Developmental Patterns   Developmentally, it has been shown that the marking of Given versus New information occurs from the outset in language development, even at the one- and two-word stages (Greenfield & Smith, 1976). From her review of the relatively sparse literature in this area, Donahue (1984) reported that devices for signaling the Given/New distinction, such as pronominalization and the use of definite/indefinite articles, develop in the preschool years.

Children who are 6 and 7 years old have been observed to use cohesive ties in oral and written stories in the following developmental order, from first to last acquired: personal pronouns, demonstratives, and comparatives (Haslett, 1983). It was found that 7-year-olds used significantly more personal pronouns, demonstratives, and other forms of deixis, such as *here, now*, and *then*, than did 6-year-olds, with concomitant reduction in the frequency of the use of *the*. In storytelling, these young children used significantly more endophoric pronouns (referring to textual antecedents) than exophoric (external to the text) references, demonstrating evident mastery of the narrative genre of discourse. They also used significantly more anaphoric than cataphoric pronouns.

More complex strategies for encoding New information, such as cleft and pseudocleft sentences, are acquired throughout the elementary school years. Cleft constructions present New information at the beginning of sentences, as in, "It was the prisoner who started the riot." Pseudocleft constructions present New information at the end of sentences, as in, "The one who started the riot was the prisoner." It is of particular interest that over 90% of school-age children studied by Hornby (1971) correctly marked New information in syntactic structure, but only the older subjects were likely to correctly produce such syntactically complex sentence types as clefts, pseudoclefts, and passives to signal the Given/New contrast. Comprehension of these devices, however, apparently emerges later, with research evidence suggesting that a fully adult level of comprehension of certain structures (e.g., contrastively stressed passive and cleft sentences) has not been acquired by many 12-year-old children (Donahue, 1984).

Memory and Discourse Structures

It has been proposed that superordinate propositions—that is, those semantic units high in the structure of the text base—are most likely to be recalled because they tend to be processed most frequently in terms of argument repetition in related micropropositions (Kintsch & van Dijk, 1978). These superordinate propositions, because they are thematically central or salient, must be held repeatedly in short-term memory to assure continuity of text. Since retrieval of a proposition depends on the strength of its connections with a macroproposition, less relevant information appears to be more readily forgotten (Kintsch, 1982).

Within short-term memory constraints, text appears to be processed most efficiently in a series of cycles; a few propositions are put into working memory, with one proposition chosen to serve as a superordinate. The short-term memory buffer would retain this subset of propositions for connection to the next set of propositions. Short-term memory is then purged, and a new set of propositions is entered. If any of these new propositions cannot be connected to those in the buffer or to each other, a reinstatement search into long-term memory is activated to find a proposition that shares an argument. If a linking proposition is found, it is reinstated into short-term memory, and a coherent connection is made. Otherwise, an inference bridge is constructed. The recency of antecedents facilitates coherence. Problems arise with greater distance between propositions that share arguments (O'Brien, 1987; van Dijk & Kintsch, 1983).

Functions of Coreference and Knowledge-Based Organization on Coherence   The distance effect may be more relevant when micropropositional processing is the focus, in contrast to processing at the macrostructural level. Cirilo (1981) studied the effects of local coreference on a micropropositional task, on a task requiring both high-level macrostructural and local micropropositional processing, and on a task focusing only on macrostructure. That is, the experimental tasks examined results of processing for global meaning and/or detail.

Interpretation of the findings led to the conclusion that textual coherence may not be regarded as a unitary concept. In situations requiring processing at the *local* coherence level, ties between sentences and/or propositions are essential. Globally, however, coherence pertains to the macrostructure, with relatively little processing of specific targets and their precursors. Comparing results of the varying experimental conditions, Cirilo (1981) explored the issue of possible competition for limited resources if processing was required simultaneously at both the micropropositional and macrostructural levels. No such interfering interaction was found. Therefore, it was suggested that, since the two levels of processing apparently cooccur, referential coherence is but one of the contributors to the construction of a text's macrostructure.

Increasing doubt has been cast on the overriding importance of coreference in memory for text. Results of experimentation provide evidence supporting the hypothesis that text is represented in memory as an integrated network rather than as a hierarchical structure based on coreference (O'Brien, 1987). It was found that a search for an antecedent referent was not always necessary, because of readers' use of knowledge-based relations to draw low-level inferences. Hierarchical organization and coreference do not take into account such inferential and elaborative processing. O'Brien (1987) concluded that hierarchies based on coreference are only approximations of the text organization. This point of view holds that knowledge-based relations may be more important to coherence than coreference in memory for text, in that the number of possible connections, determined by varying bodies of world knowledge, would provide an increase in the number of possible retrieval routes.

Under different experimental conditions of randomized order of sentences in stories and descriptive passages, Garnham, Oakhill, and Johnson-Laird (1982) found that, although the reinsertion of referents for anaphoric pronouns in nonconsecutive sentences facilitated coherence, the ability to make necessary bridging inferences was implicated. "We predicted that the skilled comprehenders would benefit more from the restoration of referential continuity in the randomized stories since the skilled comprehenders would be able to exercise their greater inferential skills in carrying out the required 'bridging' inferences" (p. 39). Their results demonstrated that only the skilled comprehenders were able to avail themselves of the restored referential continuity in the randomized passages. It would thus appear that coherence, while facilitated by coreference in the text, may require the complementary process of inference in the comprehension of and memory for various types of discourse passages.

Global Coherence and Macrostrategies   Local connections between contiguous sentences, in the absence of global coherence, may lead to chainings whose meaning has no relevance to the macrostructure. van Dijk (1985) makes this point through the following example:

> Eleanor is a very bright student.
> She excels in foreign languages.
> Foreign languages are not learned as frequently in the U.S. as in other countries.
> Other countries have many multilingual citizens.
>
> The macrostructure of a discourse defines its local coherence. Without such global coherence, there would be no overall control upon the local connections and continuations. (van Dijk, 1985, p. 115)

Sequences of propositions of the text are thus mapped onto more abstract sequences of macropropositions at a global level of meaning. Propositions may be both explicitly stated in the text and implicit in the form of given or inferred information. Processing through a hierarchy of macropropositions that subsume large sequences of semantic structures allows for the management of the overall meaning of the discourse at the macrostructure level even after semantic details are no longer accessible (van Dijk & Kintsch, 1983).

The underlying macrostructure in an extended unit is frequently expressed by such devices as titles, headings, summaries, and overall statements of purpose. Language users are believed to benefit from available information about the macrostructure in their strategies for predicting meaning of sequences of propositions. Hypothesized meaning may be inferred in bottom-up processing of textual, contextual, and world knowledge. "Once inferred in this bottom-up manner, a hypothesized macroproposition may be used as a top-down device to understand subsequent sentences, which, of course, also provide a check on the correctness of the hypothesis" (van Dijk & Kintsch, 1983, p. 196). It is acknowledged that all types of discourse are not equally predictable.

COMPREHENSION OF TYPES OF DISCOURSE

Comprehension of text is closely related to memory in that it involves accessing the stored knowledge base. Kintsch (1982) conceptualized the interaction between comprehension and memory as follows. In working memory, limited capacity is enhanced by rapid recognition of patterns of input bound to a large store of information from semantic memory; thus, information accessed from the stored knowledge base interacts with information from current text held in short-term memory without overburdening its limited capacity.

Comprehension of a complex network of textual sentences appears to involve, at least in part, analysis of Given and New components in the construction of an integrated meaning. Haviland and Clark (1974) suggested that the search for antecedents in the use of the Given-New strategy exploits the redundancy of linguistically encoded information. "As Given information, it serves as an address directing the listener [reader] to where new information should be stored. And as such, of course, it is not really redundant at all" (p. 520). Research has provided evidence in support of the notion that the closer the antecedent referents are to the present propositions, the faster is the comprehension or resolution of interpretations. "Thus, the more likely it is that referents must be linked on the basis of a reinstatement match, the longer it will take to understand the current sentence" (G.H. Bower & Cirilo, 1985, p. 88).

In retrieval of text, meaning construction is facilitated by the hierarchical macrostructure, in that one proposition serves as a cue to the next one via their association to the superordinate node. These associations are thought to be strongly established because superordinates were constructed from subordinate propositions. Both comprehension and retrieval are facilitated by top-down processing from such high-level superordinate macropropositions as discourse title or descriptive topic through lower level macropropositions to associated micropropositions.

Two well-known examples of the effects of high-level processing on comprehension and recall are the studies by Bransford and Johnson (1972) and by Dooling and Lackman (1971) in which the same passage, containing nonspecified, ambiguous information, was presented to groups of subjects under two different conditions. One group listened to the passage without any information about its topic. The other group was informed about the topic in advance of passage presentation. A part of the experimental passage from the Dooling and Lackman (1971) study is as follows:

> With hocked gems financing him, our hero bravely defied all scornful laughter that tried to prevent his scheme. "Your eyes deceive you," he had said, "an egg not a table correctly typifies this unexplored planet."

The title provided to one group was "Christopher Columbus Discovering America." Results demonstrated marked differences between comprehension and recall in the two groups. Subjects who were given the topic in advance performed significantly better in comprehension and recall than those who were not so informed. From these studies, it is apparent that knowledge of a theme prior to or during the course of processing a passage may activate appropriate memory structures into which the input can be integrated for enhancement of comprehension and recall.

Schemas, Scripts, and Frames

The terms *schemas, scripts*, and *frames* have been used by scholars in psychology, linguistics, and anthropology to refer to various aspects of knowledge structure stored in semantic memory and accessed to facilitate comprehension (Schank & Abelson, 1977). In their origin, they are essentially formalisms used in theories of artificial intelligence as constructions for representing knowledge. Tannen (1979) described the function of schematic knowledge as follows: "based on one's experience of the world in a given culture (or combination of cultures) one organizes knowledge about the world and uses this knowledge to predict interpretations and relationships regarding new information, events, and experiences" (p. 138). The terms differ in their application to knowledge domains.

A *schema* was characterized by Winograd (1977) as a description of complex objects, situations, processes, and so forth that goes beyond a dictionary definition. That is, it is regarded as an economical structure for storing knowledge that can be used in reasoning. Any discourse unit may contain schemas at different levels of abstraction, recursively embedded. Schema theories argue

> that any model of language understanding must be based on a model of a reasoning process in which each utterance is interpreted in light of the schemas currently activated and is used to activate new schemas which will affect the interpretation of subsequent utterances. (Winograd, 1977, p. 76)

Although the term *schema* has been used by some psychologists as a representation for the basic building blocks of cognition, Mandler (1984) preferred to narrow its scope to those structures that organize spatial/temporal knowledge about objects, events, and places (*schema* and *script* have been used interchangeably by some psychologists for sequentially organized knowledge). Mandler differentiated types of schemas activated in various discourse functions, among which are event schemas, scene schemas, and story schemas.

Event schemas include generalized knowledge about what happens in a given situation and possible orders in which individual events may occur in a sequence of events. An event schema consists of part-whole relations; for example, a birthday cake is part of the event schema of a birthday party. *Scene schemas*, including scripts, contain hierarchical knowledge about particular places that consists of collections of information rather than class inclusion. For example, in a scene schema of a room, the parts are organized as an inventory (e.g., walls, ceiling, windows, doors) in terms of spatial relations (e.g., next to, above, below). *Story schemas* consist of the stored set of expectations about the ways stories are constructed. A distinction is drawn between story schemas and story grammars, which are discussed below.

C.P. Bloom (1988) investigated the memory effects of imposed shifts in perspective during reading of the same stories by two groups of subjects. The focus of the perspective shifts was on event schemata within the story passages. One finding was evidence in support of the role of schemas as "sets of expectancies that help to direct subjects' processing and retrieval of information, rather than memory structures with specific slots to be filled" (p. 316). Subjects who processed the same information through two different schemas actually had the experience of additional processing of the information, thereby retaining information from both perspectives rather than substituting one for the other during recall. It is suggested that readers may employ a number of event schemas during the encoding of specific units in a story without using the story schema at the time of encoding, but that the story schema might be invoked during recall to help organize output. This issue is explored further below.

Scripts and *frames* refer to more stereotypical knowledge about specific familiar routines and situations that serve as "structures of expectations" (Tannen, 1979, p. 138). That is, they are instances of conventionalized knowledge that make relatively light demands on processing capacity, because they are activated as preprocessed entities. For example, in the comprehension of a story about the introduction in a bar of two characters who eventually fall in love, the well-learned routines/frames about Meeting, Introduction, Falling in Love, and Bar are invoked to foster relatively automatic construction of the meaning (van Dijk, 1977).

These memory structures may pertain to the various domains of world knowledge stored in semantic memory, activated during any comprehension activity, or they may refer more specifically to schematic structures of different types of discourse. Regarding the first type of stored knowledge, the reader will recall Kintsch's (1988) more recent conceptualization of a less structured, more flexible semantic memory than that represented by schema theory. However, it is generally agreed that each of the variety of discourse types exhibits its own conventionalized schematic structure, knowledge of which is believed to be invoked as a powerful aid in top-down processing (van Dijk & Kintsch, 1983). For example, stories have their own superstructure in contrast to that of expository prose. Some key concepts relevant to comprehension and recall in each of these areas of research and theory are examined.

Narrative Discourse and Story Structure

"A narrative refers to a series of real or fictional actions or events that take place in the past relative to the time of the narrative" (Gulich & Quasthoff, 1985, p. 170). Narratives are specified by certain formal characteristics of a macrostructure that, according to Gulich and Quasthoff (1985), lends itself readily to analysis because of its highly regular and relatively simple structure.

Story grammars have been constructed as rule systems, "devised for the purpose of describing the regularities found in one kind of text" (Mandler, 1984, p. 18). The structural descriptions have been analogous to a syntax of plot organization, believed to guide comprehension and facilitate recall (Thorndyke, 1977). That is, narratives have their own internal structure (as do sentences) that permits readers/listeners to generate expectancies. "The underlying assumption is that insofar as people are able to identify a particular story as an example of a general, previously learned organizational framework, they use that framework to comprehend and encode the information in a particular text" (Thorndyke, 1977, p. 79).

Example of Story Grammars   A number of investigators have devised story grammars for analysis of comprehension, recall, and generation of adult and child subjects' processing of stories (Mandler, 1984; N. Stein & Glenn, 1979; Thorndyke, 1977). The following example is illustrative of categories of information and relations among such categories generally included in extant story grammars, allowing for some variations in terminology.

Summary of Grammatical Rules

1. Story — ALLOW (Setting, Episode System)
2. Setting — States; Actions
3. Episode System — AND
                             THEN
                             CAUSE
4. Episode — INITIATE (Initiating Event, Responses)
5. Initiating Event — Natural Occurrence(s)
                             Actions(s)
                             Internal Events
6. Response — MOTIVATE (Internal Response, Plan Sequence)
7. Internal Response — Goal(s)
                             Affects(s)
                             Cognition(s)
8. Plan Sequence — INITIATE (Internal Plan, Plan Application)
9. Internal Plan — Cognition(s)
                             Subgoal(s)

10. Plan Application — RESULT (Attempt, Resolution)
11. Attempt — (Action(s))
12. Resolution — INITIATE (Direct Consequences, Reaction)
13. Direct Consequence — Natural Occurrence(s)
                        Action(s)
                        End State(s)
14. Reaction — Affect(s)
              Cognition(s)
              Action(s)

Intra-category connectors:

AND: includes simultaneous or a temporal relation.
THEN: includes temporal but not direct causal relations.
CAUSE: includes temporal relations which are causal in nature. (N. Stein & Glenn, 1979, p. 60)

It is maintained by Gulich and Quasthoff (1985) that story grammars serve the following macrostructure functions:

1. Based on empirical analysis of recall and summarization of a large corpus of texts, they lay claim to the cognitive reality of predicting processing regularities.
2. They are analogous to rule systems for sentence grammars in that they exemplify structural categories and generative capability.

Research on Processing Narratives   Mandler (1984) reported on results of reviewed investigations of the psychological validity of a story schema. The prediction that stories constructed in canonical form (i.e., having all categories in the expected order) would be better recalled than those either missing components or consisting of a mixed order of categories was confirmed in numerous studies cited. Furthermore, material central to the story was more likely to be recalled than peripheral elaborations. This finding is interpreted as evidence that the components included in a story grammar do constitute the gist of the story and provide a reasonable representation of the story's essential structure (Mandler, 1984).

In a study of adult subjects' processing of narrative discourse, comprehensibility and recall of content were found to be functions of the amount of inherent plot structure, independent of passage content (Thorndyke, 1977). Subjects tended to recall information corresponding to high-level organizational elements rather than low-level detail. The internal structure of the narrative appears to influence the generation of reader/listener expectations based on knowledge of implicit causal relations, underlying goals, and character motivations.

Studies of school-age children's recall of stories have demonstrated that, among the categories of information in a story schema, certain ones tend to be more salient and more frequently recalled or self-generated than others. In recalled stories of first- and fifth-grade subjects, major settings, consequences, and initiating events were the most frequently occurring categories, with the remainder occurring in the following order of frequency: attempts, reactions, minor settings, and internal responses (N. Stein & Glenn, 1979). In spontaneously generated stories of children ranging in age from 8;0 to 13;11 years, the following categories were likely to be included in the order of mention: attempt, initiating events or responses, and direct consequences (Roth & Spekman, 1986).

N. Stein and Glenn (1979) reported that even 6-year-old children are capable of organizing temporally sequenced information in simply constructed stories. Children younger than 6 years old have been observed to have difficulty in recalling temporal order of a pictured narrative series; however, when provided with a verbal description of causal relations existing between the pictured events, recall of correctly ordered information improved significantly (A.L. Brown, 1975).

Early Development of Narrative Abilities   The ability to generate narrative has been found to develop in children at the preschool and early elementary school levels through a progression of stages. Westby (1989) provided an account of the conceptual development and schema knowledge underlying the merging elaboration of narrative structure at advancing age levels. For example, in the preschool to early elementary school period, narratives progress through the following stages:

> Labeling characters, actions, and objects without expression of interrelations among them
> Ordering sequences of actions chronologically on the basis of perception without the realization of further interrelationships such as causality
> Chaining of actions/events that cause other events without evidence of planning
> Using abbreviated episodes, including causes, effects, goals, and so forth, with planning implicit rather than explicitly stated
> Using complete episodes, including expression of goals and intentions, plus planning, consequences, and intermediate components

Universal Types of Narratives   In addition to stories, which are fictionalized accounts of events with goal-directed plots, three types of nonfictional narratives are described by Heath (1986b): recounts, event casts, and accounts. "All these narrative forms bring to consciousness past or imagined experience and require gestalt-level processes of linking similarities and dissimilarities across space and time" (p. 88).

Recounts   This narrative form reports past events of the speaker's experience delivered with consecutive temporal ordering of the components. These narratives are generally in response to requests by others (e.g., teachers or parents) rather than volunteered. The structure may vary according to cultural expectations or level of maturity, employing one of two basic forms:

> *Paratactic form*, in which components are related in a coordinate manner with little imposed organization indicating logical relations or relative importance.
> *Hypotactic form*, making causal and temporal relations explicit through such linguistic devices as grammatical structure and conjunctions.

Event Casts   This form of narrative accompanies current activities or plans for future events. It is used to obtain some result (e.g., how some play activity will be implemented). Coordination and subordination of components that indicate "hypothetical connectedness" (Heath, 1986b, p. 89) must be included.

Accounts   In contrast to recounts, accounts are motivated by the individual's desire to verbally share experiences with others. That is, accounts are spontaneously initiated by the speaker, rather than given as responses to external requests for information. For the most part, adults do not shape the structure of children's accounts, "and children must therefore internalize the norms of these narratives, recognizing that each account must carry within it a predictable progression that allows the listener to anticipate what is coming" (Heath, 1986b, p. 89).

Comprehension of Narratives   Kintsch (1982) suggested that narratives are probably easier to understand than other types of discourse (e.g., expository) because of both the language user's accumulated knowledge of story structure and the rather universal experience with human interactions that form the content of most narratives. It has been found in a study with kindergarten-age children that the same content was more successfully processed following its presentation in a narrative style than in an expository passage (Freedle & Hale, 1979). These authors controlled exclusively for verb tense in this study, with the major difference between the two passages residing in the use of past tense for narratives in contrast to the use of tense signaling habitual state or the use of modals in the expository form. Otherwise all components present in the narrative form were preserved in the expository version. While demonstrating an experimental procedure for effecting the development of ability to process expository prose in immature children, the results do not disconfirm the greater difficulty of expository versus narrative prose, which is in all likelihood attributable to factors other than verb tense.

Expository Discourse

The universe of discourse was analyzed by Moffett (1968) in terms of levels of abstraction, conceptualized as follows:

> The lowest level of abstraction is reflected in sensory reporting; that is, verbalization of what *is happening*.
> The next level of abstraction in discourse is narration of what *has happened*.
> The next level of abstraction is generalizations about what *happens*.
> The highest level of abstraction is theorizing about what *may happen*.

In general, narration is more closely tied to experience in its sensorimotor and affective manifestations, whereas essays (or other forms of expository discourse) tend to be more distanced from perception, with concomitant increased reliance on memory and reasoning.

The comprehension and production of expository prose in monologic form place the heaviest demands on the processing resources of the language user. Within the perspecitve of this book, the processing of the literate language of education, which assumes a central role in present concerns, is largely expository in nature. Moreover, much of expository prose involved in academic tasks is in the written modality. Similarly, research in this type of discourse tends to be overwhelmingly devoted to reading or writing. Therefore, aspects of expository prose are examined predominantly, although not exclusively, in the written form.

Expository prose is frequently in the form of an extended logical essay in which propositions are considered in the effort to determine all relevant implications during the construction of a coherent text (D.R. Olson, 1977b). This monologic development of a theme is frequently characterized by a density of exposition requiring intricate antecedent referencing and inferencing. Syntax is frequently more complex and compressed (A. Rubin, 1980). It has also been pointed out that expository text is usually composed of information that is novel to the reader, making it less likely that available schematic knowledge can be readily applied in comprehension (Westby, 1989). In contrast to the processing of narratives through the use of well-learned story grammar structure, expository prose varies widely in organizational structure.

> Because the content schema and text grammar are generally not available to the student prior to the first reading of an expository text, processing of expository texts is much more a bottom-up pro-

cess than the top-down processing used in comprehending narrative texts. . . . Comprehending expository texts requires that readers use the individual facts of the text to construct a content schema, a text grammar or macrostructure, and the coherence relations among the sentences of the text. (Westby, 1989, p. 203)

In text composition at the level of low formal operations (in contrast to the level of concrete operations), Scinto (1986) observed that

the linkage of compositional units is achieved not only by thematic iteration but also involves the concatenation of thematic and rhematic material into more complex compositional nets. At this stage the entire previous composition, not simply immediately prior elements, appears to be available to the subject. (p. 152)

This description would seem to implicate processing at the global level of the macrostructure in conjunction with local coherence. The sensitivity of the language user to discourse organization has been studied in terms of effectiveness of comprehension and recall. Meyer (1975, 1977) provided examples of the rhetorical relations that may serve as the high-level organizational structural patterns of expository prose passages; for example:

Problem—solution
Question—answer
Cause—effect
Generalization—specific supportive detail
Explanation
Disjunction—comparison/contrast

In her study Meyer found that the structure of the prose itself appeared to be related to comprehension and recall of content, and that subjects more sensitive to the structure of the text were significantly superior in comprehension and recall.

Spiro (1980) took issue with the assertion that the organization of meaning within the text determines comprehension. Rather, he maintained that superordinate notions of theme are *constructed* by the listener/reader, and that such constructions are determined by prior knowledge, attitudinal factors influencing what is accepted or rejected, and focus of attention on particular aspects to satisfy pragmatic purposes.

PRAGMATIC ASPECTS OF DISCOURSE PROCESSING

The concerns encompassed in the field of pragmatics cover a wide range of disparate functions that extend beyond those immediately relevant to the focus of this chapter. Indeed, there has been some expression of discontent with what Ferraro (1985) has labeled the hodgepodge approach, "a sort of residual category into which is lumped all that cannot be labeled as phonological, syntactic or semantic in a straightforward fashion" (p. 138). From his point of view, pragmatics is regarded as the structure and implementation of a *core of intentions*, with a network of means-ends relationships among the constituents of a text presented in a functionally coherent way aimed at achieving the overarching *goal* of the discourse. For example, the repertoire of speech acts selected to achieve the goal of persuasion may include proving, reminding, and suggesting.

The intentions most immediate to the focus in this chapter are those linked most closely to academic versus all social functions. Even within this domain, space constraints limit this discussion to the more general interactions between discourse processing and contextual or interpersonal/intrapersonal variables, reserving for Chapter 5 exploration of specific pragmatic functions within the classroom. Thus, interpreting discourse, within these limits, is conceived of as involving three essential components: the text, the context, and the language user (Haslett, 1987).

The context or situation determines the potential for various communicative options, but the language user's motives, purposes, age, sex, social status, experience, and so forth will strongly influence the selection among those options. Other factors that may influence the mode as well as the content of discourse are participants' moods, willingness to take risks, and relationships in time and space (Dudley-Marling & Rhodes, 1987). The communicative strategies chosen as most appropriate are based on "best estimates" about what maximizes effectiveness in a particular situation.

In text comprehension, it is suggested that working hypotheses are formed not solely about the structure and meaning of a text fragment, but also about the language user's intent and knowledge. These hypotheses may be confirmed or disconfirmed in light of subsequent processing (van Dijk & Kintsch, 1983). For example, interpretation of particular assertions in a text may be altered in light of further knowledge about the beliefs, motives, values, and so forth of the language user. Such factors, as maintained by Spiro (1980) above, may determine how much attention is paid to particular topics and the importance accorded to certain ideas in interpreting a text, regardless of the top-down structure imposed by the message sender. Thus, in contrast to discourse analysis, which presumes constancy of structure internal to the text, functional analysis explores the interaction among text and such variables as situational characteristics and individual differences (Haslett, 1987).

Because the primary concern in this volume is discourse in the educational setting, a major emphasis is placed on processing the language of literacy, written and oral. From a pragmatic perspective, each execution of a written language product is a social event in that it entails a transaction between the writer and the intended reader within a particular language context (Dudley-Marling & Rhodes, 1987). These authors discussed the following elements of the language context that affect language use: purpose, content, type of discourse, participant characteristics, setting, activity, and speech community.

Purpose The vocabulary, syntactic structure, and mode of discourse are chosen for appropriateness to various purposes (e.g., record keeping, personal communication, exploration of ideas). The choice of modality and style may influence content; for example, written language is regarded as facilitative to thought: "Ideas can be generated and developed in the interaction between the writer and what is being written that would not be possible if the ideas were left to flower and perhaps fade in the transcience of the mind" (Smith, 1982, p. 16). This interaction between the writer and the composition of expository prose is similarly viewed by Scinto (1986) as stimulating to cognitive development: "It is perhaps the sustained intersentential organization of text and the construction strategies . . . that best demonstrate the impact of written language on elaborated thought or higher level thinking" (p. 167).

Content The subject matter will determine the style of discourse. Discussion of a scholarly topic, such as physics, will require a more formal style than discussion of a recreational pastime.

Type of discourse A letter will differ in its style from a term paper.

Participant characteristics   In addition to other characteristics, relative status between message sender and receiver will influence form and content; for example, a memorandum to the chairman of the board would differ in degree of formality from a note to a colleague.

Setting   Language used in the classroom will differ from language used in the schoolyard.

Activity   Written communication requires greater explicitness than face-to-face conversation.

Speech community   Different communities share different sets of rules governing the form and use of language. Discourse processing is generally most effective when participants "share understandings of certain rules for encoding meanings as well as agreement about how the language context affects meaning and use" (Dudley-Marling & Rhodes, 1987, p. 43).

An example of disparate understandings across cultures is described by Nix and Schwarz (1979). They examined difficulties experienced by minority students in their interaction with mainstream reading material. Using an interview technique, they secured oral accounts justifying multiple choice responses to comprehension questions. The following passage is an example of the experimental material:

> Sally loved animals. She brought home every stray animal that she could find, no matter what it looked like. Her mother declared that she adopted any animal as long as it was _____.
>
> A.   lively   B.   alive   C.   large   D.   lame (p. 186)

The most frequent choice was *lively* rather than the targeted response *alive*. The basis for this choice was an implication that the verb *declare* involves instructing someone what to do, together with a statement by the participant that his/her mother preferred lively dogs.

> Whereas in the TN [target network] the answer is knit relatively closely into the context of the rest of the paragraph, in the PN [participant network] the answer is knit into a portion of the paragraph plus a personal set of experiences of the particpant. (Nix & Schwarz, 1979, p. 189)

This processing pattern may be interpreted within the foregoing levels of abstraction posited by Moffett (1968). That is, the passage required a response at the level of generalization, whereas the response was made at the more concrete level of particularized personal experience. The present author has observed this tendency frequently in the written output of college students referred to a remedial writing program. For example, if an assigned essay topic was education, instead of writing at a level of generalization appropriate for expository prose about the nature of education or problems exhibited in education or advances in education, these students tended to resort to narrations about their own personal educational experiences or their parents' expectations of them.

The above examples illustrate possible sources of interference with optimal educational discourse processing, receptively and expressively, because of apparent differences in selection of what is relevant and/or appropriate to the reading or writing of passages in the literate style of mainstream culture. It is difficult to cleanly separate the pragmatic from the cognitive aspects of educational discourse processing. Scinto (1986) strongly suggested that the mastery of what he termed *scholarized language* makes a significant contribution to the later phases of cognitive development:

> As the child moves through phases of development there is a progressive differentiation of self from the surrounding environment. An integral part of this differentiation is a progressive distancing of the communicative system from the individual, from gesture to spoken language, and finally to written language. (p. 168)

DISCOURSE IN THE CLASSROOM

A study by D. Edwards and Mercer (1989) that observed and analyzed discourse in the classroom provides a transition from the largely theoretical approach to discourse processing in this chapter to its application to education. In what seems to be a highly effective process of teacher-student interaction, the following potent discursive devices were used by the teacher to reactivate important aspects of shared knowledge and experience from prior class sessions:

> Introduction of understandings or versions of events via presupposition and implication
> Defining these understandings as Given, not open to question
> Reconstructive paraphrasing to establish what was to serve as common knowledge for subsequent teaching and learning

"What develops between teacher and pupil might be conceived of as a collective memory, a joint version of things encoded symbolically, in which shared understandings become established through the development of a common language and a common discursive context" (D. Edwards & Mercer, 1989, p. 92).

From this perspective, once again, it is suggested that through the literate language of educational discourse, the teacher's skillful use of the discursive process helps in important ways to advance children's cognitive development beyond what might be assumed to develop spontaneously in a stage-wise progression.

SUMMARY

Language is processed through the structure of sentences embedded in the context of connected units of discourse. At both the macro- and micro-levels, discourse processing entails the construction of coherence among propositions and the use of cohesive devices to signal relations among ideas. Comprehension of and memory for discourse content are influenced by the use of and sensitivity to structure. Narrative and expository discourse place different receptive and expressive processing demands on the language user. Both of these discourse styles are intimately involved in education and, to an extent, may contribute to some aspects of cognitive development.

5 / Language of the Classroom

Betty H. Bunce

"Gimme a pencil."

"Turn to page 21 and do the first 10 problems."

"What is the capital of Argentina?"

"It's time to listen."

"Alaska is a state rich in natural resources. Many of these resources are buried beneath the frozen ground."

Conversations, oral and written instructions, worksheets, questions, discussions, lectures, stories, textbook chapters, story writing, and essay writing are all examples of classroom language events. This wide variability of language use makes the study of classroom discourse very complex. Adding to this complexity is the fact that many different types of language use can occur within a short time period. For example, there can be rapid shifting back and forth between social and instructional discourse and between oral and written language.

The classroom is also unique in that a basic purpose of the school, the development of literacy skills, is accomplished through communication. A variety of language skills and knowledge is needed to achieve this literacy development. Some of these language skills include metalinguistic skills, comprehension monitoring, classroom pragmatic and discourse skills, and specific vocabulary necessary for academic content areas (Van Kleeck & Richardson, 1988). Van Kleeck and Richardson also cited the role of language in the formation of concepts, in reasoning, and in learning strategies and study skills. Thus, language is not only part of the content to be learned, but also the tool for that learning. In addition, much of the learning is achieved through the spoken medium. Finally, the classroom is also a unique social institution where one person, the teacher, is responsible for controlling the behavior and learning of 20–30 other people.

Language in the classroom therefore includes a wide range of functions, content, form, and discourse interactions. Factors contributing to this variability include contrasts between social and academic functions, oral and written style, and primary linguistic versus metalinguistic task demands. Further variability occurs as a result of the teacher's philosophy of teaching and interactional style. The students' ability to understand the pragmatics of the classroom interactions and appropriately respond also affects the variability of classroom language. Language in the classroom also imposes multilevel demands on participants that may be implicit as well as explicit. Being able to succeed in the classroom depends, then, on the students' and teachers' ability to effectively understand and use all of these different types of language skills and processes.

In order to address some of these issues, characteristics of classroom language, per se, are presented first. The discussion includes: 1) similarities and differences between social and instructional discourse; 2) similarities and differences between oral and written language; and 3) metalinguistic, metacognitive, and metapragmatic skills needed in the classroom. Next, the focus is on classroom discourse, or the use of language by teachers and students within the classroom setting. This discussion includes: 1) instructional conversations, 2) use of questions, 3) teaching and learning styles, and 4) hidden complexities in classroom discourse. Finally, new trends in the classroom involving the use of whole language and peer learning philosophies and their effect on classroom language are briefly discussed.

CHARACTERISTICS OF CLASSROOM LANGUAGE

Social Discourse Versus Instructional Discourse

Reflection on language in the classroom often conjures up a picture of a teacher talking and students listening, or of a teacher questioning and students answering. Although this scene may be prevalent in many classrooms, the classroom is also a social setting. Therefore, both social and instructional dialogues occur. There are several features that are common to both social and instructional discourse. Each involves senders and receivers, each involves "something" to be communicated, and each has certain conventions involved in the communication of that knowledge. However, there are several differences between social and instructional discourse, including different functions, forms, content, and rules for interacting. There are also differences in the number of participants usually involved. For example, in social discourse a dyad or triad may be customary, whereas in instructional discourse there may be one teacher (speaker) to 30 students (listeners).

The purpose of *social discourse* is everyday social interaction. Form and content features of social discourse include the use of casual language, starts and stops in regard to fluency, and ongoing composition. The language used in social discourse is said to be contextualized, that is, embedded in a context in which there are many extralinguistic supports for meaning. These extralinguistic supports may include the setting, the shared knowledge between the sender and receiver, the use of gesture, and the use of suprasegmental features such as intonation, pause, and stress. Much use of personalized language occurs (e.g., use of pronouns *I*, *you*, and *me*, and personalized slang). For example, the comment "Did ya see that move?" would be completely understood not only in regard to who performed the action but also to what was done, as long as the participants witnessed the same event and/or had shared knowledge of the event. The event might be observing a young man ask a girl out on a date or someone make a slam-dunk at a basketball game. The context of the event would provide the necessary support for understanding the comment.

The participants in social discourse usually have equal status and equal responsibility for continuing the interaction. Social discourse may be oral or written. Spontaneous conversations and "jive" are examples of oral social discourse. Notes and personal letters are examples of written social discourse.

The purpose or function of *instructional discourse* is to transmit and/or demonstrate knowledge. Form and content features of instructional discourse include more formal language, more reliance on linguistic cues to signal Given/New information, less redundancy, and, in general, less personalized language than is true of social discourse. Instructional discourse thus utilizes decontextualized language. In order for a written comment (e.g., "That was a good move") to be understood, other information would need to be provided ("After Jim made a hook shot, John commented to Mary, 'That was a good move.' "). Making meaning explicit through the use of linguistic factors requires utilizing appropriate vocabulary, grammar, and organized discourse structures. Instructional language, particularly of textbooks, is often highly decontextualized.

Participants in oral instructional discourse usually do not have the same status and do not have the same responsibility for continuing the interaction. The teacher usually controls the pace, who participates, and much of the content of the interaction. To some extent, the teacher's control of the interaction also occurs for written language. It is the teacher who assigns what is to be read or written within the classroom setting.

In summary, both social and instructional language occur within any given day in every classroom. Some of the variability in language of the classroom, therefore, is due to its function, social or instructional. Other variability is due to mode of production, either oral or written.

Oral Versus Written Language

Oral and written language are similar in many ways. For example, each involves arbitrary symbols and rule-governed combinations of these symbols to represent concepts (Owens, 1984). Both oral and written language are used to communicate. Each includes vocabulary, syntax, grammar, and discourse structure. Each also has a means of being produced, a sound system for oral language and an orthographic system for written language.

However, there are a variety of ways that oral language differs from written language. Several scholars (Danielewicz, 1984; D. Olson, 1977a; Westby, 1985) have delineated an oral-literate language continuum involving a range from spontaneous spoken language to expository written language. For example, Westby (1985) proposed a continuum with orality at one end and literacy at the other. Asking for something or telling someone to do something would be at the orality end, and reading or writing a story would be at the literacy end. Intermediate stages would include oral description of a personal experience, written personal notes, listening to or giving lectures, and writing a report. The concept of a continuum highlights the interconnections and transitions between different language uses.

Other scholars (e.g., A. Rubin, 1980; D.L. Rubin, 1987) used dichotomies to describe these differences. A. Rubin (1980) used medium and message dimensions to contrast oral language experiences and written language of stories and texts. Under medium dimensions he included features of modality (written or oral production), interaction and involvement of participants, spatial and temporal commonality, and concreteness of referents. Under message dimensions, differences in topic, function, and structure of oral (social) language and literate language are discussed. D.L. Rubin (1987), in his discussion of the divergence of oral and written language, included many of the same differences organized under production, context, and style parameters.

This section discusses general differences between oral and written language, focusing on physical/production factors, contextual factors, and content and functional factors. The effect of these differences on grammatical structure is then discussed. Finally, the concepts of implicitness and explicitness are examined in relation to oral and written language, and the language used in textbooks is addressed.

Production Factors   For most people, production of oral language is usually effortless; the message is fleeting and sequenced in time. The production is through the mouth and a sound system is employed. In English, there are approximately 44 phonemes, or minimal sound units that carry meaning (Perera, 1984). Unless a recording or transcription is made, there is no permanent record of the production. Also, the sender and receiver of the communication are often in face-to-face contact, with the speaker controlling the rate at which the message is produced and received by the listener. Feedback from the listener may or may not change the speaker's productions.

In oral language a range of fluency is allowed. For example, hesitations, repetitions, and filled pauses occur along with interjections such as "oh" or "well" or rhetorical questions such as "You know?" or "O.K.?" Although these features could be interruptive to the communication, they often are not. The time taken up with such features is often used by the listener in processing the information provided. Also, different pronunciations of words are allowed. As A. Rubin (1980) noted, a salient aspect of spoken language is the use of prosodic features such as intonation, stress, and rhythm. These features are important in signaling or organizing the discourse. Pauses often occur at syntactic junctures, and emphasis on a particular word(s) provides clues to meaning.

In contrast to oral language, written language requires more effort to be produced. D.L. Rubin (1987) underscored this difficulty by noting that, "no one is a native speaker of writing" (p. 3). An orthographic system must be learned that allows a permanent message to be produced by the hand. In English, only 26 alphabet letters are used to represent the 44 phonemes. Vowel letters represent more than one sound; also, some consonant combinations, such as *ch*, are used to represent a sound different from either of the single letters. The written record makes spatial rather than temporal sequencing important. It is possible to go back to a word, sentence, or paragraph and rewrite (or reread). Also, the reader is not at the mercy of the writer in regard to the rate at which the message is received. The reader can read as rapidly or as slowly as he/she desires. In addition, there is usually physical separation between the sender and receiver. Immediate communication to a receiver, therefore, does not usually take place.

Although prosodic features are not available in written language, there are alternative conventions that help compensate (A. Rubin, 1980). First, written language segments the message for the receiver into words and sentences. Second, additional segmenting into paragraphs, sections, or chapters provides further structure for the written text. Third, the use of format features such as punctuation, underlining, boldface, and italic markings provides a means for emphasizing content or providing structural cues. The reader is able to absorb the message at his/her own speed.

Contextual Factors   In oral language there is dynamic shifting between roles of sender and receiver (speaker and listener). The speaker/listener(s) share the same temporal and, to some degree, spatial context. There is a rapid rate of composing on the part of the sender. The rate of receiving the message corresponds to the rate of production. Immediate feedback is available and breakdowns in communication can be immediately repaired. Prosodic features such as intonation and stress may also change the meaning of the verbal productions. For example, sarcastic intonation accompanying a statement such as, "Well, I really like that," changes the statement from a positive one to a negative one. Also, nonverbal communication can and does take place at the same time that verbal communication is occurring.

Communication of an oral message depends not only on linguistic factors, but also on nonverbal factors such as gestures and information shared between the participants. These nonverbal factors can have a major impact on what is communicated. For example, a point, a nod, or some other gesture can provide the necessary support for a deictic term such as *that* or *there*. (Deictic terms are by themselves empty of meaning; their interpretation depends on other factors, such as location of speaker.) In addition, the participants in a conversation may know each other well and therefore not have to make explicit many of their references. Also, the setting itself can make verbal descriptions unnecessary.

In written language, there is no bidirectional interchange between participants. Instead, writing involves an extended monologue the audience for which may not be known to the writer. Because of the permanence of the written product, there can be wide variation in time and space between the sender and receiver(s). Feedback from the receiver is usually not available or is delayed. The sender (writer) must anticipate the receivers' (readers') responses or difficulties with the subject matter in order to communicate effectively. Phelps-Gunn and Phelps-Terasaki (1982) suggested that the writer must have a "sense of audience" so that the appropriate amount and degree of information needed by the reader is produced (p. 3). Instantaneous repairs of communication breakdowns are not possible.

Production of writing may extend over a long period of time, with the author frequently able to amend or revise the content and form of the message before it is presented to an audience. The rate of the writer's production is not related to the rate at which the reader reads the product. A writer may take a year to write what a reader reads in a few hours. Also, nonlinguistic environmental factors make little contribution to the communication. Linguistic means and extralinguistic conventions such as punctuation are used to provide the necessary context for communicating the message. These conventions may need to be explicitly taught.

Content and Functional Factors   Although speech can be written down and written language can be read aloud, the content and functions of oral and written language can be quite different. Oral language is active, practical, and concerned with the listener, whereas written language is reflective and often concerned with logical relations (Phelps-Gunn & Phelps-

Terasaki, 1982). A primary function of oral language is social discourse. Casual conversations, requests for objects and actions, and discussions of everyday objects and situations often involving the here and now are prevalent. Maintaining human relationships is also a major aspect of social discourse. The vocabulary used to reflect these functions may be less formal. Non-specific words and phrases such as "give me that" or "one of those," deictic terms such as "over there," slang, and jargon all may be appropriate in oral speech.

Written language functions include recording facts, ideas, and information. Written language allows a permanent record to be kept providing access for future generations to thoughts, facts, and stories of previous civilizations. Written language also allows ideas to be explored and developed. It can serve as an extension of thinking or a means of clarifying one's ideas. Written language, therefore, is an important intellectual tool because it allows information to be accumulated, distributed, and analyzed. Expository writing often serves a teaching function. Textbooks and "how-to" books are particularly written to transmit specific information. Written language, particularly of textbooks, is characterized by use of specific vocabulary terms. There is also much less use of deictic terms and slang than is found in oral language.

Written language also serves a particular function in the development of literature. Through written language many literary genres are available, such as novels, poetry, and short stories. Written language allows the reader access to narratives without regard to the presence of a storyteller (see Westby, 1985, for a description of oral narratives as a transition to literate language).

Grammatical Structures   The production, contextual, content, and functional differences between oral and written language lead to differences in grammatical structure. In oral language the ongoing, spontaneous speech allows for little planning; therefore there usually is a high level of redundancy. There is also a high tolerance for false starts, pauses, and hesitations. It is often impossible to write down exactly oral productions as sentences. Grammatical conventions such as coordination, repetition, and rephrasing often occur (Perera, 1984). Use of these grammatical devices leads to low lexical density. That is, the words carrying most of the meaning are spaced apart. For example, in the statement, "And she said that the report was ready, and it wasn't and then, and then she said she would finish all the work and the report would be ready when I got there and then it wasn't, and she, she still had to do . . . uh . . . make the title page," the utterances are tied together through the use of "and." There is little use of subordinate clauses and much of the content is repeated or rephrased. The lack of variety in sentence structure that often occurs in oral speech may be unnoticed because of the different stress and intonation patterns that may be used.

Writing is not just talk written down; rather, it has a different base in linguistic and structural elaboration (Phelps-Gunn & Phelps-Terasaki, 1982). In written language, there is more time for planning. This leads to less redundancy and more lexical density. Many more subordinate clauses may be used. For example, the spoken statement above could be written as "Although she said the report was ready, she had not finished the title page when I got there," using less than half the number of words to express the same content. Cohesion among and between sentences is achieved through the use of linguistic devices rather than intonation and stress. These devices may include terms such as *although, because, so,* and *therefore* or may involve reference back to a previous item (see Halliday & Hasan, 1976, for descriptions of types of cohesive ties).

Perera (1984) listed some of the grammatical structures that may be used to decrease repetition and to increase lexical information within written language. These include:

1. Nonfinite subordinate clauses (e.g., *"Walking through the mountains*, she found several different kinds of animal tracks"). In oral language finite subordinate clauses are more likely to be used (*"When she was walking through the mountains . . . "*).

2. Verbless subordinate clauses (e.g., *"When very cold*, the chemical change occurs"). In oral language the phrase would more often be *"When it is very cold . . . "*

3. Ellipsis or the omission of a common element within a sentence or between sentences (e.g., "The Mazda is made in Japan and the Ford [is made] in America," or "The flowers were white. There were a dozen [flowers]").

4. Use of a whole clause as the subject of the sentence (e.g., *"The extension of curfew on Saturday nights* has meant a rise in the number of teenage accidents"). In oral language a shorter noun phrase would be more likely ("The *curfew on Saturday nights* has been extended and this has meant a rise in the number of teenage accidents"). The addition of several adjectives to the noun phrase also adds to the lexical density. For example, "The blue, old-fashioned, Pontiac car, sitting in the driveway, was my grandfather's" would more likely be a written than an oral statement.

In written language, therefore, redundancy is low and lexical density is high. Meaning is made explicit through linguistic means rather than through nonlinguistic context.

Implicitness Versus Explicitness   Several scholars have begun to challenge the concept of oral language being implicit and written language being explicit (Mazzie, 1987; Prince, 1981; Tannen, 1982). They suggested that the relative degree of implicitness and explicitness in any communication may depend more on the genre and communicative goals than on the modality used. In Prince's studies (1981), the written samples were found to contain more inferred (implicit) information than did the oral samples. Prince also suggested that the explicitness of written or oral productions depended on what assumptions the writer/speaker made about the reader/listener's background knowledge of the topic. The writer/speaker would presumably be more explicit if the audience were judged to be unfamiliar with the topic.

Mazzie (1987) investigated the concept that explicitness was a function of content and/or the relationship between participants rather than a function of oral or written modality. She had students address a real or an imagined audience in spoken or written form with either a narrative or an abstract logic task (explanation of a number system). She found that the oral texts as a whole did not contain more inferred information. She also noted that the abstract texts had three times the amount of inferred information when compared with the corresponding narrative texts (e.g., written explanation of number system to real audience versus written narrative to real audience, or oral explanation of number system versus oral narrative). Thus, it was content that appeared to control level of explicitness. Again, levels of abstraction and assumptions regarding shared knowledge of the participants appeared to interact in determining the level of explicitness.

It may be that there are different kinds of implicit and explicit knowledge. For example, in narratives, implicit knowledge may involve a general knowledge of story grammar or typical happenings in a particular culture. It may also involve understanding and remembering what pronouns refer to which people and what events. For expository texts, the implicit knowledge may be based on knowledge of logic or conventions. McCutchen (1987) examined the effect of discourse form (narrative or expository) and production modality (spoken or written) on implicitness and explicitness. Each of her subjects produced eight texts, four essays and four narratives, with two spoken and two written texts for each type. Analysis focused on structured elaboration and coherence. Coherence was evaluated not only at a surface level, where relations between text itself (cohesive ties) were examined, but also at a conceptual level involving logical underlying information. Each text was divided into independent clause units. Successive clause units were then examined for the connections linking them back to other clauses in the text. The results indicated that oral texts were more elaborated than written texts. Narratives, whether oral or written, contained proportionally more coherent clauses and inference ties than did essays. The author suggested that the inference ties reflected the reliance on real-world knowledge in narratives. Essays rely more on logical arguments rather than on inferences; therefore, the relationships must be explicitly marked. In this study, written essays contained the highest level of explicit ties. The author suggested that expository texts may demand more reorganization of the knowledge base, whereas narratives require access to existing information. Therefore, in comparing implicit/explicit knowledge, the type of discourse is an important factor to consider. The implicitness/explicitness may be describing different aspects of the content depending on discourse type.

Language of Textbooks   As the student progresses through school, more of the language of the classroom involves the language of textbooks. Familiarity with story grammar or typical patterns and knowledge of common factors can help in understanding written narratives. No such support is present for expository texts, at least initially. As students become familiar with formats such as advance organizers, chapter outlines, headings, and elaborated sentences, they may be able to use these devices to access new textbook knowledge more easily. Textbook formats and conventions (e.g., top of a map is north, boldface words are important, headings signal information to come) usually must be explicitly taught.

Features of textbook language include usage of technical or less common vocabulary. For example, when presented with the sentence, "Scientists use a liquid taken from cattle and hogs as a medication to help control a disease called diabetes," students may be unfamiliar with the terms *liquid* or *medication*. Words with multiple meanings may be a source of difficulty for some students. Also, students may be unfamiliar with techniques that are used in textbooks to explain new terms. For example, a definition or restatement might be placed in parentheses or set off by commas (e.g., "Pasteur worked with the bacteria that had been found to cause anthrax, an often fatal disease of sheep").

Another feature of textbook language is the use of unfamiliar sentence patterns, ones not often used in oral language. Some of these patterns include: 1) *altered word order* (e.g., "Contained in the cytoplasm are the highly organized structures called organelles" versus "The organelles are highly organized structures contained in the cytoplasm"); 2) *ellipsis* (e.g., "Mary saw the student wanted by the police" versus "Mary saw the student who was wanted by the police"); and 3) *extended noun phrases as subjects of sentences* (e.g., "Why this is so is unknown," or "That Alaska is twice as large as Texas is difficult to imagine"). Complex sentences involving subordinate clauses are also common in textbooks.

Textbook language, then, includes the features mentioned above pertaining to written language. Complex and unfamiliar sentence patterns may be used. Specific and often specialized vocabulary is employed. In addition, special format features such as headings, advance organizers, and italicized words may be present.

Meta-skills Needed in the Classroom

L. Miller (1990) suggested that language competence develops on two levels. Her level I processes include semantics, syntax and morphology, phonology, and basic pragmatics. Level II processes include metalinguistic awareness, discourse knowledge, and higher level pragmatics. N.W. Nelson (1989) referred to these level II processes as "meta-skills" (p. 177). Under this title, she included *metalinguistic* skills, which involve talking about and manipulating linguistic symbols; *metacognitive* skills, which involve monitoring thinking and comprehension; and *metapragmatic* skills, which involve recognizing the rules of interaction.

Although social and instructional discourse place differential demands on students, some of the "meta" demands may be similar. For example, in each case the student will need to make judgments on when and how to enter the conversation and on what linguistic forms to use (Shuy, 1988). In addition, comprehension monitoring or the ability to notice (and respond) when messages are difficult to understand is needed for both social and instructional discourse (Dollaghan, 1987).

It may be that the differences in the metalinguistic, metacognitive, and metapragmatic demands between social and instructional discourse are in the degree of complexity required rather than the kind of skill needed. Nevertheless, the metacognitive and metalinguistic skills needed for instructional discourse form a major part of the school curriculum. Much of becoming literate involves thinking, talking, and manipulating and judging linguistic symbols. Students must be able to do this when reading, writing, speaking, and listening. The students must also learn to use, judge, and manipulate different rule systems involving different linguistic levels, including sounds, syllables, words, phrases, sentences, and texts (N.W. Nelson, 1989). Metalinguistic skills are involved in such diverse tasks as being able to segment words into sound units, determine whether two words contain the same sound, locate or describe a particular syntactic form, and determine which words are equivalent in meaning. The ability to segment a sentence into component parts, recognize multiple meanings of words, summarize main and supporting ideas of a given text, or evaluate the importance of an idea or concept all demand metacognitive and metalinguistic skills. Students also need to be able to generalize knowledge learned in one lesson to other lessons, formats, or content areas. Part of this ability involves making judgments of appropriateness of application of the knowledge to other areas.

Metalinguistic Skills in the Classroom   Wallach and Miller (1988) described metalinguistic skills as those involving "the ability to make conscious judgments about one's language" (p. 9). Another way to define metalinguistic skills is as the ability to think about language as an object to study or manipulate. Metalinguistic skill is the ability to recognize the arbitrariness of language and to focus on how and why language works the way it does (Van Kleeck, 1984a). Thus, it involves knowingly manipulating aspects of language. A child might correctly employ a particular linguistic rule without being conscious of his or her usage. That is, a child might be able to form the past tense of a verb correctly but not be able to describe the linguistic rule for doing so. An older child might be able to provide a general rule for forming past tense endings. The older child is consciously using metalinguistic skills to discern and explain linguistic patterns; the younger child is not yet capable of making these judgments.

Metalinguistic skills are developmental. Wallach and Miller (1988) provided a developmental sequence from ages 1½ to 2 years through age 10 and older. They divide the sequence of development into four stages. Sample metalinguistic skills learned during stage one (ages 1½–2) include distinguishing print from nonprint and recognizing some printed symbols (brand names, signs, or symbols). During stage two (ages 2–6), the child can play with sounds of the language, note word boundaries, correct his or her own speech and language, and separate words into syllables. During stage three (ages 6–10), the child is able to segment syllables and words into sounds, resequence language elements, form judgments regarding grammatical correctness, and recognize ambiguity. The ambiguity may occur at the word level (e.g., *pale* versus *pail* or *greenhouse* versus *green house*) or at the phrase level (e.g., "Flying airplanes can be *scary*" meaning either that being a pilot is scary or that airplanes that are flying are scary). The 6- to 10-year-old child also is beginning to recognize that some words have more than one meaning (e.g., *hard*—actual physical hardness or something is mentally tough; *block*—walk around a block, or block someone in football). By stage four (age 10 and older), the child can understand figurative language and is able to manipulate grammatical structures to fit contexts.

Van Kleeck (1984a) noted that two categories of metalinguistic skills that are important to communication are those involved in recognizing and correcting speech-language errors and those involved in adapting to the needs of the listener. Other types of metalinguistic abilities may be more directly related to literacy skills. These include being able to recognize sound-symbol relationships, word meanings, and grammatical relationships. It may be that these metalinguistic skills are a prerequisite for learning to read (V.A. Mann, 1984; Ryan, 1980), or that these skills develop as a consequence of learning to read (Read, 1978), or that there is an interaction between metalinguistic skills and reading (Catts, 1989; Ehri, 1979). Catts (1989), in his review of studies concerning the relationship between phonological awareness and reading ability, reported that some aspects of phonological awareness appear to be a consequence of learning to read whereas other aspects develop independently.

Metacognitive Skills in the Classroom   One of the most important metacognitive skills used in the classroom is the ability to monitor one's comprehension of both written and spoken language. Dollaghan (1987) emphasized the difference between comprehending a message and monitoring the comprehension of the message. Comprehending is understanding the message, whereas monitoring comprehension is actively recognizing whether or not the message is understood. She then described two abilities required in comprehension monitoring. First, the failure to comprehend must be detected. Second, the appropriate reaction or response to the comprehension breakdown must be made. In the classroom, the student (or teacher) must identify when the message is not understood and then react by asking clarification questions, rereading instructions or content, or in some way repairing the breakdown. Dollaghan proposed a comprehension monitoring model that includes various paths a listener may take in detecting or failing to detect a comprehension difficulty. Part of this model includes the listener's success (or failure) in constructing and evaluating an appropriate representation of the speaker's meaning.

Some studies have indicated that children as young as 2 years old show evidence of the ability to monitor their comprehension (e.g., Pea, 1982). However, other studies have indicated that children as old as 12 can have difficulty in recognizing when they have failed to identify contradictions in a message (Markman, 1979). Dollaghan (1987) suggested that comprehension monitoring is not a single skill; rather, the necessary factors develop over a period of time and are related to both message and listener variables.

One of the variables is the listener's ability to identify the relevant features of the message. For example, if the crucial identifying factor of a message is to choose the "red" item from a choice of several colors, it does not matter if the listener does not know the precise label of the item. However, if there are several red items, then the listener must know the name of the item, and the term *red* is no longer the relevant discriminating factor. Comparison skills are important in identifying relevant features of a message (Bunce, 1989).

This ability to identify the relevant features of a message may also depend on the number of message variables, such as the amount of information contained in the message and/or response array. Familiarity of the context can also be a factor in identifying the relevant features of the message. The complexity and degree of abstractness of the message, then, are important variables in comprehension monitoring.

The ability to attend to relevant features is an important aspect of learning in the classroom. It is particularly important when following or giving directions. Sometimes directions can be ambiguous, and children (or adults) need to make the right assumptions in order to follow them. Donahue (1985) found that comprehension monitoring can be a difficult task for some children. Again, the complexity of the message and degree of abstractness involved may be factors in the children's failure to recognize their lack of comprehension. The failure may also be due to the students' fitting the message into their own frame of reference and not recognizing that the reference is not the appropriate one. This situation may have a great effect in the classroom because the students do not provide the teacher with appropriate feedback that the instructions were not understood. The teacher then does not provide the necessary clarification. Additionally, it may be that the students do recognize that they failed to comprehend, but do not ask for clarification because of social reasons. They do not want to appear "stupid" in front of classmates or to be singled out as different. In any case, monitoring of comprehension is an important classroom language skill, and difficulties in this area need to be addressed.

Metacognitive skills are also important in relation to a student's ability to comprehend information containing varying degrees of abstractness. Some of the abstractness of a message may be due to the language used and/or complexity of concepts presented. Blank, Rose, and Berlin (1978), in their book on the language of learning, have delineated four levels of abstraction based on "perceptual-language distance" (p. 17), that is, how closely language and perception match and how much they differ. Although originally designed for analyzing the language of learning in the preschool years, the analysis also has implications for language used in elementary classrooms.

> *Level 1*: "Language Matching Perception"—involves identifying, labeling, and, in general, matching language to everyday objects and events. At this level, the teacher may ask the child such questions as "What is this?" or request the child to "show me the _____." Learning new vocabulary words (written or spoken) would be an example at the elementary school level.
>
> *Level 2*: "Selective Analysis of Perception"—requires the child to focus on specific aspects of an object or event and integrate components. Typical questions or requests might include, "What is happening?", or "Complete the following sentence . . . " The cloze procedure (i.e., fill in the blank) and description tasks are often used in worksheet activities in elementary school classrooms.
>
> *Level 3*: "Reordering Perception"—the child must reorder or restructure his/her perception in response to constraints imposed by language. The child may have to exclude certain items, place items in a sequence, assume the role of another, and so forth.

Typical teacher questions or requests at this level would include, "Find the things that are not _____," "Which one comes first? What is next?" or "What would he say?" Again, these types of questions form the basis for many of the classroom activities.

Level 4: "Reasoning About Perception"—the child must go beyond the immediate perception and focus on logical relationships between objects and events. Prediction, explanations, and problem solving are all examples of this level of abstraction.

Metalinguistic and metacognitive skills are particularly important as the student advances in his or her schooling. Without the ability to deal effectively with abstractness in classroom language, the student will experience increasing difficulty in learning.

Metapragmatic Skills in the Classroom   Students must also learn to function within the classroom rule system. Tattersall and Creaghead (1985) suggested that teachers have certain basic expectations involving a child's ability to function in an elementary classroom. Some of the expectations involve language and interaction skills. For example, students need to know when to talk and, sometimes more importantly, when to listen. They need to be able to share, make requests, ask appropriate questions, take turns, and understand rules. There is the expectation that children should be able to work in a group, stay on task, and follow directions.

N.W. Nelson (1989) described the school culture curriculum as being a set of implicit and explicit rules for appropriate interaction in the classroom. Other than some discussion of a few class rules, this curriculum is often not overtly addressed. Knowing how to get things done in the classroom is part of what Wilkinson and Milosky (1987) called the "hidden curriculum." Research is only beginning to be done in the area of metapragmatics, particularly in the classroom setting.

Summary of Characteristics of Classroom Language

Analyzing language in written text, in conversations, and in instructional discourse demonstrates that different language forms, functions, and content are involved. The shift back and forth between the various language uses in the classroom can be facilitated if recognition is given to these differences. Table 1 provides a summary of the types of linguistic form, content, purpose, and interaction in discourse involving both oral and written language and according to social (contextualized) or instructional (decontextualized) functions. The vertical axis of the matrix forms a contextualized-decontextualized continuum. The horizontal axis is an oral-written language continuum. The matrix thus has oral-contextualized, oral-decontextualized, written-contextualized and written-decontextualized sections.

In oral-contextualized language, production can consist of incomplete, sometimes repetitive syntactic structures and use of implicit subjects, many pronouns, and nonspecific vocabulary. The purposes of this language can range from conveying information to establishing and maintaining interpersonal relationships. Most often the conversation is about everyday situations, often concerning the "here and now." The participants, whether speaker or listener, are both responsible for the success of the communication. "You know . . . uh . . . he was here the other day" may be a perfectly comprehensible statement in a conversational interaction.

Personal letters or notes are an example of the type of language production represented by the written-contextualized language section of the matrix. The language of personal notes or letters usually involves short idea units and use of implicit subjects and nonspecific and/or slang vocabulary. The purpose may be less communication of information and more establish-

Table 1. Types of language/discourse in the classroom

Cognitively Undemanding	
Oral	**Written**
Contextualized (e.g., conversational speech)	**Contextualized** (e.g., personal letters and notes)
Form	Form
Familiar words	Familiar words
Nonspecific vocabulary	Nonspecific vocabulary
Many pronouns	Many pronouns
Repetitive syntax	Repetitive syntax
Short ideas units	Short ideas units
Cohesion based on intonation	Content
Content	Everyday situations
Everyday objects and situations	Specific personal information
Meaning from context	Purpose
Purpose	Social communication
Request/command	Messages
Social interaction	Reminders
Interaction	Invitations
Equal responsibility	Interaction
Often a dialogue	Writer responsible
Feedback present	Feedback not present
Shared knowledge and setting	Shared knowledge
Decontextualized (e.g., formal lectures and class presentations)	**Decontextualized** (e.g., written reports and textbooks)
Form	Form
Specific vocabulary	Specific vocabulary
Elaborated syntax	Unfamiliar words
Cohesion based on linguistic markers as well as intonation	Elaborated syntax
Content	Cohesion based on linguistic markers
Abstract ideas/situations: "there and then" rather than "here and now"	Content
Planned, organized topics	Abstract ideas and situations
Meaning may be inferred	"There and then" topics
Instructions	Meaning and conclusions inferred from text
Purpose	Purpose
Teach/learn	Teach/learn
Regulate thinking/behavior	Reflect/plan
Construct reality	Regulate thinking
Interaction	Construct reality
Unequal responsibility (teacher controlled)	Interaction
	No feedback present
	Less shared knowledge
Cognitively Demanding	

ing and maintaining interpersonal relationships. Again, there is usually a history of shared knowledge between participants, so even if there is no face-to-face feedback, the writer can usually predict the reader's response to the communication. Journal writing is a classroom example of written-contextualized language. Written-contextualized language is probably used less often in the classroom than oral-contextualized language and/or oral- and written-decontextualized language.

A teacher's lecture is an example of the language production represented by the oral-decontextualized section of the matrix. In this case, elaborated syntax employing specific vo-cabulary is often used. Cohesion can involve both linguistic markers (e.g., *because*, *although*, *first*) and intonation. The content often involves abstract concepts or information and may be presented in a structured, planned manner. The meaning of the discourse may be constructed through linguistic means. Content may also be focused on providing instructions on how to complete a task. The purpose of the communication is to instruct, inform, or regulate thinking. There is unequal responsibility of the participants, with the teacher controlling the interaction and content. Although the teacher's lecture is produced orally, the structure and organization are similar to those of written language. The language represented by this cell of the matrix is particularly important in educational settings because spoken language is the medium by which much teaching takes place. It is also within the spoken language medium that learners demonstrate much of their knowledge.

A textbook chapter is an example of the language production represented by the final cell of the matrix, written-decontextualized language. Here, again, specific vocabulary and elaborated syntax are used. Subordinate clauses are prevalent. Cohesion is based on linguistic markers and on punctuation. The content of the text involves ideas and situations that often involve "there and then" topics. For example, a history text might present information about various cultures existing several hundred years ago, or a science text might discuss theories concerning elements that cannot be seen. The purpose of an expository text is to inform and to help structure thinking. Less shared knowledge would be expected; therefore, the writer would need to present the information in an explicit, succinct manner.

Higher level language processes involving metalinguistic, metacognitive, and metapragmatic skills also permeate classroom language. These skills are particularly important in the development of literacy. Students need to be able to recognize sound–symbol relationships, word meanings, and grammatical relationships. They need to be able to knowingly manipulate various aspects of language both orally and in writing. Students also must be able to monitor their comprehension of both written and spoken language. Finally, they need to be able to recognize and operate within the rules of the classroom.

CLASSROOM DISCOURSE

Teacher–child(ren) discourse is extremely important in our educational system because classroom communication is central to the learning process (Cazden, 1988). Spoken language is the primary medium used by teachers to teach and by learners to demonstrate their knowledge. Spoken language is also the primary medium for maintenance of classroom discipline. The discourse interaction between a teacher and a group of students is a developing, interactive process (Bloome & Knott, 1985; Green, Weade, & Graham, 1988). Bloome and Knott (1985) described the communicative content of classroom lessons as neither given nor prescribed but rather constructed through the face-to-face interaction of teaches and students. As students and teachers accommodate to each other, they work together to achieve curricular goals and to develop daily routines that facilitate classroom activities. Each class develops its own communicative system and routines. Each class also has multiple levels of discourse between participants, including teacher-student, student-student, and teacher–whole class interactions. This section focuses on: 1) the features of classroom conversations and interaction formats, 2) the use of questions, 3) teaching and learning styles, and 4) hidden complexities in classroom discourse.

Classroom Conversations

Dore (1979) described three major categories of conversational functions: conveying content, regulating conversation, and expressing attitude. Within these categories, Dore set up an elaborate taxonomy that divides into 35 conversational acts. N.W. Nelson (1984) presented a summary of Dore's taxonomy and provided classroom discourse examples.

Under the *convey content* category are the initiate and response functions. The *initiate* function subdivides into three classes: requestive, assertive, and performative. Soliciting information and action are the particular conversational acts making up the requestive class. In the classroom, a teacher might ask for information ("Where is the _____?") or for an action ("Let's get out our pencils . . . "). Under the assertive class, identification and explanation of perceived phenomena are important features (e.g., the teacher might note, "The two words are spelled alike but pronounced differently"). The performative class is concerned with claims, jokes, protests, and warnings (e.g., "No, you have the wrong page"). In the *response* function of the convey content category, the major conversational acts are supplying solicited or additional information, or acknowledging the initiation (e.g., "No, that is not correct," or "The right answer will be on page 20," or "That's right").

The second major category of Dore's (1979) conversational functions is those that *regulate conversation*. Factors under the regulative function included attention getters, speaker selection, rhetorical or clarification questions, and politeness markers. Classroom examples might include, "Judy, it's your turn," or "I wonder how the switch works, John." The final major category is conversational functions that *express attitude*. The expressive function involves exclamations and repetitions (e.g., "Oh! That was too bad!").

N.W. Nelson (1984), in applying Dore's taxonomy to her classroom discourse data, found that she could identify many conversational acts; however, she had some difficulty in using some of Dore's categories. One reason was the inequality of the power of the participants in controlling the interaction. Dore set up his taxonomy to analyze dyadic conversations that usually occurred between participants having equal conversational rights. There was usually equal opportunity for turn taking involving initiations and responses from all participants. However, this equality turn taking is not true of classroom conversations. In the classroom, N.W. Nelson found that the regulatory functions included language used to manage classroom routines and behavior as well as who participates in classroom conversations, aspects not considered in Dore's taxonomy.

When teachers speak, they usually: 1) ask questions, 2) provide background structure to set the context for the lesson, 3) react to the behavior of the students, and/or 4) extend a previous exchange (Berlin, Blank, & Rose, 1980). The teacher controls, to a great extent, the content of the conversations and the amount of student participation. Teacher–whole class interactions tend to occur with greater frequency than teacher–student or student–student interactions. For example, it has been estimated that elementary children spend 50% of their time listening to teachers, and high school students may spend up to 90% of class time listening to their teachers (Griffin & Hannah, 1960). In addition, the form used by the teacher may not reflect the intent. For example, the teacher might use a request form or an assertion but the intent may be regulatory (e.g., "Would everyone please line up?" is an order, not a question of choice; "Somebody's talking" means it is time to be quiet).

N.W. Nelson (1984) also found that there were differences between teachers in various grade levels in their use of various conversational functions. She analyzed discourse samples from first-, third-, and sixth-grade teachers. First-grade teachers used a high number of regulative statements. The statements were used to direct the attention of the students and to control their behavior. Many of the regulative statements dealt with classroom organization and transitions between activities. The statements often were phrased as assertives but they had an implied action request (e.g., "The Helper of the Day needs to get out the . . ."). Other common regulative statements used by first-grade teachers included those that focused on maintaining the students' attention by placing value on it (e.g., "_____ is a good listener.") and those that focused directly on behavior (e.g., "Push your chairs in, please."). Nelson noted that the content of instructions provided by first-grade teachers primarily focused on "how to do" various activities. The primary focus was on teaching of reading and math skills.

By third grade, teachers still use language to control students' behavior; however, there is more reliance on written instructions. The students are also expected to be able to work independently. Much of the instruction still focuses on teaching of reading and math; however, there is increased importance of content area subjects. There is also an increased usage of metalinguistic skills. By sixth grade, 50% of class time is still spent on organizational matters. However, the emphasis has shifted from instruction in reading to the use of reading as a tool for learning. Newly read material is increasingly related to previously read information (e.g., "Do you remember reading . . . This is another example").

N.W. Nelson (1985) further analyzed the discourse of first-, third- and sixth-grade teachers by studying its syntactical complexity. She found that first- and third-grade teachers used many simple sentences, whereas sixth-grade teachers often used complex syntactic structures. First-grade teachers also used a slower speaking rate than did third- or sixth-grade teachers. Third-grade teachers used a rate comparable to sixth-grade teachers but used sentence structure similar to first-grade teachers. Although sixth-grade teachers used a faster rate and more complex sentence structure, they also employed more hesitations. It may be that they were pausing because of difficulties in formulating the complex sentences. It also could be that the hesitations and restatements were due to (nonverbal) feedback from students indicating difficulty in understanding. In summary, it appears that there are variations in teacher discourse as students advance in their schooling. However, classroom conversation still revolves around language of the curriculum, language of control, and language for social use.

Many of the classroom conversations involving social use take place between students and occur without the teacher's acknowledgment. Even when the teacher allows social talk, there is usually a signal or boundary for it. The end of the time for socializing might be signaled with a phrase such as "Now it's time to work," "Quiet, please," or "Now, as we were saying yesterday. . . . " Social talk between teachers and students also has boundaries. The teacher again refocuses back to the topic after a short period of interaction.

Although each teacher has his or her own teaching style and routine for completing classroom activities, several scholars (Cazden, 1988; Heath, 1983; N.W. Nelson, 1985; Tenenberg, 1988) have identified a special instructional dialogue typically found in the classroom. This instructional dialogue consists of a teacher *initiation* (or solicitation), a child *response*, and then a teacher *evaluation* of (or reaction to) the response (IRE) interactional pattern. For example, the interaction might happen as follows:

> Teacher: "What time is it?" (I)
> Student: "Two o'clock." (R)
> Teacher: "That's right." (E)

If the same question occurred outside of the classroom, the first speaker's response might be "Thanks" or "That late!" rather than an evaluative response. Outside the classroom the question would be a real request for information.

This interactional pattern is also referred to as the test question or known question format (Heath, 1986a). The teacher knows the answer to the question and is testing whether the student has the same knowledge. For some children, the test question format is familiar. Their parents may use a similar format, particularly when looking at books with the child. As they look at a picture in the book, they ask the child, "What's this?", and then evaluate the child's labeling responses. However, for other children this interactive format may be unfamiliar. Only "real" questions may be used in their culture (see Heath, 1983, for a description of different cultural styles of language and learning and Iglesias, 1985, for a description of cultural conflict in the classroom). For these children, adjustment to this type of instructional dialogue may take time.

Cazden (1988) reported on extension of the basic IRE interactional pattern. First, an overall discourse unit may contain more than one basic IRE pattern. Second, there may occur optional patterns that are based on the students' knowledge, to which the student(s) may add additional information. In another variation, the initiation and response portions of the basic IRE pattern are used but the evaluation component is missing. Mehan observed Cazden's class (Cazden, 1988) and suggested that a larger unit of analysis was needed. He noted that the basic pattern plus optional sequences occurring in relation to a particular topic formed a natural unit, which he labeled a topically related set (TRS). Such units allow for basic and optional patterns to occur in some type of order. Evaluation occurs at the end of each set but does not necessarily occur after each student response. There may be nonverbal as well as verbal cues delineating the boundaries of a topically related set. For example, in beginning a topic, the teacher may use posture or gesture to orient the class toward the materials. Verbally the teacher may cue the beginning by saying "Now . . . ," or "Here we have . . . ," or using some other opening/orienting word or phrase.

Students as well as teachers have a role in development of a topic. Heyman (1986) investigated how teacher and students jointly determine topics of the day's lessons. He found that what is structured, attended to, and expected depends on the teaching style of the teacher and the interaction between the students and teacher. Heyman suggested that lessons are "joint accomplishment of meaning" by the teachers and students (p. 41). Successful teaching, therefore, needs to create a sense of shared context.

Use of Questions

Much of the development of the shared context between teachers and students revolves around the questions utilized in the classroom. Shuy (1988) suggested that the majority of teacher-student exchanges involve questions. Shuy and colleagues (see Green & Harker, 1988, for a multiperspective analysis of classroom discourse) analyzed the discourse of six language arts lessons in each of six classrooms over a 4-week period at the beginning of the school year.

Shuy reported that of the 1,952 utterances by six teachers in his sample of 12 lessons, 597 were questions. However, some of the question forms served a directive function rather than a question function. When the directive questions were deleted, the average was one question per 4.4 teacher utterances.

In describing the lessons observed, Shuy (1988) reported that most of the lessons contained four parts: "attention, focus, process, and transition out" (p. 120). He also noted that questions were used differently by different teachers during these four lesson parts. One teacher used one ninth of her questions in the attention and transition out parts of the lessons, whereas another teacher had no questions during these parts. One fifth of the total questions used by the other four teachers occurred during these opening and closing sections of the lesson.

However, the more important issue is not necessarily the number of questions used, but the kind of questions used. Open-ended questions are good indicators of what a student knows because they do not set limits on the expected answer. This type of question usually results in a self-generated response rather than a teacher-influenced answer. These questions are more "real" in that the specific response is not known by the teacher. The form of the open-ended question may vary. Examples of open-ended questions include: "Tell me about the _____" (imperative used as an open-ended question), "What do you know about the _____?" (*wh*-question), and "Can you tell me about _____?" (yes/no question).

In contrast, closed-ended questions (known questions) are those to which the teacher expects a specific response, which often consists of one or two specific words. The closed-ended questions often require restricted, right/wrong, one-word responses. Examples include: "What color is this?" (*wh*- questions), "Is it red or blue?" (yes/no questions), and "Iron is the leading export, isn't it?" (tag questions).

In general, imperative open-ended questions require the most self-generated responses. *What, where, which one*, and other such *wh*- questions, whether open- or closed-ended, usually narrow the focus more and thereby reduce the range of the response. Yes/no questions reduce the range of response even more. Students have a 50% chance of being correct whether they know the answer or not. Tag questions require the least amount of self-generated response and place the greatest limits on the possibility of being wrong. Shuy (1988) suggested that a good probing strategy for teachers is to start with open-ended questions and move down to *wh*-, yes/no, and finally tag questions.

In Shuy's (1988) analysis of six elementary teachers during the first 4 weeks of school, he found no use of open-ended questions. Four of the teachers tended to ask the same type of questions over and over, either *wh*- or yes/no questions. The other two teachers varied their question types. The variation was similar to that found in natural conversations, with a general trend of asking *wh*- questions, then yes/no, and finally tag questions. Tenenberg (1988), in his analysis of later lessons in the same classrooms, did find use of open-ended questions, particularly during inquiry lessons. Tenenberg believes that the question cycle utilized depended on the instructional model used. In some classrooms, questions were used as a means of control, and bids for opportunities to respond were tightly regulated. Hands had to be raised, and students had a short turn and were to provide the "correct" answer. In other classrooms, there was less emphasis on maintaining control and more interest in generating student response to content.

Blank and White (1986) suggested that, although open-ended, divergent questions can be used effectively to stimulate a student's thinking, use of these questions assumes that the child can comprehend the question form. Sometimes the student's failure to respond correctly may not be lack of knowledge of content, but rather failure to understand the question. The level of abstractness of the questions as well as the content must be considered. Dropping to a question at a lower level in the sequence suggested by Shuy (1988) may be helpful to the student. An alternative is to consider Blank et al.'s (1978) levels of abstractness, and vary the questions asked in regard to closeness to or distance from perception. A *why* question might be asked initially. If an incorrect response is given, the teacher uses a simplification technique that focuses the child on the appropriate response. At the end of the sequence the original question is repeated with the child now being able to respond correctly.

Questions remain an important element of classroom language. However, there should be recognition that questions have a variety of functions. Sometimes the function of the question may not be to probe the students' knowledge. Tag questions may be used as a way of getting children to become involved, or rhetorical questions might be used to focus attention. In addition, not all types of questions are equally familiar to all children or equally effective in advancing learning. There also needs to be an awareness of possible "misuse" of questions in the classroom (Blank & White, 1986, p. 1).

Questions are also an important part of the language of textbooks. N.M. Sanders (1973) found several question types in textbooks, reading books, and workbooks. Among these were memory questions, translations, and interpretation questions. Memory questions involve the recognition or recall of information given in a passage.

> Facts: "Who did _____?"
> Definitions of terms: "What is meant by _____?"
> Generalizations: "In what three ways do _____ resemble _____?"
> Values: "What kind of man was _____?"

Translations involve the expression of an idea in a different form (e.g., "What does the author mean by the phrase _____?"). Interpretation questions involve perception of relationships:

> Comparison: "How is _____ like _____?"
> Implications: "What will _____ lead to?"
> Induction: "What facts in the story support the idea that _____?"
> Quantitative thinking: "How much has _____ increased?"
> Cause and effect: "What was the result of _____ on _____?"

It is apparent that most of the questions found in textbooks are open-ended *wh-* questions. Therefore children must develop the ability to produce self-generated responses to higher level, more abstract questions in order to perform classwork successfully. This ability is enhanced to some degree by the fact that students are working with a written text; it is possible for them to return to pertinent passages and reread them to extract salient information. A comparable open-ended question in oral classroom discourse does not provide such an opportunity.

Teaching and Learning Styles

A comprehensive discussion of teaching and learning styles is beyond the scope of this chapter. However, it is important to acknowledge that there are individual differences in both teaching styles and learning styles. For example, some teachers view their role as transmitting knowledge, whereas others view their role as facilitating learning (see Cummins, 1984, for a comparison of teaching styles and Heath, 1983, for a description of cultural styles of language and learning). These different philosophies will lead to different techniques for teaching and for classroom control. For example, a quiet, "listening" classroom would be important for a teacher who views his or her role as transmitting knowledge. More verbal interchanges between teacher and student(s) and among students would be fostered in a classroom in which the teacher views his or her role as facilitory. Students would be expected to take an active role in their own learning (see Tharp & Gallimore, 1988, for a discussion of teaching and learning in a social context).

Morine-Dershimer (1988) compared various analyses of the six classrooms studied by Shuy (1988) in order to identify language and teacher factors that may contribute to pupil success. She observed that teachers who used language that focused on the content of the lesson rather than management of the lesson had students who were more successful in their learning. In comparing the two teachers who were at opposite ends of the continuum regarding use of management versus informational language, Morine-Dershimer found that both teachers used similar levels of management language at the beginning of the school year; however, only one continued to focus on management issues after the first month.

Student learning styles also have an effect on student-teacher discourse. Carbo, Dunn, and Dunn (1986) discussed using a student's favored learning style in teaching reading. They suggested investigating whether a student is a global or an analytical learner and under what conditions the student learns best (noisy/quiet environment, motivational factors, group/independent learner, etc.).

B. McCarthy (1980), in her 4Mat model, described four learning styles:

Type 1 learners learn through a combination of feeling and watching and frequently ask "why" questions. Teachers need to provide reasons.

Type 2 learners are analytical and prefer to learn by watching and thinking through concepts. They prefer facts and often ask "what" questions.

Type 3 learners prefer to learn by doing, and their favorite question is "how?"

Type 4 learners are interested in self-discovery and ask "if" or "what if."

McCarthy suggested that many teachers tend to teach in an analytical-sequential manner that is appropriate for type 2 learners. She advocated recognition of diversity in learning styles and proposed that teachers should expose children to multiple instructional techniques, as well as maintain support for the child's primary style. Teacher presentation for each of the learning styles is determined as much by the language used to present material as by the materials themselves.

Hidden Complexities in Classroom Discourse

Berlin et al. (1980) delineated several hidden complexities in the language of instruction. They noted that there may be a range of complexity in the structure of a teacher's spoken language. Children accustomed to a direct request may not be aware that a polite question is really an indirect request or demand even if phrased in the form of a question. Also, elaborate use of subordinate clauses, particularly those involving time sequences, may be confusing to some children (e.g., "Before you do your math, be sure to finish your reading assignment."). Berlin et al. suggested that teachers analyze the level of abstraction of various forms of questions so that they are aware of the complexity of some of their question/requests. Berlin et al. employ the perception-language distance factors previously discussed as one way to identify and modify the complexity of instructional language.

Both Cazden (1988) and N.W. Nelson (1984), have noted that many of the decisions teachers make regarding appropriate discourse styles and content depend on largely subconscious processes. Recognizing these processes and making them explicit may be important for children who are not successful in classroom interactions. It may be necessary for some children to be explicitly taught some of the "unwritten" classroom rules.

One of the first unwritten interaction rules to examine is how teachers and students formulate topics to achieve meaning. The opening of a topic may be achieved in various ways. In some classrooms, the teacher will indicate a new topic by making statements such as, "OK, boys and girls, what I want you to do is . . . ," or "Now, let's look at . . . ," or "Yesterday, we looked at . . . , now we need to do . . . " All of these types of sentences are signals that a new topic has begun and that the whole class or group is now to be involved. Within this opening statement, some teachers will provide information regarding what was already supposed to be accomplished, what is expected now, and even what is expected in the future. Other teachers are more opaque in their expectations and the students must "guess" what is wanted.

For example, if the topic is current events, a teacher might open with "What has been happening in the news?" This is a signal to the students to provide newsworthy comments. However, if the teacher has in mind a certain news event and a student provides an alternate story, a mismatch in communication may occur. How the negotiation for topic might proceed would depend on several factors. Some of these factors include how committed the teacher and student were to the topic, how dominant the teacher was, and the ability of the students to recognize unfavorable comments and modify them. For example, if a student responded with a local issue concerning zoning when the teacher was expecting a topic concerning international news, the scenario could go several ways:

> Teacher: "What has been happening in the news?"
> Student A: "Well, the city agreed to change the zoning so the new mall can be built."
> Teacher: "Yeah, that's right. Does anyone else have any news?"
> Student B: "Well, the drug lords in Colombia are fighting against the government."
> Teacher: "Do you think the government will be able to stop the flow of drugs?"
> Student B: . . .

The teacher's response indicates to the class that the news item worthy of discussion was the international topic of drugs, not the local zoning story. However, if the teacher or other students had provided a follow-up comment to the first story, then a different topic formulation would have occurred.

Other kinds of subtle, "unwritten" interaction cues occur because a particular utterance may be multifunctional (Cazden, 1988). For example, "That's a good one" in response to a child's answer may signal approval of that child's thought, but may also indicate to the students that other answers or ideas are also appropriate and should be made.

Another "unwritten" interaction rule involves timing of entry into a conversation (Silliman, 1984; Silliman & Lamanna, 1986). Being able to gain entry into the ongoing discourse within the classroom is important for both personal and academic reasons. It is important for students to be able to ask questions when they do not understand, make requests for needed items, and join in discussions. However, asking questions or making comments at the wrong time can be particularly disruptive to the classroom conversational flow and to the teaching/learning that is occurring. Other problems with timing of an interaction include delays in responding and excessive need for repetition. Successful entry into classroom conversations may involve recognition of the end of a topically related set (Cazden, 1988). Difficulty with timing of a bid for attention may be due to differences between school culture and home culture interaction patterns, or to mismatches in teaching and learning styles, or to lack of awareness of subtle pragmatic cues indicating appropriateness or inappropriateness of the initiations/responses.

Donahue (1985) suggested that some children in a classroom appear to be "out of sync" with the rest of the class. They may ask a needed question, but at the wrong time. They also may not ask for clarification when messages are unclear or ambiguous. It may be that some children do not recognize ambiguity and therefore fail to realize that they did not understand. Some children also may treat rhetorical questions as real and not understand that teachers might view this as rude behavior (e.g., "Why can't you finish your work on time?"—"Because I'm tired," or "I forgot"). Other factors disruptive to classroom discourse include providing irrelevant responses and having poor topic maintenance. Whatever the reason, there may be some children who have difficulty communicating in the classroom.

NEW TRENDS IN CLASSROOM LANGUAGE

Information on language in the classroom and classroom interaction patterns presented thus far in the chapter has been based on studies of classrooms primarily organized along traditional lines. However, there are new trends in educational organization and philosophy that may have major effects on language use in the classroom. Two of these trends involve the whole language philosophy and the use of cooperative learning in the classroom.

The Whole Language Philosophy

In recent years, a new educational philosophy involving language and literacy learning has developed. The term used to designate this philosophy is *whole language* (see Manning & Manning, 1989, for a collected series of articles describing whole language activities and research). A variety of scholars (Altwerger, Edelsky, & Flores, 1987; Goodman, 1986; Goodman & Goodman, 1979; Graves, 1987; Graves & Hansen, 1983; Harste & Burke, 1980) have described children's development of reading and writing skills within a whole language orientation.

According to Altwerger et al. (1987), the whole language philosophy is a set of beliefs that includes the following assumptions:

> . . . (a) language is for making meanings, for accomplishing purposes; (b) written language is language—thus what is true for language in general is true for written language; (c) the cueing systems of language (phonology in oral, orthography in written language, morphology, syntax, semantics, pragmatics) are always simultaneously present and interacting in any instance of language in use; (d) language use always occurs in a situation; and (e) situations are critical to meaning-making. (p. 144)

The major premise is that a model of acquisition of language, both oral and written, is developed through real use, not practice exercises. The main consideration in classroom reading and writing, then, is that the activities be real reading and writing, not worksheet exercises in reading and writing. Although little use is made of materials written specifically to teach reading or writing, whole language classrooms are rich in the variety of print available to the students. Literature, directions, notes from home, social studies and science texts, and children's and teacher's writing make up just some of these print events.

The whole language view of reading and writing is one of constructing meaning, of focusing on texts within situations. Word boundaries and lexical features, sounds/letters, syntax, semantics, and pragmatics are just some of the cues to the construction of meaning. A major goal of the whole language philosophy is to help children use the interrelationships among cueing systems to achieve meaning in their reading and writing.

Implementation of the whole language philosophy has implications for classroom organization and for language used in the classroom. There may not be reading groups with the teacher directing groups of children who are reading the same story while other children are busy with individual worksheets. Instead, there may be some children reading (real literature), some writing, and some conversing about what they read and/or wrote. There may be many more opportunities for child–child interactions than is true of the traditional elementary classroom organization. There may also be regular opportunities for child-children discussions, particularly as children read their own writing to classmates. The "author's chair" (Graves & Hansen, 1983), where the child writer reads and discusses his or her work with classmates, is a common feature in many whole language classrooms.

There also may be more opportunities for one teacher–one child interactions rather than one teacher–30 children lectures/discussions. This means that a child might have several turns when talking to the teacher about his/her reading or writing. This is in contrast to teacher-children interchanges in which a child may have only one turn, a response, to a teacher's initiation.

Finally, there may be more language generated by students in whole language classrooms than by those attending traditionally organized classes. For example, much of what students read, write, or talk about may be stories or essays created by classmates or themselves rather than stories or writing from commercial publishers. All of these factors will affect the amount and kind of language used in the classroom and the way it is used.

Cooperative Learning

Another educational trend in recent years that complements the whole language philosophy is the use of cooperative learning instructional methods. Cooperative learning methods (e.g., Sharan, 1980; Slavin, 1983) are structured, systematic strategies that can be used at any grade level. The teacher assigns the students to four- to- six-member learning groups. Each group is composed of high-, average-, and low-achieving students. Members of each heterogeneous group then work together toward a common goal (see S. Kagan, 1985, and Slavin, 1985, for reviews of sample tasks and methods used in cooperative learning). Sample activities might include researching, organizing information on a specific topic, or solving a specific problem. Group members would each have specific and unique responsibilities in completing the task. Another activity might include joint completion of a worksheet or joint writing of a poem or story.

Much of the research on cooperative learning has focused on comparison of academic achievement of those involved in cooperative learning and those in more traditional classrooms. For example, Slavin (1985) reviewed 46 field experiments in elementary and secondary schools that studied the effect of cooperative learning on student learning. In 29 of the studies students in the cooperative learning classroom showed significant improvement in academic achievement versus a control group of students. In 15 of the studies, no differences between the experimental and control groups were found. In two studies, there were significant differences that favored the control group. The most successful method for increasing student achievement was rewarding the groups on the basis of the sum of individual test scores. Slavin suggested that it is equally important to have both individual accountability and group reward. Slavin also reported that most studies show that high, average, and low achievers gain equally from the cooperative experience.

There has been little research on the effect cooperative learning has had on language use in the classroom. However, there are several possible effects that could occur in classrooms where cooperative learning is used. First, it is likely that oral language use by students would increase. Cooperative learning requires student–student talking and shared learning, whereas in traditional classrooms individual students often are supposed to be quiet and listen to the teacher or to work alone without talking. There would also be less teacher-directed talking, at least while group work was occurring. It is also possible that sustained conversations would occur because the students would have more opportunities to respond several times to each other. This is in contrast to the instructional conversation described earlier in which the teacher initiates, the student responds, and the teacher evaluates.

It is also possible that metalinguistic and metacognitive skills would be facilitated as students talk about what they know and how they know it. Problem-solving activities in which the students must explain their strategies also focus the students on how they know what they know. Webb (1985), in her review, found that providing explanations to another person was consistently and positively related to achievement for both the provider and the person receiving the information. Just providing an answer was not helpful. Much more research is needed on the effects of the whole language and cooperative learning philosophies on classroom interaction, language, and academic achievement of students, because additional complexity of language use in the classroom will occur with the increased use of child–child instructional dialogues.

CONCLUSION

Teacher–child(ren) and children–children discourse involves different types of interactions depending on whether the purpose of the interaction is instructional or social. Classroom instructional conversations often involve an initiation by the teacher, a response by a child, and an evaluation by the teacher. Question use is a very important aspect of classroom conversations. A variety of types of questions are employed, including closed-ended or test questions and open-ended or divergent questions. Controlling behavior of students is also a factor in classroom discourse and may be accomplished through verbal and nonverbal means. Teaching and learning styles also affect classroom discourse, particularly with regard to utilization of whole language and cooperative learning philosophies.

Table 2 summarizes some of the features of classroom discourse involving both social and instructional discourse. Some of the features of social discourse include the use of: 1) initiation-response (IR) conversations, 2) reciprocal turntaking, and 3) real questions rather than questions designed to test knowledge. The status of the participants is usually equal or the inequality is not stressed. The responsibility of the participants to maintain the conversation

Table 2.   Features of classroom discourse

	Social	Instructional	Child–child instructional
Interactions	Initiation-response (IR)	Initiation-response-evaluation (IRE)	Initiation-response-evaluation (IRE)
Turn taking	Reciprocal	Teacher dominated	Reciprocal
Status	Equal	Unequal	Peer
Knowledge base	Equal	Unequal	May or may not be equal
Questions	"Real"	Test	Test

through each one adding new knowledge is also equal. Each participant in social discourse, therefore, is viewed as equally responsible for maintaining the interaction.

Instructional discourse involves the use of: 1) initiation-response-evaluation (IRE) conversations; 2) teacher-dominated turn taking, in which the teacher initiates and the children take turns responding; and 3) many kinds of teacher questions and requests that test student knowledge. The status of the participants is unequal, with the teacher controlling the pace, participants, and content of the conversations. The knowledge base is also unequal in instructional conversations, with the teacher having the responsibility to impart knowledge to the students. The teacher is also the judge of appropriate student responses.

However, with the advent of cooperative learning procedures, there may be some changes in classroom discourse. For example, child–child instructional discourse may blend some of the features of social and instructional discourse. In child–child instructional discourse there may still may be reciprocal turn taking and equal status of participants that are similar to those found in social discourse. However, there may also be use of test questions and instructional conversations (IRE) that are similar to those found in teacher–child instructional discourse.

Language of the classroom involves social and instructional discourse within oral and written modalities. Language of the classroom also involves knowledge and use of metalinguistic, metacognitive, and metapragmatic skills. Teachers' and students' awareness of the different types of language and the assumptions underlying their uses is critical to learning. Teachers' and students' skill in classroom discourse is also crucial to children's learning. Language, literacy, and learning are intertwined, with language functioning both as a tool for learning and as content to be learned. As Butler (1984) noted, children's achievement in school has much to do with their ability to deal with the language of the classroom.

II / THE NATURE OF LEARNING DISABILITIES

Neuropsychology is the scientific study of the relationship between brain function and behavior. As such, neuropsychology, in the generic sense, is an interdisciplinary knowledge area embracing many contributing disciplines and professions. (American Speech-Language-Hearing Association, 1990, p. 3)

Neuropsychology has occupied an influential position in theory and research in the field of learning disabilities. The original source of much of the vast body of neuropsychological data has been the study of neuropathology, largely in adults. It has been noted, however, that important differences exist between adult and child pathology, in that brain damage in children is likely to be generalized whereas adult lesions tend to be localized (Obrzut & Hund, 1986). Furthermore, in contrast to the relatively static adult brain, the child's brain is evolving in its cognitive and behavioral capacities.

Central to neuropsychology across age groups is the phenomenon of hemispheric asymmetry and specialization of function. Figure 1 contains a diagrammatic sketch of the left and right hemispheres and designation of some of their specialized functions. The left hemisphere is generally believed to be dominant for certain language functions and the right hemisphere, while nondominant for these language functions, is believed dominant for visual-spatial and nonverbal auditory processing. These aspects of cerebral structure and function have been the focus of study in populations without as well as with documented neuropathology. While there is substantial agreement among theorists about certain aspects of hemispheric specialization and related cognitive/linguistic functions, diverse views abound on many issues awaiting fur-

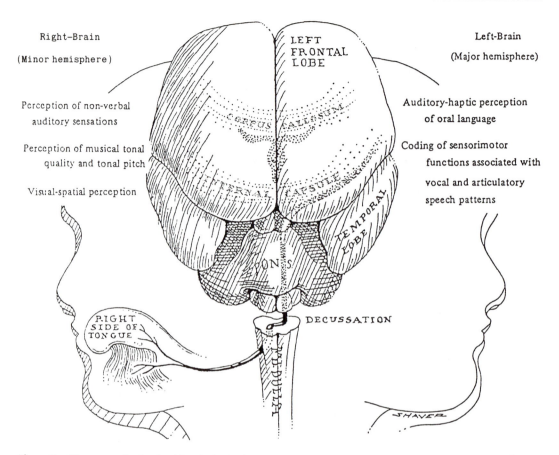

Right–Brain

(Minor hemisphere)

Perception of non-verbal
auditory sensations

Perception of musical tonal
quality and tonal pitch

Visual-spatial perception

LEFT
FRONTAL
LOBE

Left-Brain

(Major hemisphere)

Auditory-haptic perception
of oral language

Coding of sensorimotor
functions associated with
vocal and articulatory
speech patterns

RIGHT
SIDE OF
TONGUE

DECUSSATION

Figure 1. Diagrammatic sketch of hemispheric dominance designating functions of major (left) and minor (right) hemispheres. (From Berry, M. F. [1980]. *Teaching linguistically handicapped children* [p. 50]. Englewood Cliffs, NJ: Prentice-Hall, Inc.; reprinted by permission.)

ther resolution through continued research. Within the past 2 decades, intensified efforts to understand the nature of learning disabilities have further spurred investigation of brain–behavior relationship as relevant to cognitive information processing. This chapter surveys the prominent theories and research most pertinent to language-related learning disabilities.

DEFINITIONS OF TERMS (Hiscock, 1983)

Cerebral lateralization signifies qualitative or quantitative differences between the functions of the left and right hemispheres. Lateralization of higher level cognitive or linguistic function cannot be measured directly. Rather, it is inferred from anatomical, physiological, or behavioral asymmetries.

Cerebral dominance may be accounted for by lateralization of function to one hemisphere: 1) to the extent that that hemisphere assumes *control* of that function, or 2) to the extent that that hemisphere *inhibits interference* from the other hemisphere.

Laterality refers to behavioral sidedness of the hand, foot, eye, or ear. Laterality may be measured directly. However, extrapolation of results of such measurements to brain organization for higher level functions is still inferential. "There is no theoretical basis for relating some measures of laterality to cerebral lateralization, and the relevance of other laterality measures is limited" (Hiscock, 1983, p. 26).

HEMISPHERIC SPECIALIZATION: THEORETICAL ISSUES

Masland (1975) expressed a widely accepted view of hemispheric specialization:

> That language functions are centered in the left side of the brain, and that some special skills having to do with pattern recognition, spatial orientation, and body image appear to be mediated more effectively in the right hemisphere has been known for many years. (p. 4)

However, this view has been subjected to challenge and revision, partly because of its apparent oversimplification and partly because of insufficient scientific evidence. Masland (1975) himself and others (Hartlage & Telzrow, 1983) have modified and extended the description of hemispheric functions as follows:

> e.g. left hemisphere function involves analysis and direction of sequential events; right hemisphere functions involve processing of simultaneous information. (Masland, 1975, p. 17)

Successive (Sequential) and Simultaneous Processing

Luria (1980) conceptualized information processing as either simultaneous or successive, cutting across verbal and nonverbal modes. Das and Varnhagen (1986) summarized the characteristics of these two modes of processing as follows:

> Simultaneous processing involves a quasi spatial organization of units of information that are all immediately accessible in relation to each other.
>
> Successive processing involves synthesis of information temporally and linearly organized, so that each unit may be surveyed in a serial relation within a sequence.

Das and Varnhagen (1986) further blurred a sharp dichotomization of hemispheric function in terms of language when they interpreted Luria's neuropsycholinguistic theory and their own research findings as support for the following assumptions. Successive processing is important in processing the syntactic structure and *contextual* grammatical aspects of language; lesions in the frontotemporal area are believed causal to deficits in receptive and/or expressive abilities involving "automatized organized speech" such as sentence structure (p. 133). Thus, successive (sequential) processing is related to those linear aspects of language believed to be controlled by the left hemisphere. Simultaneous processing, involving spatial-conceptual relationships, is important for the *logical* grammatical aspects of language; lesions in the parieto-occipital sections of the speech area are believed to cause difficulty in the comprehension of sentences containing comparisons or spatial prepositional constructions. Thus, simultaneous processing is related to the visual-spatial modality and the comprehension of spatial-conceptual relationships. These functions are believed to be controlled by the right hemisphere.

Brain–Behavior Relationships

Much of recent neuropsychological research has been directed at establishing brain-behavior relationships. Application of these concepts to differences in cognitive style, while appealing,

continues to be speculative. Although, behaviorally, different individuals do manifest variations in strengths and weaknesses that appear to reflect hemispheric specialization, "there is no
intellectual activity that is known to depend substantially on the activity of the right hemisphere, as verbal processes are known to depend on the left" (Hiscock & Kinsbourne, 1987,
p. 139). Even the consignment of all language functions exclusively to the left hemisphere is
questionable (Pirozzolo & Papanicolaou, 1986). Masland (1975) reported on evidence that
each hemisphere, despite inherent asymmetries, does appear to have a potential to subserve all
cortical functions. At issue here is the concept of absolute qualitative versus relative quantitative differences between the two hemispheres' assumption of functional dominance (Hiscock
& Kinsbourne, 1987).

Differences in Cognitive Style

The reality of individual differences in cognitive style is not generally contested. What is at
issue is the claim that such differences are demonstrably related to particular patterns of cerebral organization. In fact, the directionality of such a relationship is still undetermined.

> Is cognitive style developed as a result of a specific, invariant cerebral organization or is cerebral
> organization molded by cognitive tasks and developed strategies? It is most likely that the brain
> operates bidirectionally. Cognitive and neural substrates are not separable into discrete entities.
> (L.J. Martin, 1986, p. 435)

Interactions Between Function and Structure

There is mounting evidence that neural structural development is responsive to functional variables. For example, research in the visual area suggests facilitation of visual cortex development through postnatal exposure to visual patterns (Willis & Widerstrom, 1986). "The infant's
fixation behavior may stimulate cortical development by exposing the central retina to salient
patterns" (p. 45). Review of prenatal and postnatal neurological development attests to a dynamic interaction between neurological structures and functions, including susceptibility to
environmental factors. Willis and Widerstrom (1986) suggested that differential functioning
may influence maturation in terms of rate or maintenance of system integrity.

The biological preprogramming of the human brain for language acquisition is virtually
unquestioned. S. Campbell and Whitaker (1986) reported clear evidence of early left hemisphere specialization for language and completion of cortical maturation by 5 years of age.
However, it is acknowledged that cortical maturation alone has not been found to correlate with
ongoing development of linguistic complexity.

With particular reference to our concerns with language-related learning disabilities,
Caplan and Kinsbourne (1982) questioned whether the manifestation of less than expected
asymmetry in the performance of certain neuropsychological tests may be more accurately
attributed to the prevalence of a relatively less verbal cognitive style than to anomalous brain
organization. However, this question leaves unanswered another question about the causation
of depressed verbal abilities in the population with learning disabilities.

ETIOLOGICAL THEORIES ABOUT LANGUAGE/LEARNING DISABILITIES

A relationship between distinctive patterns of cognitive deficit often observed in the population
of individuals with learning disabilities and equally distinctive abnormalities of brain function
is, as yet, undemonstrated (Rutter, 1984). It has been observed that many children with learn-

ing disabilities manifest a spatial, holistic style of information processing and may even have above-average nonverbal abilities. Hiscock and Kinsbourne (1987) stressed the fact that these abilities may be compensatory for verbal weaknesses, but are to be regarded as metaphors rather than clear-cut evidence of right hemispheric function. The point being made is that cognitive style lies at the behavioral level and cannot be assumed to reflect physiological or anatomical characteristics in the absence of evidence from the neurological domain. Both of these authors, in their separate and joint publications, argue against theories of anomalous brain organization, favoring instead hypotheses about genetic diversity, delayed neurological maturation, or various types/degrees of brain pathology or maladaptive processing.

Genetic Diversity Hypothesis

Selective deficits in academic performance may result from genetic diversity. In the absence of any evidence of brain damage, certain groups of individuals with learning disabilities have been characterized as having "genetic" or "constitutional" types of specific dyslexia (Masland, 1975). It has been speculated that, in a normally structured brain, a particular function (e.g., quality/quantity of neurotransmitters) may have lagged as a result of imperfect genetic programming (Kinsbourne, 1983a).

The demarcation between normal variation and abnormal maturational delay is blurred by the hypothesized existence of a critical period for development of various neural structures. Studies of early stages of fetal development reveal that the right hemisphere matures more rapidly than the left (Rosen, Sherman, & Galaburda, 1986). If developmental rate goes awry during such a critical period, it is suggested that the child might be biased toward preferring a spatial rather than linguistic processing strategy (L.J. Martin, 1986).

Delay/Deficit Hypothesis

Kinsbourne (1983a) postulated that a child's inability to perform age-appropriately on some cognitive dimension may reflect subtle damage resulting from the many factors to which the developing brain is vulnerable. Rosen et al. (1986) suggested that the biological factors controlling asymmetrical hemispheric developmental rates may render either hemisphere more vulnerable to attack by pathological agents during critical periods of maturation.

The effects of such possible disruption of normal neural maturation tend to be manifested in behavior similar to that of a younger normal child. While development does continue, ultimate full maturation is not inevitable: "the gradient of development may be such that the gap between normal and delayed function does not close and may even widen" (Kinsbourne, 1983a, p. 4).

Hemispheric Damage Hypothesis

Early left hemisphere damage may be compensated for by right hemisphere function, resulting in an absence of gross language deficits or specific reading and writing deficits. Indeed, studies of children who have undergone hemispherectomy or hemidecortication have reported that apparently normal language function develops in the presence of total or near-total incapacitation of the dominant hemisphere (Dennis, 1983; Pirozollo & Papanicolaou, 1986). On closer inspection, however, these investigators reported depressed abilities in some aspects of both verbal and visual-spatial skills.

Verbal Abilities of Hemidecordicates   Analysis by Dennis and colleagues of the behavior of three children who had either the right or the left hemisphere of their brains removed in infancy to control intractable seizures revealed some different patterns of verbal strengths and weaknesses during the school years. Possession of only the left hemisphere (right hemidecorticate) was related to: 1) superior performance in sound analysis skills on nonsense material, 2) superior knowledge of permissible letter sequences in English, 3) superior performance in matching sound and letter patterns, and 4) greater automatic use of sentence structure in decoding written text (Dennis, 1983).

An earlier study of these subjects (Dennis & Kohn, 1975) reported that left hemidecorticates (those possessing only the right hemisphere) manifested numerous deficits in syntactic abilities involved in metalinguistic tasks and in integrating semantic and syntactic information. In contrast, in the higher order skills of reading comprehension, no clear hemispheric difference was found between left and right hemidecorticates' performance on such variables as making inferences or recalling the gist of a story. Nevertheless, possession of only a right hemisphere was related to some deficits in discrimination of fine details or integration of information across sentence boundaries (Dennis, 1983).

In a subsequent study of the same subjects during adolescence (Newman, Lovett, & Dennis, 1986), differences were determined in discourse skills. The subject possessing only the left hemisphere was superior to those possessing only right hemispheres in effective use of pronominal reference to maintain story cohesion. Those possessing only the right hemisphere resorted to more frequent repetition of referents (i.e., excessive reintroduction of Given information) and, conversely, less frequent provision of referents as links to pronouns (excessive presupposition of information possessed by the message receiver without provision of the "anchor"). Newman et al. interpreted their findings as evidence of a pragmatic deficit in the left hemidecorticates, rather than grammatical deficiencies.

Nonetheless, they have admitted the possibility that the use of anaphoric reference does depend to a considerable extent on syntactic ability, in which the isolated left hemisphere had been found to have a demonstrable superiority. Their observation that the subject possessing only the left hemisphere "was able to keep a particular referent 'on stage' through a chain of anaphoric reference to it" (Newman et al., 1986, p. 40) is suggestive of the proposed sequential processing specialization attributed to the language-dominant hemisphere. Thus, the distinction between syntactic and pragmatic components is not clear cut. Furthermore, all of the results of these studies (overly abbreviated here) do seem to refute sharp dichotomization of language/nonlanguage functions as a whole to the left versus the right hemisphere.

Bihemispheric Dysfunction   Other theories of interhemispheric function take into account the effects of unilateral and bilateral damage in children with language disorders and concomitant learning disabilities. Bashir, Kuban, Kleinman, and Scavuzzo (1983) reported on results of studies that point to bihemispheric dysfunction in cases of either direct damage to both hemispheres or damage to one hemisphere related to dysfunction on the contralateral side. They suggested that greater damage to the left hemisphere may result in the right hemisphere's assumption of compensatory control of language. However, limited damage to the left hemisphere may be of insufficient degree to cause such a compensatory shift to the right hemisphere.

What must be kept in mind is the lack of sufficient evidence that functions of undamaged portions of the brain in the presence of damage to other parts are identical to functions of the normally intact brain. That is, further research on interhemispheric functions, in the absence of observable damage, is essential for support or refutation of extant theories of maladaptive cognitive processing in language/learning disabilities.

Maladaptive Processing Hypothesis

According to Kinsbourne (1970, 1983a), efficient function in neural systems is believed to be related to selectivity of focal activation and inhibition of irrelevant circuitry. Greater cognitive skill is therefore assumed to correspond to more sharply defined focal activation of appropriate portions of the brain. The degree to which relevant parts of the cortex are maximally activated is thought to be determined by brain stem selector mechanisms.

> A relative blurring or dispersion of this brain stem 'selector' influence might lead to an inability to put certain parts of the cortex to work with maximum intensity, thus imposing a ceiling on what can be accomplished when problem solving in the relevant mode. (Kinsbourne, 1983a, p. 9)

From this perspective, it is assumed that, when language activity becomes relevant, selective activation of the language territory of the left hemisphere creates a verbal set. Failure to selectively activate such functions when a mental verbal set is required may result in language or reading difficulties. In some cases, then, the difficulties are attributed not to structural abnormality, but to anomalous processing strategies.

Proposing a more flexible model of language-related learning disabilities, Kershner (1983) suggested a combination of reduced left hemisphere processing capacity and a right hemisphere attentional bias. In light of results of experimentation that has apparently reversed the expected language lateralization in subjects with learning disabilities under controlled conditions, Kershner (1983) reasoned that we cannot preclude a potential for linguistic processing in the right hemisphere. He characterized language-related learning disability in terms of maladaptive allocation of resources during the "simultaneous processing of linguistic information between hemispheres" (p. 71). The significant questions, then, are not whether dominance develops or where language is located, but, rather, does a child with learning disabilities differ from a child without such disabilities with respect to intrahemispheric and interhemispheric resource availability (arousal, effort), resource allocation (selective activation, resource competition), or hemispheric processing efficiency (capacity)?

RESEARCH SOURCES FOR PROCESSING HYPOTHESES

Hypotheses about hemispheric processing in individuals with learning disabilities have emerged from a large body of research that generally falls into three main categories: psychometric studies, behavioral laterality studies, and direct observation of brain structure and functions. Psychometric research employs batteries of tests designed to examine patterns of cognitive, linguistic, and sensorimotor abilities reflecting assumed left and right hemispheric functions. Subtyping research falls within this category because it attempts to find differentiable, homogeneous patterns within the larger heterogeneous group of disabilities. Behavioral laterality research studies sensory or motor performance on such tasks as dichotic listening or finger tapping while performing simultaneous verbal or visual tasks. From results, higher level patterns of cerebral function are inferred. Direct observation of brain structure and function is conducted through computerized technology or postmortem analysis. Samples of research in each category are provided here.

Psychometric Studies

Despite the cautionary notes sounded by some scholars about the hypothetical relation between patterns of cognitive style and hemispheric specialization, much of psychometric research design and interpretation assumes the existence of such a relationship. The verbal versus visual-spatial dichotomy has served as the foundation for research aimed at: 1) differentiating subjects with learning disabilities from those without such disabilities, 2) identifying subtypes of learning disabilities, and 3) demonstrating developmental changes in cognitive abilities attributed, in some cases, to maturational changes in hemispheric systems. The interpretations of these investigators are reported in their terms, one of which is the frequent use of the label *dyslexia* for reading disability.

Studies of Cognitive Style   A considerable body of research employing neuropsychological test batteries has demonstrated a cognitive style in subjects with learning disabilities that reflects relatively depressed verbal-sequential processing in the presence of superior visual-spatial–simultaneous processing (Bow, 1988; H.W. Gordon, 1983; Rourke, 1983, 1985; Rourke, Fisk, & Strang, 1986; Sinatra, 1989; Witelson, 1976). In one of the earlier studies, Witelson (1976) reasoned that, since the literature had provided substantial evidence for inferring left hemisphere lateralization for language in dyslexia, some abnormality in right hemispheric processing may contribute to the disorder. She selected a group of procedures designed to examine visual-spatial processing free of verbal encoding and verbal processing in the auditory and visual modalities. A total of 85 right-handed boys with dyslexia and 156 normally achieving boys were tested over a period of 5 years.

In summarized form, results demonstrated the expected patterns of asymmetries for subjects without dyslexia but a different pattern for subjects with dyslexia. Although left hemisphere specialization for language was exhibited by subjects with dyslexia, the level of performance was markedly inferior to that of controls. On visual-spatial processing tasks, normally achieving subjects showed the expected pattern of inferred right hemisphere specialization. Subjects with dyslexia, however, appeared to have bilateral spatial representation. On the bilateral visual-verbal task, they tended to employ spatial-holistic strategies more than did control subjects, demonstrating a greater reliance on processes ascribed to the right hemisphere.

Similar findings have been reported from other studies using batteries of tests designed to assess hemispheric functions in subjects with and without known pathologies (H.W. Gordon, 1983; Pirozzolo & Rayner, 1979). H.W. Gordon (1983) found that 105 out of 108 subjects with learning disabilities performed better on tests of right hemisphere function than on tests of left hemisphere function. Performance on right hemisphere tests was above average by 0.5 standard deviation. Performance on left hemisphere tests was below average by 0.5 standard deviation. H.W. Gordon (1983) speculated that children with learning disabilities are locked into a right brain mode of processing, using this mode whether or not it is conducive to the task at hand.

Rourke (1983) reported on a series of studies demonstrating a clear-cut differentiation of skills in subjects with and without learning disabilities (ages 9–14 years) based on Verbal and Performance scores on the WISC (Wechsler, 1949). Subjects with high verbal scores were markedly superior in such tasks as word recognition, spelling, speech sound perception, and auditory discrimination. Subjects with high performance scores were superior in short-term visual memory and visual-spatial sequencing.

Hypotheses About Hemispheric Dysfunction in Language-Related Learning Disabilities From a group of these studies conducted during the late 1970s and early 1980s, the following hypotheses have been advanced about the nature of the dysfunction underlying reading/learning disabilities (Denckla, Rudel, & Broman, 1980; H.W. Gordon, 1983; Pirozzolo, Dunn, & Zetusky, 1983; Pirozzolo & Rayner, 1979; Witelson, 1976):

1. A bilateral representation of spatial processing may interfere with left hemisphere processing of language.
2. An inferior or dysfunctional left hemisphere in some way is causal to lack of right hemisphere specialization for spatial processing.
3. Interaction between an inferior left hemisphere and a superior right hemisphere may occur.

In regard to the latter hypothesis, it has been suggested that individuals with auditory-linguistic dyslexia "suffer from pathologically slow transmission of linguistic information within the left hemisphere, and thus auditory-linguistic dyslexia can be said to resemble an aphasic disorder" (Pirozzolo et al., 1983, p. 45).

Longitudinal Studies Longitudinal studies have revealed that persons with some types of reading deficits eventually overcome deficits in neuropsychological abilities somewhere around 9 years of age, particularly in those functions presumed to be subserved by the right hemisphere (Nichols, Inglis, Lawson, & MacKay, 1988; Rourke, 1983). For adults with learning disabilities tested on the Wechsler Adult Intelligence Scale (WAIS) (Wechsler, 1955), scores on the Similarities subtest were significantly higher than earlier WISC–R scores by these same subjects with learning disabilities (Sinatra, 1989). The author interpreted performance on the Similarities subtest as a reflection of the holistic processing generally attributed to the right hemisphere.

In those persons who do not overcome reading deficits, the abilities implicated in continued deficits are those believed to be subserved by the left hemisphere. The verbal-sequential processing abilities of these persons have been reported to decline over time in comparison with peers who do not have a learning disability (Nichols et al., 1988; Rourke, 1983; Sinatra, 1989). In adults with learning disabilities who had demonstrated primary linguistic deficits during childhood, a pervasive impairment continued to depress general learning abilities (Spreen & Haaf, 1986), with academic performance in one sample below the mean educational level of 10.5 years (McCue, Shelly, & Goldstein, 1986). Although performance on a neuropsychological test battery by this latter group fell within the normal to mildly impaired range, relative impairment was demonstrated in certain aspects of language, attention, and motor abilities, with better results on tasks involving nonverbal abilities.

In studies of acquired knowledge by adults with reading disability manifesting continued verbal deficits, depressed performance has been attributed to low sequential processing abilities, thereby inferring inferior left hemispheric function. Sinatra (1989) reported that these individuals showed a strong preference, vocationally and avocationally, for nonverbal, manipulational three-dimension activities, with infrequent use of written language as a mode of expression and learning, probably because of their poor skills in this area. A function-structure relationship is conjectured in the observed decline of verbal skills over time.

It may be that, because there is a deficit of verbal ability in such children, they come to rely more heavily on nonverbal ability. Such exercise of one kind of ability at the expense of the other may lead to its greater development and even its overdevelopment. (Nichols et al., 1988, p. 508)

An Attentional Deficit Hypothesis   There is little reason to doubt that important differences between people with and without learning disabilities do exist in cognitive style and in the skills ascribed to left and right brain functions. There is not, however, universal agreement about the cause of these differences. While acknowledging the potentially interfering role of bilateral spatial representation to the detriment of linguistic processing in the left hemisphere, Obrzut, Hynd, and Boliek (1986) are inclined to attribute the observed patterns to attentional variables rather than to anomalies of cerebral specialization.

It has been suggested that a mechanism may have developed in normal children that suppresses information from a nondominant hemisphere during the processing of information in the dominant hemisphere. If individuals with learning disabilities have not established such a mechanism for reciprocal inhibition, they may have a tendency to direct attention to stimuli presented to either perceptual field (Hiscock & Hinsbourne, 1987; Obrzut & Boliek, 1986). While average or above average visual-spatial skills in individuals with learning disabilities are quite uniformly reported in the literature, questions still remain regarding interpretation of these data in terms of neurophysiological implications for information processing (Obrzut, 1989).

Subtyping Research   In view of the evidence refuting the homogeneity of learning disability as a unitary entity, numerous investigations have attempted to identify subtypes demonstrating common patterns of strengths and weaknesses. Certain research techniques have

> yielded rather compelling evidence that at least a majority of learning disabled children can be classified reliably into clinically meaningful subtypes based on statistical analysis of their performance on a wide variety of measures known to be sensitive to the functional integrity of the brain. (J.L. Fisk & Rourke, 1983, p. 530)

In his review of methods used in subtyping research, J.M. McKinney (1985) differentiated between early and more recent approaches to classification. Most of the studies conducted throughout the 1970s (e.g., Boder, 1971; Denckla, 1972; Mattis, French, & Rapin, 1975) tended to use an inferential approach wherein theoretical assumptions determined a priori criteria for decisions about the use of diagnostic test results in assignment of subjects to groups. Mattis et al. (1975) reported learning disability subtypes of Linguistic, Visuospatial, and Graphomotor. Denckla (1972) had classified subjects on the basis of extended neurological examination as having Specific Language Disability, Specific Visuospatial Disability, and the Dyscontrol Syndrome. (Boder's [1971] subtypes are included in the section on reading disability subtypes below.)

In later studies, investigators resorted to established empirical methods, such as factor analysis and hierarchical cluster techniques, for deriving subtypes. Results of these studies are presented in summarized form.

Learning Disability Subtypes   Rourke and Finlayson (1978) used the WISC (1949) to study the visual and verbal abilities of 9- to 14-year-old students with learning disabilities and analyzed the neuropsychological significance of variations in these abilities on academic performance. Subjects clustered into three groups: 1) uniformly deficient in reading, spelling, and arithmetic; 2) good in arithmetic but poor in reading and spelling; and 3) good in reading and spelling but poor in arithmetic. Group 1 was superior to Group 3 on visual-perceptual and visual-spatial skills. Group 2 was superior to Group 3 on visual-perceptual and visual-spatial skills. Group 3 was superior to Group 1 and 2 on verbal- and auditory-perceptual abilities. Group 3 exceeded Group 2 on all 10 measures of these abilities in the WISC. In Group 2, 14 out of 15 subjects had lower Verbal IQs than Performance IQs.

Fletcher (1985) studied a group of 9- to 12-year-old students with learning disabilities employing similar methods in the same research program. Subjects again clustered into three groups: Group 1 subjects were impaired in both verbal and visual tasks, those in Group 2 had better spatial but poorer verbal skills, and those in Group 3 had better verbal but poorer spatial skills. It has been assumed that these patterns in both neuropsychological abilities and academic achievement were likely to reflect relatively dysfunctional left or right hemispheres. "The emergence of these subgroups in the absence of a priori assumptions concerning the nature of the learning disabilities further highlights the importance of these academic patterns" (Fletcher, 1985, p. 197).

A later study in the Rourke research program (Ozols & Rourke, 1988) replicated the methods with 45 children 7–8 years old with learning disabilities. Subjects clustered into three groups:

> Group 1 was evenly deficient in reading, spelling, and arithmetic.
>
> Group 2 was deficient in reading and spelling with significantly higher (although impaired) arithmetic skills.
>
> Group 3 was average or above average in reading and spelling but significantly deficient in arithmetic (one grade level below reading and spelling scores).

On the neuropsychological battery, Group 3 performed significantly better than Groups 1 and 2 on auditory-perceptual/linguistic measures and significantly more poorly on visual-perceptual measures. Groups 1 and 2 demonstrated significant deficits on the language-related measures in comparison to group 3 and to the normally developing population. These results replicated patterns revealed in the Rourke and Finlayson's (1978) study of older subjects.

J.M. McKinney, Short, and Feagans (1985) examined 55 first- and second-grade children identified by schools as having learning disabilities on a battery of experimental tasks that assessed aspects of linguistic and perceptual development and on selected subtests of the WISC–R. Results were subjected to a hierarchical cluster analysis that yielded six subtypes. Only three of the six subtypes showed significant linguistic or perceptual deficits. Of those three displaying atypical patterns, one group demonstrated severe language impairment and two groups were characterized by mixed deficits—that is, deficits in both linguistic and perceptual areas. No group was found with perceptual deficits and intact linguistic abilities. In the third year of a longitudinal study, the originally identified subgroups were differentiated on measures of reading ability. The children with normal-appearing profiles having marginal perceptual or language deficits performed better than those in the subtypes identified with atypical language and perceptual profiles, but not as well as matched normally achieving controls.

One subtype that has been frequently reported in the literature on learning disabilities has been a pattern of depressed scores on a particular group of WISC subtests: Arithmetic, Coding, Information, and Digit Span (ACID). Arithmetic, Digit Span, and Coding are believed to require the mental manipulation of symbols and attentional alertness (Rourke et al., 1986). The ACID pattern had been regarded as predictive of poor performance in reading, spelling, and

arithmetic. Joshko and Rourke (1985) found at least two definable subgroups of children manifesting the ACID pattern—1) those with poor immediate auditory verbal memory problems, and
2) those with poor visual imagery—thus contraindicating a unitary approach to remediation.

Reading Disability Subtypes   Boder's (1971) classification of developmental dyslexia
into three types has continued to be cited over the past 2 decades. The subtypes were derived
by analyzing patterns of reading and spelling jointly, observing both assets and deficits:

> Group 1. Dysphonetic Dyslexia—*Reading-spelling pattern* reflects primary deficit in symbol-
> sound (grapheme-phoneme) integration and the ability to develop skills in phonetic word
> analysis-synthesis.
> Group 2. Dyseidetic Dyslexia—*Reading-spelling pattern* reflects primary deficit in the ability to
> perceive letters and whole words as configurations, or visual Gestalts.
> Group 3. Mixed Dysphonetic Dyseidetic Dyslexia-Alexia—*Reading-spelling pattern* reflects pri-
> mary deficits both in ability to develop word analysis skills and whole words as visual Ges-
> talts. (Boder, 1971, p. 199)

These subtypes were derived by the earlier clinical-inferential method reported above by J.M.
McKinney (1985). Fletcher (1985) has noted that Boder's research and findings have been
criticized because of internal validity problems.

Satz and Morris (1981) studied fifth-grade students with significantly low scores on the
Wide Range Achievement Test Reading and Spelling Subtests. Hierarchical cluster analysis
yielded five learning disability subtypes:

> Group 1 had a global language impairment with strengths in visual-motor integration.
> Group 2 had specific language impairment on verbal fluency (naming disorder).
> Group 3 was deficient on language *and* visual-perceptual measures (mixed).
> Group 4 was impaired in visual-perceptual-motor skills but not in language.
> Group 5 had no neuropsychological impairment.

A group of studies has been conducted by Lyon and his associates. Lyon and Watson
(1981) studied the performance of 11- to 12-year-old students with reading disability on tests of
word recognition and comprehension and a battery of language and perceptual measures.
Cluster analysis of results yielded six subtypes:

> Group 1, the poorest readers, had a combination of poor auditory and visual skills.
> Group 2 had similarly mixed deficits but to a milder degree.
> Group 3 had a primary language disorder with a notable lack of proficiency in phonics.
> Group 4 had deficits in visual perception but not in language, and included the largest
> membership of all the subtypes.
> Group 5 had deficits that resembled an aphasic pattern of inability to remember and
> correctly sequence auditory verbal information, resulting in deficits in syntactic,
> sound blending, and reading behaviors.
> Group 6 had normal neuropsychological profiles.

Lyon and Watson (1981) found the large membership in Group 4 surprising "since visuospatial
disorders are reported to occur much more frequently in younger children" (p. 260).

A study by Lyon, Stewart, and Freedman (1982) compared 75 younger children with
identified learning/reading disabilities (ages 6–9 years) with 42 normally achieving controls
on a battery of 10 language and visual-perceptual tests. The Woodcock Reading Test (Wood-

cock, 1973) was administered to the subjects with reading disability. Multiple cluster analyses yielded five subgroups:

Group 1 had deficits in all visual areas tested within a context of language strengths, resembling the Visual-Perceptual-Motor subtype reported by Satz and Morris (1981) and the Dyseidetic Group described by Boder (1973). Oral reading of single words was deficient, but relative strengths were observed in reading and comprehending contextual material.

Group 2 had deficits in a variety of language skills, with strengths in visual-perceptual skills. Reading scores on comprehension were lower than measures of oral reading and word decoding. This group resembled the Dysphonetic Group described by Boder (1973) and the Naming Disorder subtype reported by Satz and Morris (1981).

Group 3 had a normal neuropsychological profile. Although they scored higher than other subgroups on reading, they scored below normal.

Group 4, the poorest readers, exhibited difficulty in both language and visual information processing.

Group 5 had deficits in specific language skills and an array of visual skills, resembling Boder's (1971) Dysphonetic and Dyseidetic combination and Satz and Morris' (1981) Mixed Deficit subtype. Reading was impaired by difficulties in both recognition of phonetically irregular (sight) words and decoding of phonetically regular words.

In a later study, Lyon (1985b) examined the responses of subtypes to a phonics-based reading/writing instruction program. External validity of the subtypes was secured on the basis of the difference in gains made by the subtypes. Students in the subtypes exhibiting deficits in auditory memory, sound blending, and auditory comprehension did not benefit from the synthetic phonics approach. Those with measured strengths in auditory discrimination, auditory and visual memory, and sound blending made marked gains from the instructional program.

It is acknowledged that the process of subtyping is not problem free. Boundaries between groups are not always clearly defined or maintained over time. A number of scholars have observed that diversity in results is likely due to variations in procedures emerging from different theoretical perspectives (Lyon, 1985a; J.M. McKinney, 1985; Morris, Blashfield, & Satz, 1986). Morris et al. (1986) have suggested that some of the inconsistencies found in research on subtyping reading disabilities may be explained by differences in subject samples. Among these differences in subjects is the factor of age or developmental level. That is, certain types of disability may be manifested at a particular stage of development but not necessarily at another stage.

Over the past two decades, Satz and his associates have advanced the hypothesis that, because sensorimotor development in the brain precedes language maturation, younger children with dyslexia would tend to manifest visual-motor deficits, and older children with dyslexia would be likely to exhibit language deficits. These hypotheses were partially supported by results of a study of children in age groups 7–8 years and 11–12 years (Satz, Rardin, & Ross, 1971).

In a longitudinal study of 80 second-grade children with reading disability and matched controls, Morris et al. (1986) used cluster analysis of results of a neuropsychological test battery to derive subtypes. Subjects were reexamined in fifth grade on the same measures of verbal-conceptual and sensory-perceptual abilities. Results of cluster analysis yielded three types of poor readers and two types of good readers. The poor readers were described as follows:

> Type A had poor verbal skills with increasing strengths in visual-perceptual and motor skills as they matured. These children demonstrated poor academic achievement.
>
> Type B had average verbal-conceptual abilities in second grade but were measured as deficient in these skills in fifth grade. Visual-perceptual-motor abilities were poor across the period studied. This group manifested below-average academic achievement.
>
> Type C was below average on all measures at initial testing and showed a mild weakening across verbal, perceptual, and motor abilities with advancing age.

Morris et al. (1986) commented that Types A and B "showed a clear dissociation between the development of their verbal and visual-perceptual-motor abilities" (p. 387). They interpreted their findings as support for the theory that early deficits in visual-perceptual-motor abilities and later language deficits differentially determine reading disability at these different stages.

Inspection of the subtype descriptions reported above by other investigators for different age levels casts some doubt on these assumptions. For example, Lyon and Watson (1981) called attention to the fact that, in their older subjects (11–12 years), the largest subtype group of subjects with reading disability exhibited deficits in visual-perceptual abilities but not in language. In their study of younger children with reading disability (6–9 years), Lyon et al. (1982) found that the expected pattern of a significantly higher incidence of sensorimotor and visual-motor deficiencies did not obtain. "Conversely, our data indicated that language-related deficits were associated with the reading problems in approximately 52% of the [learning disabled readers] sample" (p. 361).

Although two of their subtypes manifesting primarily visual-perceptual deficits had the youngest mean age, and one of the two older groups contained subjects demonstrating impairment in receptive and expressive language, Lyon et al. (1982) pointed out that *all* of their subjects were within the age range that, according to the developmental lag theory proposed by Satz and his colleagues, should have a significantly higher incidence of sensorimotor and visual-motor deficiencies. It is also noteworthy that, among first- and second-grade subjects with learning disabilities studied by J.M. McKinney et al. (1985), no subtype was found that had perceptual deficits in conjunction with intact language skills.

Bakker (1992) applied a modification of the developmental theory to his ongoing research on the relative influences of perceptual and linguistic influences on reading disability:

> Learning to read implies a developmentally changing balance of perceptual and linguistic investment which at the cerebral level is paralleled by a developmentally changing balance of right- and left-hemisphere subservience. The balance dips to the right- and left-hemispheric reading control during the initial and advanced stages of the learning to read process respectively. (p. 103)

The type of experimental procedures used in his study are discussed in the next section. However, the results are included here because of their relevance to the subject of reading disability subtypes.

In a longitudinal study starting with kindergarten children, Bakker (1992) studied the measured dichotic listening responses and Word Response Potential (a measure of brain activity) during the initial and subsequent stages of reading. A larger right temporal amplitude was observed in years 1 and 2, and a larger left temporal amplitude was observed in years 3 and 4. Subsequent studies differentiated between two types of dyslexia:

> P type, individuals who relied excessively on perceptual processing, resulting in halting, fragmented reading, presumably those who "failed to shift from predominant right- to predominant left-hemisphere mediation of reading" (p. 106).
>
> L type, individuals who shifted too early to language processing, thereby making more errors in precision of word decoding, presumably showing "predominantly left-hemisphere control of reading from the onset of the learning to read process" (p. 106).

Hynd (1992), commenting on Bakker's Balance Model, concluded that "The evidence of involvement of the right hemisphere in early reading is not conclusive" (p. 111). As an alternative, he postulated that in early reading it is likely that regions in both hemispheres may be involved, with increasing involvement of the left central language area as linguistic processing becomes more automatized.

Over the past 2 decades, the role of perception in reading acquisition has been deemphasized as a consequence of the voluminous body of research literature presenting evidence of a crucial relationship between language factors and reading acquisition (see Chapter 7). One of the subtyping studies narrowed the focus of its investigation to language abilities and disabilities in young children. Feagans and Appelbaum (1986) used hierarchical cluster analysis to identify language subtypes among 6- and 7-year-old children with learning disabilities. Abilities assessed were syntax, semantics, narrative discourse, verbal fluency, and linguistic complexity in paraphrased stories. Six subtypes were identified:

> Group 1 had normal syntactic and semantic skills with below-normal performance on comprehending and producing narratives.
>
> Group 2 was superior in vocabulary, with poor skills in all other areas measured.
>
> Group 3 was hyperverbal in terms of quantity and complexity of output but deficient in meaning and substance.
>
> Group 4 had narrative skills that were superior to their measured skills in syntax and semantics.
>
> Group 5 had superior narrative skills and verbal output.
>
> Group 6 had average narrative skills and high syntactic and semantic scores.

These subtypes were externally validated on a number of variables, one of which was academic achievement over a 3-year period. Groups 1, 2, and 6 had the poorest outcome. Groups 4 and 5, characterized by good narrative skills, had fewer academic problems over the 3-year period, thereby demonstrating a possible relationship between the ability to comprehend and produce narrative discourse and reading ability.

The long-term effects of language deficits may be generalized to learning disability throughout the life span. In a longitudinal study into adulthood, only two subtypes could be clearly identified: visual-spatial and graphomotor. Those subjects manifesting linguistic deficits could not be separated from other subjects with deficits into a distinct cluster, since they appeared in clusters characterized by overall low performance, "perhaps suggesting a poor long-term outcome" (Spreen & Haaf, 1986, p. 179).

Two recent studies have called into question diagnostic practice based on subtypes revealed by analysis of WISC–R results and/or other verbal/nonverbal neuropsychological test batteries. In their study of the profiles of 119 children classified by schools as having learning disabilities, Holcomb, Hardesty, Adams, and Ponder (1987) found six subtypes based on analysis of WISC–R results. Only two of the six groups manifested the discrepancy between language and visual-spatial skills regarded as one possible characteristic of learning disability. Type A showed low verbal and high performance scores with an overall verbal-performance difference of 18 points. These children were described as having average spatial ability, below-average sequencing skills, and very low scores on verbal conceptualization and acquired knowledge. Type C demonstrated the ACID profile, with attentional and sequencing deficits. The remaining "subtypes" did not meet the criteria for classification as having learning disabilities.

It has also been found that the batteries of neurospsychological tests reveal inherent differences in learning style in populations of children with and without impairment (Shinn-Streicker, 1986). In this study there was no differential clustering of children with and without handicaps on the following patterns:

> Higher scores on visual than verbal tasks occurred in 50% of subjects with handicaps and 50% of those without.
> Higher scores on verbal than visual tasks occurred in 58% of subjects with handicaps and 42% of those without.

It would appear that group differences in cognitive style, while valuable in individual assessment and treatment of learning disabilities, may not, in and of themselves, be diagnostic of the classification of a learning disability, in that the patterns of asymmetry attributed to this population are not unique to this group of individuals.

The issues of classification and etiology remain problematic, with inconclusive evidence of neural integrity in children with learning disabilities. In most of the neuropsychological subtyping studies, comparisons have been made with normally developing controls. Pursuing a different research direction, Arffa, Fitzhugh-Bell, and Black (1989) examined 24 subjects classified by schools as having learning disabilities (mean age = 10.4 years) and 36 children with documented brain damage (mean ages across types of trauma ranging from 7.4 to 10.3 years). The two groups were administered a comprehensive battery of neuropsychological tests measuring auditory verbal, sequencing/visual-motor, visual-spatial, visual-conceptual, motor, spatial, tactile, and sensory skill areas. The standard scores were submitted to a factor analysis to derive clusters of subjects across groups.

Results revealed five clusters with dissimilar numerical membership. However, "of the five clusters of subjects no single cluster was composed of either [learning disabled] or [brain damaged] subjects" (p. 636). That is, on the measures used in this study, many similarities were demonstrated by the two groups, but the clusters differed in patterns of deficit and degrees of severity.

> Group 1 included almost half of the subjects with learning disabilities and two thirds of subjects with brain damage. Deficits were regarded as mild since all scores fell within 1 standard deviation below the mean.
> Group 2 consisted primarily of subjects with brain damage. Performance was generally

more depressed, with marked deficits in auditory and visual processing, sequencing and fine motor and tactile skills.

Group 3 contained more subjects with learning disabilities than did Group 2. Whereas most scores fell within 1 standard deviation from the mean, some specific areas showed markedly contrasting strengths and weaknesses. Among the areas of significant weakness were auditory discrimination, sequencing/visual-motor, tactile perception, and visual-conceptual skills.

Because both types of subjects were included within all factors, the authors suggested that "there may be similarities in functional neuropsychological organization in both groups (Arffa et al., p. 638). Therefore, they concluded that there is a need to continue research into possible neuropathology in at least a subset of children with learning disabilities and into comparative neuropsychology over time to identify children with possible organic anomalies or developmental delay.

Behavioral Laterality

Behavioral laterality studies have investigated preferred handedness, footedness, and eyedness. Evidence for a relationship between such measures and academic achievement is weak or nonexistent (Obrzut et al., 1986). Studies of inferred lateralization of function using dichotic listening and visual half-field techniques have produced interesting, although equivocal, results. Dual-task or time-sharing techniques have been fruitful in their contribution of evidence about hemispheric specialization and resource allocation. Research employing these experimental techniques is briefly reviewed.

Dichotic Listening Studies   Dichotic listening has been widely used clinically and in research in efforts to ascertain functional lateralization. The procedure permits observation of which ear is better able to use its respective input of auditory verbal information for successful encoding, retention, and recall under conditions of simultaneous presentation of verbal material to both ears. A right ear advantage is interpreted as a direct indication of the lateralized function of language to the left hemisphere. A left ear advantage or lack of ear advantage has been viewed as a possible indication of failure to establish optimal left hemispheric dominance for language or faulty transfer of information between the hemispheres (Kershner, 1983).

The literature on dichotic listening studies is too vast and controversial to be reported in extensive detail within the constraints of this chapter. Selected reports, reviews, and evaluations of the research in this area have been drawn from the literature. Results of dichotic listening studies have been conflicting and therefore equivocal, with mixed patterns reported in terms of the existence/nonexistence of a right ear advantage and in terms of the magnitude of the difference between left and right ear performance in subjects with and without learning disabilities (Bryden, 1982; Obrzut et al., 1986). While recent research is viewed by some scholars as suggestive of a relationship between possibly incomplete lateralization of hemispheric function and learning/reading disabilities, it has not been judged sufficiently strong to be diagnostic or predictive: "Some children with perfectly normal functional lateralization become poor readers, whereas others with poorly lateralized verbal and spatial processes overcome this difficulty and become quite skilled at reading and language" (Bryden, 1982, p. 254).

In a review of 15 studies of reading disability and laterality, Satz (1977) did not find evidence of a clear relationship between the two measures, nor were results of dichotic listening found to be a valuable predictor of reading disability. A right ear advantage in good *and* poor readers was reported in many studies. In addition, it has been reported in several studies that the right ear advantage for children with learning disabilities processing verbal material dichotically was abnormally large (Hynd & Obrzut, 1981; Kershner, 1983).

In some studies reviewed by Obrzut et al. (1986), children with learning disabilities showed the expected right ear advantage for language but recalled less information from both sides of space (i.e., regardless of whether information input came from the left or right side of the external environment) than did children without such disabilities. Parenthetically, it should be noted that some evidence has been cited in support of the theory that a right ear advantage may indeed be a right side of space advantage rather than a demonstration of the functional prepotency of the contralateral auditory pathway (Hiscock & Kinsbourne, 1987).

Difficulty in establishing the validity of such laterality measures is related to the fact that about 95% of right-handed people have left hemispheric speech representation. It is estimated, however, that only 70% of a representative sample of right-handers demonstrate a right ear preference on dichotic listening tasks (Satz, 1977). Thus, a conditional probability of predicting left hemisphere language control in an individual given the presence of a right ear advantage is high (.7) but not perfect (according to Satz). However, the probability of right hemisphere language control given a left ear advantage is only .1. Therefore, prediction of right hemispheric speech representation would be wrong 90% of the time. Since an extraordinarily precise laterality measure would be required to classify people for hemispheric language specialization under these circumstances, Hiscock and Kinsbourne (1987) cautioned against equating anomalous performance with anomalous hemispheric specialization.

The point has been made that most lateralization studies invoke voluntary use of the peripheral nervous system in executing motor, spatial, or verbal tasks, whereas cerebral dominance is viewed as involuntary functioning of the right and left hemispheres (Obrzut & Boliek, 1986). A number of scholars have suggested that the results obtained on dichotic listening tasks may reflect factors other than, or in addition to, functional lateralization, such as strategies used in task performance, memory, rehearsal, prior experience, temporal sequencing, and attention (Bryden, 1982; Hiscock, 1983; Naylor, 1980; Obrzut et al., 1986). "In dichotic studies it may be that the variability among children of different age levels in the ability to selectively attend has contributed to what appears to be developmental trends in the establishment of cerebral dominance" (Obrzut et al., 1986, p. 453).

A recent study presented evidence that degrees of lateralization on dichotic listening tasks were task related. Kershner and Stringer (1991) examined dichotic listening effects in three groups of subjects (children with reading disability and reading-matched and age-matched controls) under three conditions: baseline, reading, and writing. Results revealed that reading increased lateralization in all three groups. Reading and writing caused a decrement in left ear recall for all groups, indicating left hemispheric lateralization during these linguistic activities. However, writing induced a decrement in right ear recall for children with reading disability. The results were interpreted to mean that lateralization is a flexible, context-related mechanism for information processing. Although baseline results indicated no significant difference between subjects with and without reading disability, a lesser degree of lateralization was observed in the results of subjects with reading disability during the writing condition. Furthermore, "In the writing condition, individual children with dyslexia who were less lateralized also were poorer in single word decoding" (Kershner & Stringer, 1991, p. 565).

These authors have speculated that, in writing, the demands of single word decoding (a well-documented deficit in individuals with reading disability) and the concurrent engagement in manual output may increase the attentional demands in a dichotic task. It was thus conjectured that children with reading disability are particularly vulnerable to task-related variations in attentional demands that involve interhemispheric shifts. For example, note taking during oral instruction may prove very difficult for these children "because of attentional demands that are fundamentally incompatible with efficient learning for them" (Kershner & Stringer, 1991, p. 566).

Directed Attention Studies A prestimulus cuing paradigm has been used to focus attention on the right or left ear during dichotic listening tasks. In a number of studies, this directed attention technique demonstrated no effects on ear advantage in children without learning disabilities, but did obtain a dramatic reversal of ear advantage in children with such disabilities. Kershner (1983) described two studies that experimentally modified the attentional demands of dichotic tasks by directing attention to either ear input. Results demonstrated a complete reversal of ear superiority in the subjects with learning disabilities, showing a left ear advantage for them, but no shift by the achieving readers. This outcome is interpreted as a refutation of the assumption that performance on a laterality task such as dichotic listening reflects fixed localization of particular hemispheric functions: "At any rate, one can be sure that a simple experimental manipulation could not have caused a rearrangement of the brain's physical features or a translocation of a localized neurological dysfunction from one place in the brain to another" (Kershner, 1983, p. 70).

Similar findings in a number of cued dichotic listening studies (Kinsbourne, 1970; Kinsbourne & Hiscock, 1981; Obrzut & Hynd, 1983; Obrzut, Hynd, Obrzut, & Pirozzolo, 1981; Obrzut, Obrzut, Bryden, & Bartels, 1985; Obrzut et al., 1986) led to the interpretation that, in children without disabilities, language dominance develops concurrently with suppression of nondominant hemispheric function during linguistic processing. It is considered possible that subjects with language-related learning disabilities have not similarly established such a reciprocal inhibitory mechanism, thereby dividing attention interhemispherically. This view hypothesizes that children with selective language/reading deficits may have brain activation patterns that render them more susceptible than children without such deficits to attentional effects in processing certain classes of auditory/visual/verbal material (Kinsbourne, 1983a; Obrzut et al., 1986). In particular, some early evidence points to a relationship between dysphonetic readers and weak lateralization on dichotic tasks, but disconfirms such a relationship in dyseidetic readers (Obrzut & Boliek, 1986).

Time-Sharing Studies A dual-task paradigm has been employed as an alternative method of examining cerebral lateralization. The assumption underlying this research technique is that two tasks processed simultaneously in the same hemisphere are not usually performed as well as a single task. For example, following the establishment of a baseline performance of finger tapping with the right or left hand, tasks such as reading or speaking, presumably controlled essentially by the left hemisphere, or solving spatial problems (assumed to be a right hemisphere task) are performed concurrently with the finger tapping. Disruptions in finger tapping rate under these time-sharing conditions are interpreted as evidence of a hemispheric competition and cortical inhibition (Kinsbourne & Hiscock, 1981; Kinsbourne & McMurray, 1975).

Stellern and his colleagues (Stellern, Collins, & Bayne, 1987; Stellern, Collins, Cossairt,

& Gutierrez, 1986) studied samples of students who ostensibly had no handicaps by using time-sharing tasks, and assessed reading and visual-spatial abilities. They found that reading disrupted right-handed tapping significantly more than left-handed tapping, implicating left hemispheric competition for processing resources. In contrast, left-handed tapping was disrupted to a significantly greater extent during the visual-spatial task, suggesting right hemisphere capacity competition. Analysis of results revealed that 49 of 76 subjects demonstrated the expected pattern of functional lateralization and that all of these subjects were classified as having good academic skills. No poor students manifested this normal pattern. Of the 27 subjects presenting the nonnormal brain organization pattern, 23 were poor students and 4 were good students.

These results led to the proposal that some slow learners may, in fact, be classifiable as having learning disabilities "because of nonnormal brain organization, which manifests itself as nonnormal language-spatial lateralization (L-L, R-R, and R-L for right handers)" (Stellern et al., 1987, p. 555). That is, either both language and spatial function were lateralized to the left hemisphere, or both were lateralized to the right hemisphere, or the expected asymmetry was reversed, with language in the right and spatial functions in the left hemispheres.

Time-sharing research on subjects with learning disabilities was reviewed by Obrzut et al. (1986). Subjects with learning disabilities were found to tap more slowly than children without such disabilities when naming of animals was introduced, with a greater reduction in right-handed than left-handed tapping (Obrzut, Hynd, Obrzut, & Leitgeb, 1980). However, Hughes and Sussman (1983) found that language-concurrent tapping tasks reduced tapping in both hands for children with and without language disorders. An interesting effect noted in the performance of children with language disorders was a reduction in language output rather than a reduced rate of finger tapping. Different groups of readers with disability have shown varying patterns of performance on a verbal-spatial time-sharing task (Dalby & Gibson, 1981):

> *Dysphonetic* subjects exhibited patterns interpreted as bilateral representation of both verbal and spatial functions.
> *Dyseidetic* subjects' performance indicated bilateral verbal representation and right lateralization of spatial function.
> *Nonspecific* subjects exhibited patterns interpreted as left lateral verbal representation and bilateral spatial representation.

These results may be regarded as providing additional support for the hypotheses about aberrant hemispheric function in individuals with learning disabilities derived from other neuropsychological studies cited above.

Thus, despite some differences in the interpretation of the various types of psychometric investigations, there is a substantial degree of convergence regarding the neuropsychological behavioral patterns of individuals with language-related learning disabilities. Recent technological advances have opened new avenues of research into the physiology and anatomy of the brain, holding promise of increased understanding of anomalous information processing.

Direct Observation of Brain Structure and Function

A number of physiological techniques have been developed for noninvasive observation of brain activity during language-related task performance. Some of these have been in use for some time, and others reflect advances in computer technology.

Electroencephalogram (EEG) Research   The study of children's cerebral function is complicated because of variability related to a number of age or metabolic factors. In their review of this literature, Hynd and Semrud-Clikeman (1989) reported results of studies showing that only 68% and 77% of children and adolescents, respectively, without disabilities had normal EEGs. Nevertheless, in comparison to results on children without reading problems, EEG abnormalities have been reported more frequently in children with severe reading problems (Pirozzolo & Hansch, 1982).

Haynes, Haynes, and Strickland-Helms (1989) have conducted a review of EEG research on subjects with learning disabilities. Their results may be summarized as follows:

1. Less alpha attenuation in boys with than without learning disabilities on language and mathematical tasks, suggesting attentional deficit.
2. Significant power differences for certain brain wave frequencies between subjects with and without learning disabilities, especially in frontal-temporal regions; discriminant analyses of EEG power spectra have reliably predicted identification of subjects as having learning disabilities or not having such disabilities.
3. Major differences between children with and without dyslexia in bifrontal, left temporal, and left posterior quadrant regions; children with dyslexia exhibited alpha wave patterns indicative of relative cortical inactivity.

"Brainwave frequencies in the alpha band (8–13 Hz) have been found to reduce in amplitude during organized information processing" (Haynes et al., 1989, p. 391).

In their own research, Haynes et al. (1989) used the EEG technique to study hemispheric processing during receptive and expressive story-telling activity. Electroencephalograms were monitored in 12 subjects with learning disabilities and 12 subjects without such disabilities (ages 8–12 years) during a baseline vigilance condition, while listening to a story without an ending, and while rehearsing the completed story for retelling. No significant differences were found between groups under any task conditions. Significant differences across groups were found related to tasks, with increased suppression of alpha waves from rest condition, to comprehension, to rehearsal, indicating greater mental activity in the expected direction.

It was noted, however, that the quality of the narratives produced by the subjects with learning disabilities was markedly inferior to that of the narratives produced by controls. Therefore, the amount of brain activity may not necessarily be an index of the quality of that activity. The authors suggested that individuals with learning disabilities may engage in inefficient modes of information processing and/or may experience difficulty in organizing information in an efficient manner for retrieval. In any event, the procedures employed in this study were admittedly relatively gross technologically. Haynes et al. (1989) urged further research of similar naturalistic language processing tasks using more sophisticated instrumentation and analysis.

Other Physiological Techniques   Other investigative techniques emerging from advances in technology have begun to yield preliminary evidence of brain-behavior patterns in reading and learning disabilities. Table 1 presents descriptors of some of these techniques, summarizations of findings, and reference citations. Although the findings of the postmortem studies noted in Table 1 are valued for their contribution of direct neuropathological evidence about cerebral anomalies associated with developmental dyslexia, they are subject to some critical evaluation. Hynd and Semrud-Clikeman (1989) took note of poor documentation of the

Table 1. Procedures for study of brain structure and function

Procedures	Functions	Results	Sources
Brain electrical activity mapping (BEAM)	Measurement of activity in specific areas of the brain during various tasks	Useful in early diagnosis of developmental dyslexia	Pirozzolo, Dunn, and Zetusky (1983)
		Patterns of activation in localized areas differentiated dyslexics from nondyslexics	Duffy, Denckla, Bartels, and Sandini (1980)
	Comparison of pre- and posttraining patterns	Relationship between improved task performance and measured brain activity	Languis and Wittrock (1986)
Auditory-evoked response (AER)	Measurement of ongoing electrical activity time-locked to onset of external auditory events	Prediction of later language development from infant responses to speech cues	Molfese and Molfese (1986)
	Measurement of hemispheric specialization	Larger left hemispheric responses to verbal stimuli; larger right hemispheric responses to nonverbal stimuli	S. Campbell and Whittaker (1986)
Event-related potential (ERP)	Reactions to repetitive, precisely timed stimuli (e.g., words and music)	Differences in latencies between responses to words and chords varied across dyslexic and nondyslexic groups	Fried, Tanguay, Boder, Doubleday, and Greensite (1981)
Regional cerebral blood flow (rCBF)	Monitoring metabolic activity during task performance	Evidence of left and right brain processing differences	O'Boyle (1986)
	Differential diagnosis of dysphonetic and dyseidetic readers compared to normally achieving readers	Different patterns of left and right brain activation during different types of reading tasks; right hemispheric activation during narrative processing	Hynd, Hynd, Sullivan, and Kingsbury (1987)
Radiological techniques: computerized tomography (CT scans); magnetic resonance imaging (MRI)	Examination of symmetry or asymmetry of left and right hemispheres in normally achieving subjects and those with dyslexia	Reversed symmetry in 42% of dyslexics	Hier, LeMay, Rosenberger, and Perlo (1978); Rosenberger and Hier (1980)
		Review of research reveals majority of right-handed subjects with dyslexia have normal asymmetry	Parkins, Roberts, Reinarz, and Varney (1987)

(continued)

Table 1.   *(continued)*

Procedures	Functions	Results	Sources
		Subgroups (subjects who are left-handed or have severe language disorders) may show reversed or symmetrical patterns	Haslam, Dalby, Johns, and Rademaker (1981)
		No evidence of brain injury in subjects with dyslexia	Hynd and Semrud-Clikeman (1989)
Postmortem studies	Study of brain tissue in subjects with history of dyslexia	No evidence of gross abnormality; symmetry rather than expected asymmetry in certain areas	Galaburda (1988, 1989); Galaburda, Sherman, Rosen, Aboitz, and Geshwind (1985); Rosen, Sherman, and Galaburda (1986)
		Reorganization of nerve cells	Duane, 1989
		Microscopic cellular abnormalities predominantly in left hemisphere areas associated with language and reading	Galaburda, Sherman, Rosen, Aboitz, and Geshwind (1985); Hynd and Semrud-Clikeman (1989); Rosen, Sherman, and Galaburda (1986)

reading disability diagnosis, which is either historical in nature or derived from inadequate testing procedures and/or interpretation. They also called attention to discrepancies between the postmortem findings and those reported from other technological studies regarding sites of abnormalities. Finally, they cautioned that results based on small numbers of subjects must continue to be viewed as tenuous.

Hynd and Semrud-Clikeman (1989) have provided a fine-grained and provocative analysis of the frequently inconsistent results of research emanating from diverse methodologies. The reader is urged to consult this primary source, whose degree of technical detail exceeds the bounds of the present chapter. According to these authors, the long-standing recognition of cognitive-linguistic deficits correlated with processes deemed essential for reading suggests some neurodevelopmental pathology or anomaly disruptive to optimal neurocognitive function. Neurodevelopmental anomalies may very well not parallel patterns characteristic of adult pathology. For example, lesions reported from the postmortem studies of developmental dyslexia were scattered rather than discretely localized. However, these anomalies did tend to cluster heavily in those areas of the left hemisphere associated with lesions in adult aphasia. These areas may be vulnerable to morphological-functional aberrations in mid- to late fetal development because of later maturation and myelinization. From Luria's (1980) neurodevelopmental perspective, the effects of lesions in certain parts of the brain will manifest themselves differently at different stages of development. This dynamic interaction between cortical functions and development must be taken into account in the interpretation of measurements of cognitive-linguistic functions involved in the acquisition of reading.

Obrzut (1989) emphasized this relationship between development and cortical-functional organization, asserting that the brain is not fully developed until early adulthood. Therefore, studies of child neuropsychology are confounded by the difficulty in predicting cortical-functional organization in children without disabilities, let alone those experiencing neurological delay or deficiency. Furthermore, the evidence from subtype studies attests to the multiplicity of neurocognitive systems pertinent to the disruption of reading acquisition.

SUMMARY

There is substantial evidence that individuals with learning disabilities manifest different cognitive styles in the processing of information critical to literacy and academic performance. While such behavioral differences are assumed to reflect specific patterns of hemispheric function, there is, as yet, insufficient scientific evidence to establish brain-behavior correspondence. Neuropsychological research does point to a maladaptive allocation of right hemispheric resources during the processing of verbal information.

Extensive research has directed its efforts at determining the neurological foundations of dyslexia. Theories about the causes of presumed dysfunction vary, ranging from genetically determined individual differences to developmental anomalies and possible neurological impairment. It is noteworthy that recent research (reported in Chapter 7) has called into question the traditional characterization of dyslexia as a discrete, immutable, biologically based disorder (Shaywitz, Escobar, Shaywitz, Fletcher, & Makuch, 1992).

Since a number of subtypes of learning disabilities have been identified, a unitary etiological theory would be problematic. Investigative procedures reflecting technological advances are producing new information about patterns of brain structure and function during information processing for specific tasks by subjects with and without disabilities.

Brain-behavior relationships are complex to a degree that defies simplistic inferences from empirical research. Within the context of a century-long debate about the nature of intelligence, Gardner (1983) argued "that there is persuasive evidence for the existence of several *relatively autonomous* human intellectual competences" (p. 8), and that certain aspects of intelligence, such as linguistic, spatial, and mathematical, are independent of each other. However, in complex, higher level cognitive-linguistic processes, such as inferencing, comprehension of figurative language, and narratives, the boundary between right and left hemispheric functions becomes blurred (Gardner, 1983).

Nevertheless, the frontiers of knowledge about information processing at different levels of complexity are being explored by technology and methods of increasing sophistication. Current neuropsychological research and theory offer exciting prospects for further understanding of both normal and aberrant information processing. With increasing insight into the nature of the cognitive-linguistic problems of learning disabilities, improvements in habilitative and rehabilitative intervention may be anticipated.

7 / Linguistic Correlates of Learning Disabilities

The language problems associated with learning disabilities reported in the literature range from a degree of severity akin to aphasia (D.J. Johnson & Myklebust, 1967) to those of sufficient subtlety to escape detection until signaled by reading and/or learning failure (L. Bloom & Lahey, 1978). They may manifest themselves as deficiencies in some systems (i.e., phonological, morphological/syntactic, semantic, and/or pragmatic) but not in others. Predominant disability may exist in either the expressive or the receptive channel, or may occur as mixed receptive-expressive disorders (Bashir et al., 1983; Wiig & Semel, 1984). Within these channels, disabling conditions may predominate in the oral or written modalities, or in both to different degrees. The nature of the problems and the degree of severity may vary within individuals across age levels and may appear to diminish or increase in reaction to different educational demands throughout grade levels (Bashir et al., 1983).

In view of the multifaceted dimensions of language, such heterogeneity is not surprising. In the present description of language problems associated with learning and reading problems, a fully detailed catalogue of all possible aspects of deficiency has not been attempted. The reader is referred to Wiig and Semel (1984) for an exhaustive compilation of observed and potential areas of language deficit in children and adolescents with learning disabilities.

The intent in this chapter is to examine research findings that document language deficits in children and adolescents with learning disabilities in a search for any discernible patterns that may further understanding of the related disabilities. Reports of research are supplemented to a limited degree with reports of clinical observations made by the present author and by others in the literature. One such observational description of the language problems associated with school performance of children with learning disabilities was provided by Sawyer (1985):

> Limited spontaneous speech flow
> Word-finding difficulties
> Occasional production of novel words and phrases (e.g., "My earsight is good")
> Use of "immature for age" grammatical forms
> Difficulty untangling the relationships in more complex sentences
> Trouble remembering information and repeating information presented orally
> Poor spelling
> Poor reading decoding and comprehension (pp. 322–324)

Another list of descriptors summarized the types of problems encountered in the caseload of a speech-language pathologist in a school for children and adolescents with learning disabilities (A. Gerber & Bryen, 1981):

> Difficulty following oral directions
> Problems with processing and recall of critical information
> Deficient comprehension of basic vocabulary and concepts used in the classroom
> Difficulty with word retrieval
> Deficient ability to categorize in verbal tasks
> Deficits in the ability to organize thought prior to succinct oral output
> Reductions in the ability to abstract and express details in a descriptive task
> Reduced ability to make simple inferences
> Reduced ability to engage in flexible thinking

General impairment of auditory memory and comprehension, including problems of
    attention

In view of the wide range of deficiencies involving the various domains of language, this
chapter considers research in the areas of syntax and morphology, phonology, semantics, and
discourse in the oral and written modalities. Incidences of the problems listed above vary with
age and grade level. Therefore, information contributing to an understanding of language-
related learning disabilities has been organized into two major sections: 1) language/learning
problems in preschool children, and 2) language/learning problems in school-age students.
Each section discusses different aspects of deficit.

LANGUAGE/LEARNING PROBLEMS IN PRESCHOOL CHILDREN

A landmark study by de Hirsch and her associates (de Hirsch et al., 1965) highlighted early
signs of delay in language and other developmental areas predictive of later reading problems.
Among the factors contributing heavily to prediction of performance by the end of second
grade was kindergarten children's expressive language ability. These investigators found that
both the richness of verbal output and the ability to integrate details into an organized narrative
were excellent prognosticators of subsequent success or failure.

Characteristics of expressive language delay in those preschool children who were regarded as at risk for later academic difficulty were described (de Hirsch, 1981) as follows:

Unintelligible speech after 4 years of age
Occasional persistence of jargon
Undifferentiated output attributed to diffused input (i.e., either word configuration or
    word meaning may be unstable)
Verbal output limited in quantity and primitive in quality
Syntax generally immature and morphology delayed

Receptively, these children seemed not to attend to all necessary information fed to them
through the auditory verbal channel and not to understand all that they did hear. In summary
fashion, de Hirsch (1981) commented:

> Linguistic deficits, even subtle ones, are red flags in terms of subsequent learning difficulties. The
> child who around the age of 4 does not like to be read to, who does not follow the story line, the
> child who has severe word-finding difficulties (which is a matter of retrieval and not to be confused
> with vocabulary), and the youngster who uses only primitively constructed sentences—all are at
> risk in terms of first grade reading. (p. 63)

Other more specific deficits in young children include difficulty learning the alphabet,
rhyming, and remembering songs, finger-play routines, numbers, color names, and days of the
week (Wiig & Semel, 1984). Denckla (1972) noted that some of these deficiencies fall within
the category of rote skills, which may manifest themselves in subaverage scores on the Digit
Span and Coding subtests of the WISC (1949).

PREDICTORS OF ACADEMIC PROBLEMS

A number of investigators have studied the relationship between early language deficits and
later reading/writing performance. Deficits or delays in various aspects of language or language-related skills during preschool or at school entrance have been found to be significantly

predictive of subsequent reading difficulties and problems with written language. Table 1 provides an overview of this research.

TYPES OF PRESCHOOL LANGUAGE PROBLEMS

Bashir and his colleagues (1983) surveyed a number of longitudinal studies that tracked preschool children with language problems into grade school. Their findings provide additional support for conclusions about the nature of these students' persistent difficulties in language-related learning (i.e., reading and writing) into later school years. Bashir et al. (1983) categorized preschool children with language impairments into four groups, all of whom are at risk for later school difficulties:

1. Those with mixed receptive and expressive disorders, including varying production problems and deficits in the comprehension of single words and certain sentence structures, particularly complex or embedded
2. Those with primarily expressive problems consisting of syntactic and morphological delays, dysnomia, poor organization and maintenance of narratives, and differences between responses in unsolicited and solicited speaking situations
3. Those with dysnomia in the absence of syntactic or morphological deficits, with possible accompanying difficulty in story telling
4. Those with phonological disorders associated with voluntary motor production and sequencing of speech sounds

Table 1. Predictive studies of the relationship between early language deficits and later academic language performance

Study	Subject age/grade at time of original assessment	Predictors	Follow-up findings
Aram, Ekelman, and Nation (1984)	3;5 to 6;11 years (N = 20)	Phonemic formulation	Significant predictor of reading at adolescence
V.A. Mann (1984)	Kindergartners (N = 44)	Speed/accuracy of letter naming; syllable and phoneme awareness; verbal memory	Excellent predictors of first-grade reading achievement
Levi, Capozzi, Fabrizi, and Sechi (1982)	3;0 years (N = 32)	Measures of semantic, syntactic, and phonological deficits	Retardation in all areas predicted reading/writing difficulty at 6–7 years more accurately than phonology alone
	6;0 years	Syntactic deficits	Highly associated with reading difficulty
Silva, McGee, and Williams (1983)	3;0 years	Comprehension deficits	45% had reading difficulty or low IQ at 7 years
	(N = 891)		
Lassman (1980)	3;0 years (N = 20, 137)	Delay on language protocol	2–3 times more likely than subjects without delay to fail written communication protocol at 8 years

These patterns have been observed with some minor variations through the present author's clinical experience with preschool children having language impairments. The following description of mixed receptive and expressive disorders may be helpful in making these generalizations more concrete:

> Manuel's speech at 3 years of age was largely jargon interspersed with recognizable words. At 3,8 years syntactic evaluation revealed an MLU [mean length of utterance] of 3.63 and emerging but delayed acquisition of age-appropriate morphology. Receptively he demonstrated great difficulty learning the directional terms "over" and "under". He also manifested processing problems in response to directions, appearing to attend to some but not all critical information. For example, when asked to point to a bird in a tree, he pointed to a bird in the sky.
>
> Subsequently, at age 4,6 intelligence testing revealed performance at age level on nonverbal tasks. Receptive and expressive vocabulary were depressed by approximately one half to one full year respectively. Echolalia in response to adult questions or directions was fairly frequent, demonstrating comprehension failure. (A. Gerber & Mastriano, 1991, p. 79)

Most of the children from this clinical group with similar problems were placed in programs for students with learning disabilities on entrance into the primary grades. All qualified for such placement because of normal intelligence and absence of impairments other than language disorder. Although the data on ultimate progress are fragmentary, academic difficulties through the first year in school were expected and experienced by those on whom there was at least partial report. Feedback received 1–2 years later also provided evidence, however, of eventual improvement in language as a result of both early intervention and maturation. (See A. Gerber and Mastriano [1991] for a description of the preschool intervention program.)

It should be stressed that all children do not mature at the same rate. de Hirsch (1981) labeled some of those who are intellectually normal but cognitively, linguistically, and/or emotionally immature the "unready children." She cited research reporting that 25% of kindergarten children are poor listeners, poor processors of linguistic input: "They understand nouns and verbs and most prepositions, but if the teacher shows them . . . boxes each containing four words and says: 'Draw a line to connect the ones that look alike', these children are at a loss" (p. 63). She went on to state that children who cannot comprehend the language encountered in early education will retreat to daydreaming and inattentiveness. "There are many youngsters who have learned *not* to listen before they are seven" (de Hirsch, 1981, p. 64).

EARLY IDENTIFICATION ISSUES

A cautionary note must be sounded about early identification of preschool children as having learning disabilities. At the most, it would seem judicious to regard them as "at risk" rather than to label them with a special education classification prior to actual academic failure, considering the possible negative effects of such labeling (Esterly & Griffin, 1987). A number of authors have emphasized the variations in preschool children's rate of maturation, acknowledging that there is an inescapable degree of hypothesizing about the relationship of early delay and future learning problems (Keogh & Becker, 1973; Keogh, Tchir, & Windeguth-Behn, 1974; A. Lewis, 1980). In numerous cases, the "at risk" status has been reportedly transitory, with predictions of later learning failure unconfirmed. It has been stressed that such predictions of school failure for the very young child "cannot take into account the range and interaction of compensatory factors available to the individual child" (A. Lewis, 1980, p. 56). One of the concerns expressed by state consultants in a nationwide survey of practices for service delivery to preschool children at risk for academic difficulties was a need for "establishment of identification criteria for children who have not begun formal education" (Esterly & Griffin, 1987, p. 573).

The above caution about early identification is not intended as a recommendation for lack of action in cases of early language deficits. To the contrary, early intervention is believed to be indispensable to fostering growth in areas of delay, in the hope of *preventing* subsequent academic failure. However, it is urged that premature categorical labeling be deferred to avoid undue stigma and possible lowering of expectations.

LANGUAGE-RELATED LEARNING PROBLEMS IN SCHOOL-AGE STUDENTS

The literature is replete with research and theory on the relationship of various aspects of language to academic learning problems, both written and oral. A general relationship between oral language ability and educational performance has been recognized by some authorities for the past half century (Loban, 1963; Orton, 1937; Van Riper, 1954). Over the past 2 decades, scholars and practitioners have been engaged in the increasingly refined delineation of the nature of deficits in specific linguistic systems that have an impact on language for learning.

The relationship between language impairment and academic learning difficulties has been demonstrated to exist throughout the school years. Table 2 presents an overview of five studies that followed the progress of students identified as having language impairment. Each study reports: 1) the age of subjects who had been diagnosed as having language impairment at the time of the initial observation (time 1), 2) the age of the same subjects at the second observation after a substantial interval (time 2), and 3) patterns of language and/or learning problems manifested by these older subjects at time 2.

This section examines some of the literature that describes deficits in syntax/morphology, phonology, semantics, and discourse processing as they relate to problems in receptive and expressive processing in reading, writing, and the oral language of education. Admittedly, these systems function interactively, but in many instances a particular aspect of language is selected for research, reflecting the investigators' current focus and/or point of view. In the interest of organizational manageability, some artificial separation must be tolerated, with the understanding that distortion is subsequently inevitable but (it is hoped) has been contained to a minimum.

SYNTACTIC/MORPHOLOGICAL PROBLEMS

Expressive Abilities

Throughout the past 2 decades, results of investigations of syntactic/morphological abilities in children with learning disabilities have been, at times, disparate. This phenomenon may be explained by: 1) possible lack of homogeneity across investigations in sample types, and 2) variations in experimental procedures. With regard to heterogeneity of student subjects, it has been noted above (and continues to be discussed below) that some subjects with learning disabilities have exhibited overt oral language impairment whereas others, demonstrating reading and writing disabilities, have not been identified as having language impairment by either formal or informal measures. The research reviewed and summarized here (Andolina, 1980; Donahue, Pearl, & Bryan, 1982; Fletcher, Satz, & Scholes, 1981; Idol-Maestas, 1980; Klecan-Aker, 1985; Minskoff, 1976; Moran, 1981a; Moran & Byrne, 1977; Semel & Wiig,

Table 2. Relationships between language impairment and later learning problems in school-age children

Studies	Ages at times 1 and 2	Findings at time 2
Stark, Bernstein, Condino, Bender, Tallal, and Catts (1984)	Time 1 mean CA[a] 6;6 Time 2 mean CA 10;3 (N = 29)	90% showed some degree of reading disability; almost 80% required remedial instruction
Strominger and Bashir (1977)	Time 1 CA 5;0 Time 2 CA 9–11 (N = 40)	38 of 40 had language-related learning problems
Aram and Nation (1980)	Time 1 mean CA 4;7 Time 2 mean CA 10;4 (N = 63)	Half had observable language problems; other half had learning problems
Aram, Ekelman, and Nation (1984)	Time 1: 3;5 to 6;11 Time 2: 13;3 to 16;10 (N = 20)	60% in learning disability class or regular education plus tutorial assistance; only 25% scored above 50th percentile in reading and spelling
King, Jones, and Lasky (1982)	Time 1 mean CA 13;10 Time 2 mean CA 20;5 (N = 50)	42% had continuing communication problems, 52% had academic problems

[a]CA, chronological age.

1975; Siegel & Ryan, 1984; Snyder & Downey, 1991; Vogel, 1975; Wiig & Roach, 1975; Wiig & Semel, 1974, 1975; Wren, 1983) includes such variations in its samples. It also reports on results emanating from the following experimental procedures used in different studies to secure and analyze samples of language:

Structured elicitation tasks
    Sentence repetition
    Sentence generation
    Location and correction of grammatical errors
    Oral cloze procedure (sentence completion)
Analysis of communicative language samples
    Responses to questions and requests for information
    Monologues on designated topics
    Generation of stories about movies or television programs
    Conversation in referential communication games
Measures for analysis
    Developmental Sentence Scoring (DSS) (L.L. Lee, 1974)
    Mean length of utterance (MLU)
    T-units (one main clause plus attached subordinate clauses and nonclausal structures)
    Conjunction of clauses via cohesive ties
    Frequency of different parts of speech

ıdies yield the following generalizations:

1. Subjects with learning disabilities make more errors of omission, reversal, and substitution in sentence repetition than do peers without disabilities. Substitutions tend to be words from the same grammatical class. The gist of the sentence is generally retained in the presence of errors in the surface form (Minskoff, 1976; Wiig & Roach, 1975). For example:

   Stimulus: The woman carried the twelve, old heavy brown books.
   Response: The woman carried twelve old books.

   Stimulus: Jack likes french fries with hamburgers with relish and ketchup.
   Response: Jack likes hot-dogs and hamburgers with beans and ketchup.

   Stimulus: The robber that the police caught escaped easily.
   Response: The robber escaped easily. (Wiig & Semel, 1984, p. 318)

2. Children with learning disabilities are poorer than children without disabilities in detecting and correcting grammatical errors in presented sentences (Siegel & Ryan, 1984).

3. Children with reading disability made significantly more errors on a sentence completion task than do normally achieving readers (Snyder & Downey, 1991). On the oral cloze procedure, subjects with learning disabilities requested more repetitions than did subjects without disabilities in order to hold onto surrounding context before supplying the missing word (Vogel, 1975).

4. Children with learning disabilities demonstrate less mastery than children without disabilities of the morphological inflections for verb tense, plurality, and possession (Fletcher et al., 1981; Moran & Byrne, 1977; Siegel & Ryan, 1984).

5. Children and adolescents with learning disabilities produce shorter MLUs and T-units and achieve lower scores on the DSS than do peers without disabilities (Andolina, 1980; Donahue et al., 1982; Idol-Maestas, 1980; Wiig & Semel, 1975).

6. Six-year-old children with learning disabilities have been reported to demonstrate varying degrees of syntactic immaturity in contrast to peers without disabilities (Wren, 1983).

7. Children with learning disabilities have demonstrated syntactic growth across grades 2, 4, 6, and 8 in some studies. Others note a plateau effect at around grade 6 into early adolescence (Andolina, 1980; Donahue et al., 1982; Idol-Maestas, 1980).

8. The differences beteeen preadolescent subjects with and without learning disabilities on words per T-unit, clauses per T-unit, and words per clause were not statistically significant (Klecan-Aker, 1985; Moran, 1981b).

9. Of 14 parts of speech analyzed for frequency of occurrence, only two (adverbs and auxiliary verbs) differentiated groups with and without learning disabilities, and only to a 2–2.5% difference (Moran, 1981b).

10. In written language, adolescents without disabilities were superior to students with learning disabilities on mean morphemes per T-unit (a measure of productivity) but not on the percentage of complex T-units, a measure of structural mastery (Moran, 1981b). (The method of scoring ignored punctuation errors in the marking of sentence boundaries.)

11. Subjects with learning disabilities used fewer cohesive conjunctions than did subjects without disabilities, and less variation in the types of conjunctions (Moran, 1988).

Despite the evidence of developmental delay—that is, slower growth in the ultimate acquisition of mature syntax—there is evidence in a number of the samples studied of persistent patterns in what may be characterized as performance, rather than competence, deficits. It is possible that development of the ability to imitate sentences orally or generate well-formed written sentences may be impeded by such factors as a generalized verbal memory deficit, working memory limitations, word retrieval problems, deficient pragmatic/discourse skills, and a lesser inclination to verbally encode information with specificity and elaboration.

Receptive Abilities

A variety of syntactic structures have been found to contribute to comprehension problems for subjects with learning disabilities in contrast to achieving peers—for example, questions, passives, and direct-indirect object relations (Semel & Wiig, 1975) and certain types of complex sentences containing relative clauses and adverbial or infinitival complements (Byrne, 1981; Morice & Slaghuis, 1985; C.L. Stein, Cairns, & Zurif, 1984; Wallach, 1984; Wallach & Goldsmith, 1975). There is evidence suggesting that subjects with reading/learning disabilities use less mature comprehension strategies than achieving peers, relying unduly on semantic rather than syntactic knowledge in interpreting sentences (Byrne, 1981; Roth & Spekman, 1989b).

For example, poor and good 7- to 8-year-old readers did not differ in their ability to interpret sentences like "The apple that the boy is eating is red." However, poor readers were less accurate in interpreting sentences like "The cow that the monkey is scaring is yellow." In the former sentence real-world knowledge may provide the main clues to grammatical structure for children who are syntactically less mature. The latter sentence type, lacking the semantic constraints to support interpretation, requires resort to syntactic strategies for interpretation (Byrne, 1981).

Wiig and Semel (1984) presented a lengthy compilation of other potential areas of receptive syntactic and morphological problems for the child and adolescent with learning disabilities, some of which have been clinically observed by them. The extensive length and detail of this material precludes its inclusion here. Some other aspects of comprehension difficulty reported by Wren (1983) as clinically observed, although not rigorously researched, are the following:

> Difficulty with clause structure that deviates from the expected order for purpose of emphasis: "With your right hand, point to the letter A" (p. 125).
> Difficulty with certain question forms: "Which is bigger, a kitten or a cat?" (p. 125).
> Difficulty with certain forms of embedding: "Whoever wins gets a prize." (p. 126).

Syntactic Deficits and Reading Disability

Generalizations about the interaction between reported syntactic/morphological deficits and reading disabilities are problematic for at least four reasons. First, not all students with reading disability manifest any discernible language deficit. Doehring, Trites, Patel, and Fiedorowicz (1981) reported that, of their 88 subjects with reading disability (mean age, 12,3 years), only about 50% were observed to have language problems as measured in a number of areas, including syntactic usage, in which they averaged 5 years below the level expected for their age. The other 50% exhibited age-appropriate language.

Further confirmation of the absence of uniformly deficient linguistic structure in this population was secured by Roth and Spekman (1989b). Calling into question the accepted conclusion that all children with reading/learning disabilities are delayed in syntax and morphology, they selected a sample of 46 children (8;0 to 13;11 years) classified as having learning disabilities but exhibiting no oral language deficits on formal or informal observations. Systematic analysis of their sentences elicited in spontaneously generated stories, compared to those of achieving peers, revealed "nearly identical rates of *correct* usage and highly similar usage *patterns* on all measures of syntactic complexity examined" (p. 73).

Despite Roth and Spekman's challenge to the long-standing consensus that syntactic problems are widely prevalent among students with reading/learning disabilities, there is counterevidence that such problems do exist. Examples of syntactic immaturity in adolescents with learning disabilities are provided in the following sentences generated by 12- to 14-year-old subjects asked to talk about ice cream:

> I like a whole big ice cream, big ice cream, big ice cream.
> Ice cream lasts long, long, long.
> My mother has a giant bowl of ice cream and full of cake.   (Wiig & Semel, 1984, p. 316)

A second factor that must be taken into account is the age of the subjects and the stage of reading acquisition investigated. As noted above, at the early stage of schooling, significant differences were found between good and poor readers in comprehension of syntactically complex sentences (Morice & Slaghuis, 1985). It is suggested that such comprehension difficulties at school entry "preceded reading impairment and may have been instrumental in its development" (p. 154). However, those who may have mastered basic syntactic patterns adequate to meet the demands of simple constructions encountered in early reading may experience difficulty with more complex constructions found in more advanced texts (Roth & Spekman, 1989b).

Although measured syntactic/morphological deficiencies are reported to exist in samples of students with reading disability, a discrepancy does exist between degrees of severity in the two areas. It has been pointed out that the severity of the reading disability is not matched by the relatively milder impairment in oral syntax (Byrne, 1981; Glass & Perna, 1986; Kamhi & Catts, 1986; Kamhi, Catts, Mauer, Apel, & Gentry, 1988). "Linguistic maturity expressed in syntactic control is far from an infallible guide to reading skill" (Byrne, 1981, p. 210). The relatively mild impairment of higher level semantic-syntactic skills observed by Doehring et al. (1981) in their sample of students with reading disability led to the tentative conclusion that "most subjects do not have a generalized language disorder" (p. 139). However, the possible confounding effect of an interaction between syntax and semantics is another factor requiring consideration.

Glass and Perna (1986) attempted to determine the nature of relationships among deficits in syntax, vocabulary, and both auditory and reading comprehension. Correlations were found among all of these variables. However, when the effects of vocabulary were partialed out, correlations between syntax and comprehension did not reach significance. It was reasoned that syntactic development is at least partially dependent on a vocabulary large enough to allow the child to understand meanings of words in an utterance, to a level that permits informed guesses at the syntactic structure. The implication that vocabulary deficits may underlie syntactic deficits is countered by other findings demonstrating that, in the presence of superior vocabulary, syntactic deficits were apparent in a subgroup of children with learning disabilities, to a degree that interfered with processing complex sentences and stories (Feagans & Appelbaum, 1986).

It becomes increasingly apparent that the relationships among syntax, semantics, and reading continue to require investigation. At issue here is the question of deficits in discrete linguistic systems, in different groups, to different degrees, and at different stages, in contrast to a more generalized language impairment. Support does exist, empirically and theoretically, for individualized deficits in such discrete systems as syntax versus vocabulary (Kemper, 1989). While a substantial proportion of individuals diagnosed as having impaired language may exhibit deficits in all systems, caseloads of many speech-language pathologists include those with problems predominantly or exclusively in one linguistic system. For example, there are many children with delayed articulation who do not manifest problems in syntax or semantics and whose academic achievement is unremarkable. In other cases, relative impoverishment of vocabulary (for a number of possible reasons) may exist in the presence of age-appropriate syntax.

In contrast, poorer performance by children with reading disability on certain measures of syntactic ability have been found to coexist with measures of other verbal abilities (Siegel & Ryan, 1988), leading these investigators to the conclusion: "These findings clearly support the idea that reading disability represents a language disorder" (p. 34). Thus, while correlations between syntactic deficits and reading disability have been found to be positive, inferences about direct causality between the measured syntactic deficit and reading disability are not necessarily justified, since the relationship may reflect problems in other aspects of language as well (Kamhi, 1988).

One further point made by Roth and Spekman (1989b) attempts to place the research findings on syntactic deficits among individuals with reading/learning disabilities and assumptions about their significance into perspective. They asserted that statistical differences between syntactic skills in the two groups (with and without reading disability) do not necessarily represent *deficiencies*. To illustrate this distinction, subjects with reading disability in their study achieved an 86.57% correct rate on overall usage of complex sentences, in contrast to a 93.26% correct usage rate achieved by the group without disabilities. Although the difference between group performances reached significance, "a correct usage rate of nearly 87% by the [learning disabled] subjects cannot be interpreted as a syntactic deficit" (p. 76). While this interpretation is justifiable for the sample in this particular study, it is not necessarily generalizable to all samples reported in the literature, nor, perhaps, to all individuals with language-related learning disabilities.

Summary of Syntactic/Morphological Problems

From the foregoing information, it may be concluded that most individuals with language/learning disabilities who are functioning within educational settings are *not* individuals with severe dysphasia who acquire only very limited language. Rather, they appear to be those who *have* acquired language at a slower rate than "normally" achieving peers, with their upper level of language development reflecting a lesser degree of verbal proficiency. Such individuals have frequently been reported to produce less elaborated sentences that may fall short of fully encoding all possible relevant information, and they may experience difficulty comprehending some syntactic structures of high complexity. Yet there is evidence that basic, functional syntactic skills have been largely acquired over the course of the elementary school years.

Three questions demand attention in efforts to understand the nature of structural language deficits that *do* persist and their relation to academic learning (particularly reading). The first question concerns the apparent interaction between syntactic knowledge and memory. A number of the studies cited above have reported poorer performance by the subjects with language/learning disabilities on sentence repetition and/or oral cloze tasks, as well as tests of short-term memory, that seemed to implicate deficits in auditory verbal memory. A causal connection between memory deficits and syntactic deficits is not universally assumed, since it is acknowledged that linguistic knowledge may facilitate working memory in top-down information processing. Conversely, deficient linguistic knowledge may place greater demands on short-term and working memory. However, from results of research surveyed by Menyuk (1988), evidence exists that is suggestive of relations between aspects of memory and language development or use. This information is summarized in Table 3.

While accepting a description of reading disability as a language-based disorder, Kamhi (1989) sought to explain the described deficiencies in terms of underlying processing limitations. Among these limitations, he includes "inefficient regulation of information in working memory" (p. 92). Other contributing factors are believed to reflect interactions among various linguistic and cognitive processes, many of which are discussed in the remainder of the present chapter and in Chapter 8.

A second question concerns the variability in predictive power of the different aspects of language for later reading achievement. For example, syntactic development was found to be a less successful predictor than phonological ability in one study, whereas semantic/syntactic ability was reportedly more predictive in another. A distinction has been made between the possible negative effects of a syntactic lag on reading comprehension in contrast to a phonological lag detrimental to word analysis skills (Kamhi, 1989). From longitudinal studies extending into the upper age/grade levels, it does appear that, while higher level syntactic/semantic abilities continue to improve, phonological disabilities of some sort persist and appear to be closely associated with reading disability (Doehring et al., 1981). It is also possible that, although manifested syntactic deficits decrease throughout the school years, a more subtle residue may continue in the form of a reduction in metalinguistic abilities regarded as important in the reading process (Mattingly, 1972). For example, Cambourne and Rousch (1982) found that children with reading impairment were more likely than achieving peers to make errors that violated syntactic constraints in reading sentences, although spoken syntax was observed to be intact. Such deficiencies have been attributed to an underdeveloped syntactic system, cues from which aid in the effective decoding of individual words (Vellutino, 1977). These issues are discussed below.

The last question stems from the statement by Doehring et al. (1981) that the results of their study do not justify the conclusion that the reading problems were caused by the observed language deficits. "Failure to master the mechanics of reading could contribute to any or all of the language deficits that were found. The reading and language deficits must be interpreted in interactive rather than cause–effect terms" (p. 139). This view seems to fly in the face of the evidence provided by longitudinal studies of the relationship between earlier language deficits and subsequent reading acquisition. Nonetheless, it is recognized that, at more advanced levels of schooling, the interactive effects of language deficit and reading disability are likely to be reciprocal (Glass & Perna, 1986; Kamhi, 1989). That is, inadequate exposure to the language of literacy because of reading disabilities is likely to reduce input of more advanced syntactic structures that may contribute to ongoing development in language proficiency. A fuller discussion of this issue is presented later in this chapter and in Chapter 8. What is evident from the

Table 3.   Aspects of linguistic ability and memory functions

Aspects of language	Memory functions
1. Delays in development of basic syntax and morphophonology, including markers of tense, number, and location	Keeping in mind both basic syntactic and semantic relations and surface markers
2. Difficulty processing coordinated or embedded sentences	Keeping in mind relations among clausal/sentential units
3. Reductions in ability to follow oral commands containing expanded noun phrases	Storing and retrieving appropriate information in working memory
4. Developmental differences in use of anaphoric reference	Holding in mind features that differentiate referents from nonreferents

Adapted from Menyuk (1988).

foregoing discussion is that, while syntactic deficits may coexist with reading disability, the nature of that specific relationship remains unclear.

PHONOLOGICAL PROBLEMS

There has been extensive investigation of the relation between the phonological component of language and academic learning problems, with particular emphasis on reading. As was evident in the area of syntax, research is characterized by diversity in aspects selected for study, methods used, and results that frequently may be conflicting. The complexity of the phenomena being studied precludes the emergence of straightforward, unequivocal findings in all areas. Nonetheless, some important insights have been gained about probable relations between deficits in phonological processing and reading disability. Three prominent lines of research into relationships between phonological deficits and language-related learning disabilities are: 1) phonetic coding in short-term memory; 2) perception of auditory verbal material at the automatic level (i.e., out of awareness); and 3) phonological awareness, with particular emphasis on segmentation of linguistic material into its component elements.

V.A. Mann (1984) enumerated some of the manifestations of phonological problems as follows:

> Difficulty with short-term memory for verbal material, such as strings of digits, words, and even the words of spoken sentences
> Difficulty identifying spoken words partially masked by noise
> Difficulty recovering the phonetic representation of words (p. 122)

These problems and others (some of which are addressed in other sections in the present chapter) have been attributed to a basic deficiency in the use of phonetic representation in short-term memory that negatively affects reading as well as certain aspects of oral language. The reader will recall from Chapter 3 that phonemic or phonetic coding of information enhances its retention in short-term memory.

Phonetic Representation in Working Memory

I.Y. Liberman and her colleagues (I.Y. Liberman & Shankweiler, 1979; Shankweiler & Liberman, 1972) have underscored the function of phonetic representation in working memory as one important determinant of speech-language processing and reading. "The role of the phonetic representation in speech perception is to hold information about shorter segments (say, words) in short-term memory until the meaning of longer segments (say, sentences) can be extracted" (I. Y. Liberman & Shankweiler, 1979, p. 110). Much of the work done by Liberman and her associates has demonstrated that the memory deficit observed in poor readers is indeed verbal, not visual.

Research by a number of different investigators has shown that good readers are significantly better than poor readers at remembering verbally codable material, such as nonsense syllables or words. However, no significant difference has been found between the two groups in memory for non–verbally codable material, such as faces or nonsense designs. These findings have led to the conclusion that poor readers do not suffer from a generalized memory deficit, but differ only on memory for linguistic items, and that this deficit is probably restricted to the domain of phonetic representation in short-term memory (I. Y. Liberman, Mann, Shankweiler, & Werfelman, 1982; Mann & Brady, 1988; Pratt & Brady, 1988; Torgeson, 1988b; Vellutino, 1979).

One experimental procedure for examining effects of phonetic coding has demonstrated that phonetically confusable items, such as letter names that rhyme (e.g., *B C G T*), are more difficult to recall than nonconfusable items (e.g., *M R W E*) (Conrad, 1972). Reduced recall of confusable material in experimental tasks has been accepted as evidence that the stimulus information is being phonetically coded, whereas a lack of such a reduction is regarded as evidence of failure to encode material phonetically.

A sizable body of research has demonstrated that, when visual or auditory material to be remembered is phonetically confusable, recall by good readers is penalized to a greater degree than recall by poor readers. That is, good readers have been shown to encode material phonetically and, therefore, are at a memory disadvantage when items are phonetically similar. In contrast, there is substantial evidence of poor readers' failure to encode visually presented linguistic material phonetically, because results have shown a lack of penalty on their memory for phonetically confusable material (Hardy, McIntyre, Brown, & North, 1989; I. Y. Liberman & Shankweiler, 1979; Siegel & Linder, 1984; Siegel & Ryan, 1988). The implication of these findings has been that poor readers are less likely than good readers to engage in phonetic coding in short-term memory, with detrimental effects on reading-related short-term memory processes.

The general assumption that children with reading disabilities fail to use phonetic codes for short-term memory processing has been questioned, however, on the basis of evidence that the rhyming effect appears to be present only when stimulus length taxes the system. When short sequences of nonsense syllables with and without the confusability of rhyme were used, the penalizing effects of rhyme were not found (Brady, Mann, & Schmidt, 1987). Nevertheless, evidence continues to be reported that implicates *less efficient* activation of both phonetic and visual codes during the initial processing stages of confusable material (Hardy et al., 1989). It is surmised that these deficiencies during early information processing stages have a negative impact on later stages of processing for recall.

Perceptual Deficits in Phonological Processing

The use of techniques other than stimulus confusability during investigation of phonetic coding in short-term memory has produced evidence leading to a different interpretation of the phonological deficit manifested by poor readers. Brady and her colleagues (Brady, Shank-weiler, & Mann, 1983; Brady et al., 1987) reported that auditory verbal material presented under noisy listening conditions was recalled less accurately by poor than good readers, but that presented under quiet conditions was not less accurately recalled. This result was interpreted as evidence that poor readers do encode phonetically but less efficiently than good readers. Brady has ascribed the less efficient use of the phonetic code to a perceptual deficit rather than to a disinclination to employ phonetic coding per se.

It is important to keep in mind, however, that perceptual and related short-term memory deficits manifested by poor readers have been limited to linguistic material, since poor readers have not differed from good readers in their perception of nonlinguistic (environmental) sounds in a noise-masked condition (I.Y. Liberman, 1987). Speech sound perception and auditory closure, characterized as measures of phonological analysis, were the tests that most consistently differentiated between children with and without reading disabilities (Rourke et al., 1986). Summarizing a review of research on the nature of phonological problems involved in the processing of written and oral language, V.A. Mann (1984) asserted:

> it is, by now, quite clear that poor readers in the early elementary grades . . . do not suffer from a general impairment in perception, or in learning and memory, so much as from a language impairment *that specifically penalizes certain phonological processing skills.* (p. 122) [italics added for emphasis]

Phonological Processing Deficits in Reading and Language Disabilities

Other aspects of phonological processing have been examined in a series of studies by Kamhi, Catts, and their colleagues (Catts, 1986; Kamhi & Catts, 1986; Kamhi et al., 1988). These investigators have attempted to determine whether the phonological processing deficiencies observed in children with reading impairment are similar to or distinguishable from those characteristic of children with language impairment. They have compared performance of normally achieving children with that of children classified as having reading impairment but not identified as having overt language impairment, and children identified as having language but not reading impairment on a number of tasks designed to tap (among other processes) phonological perception, phonological representation, and speech production abilities. The tasks from the most recent study (Kamhi et al., 1988) that are relevant to present concerns consisted of:

> Repetition of monosyllabic consonant-vowel-consonant (CVC) nonsense words (e.g., *sar*)
> Repetition of monosyllabic CVC nonsense words in noise
> Repetition/recall of series of three CVC nonsense words
> Repetition of multisyllabic nonsense words varying in phonetic complexity (e.g., *manemem, stesafik*)

A descriptive summary of some of the results is presented in Table 4.

All three groups experienced difficulty repeating nonsense words against background noise. It is of particular interest that the children with reading disability but no overt language disorder, as well as those with identified language impairment, performed more poorly than children without disabilities on the simple task of repeating even single CVC nonsense words, thereby demonstrating phonological processing deficits in both groups with disabilities. Similarly, the children with reading disability did not differ significantly from those with language

Table 4. Group means (*M*) and standard deviations (*SD*) for four word repetition tasks

Subject group	Word repetition tasks[a]			
	Monosyllabic (25)	Noise (25)	Three-item (30)	Multisyllabic (40)
Language impairment				
M	17.6	12.5	15.8	16.3
SD	3.0	4.0	3.4	4.8
Reading impairment				
M	18.7	14.0	17.0	23.7
SD	2.9	2.4	5.0	9.7
Normal				
M	23.8	16.4	25.1	29.6
SD	1.2	2.7	2.4	7.9

Excerpted from Kamhi, Catts, Mauer, Apel, and Gentry (1988).

[a]Numbers in parentheses indicate total possible correct.

impairment in repeating strings of nonsense words, with children without disabilities performing significantly better than both groups with disabilities. Only on the repetition of multisyllabic nonsense words were the two groups with disabilities differentiated, with significantly poorer performance by children with language impairment than by those with reading disability. Children without disabilities again performed significantly better than both groups with disabilities.

Kamhi and Catts (1986) reasoned that similar phonological processing deficits underlie reading and language disability but to differing degrees of severity. They proposed as a candidate for causality some "low-level perceptual deficits in identifying and discriminating phonemes and difficulty forming accurate representations of linguistic (or linguistic-like) information" (p. 344), a tentative conclusion in agreement with the findings of Brady et al. (1983, 1987).

It was also conjectured that the greater degree of severity observed in children with language impairment may be attributed to a more specific deficit in speech programming abilities. In their more recent work, Kamhi et al. (1988) have taken into consideration the differences between reading and oral language:

> The most obvious differences are between expressive language abilities and written word recognition processes. As we have stated before, written word recognition problems are attributed primarily to difficulty processing phonological information. In contrast, expressive language problems can be caused by deficits in syntactic, semantic, phonological, or pragmatic knowledge and processes. An intriguing speculation is that the difficulty LI [language-impaired] children seem to have in programming complex phonological sequences might reflect a more basic difficulty in programming or formulating grammatically well-formed utterances. (p. 325)

It is thus conceivable that ostensibly similar performance of children with language impairment and those with reading impairment on phonological processing measures may reflect distinctly different dimensions of language disability. These complex issues are not amenable to full clarification here. The murkiness is, in part, attributable to the artificial, although logistically unavoidable, separation of the phonological component from the other components of language within the organization of this chapter. However, another factor meriting consideration is the distinction between primary linguistic and metalinguistic abilities specific to heightened phonological awareness.

Deficits in Phonological Awareness

One of the major areas of research into phonological processing deficits has been the study of the relationship between reading disability and the ability to explicitly segment units of linguistic material into their component elements.

Phoneme Segmentation   Phoneme segmentation is the ability to discern the separate sounds contained within a word, in contrast to perceiving only the holistic combination of sounds in a word associated with its meaning. An example is the ability to detemine that the word *sit*, perceived as a single unit of sound associated with the meaning of placing the body on a horizontal surface, is composed of the three phonemic segments /S/, /I/, and /T/. As reported earlier in this chapter, deficient ability to segment the syllable into its component phonemes has been associated with poor reading acquisition by children.

The studies by Kamhi and Catts (1986) and Kamhi et al. (1988) discussed above also examined as a second focus the performance of children with language impairment and those with reading impairment on a group of metalinguistic tasks in the phonological and morphological domains. For example, children were asked to segment words into phonemes, divide nonsense words into their syllabic segments, and segment sentences into their component words. Another metalinguistic task required judgments about the correctness of morphological forms in sentences, such as "They throwing the stick." Some of the results may be summarized as follows:

1. No significant group differences were found on the division of words into syllables. All performed this task with high degrees of success.
2. All groups (with and without impairment) had difficulty segmenting words into phonemes.
3. Children with reading impairment performed significantly more poorly than achieving peers on the sentence division task.
4. Both groups of children with disabilities (language and reading) made significantly more errors than did children without impairment on the test of morphological awareness.

It is of particular interest that the word repetition results described in the previous section on primary phonological processing deficits did not correlate significantly with any of the measures of phonological awareness described in the present section. Thus, it may be assumed that out-of-awareness and in-awareness tasks were tapping different phonological processing skills. Kamhi and Catts (1986) are inclined toward the belief that there are certain "phonological processing skills that are highly correlated to reading performance but vary independently of language ability" (p. 345).

Research on Phonological Awareness and Reading   More than a decade of research has investigated the relationship between phonological awareness and reading acquisition using a number of methods for studying and training subjects, with the following results:

1. Backward readers performed more poorly than age-appropriate readers on a sound categorization task involving identification of the one word out of four that did not have a common initial, medial, or final phoneme (Bradley & Bryant, 1978).

2. High correlations existed between performance on the above sound categorization task and reading and spelling achievement (Bradley & Bryant, 1983).
3. Training in sound categorization in conjunction with letter identification yielded strong support for a causal, rather than correlational, relationship between phonological awareness and reading and spelling achievement (Bradley & Bryant, 1983).
4. Training in phonemic segmentation and blending was found to be causally related to reading acquisition (Fox & Routh, 1976, 1984).
5. Ability to identify sounds and their sequential relations in syllables differentiated high- and low-ability second-grade students (Calfee, Lindamood, & Lindamood, 1973).
6. Kindergarten children who were poor at counting syllables in words were poorer readers in first grade (V.A. Mann, 1984).
7. High correlations were obtained between decoding scores (timed and untimed) and scores on a consonant deletion test of phonological awareness by poor decoders (Lenchner, Gerber, & Routh, 1990).
8. Phonemic segmentation and blending tests yielded scores that were most highly correlated with reading ability and with other measures of reading-related skills (Doehring et al., 1981).

In older school-age children with reading disability, deficits have been reported in phonemic sensitivity (Siegel & Ryan, 1988). Adults with dyslexia continue to experience problems in performing explicit phonological analyses on words to a degree of severity that is detrimental to both reading and spelling (I.Y. Liberman, 1987).

In contrast to a developmental lag across a broad spectrum of linguistic/cognitive abilities characteristic of the "garden-variety" poor reader, Stanovich (1988, 1993) has advanced a phonological core variable-difference model that attributes to individuals with dyslexia a deficit only in a specific domain (i.e., phonology). From his review of pertinent research, he concluded that lack of phonological sensitivity makes learning of phoneme–grapheme correspondences extremely difficult for anyone with dyslexia, and that characteristics of a phonological processing deficit coexist with intact abilities in other linguistic domains and intelligence.

Although the NJCLD definition of learning disabilities presumes that deficits such as those described here are intrinsic to the individual, implicating central nervous system dysfunction, Ehri (1989) has taken exception to the neurological theory of dyslexia. She has maintained that failure to develop phonological awareness and resultant lack of mastery of the orthographic system for reading and spelling are due to such environmental factors as inadequate prereading exposure to literacy and to ineffective instruction. While she has acknowledged the existence of individual variations in phonological awareness, she has cited evidence that such a deficiency is susceptible to change. From her work in training beginning readers in spelling and phonics and from other reports of training effects in the literature (e.g., Bradley & Bryant, 1983, 1985), she has concluded that deficits in phonological awareness are responsive to instruction, demonstrated by the achievement of improvement in both word reading and phonemic analysis.

It is Ehri's (1989) position that the cause of dyslexia is lack of complete knowledge of the spelling system.

> The bulk of readers' knowledge of how to divide words into phonemes develops when they learn to read and spell an alphabetic orthography, and this development is under the control of instruction.

> If instruction fails to provide beginning readers with full knowledge of the spelling system, then individual differences in rudimentary levels of phonological awareness may influence reading and spelling acquisition. (p. 364)

This viewpoint, while rejecting neurological dysfunction as the cause of dyslexia, does not refute claims that important individual differences in phonological awareness do exist and may be intrinsic to the individual.

A position similar to Ehri's (1989) has been advanced by some other authors over the years. For example, Boder (1971) asserted "when proper diagnosis is followed up with appropriate remedial programs ([D.J.] Johnson & Myklebust, 1967) the prognosis is good for overcoming the reading disability for most dyslexic children—though spelling may lag behind" (p. 293). Fletcher and Satz (1985) have pointed out that the concept of *dyslexia* is a hypothesis, and that a number of studies have demonstrated that children meeting the criteria for this assumed discrete clinical entity cannot be differentiated from other children with learning difficulties attributed to a variety of problems.

Strong support for these views has been provided by a recent study by Shaywitz et al. (1992). The results of this study have challenged the assumption that dyslexia is a biologically based disorder that is distinct from other reading difficulties. Using the criteria of a specified discrepancy between IQ (as measured by the WISC-R) and achievement (as measured by the Woodcock-Johnson Psychoeducational Battery), Shaywitz et al. (1992) found that discrepancy scores of subjects classified as having dyslexia followed a normal distribution of reading ability. That is, using a normal distribution model, the investigators predicted the incidence of dyslexia at different grade levels. Their predictions were confirmed by their findings.

A longitudinal study was conducted to determine the stability of the diagnosis of dyslexia across grades 1, 3, and 5. Shaywitz et al. examined correlations of discrepancy scores in grades 1 and 3. Results demonstrated that, although in first grade 25 children had been classified as having dyslexia and 31 third grade children were so classified, only "7 of them were identified as having dyslexia in both grades" (p. 147).

At a later stage of the study, it was found that, in third grade, 30 children were classified as having dyslexia and, in fifth grade, 24 of these subjects were so classified, "with 14 so classified in both grades" (p. 147). Shaywitz et al. (1992) concluded that the data do not support the belief that dyslexia is a discrete diagnostic entity. Rather, they maintained that "dyslexic children simply represent the lower portion of the continuum of reading capabilities" (p. 148). Furthermore, they reasoned that the variability observed in children classified as having dyslexia may be due, in part, to variations in severity (akin to hypertension or obesity), and, in part, to changes in criteria for diagnosis across grade levels. Their data revealed that "only 17% of the children classified as dyslexic in grade 1 will be so classified in grade 6" (p. 149). Whereas the interpretation of their findings calls into question the validity of a distinct biological basis for dyslexia, Shaywitz et al. (1992) recognized that children with reading disabilities who do not meet arbitrarily established criteria for dyslexia may still need and derive benefit from special services.

Familial Patterns of Phonological Deficit

There is some preliminary evidence in support of a genetically linked relationship between phonological disorders (and other frequently accompanying language problems) and reading/

learning disabilities in at least a subset of cases (B.A. Lewis, 1990; B.A. Lewis, Ekelman, & Aram, 1989; Tomblin, 1989). In studies by B.A. Lewis and her colleagues, siblings of children with severe phonological disorders demonstrated poorer performance than siblings of children without impairment on measures of both phonology and reading. Out of the 20 families of children with severe phonological disorders, 4 families showed a high incidence of speech-language problems over three consecutive generations. In addition, and of particular interest here, in these 4 families there was a markedly higher incidence of reading/learning disabilities than in the remaining 16 families. Proportions of these problems in the two groups of families are presented in Table 5.

Lewis et al. (1989) have pointed out that dyslexia was the second most frequently occurring problem among family members of subjects with phonological disorders (11 of 20 families reported serious reading problems). The question is raised about whether there is an underlying linguistic deficit common to both the phonological disorder and the reading disability or the phonological disorder promotes reading disability.

Further evidence of genetically based reading problems has been provided by R. Olson, Wise, Conners, Rack, and Fuller (1989). In a large study of identical and fraternal twins, one of each pair of whom had some degree of reading disability, it was determined that a phonological coding deficit reflecting a segmental language deficiency is due to heritable factors. The authors have admitted that there is a need for further evidence to support this hypothesis. The claim of a genetically determined deficit does not necessarily imply immutability. R. Olson et al. (1989) have asserted that even heritable phonological segmentation deficits are amenable to modification through environmental intervention, attested to by promising results from their own experimental procedures using computerized feedback of segmented words and syllables to improve phonological coding skills.

Lenchner et al. (1990) have suggested that, while phonological awareness is probably necessary for decoding in reading, it may not be sufficient. Indeed, the issue of decoding failure and reading failure has been the subject of debate. Some authorities have assigned an indispensable role to phonological decoding in reading success (Chall, 1989). Others have postulated direct access to meaning without phonological decoding, implicating higher level linguistic competencies such as semantic and syntactic knowledge (Smith, 1973). Furthermore, it has been argued that at least some reading disability stems from undue reliance on phonological decoding to the detriment of engaging the higher level processes required to access meaning (Cambourne & Rousch, 1982). However, further investigation is still required for more complete clarification of these phenomena.

Summary of Phonological Problems

There is ample evidence attesting to a number of phonological deficits in individuals with reading/learning disabilities. These deficits may differ in kind and degree among individuals and across ages, manifesting themselves in:

1. Early delay in the acquisition of a mature phonological system for speech production
2. Inferior ability to perceive and/or produce complex phonemic configurations, even through adolescence and beyond
3. Inefficient use of phonological codes in short-term memory
4. Impairment of metalinguistic awareness or phonological sensitivity, which interferes with the establishment of phoneme-grapheme correspondences in reading/spelling acquisition

Table 5. Incidence of speech-language and reading/learning disabilities in families of children with severe phonological disorders with and without hereditary patterns

Problems	Selected families (N = 4)	Remaining families (N = 16)
Speech-language problems	68%	28%
Reading disability	17.64%	2.05%
Learning disability	8.5%	1.71%

Adapted from Lewis (1990).

Certain phonological processes are believed to mediate access to words stored in the lexicon. Conversely, there is reason to believe that word knowledge and word retrieval exert a top-down influence on the bottom-up process of phonological analysis. Therefore, reading and writing disabilities may result from an interaction between phonological and semantic deficiencies.

SEMANTIC PROBLEMS

Problems in *decoding* meaning from spoken utterances and written text are at least partially attributable to deficiencies in word knowledge and in processing relationships among word meanings. Problems with *encoding* meaning into spoken utterances and written output are frequently caused by difficulty in accessing stored lexical knowledge. Bashir (1973) has suggested that, in reading acquisition, problems with retrieval of word sound patterns and word labels may be attributed to the same underlying deficit. This section examines deficits reported in individuals with learning disabilities in the areas of quality of word knowledge, word retrieval, and integration of semantic information within and across sentences.

Deficits in Word Knowledge

Laughton and Hasenstab (1986) observed that the overwhelming complexity of the entire area of semantics defies succinct description and analysis. Even a single aspect of semantics—vocabulary—eludes systematic investigation because of the constant change in knowledge base and evolving concepts, schemas, and concomitant word meanings. Decoding of word meanings involves more than determining the meaning of individual words; it also requires interpretation of relationships *between* concepts at the propositional level (L. Miller, 1984).

Deficits in semantic knowledge seriously affect competence in reading. Even after effective decoding skills are acquired in beginning reading, comprehension difficulties are likely to be experienced in the presence of an impoverished vocabulary and knowledge base. Reciprocally, this impoverishment of semantic knowledge persists in problem readers because of restrictions on the enrichment to be gained through the input of reading (Snider, 1989). The following deficiencies in word knowledge and usage have been observed in persons with learning disabilities (D.J. Johnson & Myklebust, 1967; Snider, 1989; Wiig & Semel, 1984):

Limited extent of vocabulary
Restrictions in word meanings
Difficulties with multiple word meanings
Excessive use of nonspecific terms, such as *thing* and *stuff*, as well as indefinite reference (e.g., *that* and *there*)

    Concreteness in symbolization and conceptualization
    Impoverished schematic knowledge

Research on receptive vocabulary in children with learning disabilities is fragmentary, much of it consisting of clinical reports. However, since such generalized descriptions are often based on extensive clinical observations, they are not without value.

    D.J. Johnson and Myklebust (1967) reported that word knowledge of children with learning disabilities is frequently restricted, literal, and concrete, lacking in the flexibility of multiple meanings, figurative expressions, and subtle nuances. Hoskins (1983) provided a few examples of clinically observed limitations in word meanings manifested by adults with learning disabilities but with better-than-average intelligence:

> Failure to understand the meaning of the word "nature" in the context of the phrase "The nature of the banking industry" because of narrow interpretation of the word (i.e., flowers and trees, etc.) (p. 94)
>
> Literal interpretation of the expression "barking up the wrong tree" in terms of bark on a tree (p. 94)

Wren (1983) reported observed difficulty with comprehension of certain conjunctions, such as *but*, *or*, *if*, *then*, *either*, and *neither*, although she conceded that this area has not been rigorously researched. The following findings have been revealed by more formal assessment:

> Conflicting reports of receptive vocabulary deficits in children and adolescents as measured by the Peabody Picture Vocabulary Test (Dunn, 1965; Dunn & Dunn, 1981) (Wiig & Semel, 1984)
>
> Vocabulary deficits in children with learning disabilities measured by the Test of Auditory Comprehension of Language (Carrow, 1973) (Hresko, Rosenberg, & Buchanan, 1978)
>
> Poorer performance by first-grade children with learning disabilities than by children without disabilities on the Boehm Test of Basic Concepts (Boehm, 1971), a measure of the comprehension of terms judged important for early academic success (Kavale, 1982)
>
> Significantly lower scores and slower responses by adolescents with learning disabilities than by their normally achieving peers on tasks requiring word definitions and the naming of word opposites (Wiig & Semel, 1975)
>
> Immature performance by 12-year-old subjects with learning disabilities in interpretation of ambiguous terms with multiple meanings (Wiig, Semel, & Abele, 1981)

From the admittedly sparse research available, adolescents with learning disabilities appear to be delayed in semantic development underlying word knowledge. Their apparent dependence on concrete meanings suggests that, cognitively, adolescents with learning disabilities tend to perform at the late preoperational and early concrete operational levels (Wiig, 1984). It has also been observed that many adolescents with learning disabilities have difficulty with the less familiar polysyllabic words encountered in educational material (Lenz & Hughes, 1990).

    Other studies have attempted to determine the respective influences of expressive versus receptive vocabulary deficits on academic performance. Van der Wissel (1988) found a stronger correlation between productive vocabulary deficits and school failure, with a weaker relationship demonstrated between receptive vocabulary and academic difficulty. These findings led to the conclusion that "hampered word production, not poor vocabulary, is characteristic of problem learners (van der Wissel, 1988, p. 518). This claim must be tempered in light of other research reporting a relationship between reading comprehension problems in adolescents and performance on the Woodcock-Johnson Psycho-educational Battery (Woodcock & Johnson, 1978) subtests of picture vocabulary, antonyms/synonyms, and analogies (Santos, 1989). Results on these tasks, implicating receptive vocabulary deficits, were among the best predictors of reading comprehension as measured in this study.

It is likely that the aspects of academic language selected for study may influence conclusions about the relative importance of receptive and expressive vocabulary. For example, a study of compositions written by college students with and without learning disabilities revealed that one factor differentiating the two groups was fluency of output. That is, the students with learning disabilities did not use as many words or as many different words as did their normally achieving counterparts (Gajar, 1989). The distinction between word knowledge and word retrieval deficits in expressive language tasks is not easy to establish.

Interpretation of observed deficiencies in word knowledge is not a straightforward process, since the underlying concepts, associated concepts, and features are not directly observable (N.W. Nelson, 1986a). In addition, theories about the manner in which lexical knowledge is organized continue to be debated. It has been asserted that, while "semantic memory is capable of producing categorical organization when the situation requires it . . . this does not mean that it (memory) is organized this way" (Ehrlich, 1979, p. 199). Nevertheless, it has been frequently assumed that impoverished conceptual structure and weak categorization skills are related to deficient word comprehension (Hoskins, 1983). Therefore, efforts have been made to examine semantic organization abilities of children with and without learning disabilities.

Deficiencies in Semantic Organization   Two methodologies employed in the examination of semantic organization have been categorization and word association. Results of early studies during the 1970s suggested that, while many children with learning disabilities have evidenced a basic competency in verbal categorization skills, they have demonstrated reduced ability to take advantage of such organization on difficult task performance (Cartelli, 1978; T.B. Parker, Freston, & Drew, 1975; Ring, 1976; Suiter & Potter, 1978). The basis for sorting common items into categories has been reported to be less mature in children with learning disabilities than in children without disabilities (Harris, 1979).

In normally developing children, word association patterns have been found to shift from the less mature syntagmatic response (e.g., *bicycle–fall*), reflecting sentence word order and real-world experience, to the more mature abstract paradigmatic or taxonomic association (e.g., *bicycle–car*) (K. Nelson, 1977; Petry, 1977). Studies of the associations made by children with learning disabilities have found greater frequency of syntagmatic associations and fewer paradigmatic associations than were produced by their normally achieving peers:

> Age range 7;5 to 12;3 years: The percentage of paradigmatic responses by subjects with learning disabilities was less than half the percentage produced by their normally achieving peers (Israel, 1984).

> Age range 10–13 years: Subjects with learning disabilities produced 48% paradigmatic responses, whereas subjects without disabilities produced 67% paradigmatic responses (Shilo, 1981).

It was also found that subjects with learning disabilities more frequently made use of rhyming or clang associations (14%), an immature pattern not utilized by any of their normally achieving peers (Israel, 1984). (Clang words are real or nonsense words that sound like a target or stimulus word [e.g., *house-souse*].)

A variation in methodology for examining evidence of semantic organization has been the use of controlled association. In this task, subjects are required to name as many examples of a given category as they can in 1 minute. Wiig and Semel (1975) required adolescents with and without learning disabilities to name as many foods as they could within the time limit. The fewer responses of subjects with learning disabilities were characterized by relative absence of categorical grouping, whereas normally achieving peers used associative clustering of different subcategories.

Figurative Language   Descriptions of word knowledge should not be limited to literal meanings. Based on clinical observation, Wiig and Semel (1984) noted that "Typically learning disabled children perceive and interpret only the literal, concrete meaning of the words" (p. 106) in idioms, similes, metaphors, and proverbs. Research documenting such clinical generalizations has been increasing. Studies of the comprehension of metaphors, similes, and idioms by elementary school and preadolescent children with learning disabilities has revealed a delay, manifested in a tendency to ascribe literal meanings to figurative language (Nippold, 1985, 1991; Nippold & Fey, 1983; Seidenberg & Bernstein, 1986; Strand, 1982). Examples of figurative language reported to cause difficulty in interpretation are:

> Simile: "Bob eats like a bird" (Wiig & Semel, 1984, p. 106).
> Metaphor: "She has pearly teeth" (teeth with pearls on them) (Nippold, 1985, p. 2).

Seidenberg and Bernstein (1986) reported other findings indicating that children with learning disabilities do seem to have the cognitive ability to comprehend metaphoric language. It is suggested that their poorer performance may be due to the failure to recognize the *usage* of metaphoric language and consequently to engage in the appropriate comparison activity. Still another interpretation attributed some failure to comprehend figurative language to inadequate word knowledge.

Issues in the Study of Word Knowledge   Admittedly, research on word knowledge and semantic organization in children and adolescents with and without learning disabilities remains inconclusive, with occasional conflicting evidence. In view of the complexity of the phenomenon and its relative inaccessibility to direct inspection, it is not surprising that a number of issues continue to need resolution, and a number of questions continue to remain unanswered.

Assessment of word knowledge by the traditional recognition response to pictured stimuli does appear to permit observation of automatic coding. However, some existing instruments tend to tap only restricted knowledge of mostly nouns, and such receptive vocabulary measures have not been found uniformly to correlate significantly with academic failure. Definitions as alternate means of assessing word knowledge involve metalinguistic ability to make knowledge explicit, rather than the use of tacit knowledge available for automatic semantic coding.

Word association analysis does appear to reflect developmental shifts in the ability to perform certain verbal tasks that seem related to academic achievement. However, it must be acknowledged that actual knowledge of words and the ways in which relations among words are organized in semantic memory is only inferred rather than inspected by such procedures.

K. Nelson (1977) expressed reservations about drawing conclusions regarding developmental status of semantic organization based on association or word-finding tasks, maintaining that children's responses may be determined by their perception of the task and their strategic attempts to comply with task demands. In some cases, results may be confounded by word retrieval problems.

Summary of Semantic Deficits at the Word Level   In language-related learning disabilities, there is equivocal evidence of deficits in receptive vocabulary. There is also abundant evidence of problems with the ready retrieval of words under a variety of conditions ranging from structured, confrontational tasks to spontaneous conversation in many, although not all, individuals with language-related learning disabilities. From clinical reports and preliminary research, evidence points to restricted word knowledge in terms of elaboration, abstraction, and multiple meanings.

There seems to be little reason to doubt the existence of delays and deficits in the development of enriched word meanings in many individuals with learning disabilities. What is unclear is the degree to which the deficits are manifestations of an impairment exclusively intrinsic to the individual or to some interaction between reduced verbal capacity and resultant limitations on input. That is, since in the normally developing child and adolescent receptive vocabulary growth is powerfully stimulated by reading, is it not possible that reading disability may not only reflect but also contribute to deficiencies in the semantic domain?

The deficits suggestive of reduced proficiency rather than disorder may lower the level of academic performance in the following ways:

1. Restricted word meanings tend to interfere with interpretation of sentences containing words with multiple meanings.
2. Concreteness of word meanings tends to render comprehension of abstractions problematic.
3. Limitation of vocabulary to high-frequency, familiar words is likely to impede reading of unfamiliar, multisyllabic words.
4. Underdeveloped associations among words and categorization of classes of verbal items may reduce the level of comprehension of and memory for information in texts or oral instruction.

In addition to limitations in word knowledge, problems with word retrieval have been reported in a sizeable segment of the population with language-related learning disabilities.

Word Retrieval Problems

Word retrieval problems have been described as difficulty with the recovery of the phonetic shape of items stored in the lexicon. That is, despite assumed knowledge of words, there is not ready access to their production to express meanings in spontaneous verbalization. Frequently there is delay in retrieval, substitution of other words, circumlocution (e.g., *the thing you wash up in—sink*), and/or use of gesture or pantomime or nonverbal vocalizations in the event of unsuccessful search for the desired word. Different parameters have been the focus of investigation by different researchers.

Structured Tasks   Studies of word retrieval by children and adolescents with and without learning disabilities have employed such techniques as confrontation naming of pictures; rapid naming of colors, objects, numbers, and letters; sentence completion; and naming to description (Denckla & Rudel, 1976a, 1976b; German, 1982; White, 1979; Wiig, Florence,

Kutner, Sherman, & Semel, 1977; Wiig & Semel, 1975, 1984). On all tasks, subjects with learning disabilities made more errors by substitution, association, and circumlocution and were slower in responding than controls.

German (1982) performed a detailed analysis of word substitution types of errors produced by children ages 8–11 years with and without learning disabilities. Results revealed significantly higher percentages of the following types of responses by children with learning disabilities than by their normally achieving counterparts:

> Substitution of functional attributes; e.g., rain/cloud
> Substitutions of items visually similar to the target; e.g., string/rein
> Substitution of initial sounds preceding the target word; e.g., f/f/thunb (German, 1982, p. 224)

Subjects with learning disabilities did not differ significantly from controls in the percentage of responses such as:

> Semantically related words; e.g., fork/knife
> Part substitutions; e.g. cord/drill
> "I don't know" responses (German, 1982, p. 224)

Children with learning and reading disabilities have demonstrated particularly poorer naming performance on low-frequency than high-frequency words (Denckla & Rudel, 1976a; German, 1982; Wiig & Becker-Caplan, 1984). Denckla and Rudel (1976a) noted a similarity between the prevalence of circumlocution by their subjects with dyslexia and that by adults with left hemisphere damage. This observation led them to conclude that children with dyslexia resemble individuals with dysphasia in this respect.

Reduced Speed and Accuracy of Naming   Additional evidence of reduced speed and accuracy of retrieval by children with learning disabilities was observed in their significantly slower production of color-form names in confrontation tasks compared to normally achieving peers (Denckla & Rudel, 1976b; Semel & Wiig, 1980; Wiig, Semel, & Nystrom, 1982). In some of these studies, it was found that lower performance in reading correlacted with reduced rates of speed in rapid repetitive naming. In contrast to the deficiencies noted on the combined color-form naming, subjects with learning disabilities performed at a level equivalent to normally achieving peers on confrontation naming of color or form separately. Longer response latencies were also found in subjects with learning disabilities on other tasks, such as naming opposites and giving word definitions (Wiig & Semel, 1976). In conjunction with reduced speed, subjects with learning disabilities made more errors on these tasks than did controls. While children with reading disability have been slower than children without disabilities in automatized naming of objects, colors, letters, and numbers, the order of difficulty among these classes of material was similar in both groups of children. That is, object naming was significantly slower than any of the other naming tasks. Color naming has been found to be significantly slower than naming letters and numbers among all groups.

It has been demonstrated that children manifesting word-finding difficulties in constrained, single word-naming tasks, such as the Test of Word Finding (German, 1986) also evidence word-finding difficulties in connected discourse (German & Simon, 1991). In narratives about pictures and explanations of hypothesized variations in pictured scenes and actions, children with tested word-finding deficits produced more repetitions, reformulations, substitutions, and empty words and had more frequent delays than children who tested within the normal range on single-word retrieval.

Naturalistic Samples   Analysis of word-finding problems in the more naturalistic language usage of spontaneous, self-generated stories revealed an apparent relationship between quantity of verbal output and incidence of word retrieval difficulty (German, 1987). Those children whose verbalization was judged adequate or extended in quantity exhibited more repetition, reformulation, and substitutions than those whose verbal output was limited in quantity. It appeared that the strategy of the subjects with limited output was to avoid word retrieval difficulty by omitting rather than searching for or substituting words not readily retrievable. The types of substitutions produced by the subjects exhibiting adequate-length word-finding deficits (e.g., semantic, functional, and phonemic) did not differ from those produced by the group without impairment, but the frequency of occurrence was much greater in the group with language disorders.

Word Retrieval and Word Knowledge   The assumption underlying retrieval deficiencies is that word knowledge is intact but not readily accessible. However, it is worthy of notice that frequency of word occurrence was found to be a determining factor in speed and accuracy of retrieval. Leonard and his colleagues (Kail & Leonard, 1986; Leonard, Nippold, Kail, & Hale, 1983) examined the effects of frequency on pictured-word naming by children with language impairment and language-matched and age-matched controls. All three groups named most of the pictures accurately. However, the children with language impairment were significantly slower than age-matched peers without impairment but significantly faster than language-matched (younger) subjects. Further analysis of results yielded some information about the relationship between frequency and retrieval. "The language-impaired as well as the normal children named pictures of objects with frequently occurring names more rapidly than pictures of objects with less frequently occurring names" (Leonard et al., 1983, p. 613). Two hypothetical explanations of the frequency effect are: 1) associative strength in the semantic network, and 2) distinctiveness of representations in lexical storage.

Since the children with language impairment in this study demonstrated more limited lexical knowledge than age-matched controls as evidenced by deficits on standardized tests of both expressive and receptive vocabulary, it was inferred that these children may not have known the names of the pictures well as the control subjects. Leonard et al. (1983) suggested that the slower naming times of the subjects with language impairment may be interpreted not solely as evidence of retrieval difficulty; they may also be due to lexical storage limitations. That is, words may have less distinctive, less elaborated representations in semantic memory or have fewer associative connections in the semantic network.

Effects of Training on Word Retrieval   To investigate effects of training in elaboration of word knowledge and/or retrieval strategies, McGregor and Leonard (1989) compared results of two experimental techniques on the performance of four children with word-finding problems (two experimental and two control subjects). For the experimental subjects, semantic elaboration training included both semantic enrichment and heightened phonemic awareness through rhyming similarities. Retrieval strategy training consisted of demonstrating the facilitating effects of using categorical knowledge and locational or phonemic cues in retrieval.

Among other effects, on the posttest, experimental subjects made fewer naming errors on trained words than they had on pretesting. Control subjects who had received no training in either elaboration or retrieval did not show comparable reductions in errors. The greatest benefit on posttest and maintenance by experimental subjects was derived from the combination of elaboration plus retrieval strategy training, in contrast to the effects of each method individually. These results were interpreted as consistent with the findings of Kail and Leonard (1986) that "children with word-finding problems have limitations in elaboration and, in some cases, retrieval as well" (McGregor & Leonard, 1989, p. 164).

Wing (1990) studied responses to training of 10 children with primarily expressive language deficits but apparently intact receptive abilities. In contrast to the view expressed by McGregor and Leonard (1989) that the expressive disorder of word retrieval is likely to be accompanied by some receptive deficit in word knowledge, Wing (personal communication, September, 1990) has maintained that retrieval difficulties in the presence of stored elaborated word meanings are frequently encountered in children with expressive language impairment, thus adhering to the traditional criteria for classifying word retrieval problems.

Wing's experimental training method was based on Wolf's (1982, 1984) model of word retrieval. Semantic training effects for five subjects were contrasted with the effects for five other subjects of perceptual training in phonological analysis of words and the creation of internal visual images of pictured objects. Results demonstrated significantly higher gains on naming untrained words during posttesting on the Test of Word finding (German, 1986) by the perceptually trained group than those made by the group trained in semantic elaboration. It should be noted that the differences, while significant, were small, and that neither group reached age-appropriate levels of performance.

Wing (1990) has speculated that some substitution errors made by children with word-finding problems may reflect inadequate semantic organization along with failure to inhibit production of an error word that is semantically related (e.g., *zebra* for *giraffe*; p. 155), thereby demonstrating inadequate discrimination among distinguishing attributes. Therefore, she reasoned that such children may benefit from training aimed at refining imagery and sharpening phonological analysis of labels. According to Wolf (1984), "Emphasized within lexical operations are the development and organization of semantic and phonological functions and the ability of the total system to be accessed through either the phonological or semantic pathways" (p. 92).

It is indeed likely, as Donahue (1986) has pointed out, that there may be different subtypes of word retrieval problems. While some types may be demonstrated by increased errors and/or longer latency on retrieval of less familiar words, others may reflect slow retrieval of highly familiar words. Difficulty with the automatic retrieval of familiar words is reminiscent of the retrieval problem frequently experienced by aging adults who had been formerly competent language users possessing well-developed word knowledge (Burke, Worthley, & Martin, 1988). In contrast, however, children with word retrieval problems are still developing organisms. Thus, whereas some neurological dysfunction may be presumed to disrupt access to word knowledge in both groups, the nature of these malfunctions are probably different in the young and elderly populations. Leonard and his colleagues have acknowledged the need for further research to distinguish between the roles of storage and retrieval factors in the word naming difficulties of children with language impairment.

Beyond the Word: Semantic–Syntactic Relations

The foregoing information addresses some of the issues related to isolated word meanings. However, semantic relations are usually encoded in multiword constructions both within phrases and across phrases in clauses, sentences, and intersentence discourse. Word meanings are influenced by grammatical role, modified by morphological features, and altered in different contexts as they serve communicative functions. Problems have been experienced by students with language-related learning disabilities in: understanding the meaning of questions, comprehending or retaining the meaning of all critical elements in following directions, and abstracting the meaning of linguistic concepts. Some research in each of these areas is examined.

Understanding Questions   Young children with disordered language have been found to produce significantly fewer appropriate and accurate responses to questions than do linguistically normal children across three conditions differing in contextual support (Parnell, Amerman, & Harting, 1986). Analysis of response patterns revealed that the hierarchy of difficulty reflected by children with language disorders was similar to that observed in normally developing children. Questions beginning with *what* + *be*, *where*, and *which* presented the least difficulty. Those beginning with *why*, *when*, and *what happened* created the most difficulty. Confusions in processing the meaning of particular *wh-* words were evident in some of the responses rated as inaccurate or inappropriate:

> "When do you sleep?" "In bed."
> "Who's this?" (pointing to examiner) "Your head."

Other confusions reported, largely under the conditions providing no immediate visual referential source, were as follows (ranked from least to most confusing): *what/who*, *where/when*, *what* + *be* and *what* + *do*, *who/whose*, and *why/when*.

Based on clinical observation, Wiig and Semel (1984) ranked *wh-* question terms in the following order of difficulty for children with learning disabilities: *what–who–which–where–when–why–how–whose*. They have observed that "learning disabled children may be able to answer questions formed with 'what place', 'what time' and 'in what way' even though they may not respond to questions with the expected *wh-*forms 'where', 'when' and 'how' " (p. 331).

Processing Oral Directions   Research examining the ability to process increasing amounts of semantic information in oral directions has used the Token Test (DeRenzi & Vignolo, 1962) or the Token Test for Children (TTC) (DiSimoni, 1978). The TTC, like its original adult version, consists of five parts, with each part containing more critical information that must be processed to follow the directions; for example:

1. Touch the red circle
2. Touch the big red circle
3. Touch the blue square and the green circle
4. Touch the big yellow circle and the small red square
5. Except for the green one, touch the circles (DiSimoni, 1978, pp. 27–28)

As can be seen, the first four parts merely increase the amount of information to be processed, whereas the fifth part adds grammatical complexity.

Two studies reported on the performance of preschool and school-age children with language-related learning disabilities on the TTC (Murray, Feinstein, & Blouin, 1985) and that of adolescents with learning disabilities on the Token Test (Riedlinger-Ryan & Shewan, 1984). A summarization of the findings of these studies is presented in Table 6. For the preschool group, part 1 emerged as the most significant indicator of a possible learning disability, demonstrating that either conceptual acquisition or processing abilities were delayed. Significantly lower scores on parts 3 and 4 have been interpreted not so much as an indication of failure to under-

Table 6. Patterns of difficulty on different parts of the Token Test and TTC shown by subjects with language/learning disabilities according to age group

Study	Age group	Part 1	Part 2	Part 3	Part 4	Part 5
Murray, Feinstein, and Blouin (1985)(TTC)	Preschool	X[a]				
	School-age				X	X
Riedlinger-Ryan and Shewan (1984) (Token Test)	Adolescents			X	X	X*

[a]X indicates difficulty experienced.
*Narrowly missed statistical significance.

stand the meaning of the content as an indication of difficulty with processing longer strings of words. Part 5 was the best predictor of overall scores of auditory comprehension in the population with learning disabilities. A second part of the Riedlinger-Ryan and Shewan study examined the ability to understand certain linguistic concepts. Since these concepts are described in the next section, results are reported there.

Understanding Linguistic Concepts and Relationships   Logical relationships such as comparative, passive, spatial, temporal, or familial (possessive) may be expressed by the interactive meanings of two or more critical words within sentences. Children and adolescents with learning disabilities who were tested on comprehension of these linguistic concepts showed significant delays in comparison with normally achieving peers (Reidlinger-Ryan & Shewan, 1984; Wiig, Lapointe, & Semel, 1977; Wiig & Semel, 1973, 1974). Greatest difficulty was found in interpreting familial relationships. In decreasing order of difficulty were problems with spatial, temporal-sequential, passive, and comparative relationships (Wiig & Semel, 1984). Regarding the inferred interaction between semantics and cognition, Wiig, Lapointe, and Semel (1977) interpreted performance deficiencies as follows: "The deficits were considered to reflect impairments of abstraction, generalization, simultaneous analysis and synthesis and delays in logical growth" (p. 293).

Semantic Integration   Semantic integration studies have examined the ability to abstract the meaning of individual sentences and to integrate such meanings across sentence boundaries. Semantic integration across multiple sentence boundaries also depends on working memory's capacity to hold input of discrete units long enough to establish relationships among individual sentences. Construction of integrated meanings generally involves inference in the interpretation of the gist of sentences, thereby drawing on information from long-term memory that supplements information given in the presented sentences.

Klein-Konigsberg (1984) studied children with and without learning disabilities in grades 2 through 5 on a semantic integration task. In part 1, subjects were presented with lists of sentences derived from longer, higher level combinations of propositions. For example, such four-item sentences as "The big brown bear ate the chocolate candy in the woods," or "The old farmer milked the brown cow in the barn" were decomposed into sentences containing one, two, or three of the items:

"The farmer was old."
"The bear ate the candy."
"The big bear ate the chocolate candy."

Lists of these sentences were presented in nonsequential order.

In part 2, after a 2-minute break, the following sentence types were presented for recognition and identification:

Old: same information as in the original sentences (e.g., "The bear ate the candy.")

New: same information as in the original sentences but in different forms (e.g., "The bear ate the chocolate candy.")

Noncase: information not originally presented (e.g., "The farmer ate the chocolate candy.")

Some sentence groups contained information characterized as concrete, and others were more abstract. Subjects were required to say whether they had heard the sentences during the first presentation list. Old and new sentences should both receive "yes" responses because they consisted of combined information of a sentence set, not just individual sentences previously heard.

Subjects with learning disabilities made significantly more responses than controls in which they identified as "old" sentences involving a false inference (e.g., "The farmer ate the chocolate candy in the barn"). They also made significantly more noncase errors, identifying as "old" sentences that did not contain originally presented ideas but that contained an "old" lexical item (e.g., "The cow ate the grass"). No subjects without learning disabilities produced these noncase responses. The data produced evidence that the subjects without learning disabilities did integrate information across sentence boundaries, recognizing new sentences as old ones when they contained ideas consonant with information originally presented.

Analysis of responses of subjects with learning disabilities led to the conclusion that these children did, in fact, abstract information from individual sentences as well as controls, but only up to the level of two sentence elements. They were significantly poorer in integrating information from three or four sentence elements and in integrating more abstract information, except in verbatim form. From observation of test-taking behavior, Klein-Konigsberg (1984) conjectured: "It was almost as if the [learning-disabled] children were trying to memorize each sentence" (p. 263). In summary, the subjects with learning disabilities were observed to attend to smaller units, short sentences, and individual lexical items, leading to the speculation: "Perhaps they can integrate up to a certain point, beyond which additional information is in excess of their integrative capacities" (p. 262).

Individual differences in factors influencing the ability to integrate meaning across sentence boundaries, whatever their causes may be, are likely to determine the efficiency and effectiveness of processing the larger units of discourse in its various modes. This topic is considered in the following section.

DISCOURSE PROCESSING PROBLEMS

The problems exhibited in oral and written discourse by students with learning disabilities contribute significantly to academic failure. Receptive processing of written discourse is, of course, involved in the reading comprehension deficits experienced by many of these students. Expressive production deficiencies are frequently observed in their written output. The literature is replete with reports of their difficulties with the processing of the oral language of instruction and of their inadequate oral expressive abilities in academic tasks.

:essing Problems in Written and Oral Language

ly reported deficit in academic performance of students with learning disabilities is
vith comprehension of instructional language and the subsequent recall of its content. These problems are manifested to differing degrees by different students in reading and listening. While certain processes are unique to each modality, others may be found to apply in a manner similar, although not identical, to language problems in both modes. In approaching this complex phenomenon, the attempt is made to discern patterns of deficit and potential proficiency reported in the research reviewed above and to try to interpret these patterns within the framework of existing theory.

Speed of Processing   Increased response latency by subjects with learning disabilities on a wide variety of naming and word retrieval tasks under different conditions has been reported in numerous studies cited above. The relationship between increased response latency in expressive word retrieval and retrieving the spoken equivalent of printed words during reading has been noted by Jansky and de Hirsch (1972).

The performance of individuals with reading/learning disabilities has been reported to be poorer than that of normally achieving peers on the following aspects of verbal coding:

Semantic processing of words (Howell & Manis, 1986)

Recognition of long (seven to nine letters) printed words (Shapiro, Ogden, & Lind-Blad, 1990)

Decisions about words as instances of superordinate categories and truth value of orally presented sentences (J. Kagan, 1983)

Phonemic coding (LaBuda & DeFries, 1988; Siegel & Ryan, 1984)

It has been argued that limitations on the extent to which information can be accurately and completely encoded in short-term memory in the time available determine the degree to which that information is available to interact with long-term memory (see Chapter 3). Thus, speed of verbal coding is viewed as one determinant of how the contents of long-term memory are learned, particularly in the domain of semantic knowledge. Speed of verbal coding has reportedly differentiated high-verbal from low-verbal college students (Hunt, Lunneborg, & Lewis, 1975). Since it is generally recognized that comprehension of new input is facilitated by the availability and accessibility of relevant knowledge from long-term memory, less efficient verbal decoding and encoding are seen to have overall effects on the comprehension, storage, and retrieval of verbal information.

Reading Comprehension   It is reasoned that, in the process of reading, slower, less efficient verbal coding places heavier demands on the limited capacity of working memory, thus contributing to the memory span problems frequently reported in individuals with reading/learning disabilities (Lorsbach & Gray, 1986), disrupting the formulation of phrase or sentence (Shankweiler & Liberman, 1972) and resulting in the loss of information from working memory necessary to the construction of meaning in the comprehension process.

> If the meaning of words, even words correctly read, does not come automatically as the child pronounces them, but about a second later, the reading process becomes slowed, and the child can lose more easily the coherence of the phrase or sentence he is attempting to decipher. (J. Kagan, 1983, p. 79)

An account of verbal efficiency in reading comprehension has been advanced by Perfetti (1985), emerging from the experimental work done by him and his colleagues over a decade.

Efficient reading comprehension is believed to involve rapid automatic access to word meanings in the encoding of propositions, thereby freeing up higher level resources for the integration of propositions and the process of inferencing. It is hypothesized that failure to achieve rapid, effortless processing at the level of decoding word meanings diminishes availability of resources for these higher level processes. Deficits in such high-level processes as inferencing, interpreting ambiguous sentences, and interpreting metaphoric expressions were demonstrated by high school students with learning disabilities (Santos, 1989).

It has also been observed that excessive allocation of resources to low-level decoding skills in bottom-up processing interferes with accessing of schematic knowledge by individuals with reading disability (Cambourne & Rousch, 1982; Pearson & Spiro, 1980).

> Because of the amount of effort they are apparently putting into achieving a high degree of graphophonic match, they do not have sufficient working memory left to monitor what they are producing in order to decide whether it does make semantic or symtactic sense. (Cambourne & Fousch, 1982, p. 67)

Subjects in the study by Cambourne and Rousch (1982) ranged from second to eighth graders. A study reported by Stanovich (1984) examined reading behaviors of first-grade poor and good readers to determine the extent to which context was used to facilitate word decoding. When poor readers attained a level of decoding ability achieved earlier by good readers, they appeared to

> make use of the mechanism of conscious contextual prediction. . . . This compensatory mechanism will indeed speed the processing of congruous words, but will do so at the expense of cognitive capacity. Thus, less capacity remains for the comprehending processes that tend to be very capacity demanding. (p. 15)

All of these factors probably interact to interfere with ready, ongoing comprehension through a process labeled *hysteresis* (Perfetti, 1985). This term signifies the inability of short-term memory to keep up with ongoing processing demands. That is, while the system is still working on assembling a proposition for one unit of verbal input, the next unit enters the system in the absence of available resources for processing. Perfetti (1985) noted that factors associated with reading comprehension inefficiencies may also operate, to varying degrees, in oral comprehension.

This description of hysteresis bears some similarity to one of the patterns observed by Brookshire (1974) in describing auditory verbal processing deficits manifested by aphasic subjects. *Information capacity deficit* is the term Brookshire used to describe an inability to receive and process information at the same time. Individuals with this deficit seem to take longer to process a unit of information than do those without such deficit. Therefore, while they are engaged in processing an earlier unit, they miss the next incoming segment. They tend to respond correctly to the first and last elements in a message and miss the middle parts.

The research conducted by Perfetti and his colleagues on individual differences in reading comprehension led to the "double whammy" theory:

> When we consider the less-skilled comprehender's poorer memory for sentence wording while reading or listening, we see how easily this compounds his difficulties. The poor reader is slower at getting to the point in the comprehension process beyond which exact wording is not needed, but he is also poorer at retaining exact wording. Thus, he is confronted with a double whammy— slower processing and lower tolerance (in terms of working memory), both of which combine to create more processing needs than might otherwise exist. (Perfetti & Lesgold, 1977, p. 178)

An important component of successful reading is comprehension monitoring, a process in which students with learning disabilities are reportedly less actively and less effectively engaged than readers without disabilities. This topic is covered in Chapter 8 in the section on metacognition.

Listening Comprehension   Perfetti (1987) reported that the research conducted by his group of colleagues has yielded results "consistent with the picture that poor readers, as measured by a comprehension test, are also poor at listening comprehension" (p. 365). He considered the possibility that reading problems are intimately tied to problems in the processing of oral language.

In the auditory modality, it is assumed by some theorists and practitioners that problems in language comprehension may be attributed to a central auditory processing impairment wherein some abnormality disrupts optimal processing of the signal. This assumption has been the subject of ongoing debate throughout the 1970s and 1980s. One school of thought has posited an intimate relationship between central auditory processing disorder and language/learning disabilities (J. Katz, 1977; Willeford, 1985). This position has been rejected by those favoring a top-down psycholinguistic perspective, who argue against the critical importance of bottom-up processing in accounts of language and learning (Goehl, 1983; Rees, 1983), and by those who have questioned the validity of tests used for examination of central auditory processing in children (Lovrinic, 1983; Matkin & Hook, 1983).

Despite questions about the possible relations between auditory processing deficits and language/learning disabilities, research has continued to explore aspects of the phenomenon, with refinements in experimental techniques throughout the recent past. Performance on fine-grained auditory discrimination of syllables has been found to correlate with academic success in young (6–7 years), but not older, children and with results on the Peabody Picture Vocabulary Test–Revised and the TTC (Elliott & Hammer, 1988; Elliott, Hammer, & Scholl, 1989). Both adults with learning disabilities and adolescents with histories of early language impairment demonstrated deficits in auditory processing against background noise, but no deficits in quiet conditions (Aram, Ekelman, & Nation, 1984; Elliott & Busse, 1987). (These findings are reminiscent of those results of the study by Brady et al. [1983] reported above.) Children with learning disabilities were more penalized than nondisabled controls in discriminating words against linguistic and nonlinguistic distractors in a selective attention task (R. Cherry & Kruger, 1983). It is noteworthy that the semantic distractor (a background story) interfered more with selective auditory attention than did a linguistic but nonsemantic distractor (tape of a story played backward), suggesting that language processing, rather than auditory information processing deficits, may tax the resources of children with learning disabilities to a greater extent than those of children without such disabilities in a competing verbal message task.

Despite the ongoing debate about the adequacy of auditory processing hypotheses to explain language and learning disabilities, the fact remains that many individuals with learning disabilities do manifest problems processing auditory language under certain conditions. Rees (1981) took cognizance of the fact that some individuals who experience difficulty processing linguistic information at a rapid or even a normal rate do demonstrate improved processing of auditory language at a slower rate.

Rate of Auditory Processing and Comprehension   A number of studies have demonstrated improved auditory comprehension under conditions of slowed presentation rate and insertion of pauses at phrasal boundaries for children with language/learning disabilities and adults with aphasia (T.F. Campbell & McNeil, 1985; Lasky & Chapandy, 1976; Lasky, Weidner, & Johnson, 1976; Liles, Cooker, Kass, & Carey, 1978). T.F. Campbell and McNeil (1985) argued from their data that the slowed comprehension by children with acquired language disorder was attributable not to limitations in linguistic knowledge, but rather to disruption in the processing of language. By experimentally manipulating conditions that influence allocation of attentional resources, they were led to the conclusion that the slower rate of sentence presentation "may allow even a disordered system to allocate the necessary attention to complete the task at a more adequate level" (p. 518).

While this interpretation presents fresh insights into the phenomenon of slowed auditory comprehension by individuals with language impairment, it is not possible to judge at the present time whether it is equally applicable to individuals with developmental and acquired language deficits. Regarding the population with language-related learning disabilities, questions still remain about the potentially negative effects of linguistic deficits in conjunction with processing deficits. From all of the foregoing reports of possible reductions in semantic/syntactic abilities and demonstrated deficits in phonological processing, the locus (or loci) of increased effortfulness and reduced speed of processing is not as yet clearly resolved.

Bottom-Up and Top-Down Revisited   The role of the auditory signal itself continues to be debated. From a current psycholinguistic perspective, it is maintained that auditory comprehension is not based on matching the auditory input to verbal patterns stored in the lexicon (MacWhinney, 1989). It has been demonstrated that "when the auditory signal is unclear, syntactic expectations can influence lexical activation (MacWhinney, 1989, p. 68). This represents a strong top-down processing model, in which the role of the auditory signal is not assigned overriding importance in the interpretation of message. However, Elliott and Busse (1987) pointed out that adults with learning disabilities "made good use of 'top-down' processing *provided that they perceived a sufficient portion of the acoustic speech signal*" (p. 126), thereby underscoring the role of bottom-up data.

Duchan and Katz (1983) have contrasted the roles of top-down and bottom-up processing in different aspects of auditory verbal performance. They cited particular examples in which speech-sound processing may occur with reduced support from preexisting knowledge (e.g., repeating nonsense material, mimicking utterances in a foreign language, learning the phonemic boundaries in Japanese versus English). Proposing a synthesis of top-down and bottom-up processing models, fusing language processes and auditory processes in an interactive manner, Duchan and Katz have suggested that different language processing situations may provide or demand different proportions of higher order processing and signal emphasis. They also suggested that patterns of deficit may vary among individuals with language processing problems. For example, some children with learning disabilities may depend excessively on higher order processing without sufficient signal processing. These children may tend to respond impulsively or appear to have hearing impairment. In contrast, "Those who are primarily bottom-up processors may miss the nuances conveyed from higher order knowledge. They could appear to think concretely and have difficulty making higher-level abstractions" (Duchan & Katz, 1983, p. 43).

Lasky (1983) stated, at the outset of her chapter on parameters affecting auditory processing, that "The relationships among perceptual, linguistic, and cognitive processes are not clear-cut" (p. 11). She took into account the multiplicity of internal and external variables that may contribute to effective or deficient auditory language processing. She cited evidence from electrophysiological studies reflecting different neural responses to tasks of differing degrees of difficulty as one level of analysis.

In addition to the interactive effects of presentation rate on the processing of varying dimensions of linguistic information, environmental factors such as the nature of the task, background noise, interpersonal interaction, meaningfulness and familiarity of material, and situational expectations are regarded as influential in determining effectiveness of auditory language processing. Such a comprehensive account of factors involved in the auditory processing of language may serve as a fitting conclusion to the information presented in this section.

Receptive-Expressive Problems

Within the past decade, empirical research on the oral discourse of students with learning disabilities has focused predominantly on the narrative form.

Research on Narrative Discourse Skills   Some studies have investigated comprehension and production of narratives, whereas others have focused primarily on one of these channels. Results on comprehension are examined across studies, followed by review of production studies. Finally, relevant patterns that may emerge from these analyses are considered.

Comprehension Studies   Studies of school-age children classed as having a learning disability with and without documented language impairment have indicated that these children appear to comprehend and recall stories at the factual level as well as their unimpaired peers (Feagans & Short, 1984; Merritt & Liles, 1987; Roth, 1986). They seem to have little difficulty understanding the gist of stories, thereby apparently processing adequately the order and structure of narratives.

However, less-skilled comprehenders have been observed to differ from normally achieving peers in their responses to questions requiring inference about causality. In the Merritt and Liles (1987) study, children with language impairment did not differ significantly from controls in answering factual questions. For example, testing comprehension of a story about Jim's being buried in his truck under a huge snowdrift, the following questions asked for factual information:

What was the weather like in this story?
What did Jim do with his truck when the roads got bad?

The control group was significantly better than the group with language impairment in answering questions that asked for inferential information reflecting story grammar knowledge, such as the following:

Why was it so dark in the truck?
Why did Jim worry when he discovered the door wouldn't budge?

In a study by Crais and Chapman (1987), performance of children with language-related learning disabilities on answering inference questions resembled that of younger normally achieving children. This manifestation seemed to stem from a reduced grasp of some of the relations that are implicit in story grammar structure.

Retold Stories   In one study of 93 children with reading disability, it was found that they produced significantly less content in retold stories in terms of mean number of propositions produced by 93 normally achieving controls (Snyder & Downey, 1991). Children classed as having learning disabilities with and without language impairment were observed to use story hierarchies (temporal sequencing of information as one component of narrative structure) in retold stories, but the stories of children with language impairment were less logical in sequencing events, a deficit suggesting loss of information from memory (Merritt & Liles, 1987). In response to picture stimuli depicting story events, it was found that, even following an adult model for a second trial, the narrative style and content produced by children with learning disabilities did not show noticeable improvement (Levi, Mussatti, Piredda, & Sechi, 1984). These subjects tended to describe the pictures rather than construct a narrative reflecting a grasp of story grammar. In another study requiring paraphrases of heard stories, children with reading disabilities produced fewer action units, fewer words, fewer complex sentences, and more nonreferential pronouns than the normally achieving comparison group (Feagans & Short, 1984).

From her review of research on recalled stories, Roth (1986) summarized some of the deficits observed in the performance of subjects with learning disabilities:

> Inadequate encoding of important temporal and causal relationships
> Impoverishment of significant detail
> Shorter in length
> More incorrect information

It is conceivable that the noted inadequacy of temporal and causal relationships reflects a descriptive versus narrative style. It may be inferred that, particularly in response to picture stimuli, these children tend to remain dependent on the discrete, perceptually present elements rather than engaging in the higher level cognitive operation of discerning and constructing relations among those pictured objects/events that do not exist on the perceptual level but are reflected in narrative structure.

Story Generation   Whereas children with learning disabilities without identified language impairment performed similarly to normally achieving peers in the use of all categories of story grammar (Roth & Spekman, 1986), they shared some of the characteristics of children with language impairment (Merritt & Liles, 1987) in their production of fewer complete episodes. There was a tendency to omit middle components and to use fewer propositions in the narration of episodes. It was also found that children with language impairment generated fewer story grammar components than did their normally achieving peers (Merritt & Liles, 1987).

Garnett (1986) summarized findings from a body of research on narrative discourse abilities of children with learning disabilities beyond the parameters of story grammar:

1. Impoverishment in amount of information
2. Reduced ability to distinguish more important from less important ideas
3. Pragmatic deficits evidenced by less explicit clarification of content for the listener
4. Deficits in organizational structure and cohesion
5. Inefficient memory strategies for recall

Claiming that story grammar analysis is inadequate to account for the great variety of narrative types in natural contexts, Scott (1988a) examined research on cohesion in generated stories.

Cohesion and Organization   The stories of children with language impairment are reportedly poorer in organization of their episodes and in sentence cohesion than stories of normally achieving peers. They tend to contain more inaccurate conjunctions and make less effective use of personal pronouns for reference across chains of propositions (Liles, 1985, 1987; Ripich & Griffith, 1988). Roth and Spekman (1986) provided an example of a narrative that may be structurally intact but is difficult to follow because of deficits in syntax, cohesion, and confused referents:

Proposition	Category Type
One time there was this little dog	Major Setting
All these people didn't want to buy him	Minor Setting
Well, when anybody came by and watched	Minor Setting
him do the little tricks	
They just walked off	Minor Setting
When they did that	Initiating Event
and he saw 'em	Initiating Event
he just walked out of the door	Attempt
of the place	
and then he bit his leg	Attempt
or bit his bottom	Attempt
take a little piece if his pants	Attempt
and then go back in his cage	Direct Consequence
and put it down	Direct Consequence

(Roth & Spekman, 1986, p. 21)

With reference to cohesion, Liles found that the pattern was not uniform across all subjects with language disorders. Some, described as good comprehenders, appeared to understand the logical relationships connecting the episodes but were inferior to controls in organizing the episodic information. Others (poor comprehenders) did not appear to understand how episodes were conjoined. This deficit had been manifested in the inferior performance of this latter group in answering questions involving knowledge of the relationships contained in the story grammer. Liles (1987) concluded that "the higher order level of episode organization is separate but not distinct from the cohesion of separate sentences" (p. 193).

Patterns of Difficulty in Narrative Discourse Skills   Results of research appear to demonstrate certain effects of language/learning disabilities on the comprehension and production of narrative discourse. A summarization of the research findings is provided in Table 7. Some patterns of difficulty have emerged from a review of these findings.

Norris and Bruning (1988) point out that, even at the kindergarten and first-grade levels, low and high achievers are differentiated by:

Ability to develop a theme
Ability to maintain coherence within their narratives
Use of cohesive ties
Use of reference to establish connections
The number of propositions produced

While both groups appear to be developing the ability to employ decontextualized language, high achievers tend to manifest greater sophistication in its use. It is apparent that individuals vary in their awareness of organization and/or ability to encode relationships within the organization.

The possibility does exist that *sensitivity* to organization may be inadequate in some individuals with learning disabilities. Children with learning disabilities have been observed to be

Table 7. Summary of narrative abilities of children with learning disabilities (LD), reading disability (RD), and/or language impairment (LI)

Type of disorder	Descriptors	Evaluation
	Story Comprehension	
LD, no LI	Comprehension of factual information and gist with and without contextual support	No deficit
LD + LI	Response to inferential questions reflecting relations implicit in story structure	Deficit
	Retold Stories	
LD + LI	Use of story hierarchies	No deficit
	Logical sequencing of events	Deficit
RD	Amount of content (number of words and action units)	Deficit
	Sentence complexity	Deficit
	Use of referential pronouns	Deficit
	Generated Stories	
LD, no LI	Use of story grammar categories	No deficit
	Syntactic complexity	No deficit
LI	Number of complete episodes	Deficit
	Organization	Deficit
LD + LI	Cohesion	Deficit[a]

From studies by Crais and Chapman (1987), Feagans and Short (1984), Liles (1985, 1987), Merritt and Liles (1987), Ripich and Griffith (1988), and Roth and Spekman (1986).

[a]Good and poor comprehenders differed, with good comprehenders showing better cohesion than poor comprehenders.

significantly inferior to controls in detecting the difference between presented passages that were organized and those that were disorganized. When required to reorganize the disorganized passages, subjects without learning disabilities were significantly superior to subjects with learning disabilities. On a recall task, subjects with learning disabilities recalled significantly less content. Since the subjects with learning disabilities did demonstrate significant improvement after a training period, the authors concluded that these children must have possessed some rudimentary idea about passage organization (Wong & Wilson, 1984).

The interaction between organizational ability and cohesion remains unclear. As noted above, Liles (1987) observed that points of difficulty in narrative organization may be indicated by inaccurate cohesion at episode boundaries, but such misuse of cohesive ties does not specify the nature of the particular difficulty responsible for the problem.

For further enlightenment about this aspect of discourse in the student with language deficiencies, cohesion in the production of the three hemidecorticate children described in Chapter 6 is briefly analyzed. Newman et al. (1986) found that the adolescent who had undergone a right hemispherectomy as a young child used anaphoric pronominal reference in narrative in a manner similar to that represented in the original story. His frequent production of pronominalized referents and chains of anaphoric reference sustained cohesion and demonstrated his ability to keep a particular referent "on stage" in the listener's short-term memory.

In contrast, the two individuals who had undergone left hemispherectomy as young children produced fewer personal pronouns and resorted to more frequent reinstatement of the nominalized referents. This difference in performance between individuals with only a left or right hemisphere is described by Newman et al. (1986) as a possible difference in pragmatic (versus semantic or syntactic) competence in terms of the use of Given and New information. A summary of the contrast between the performance of left and right hemidecorticates is presented in Figure 1.

The foregoing account provides some valuable illumination of possible neuropsychological factors underlying but one of a number of skills involved in the construction and comprehension of narratives.

Oral and Written Narrative Skills in Students with Learning Disabilities   To this point the consideration of differences and deficits in the discourse skills of individuals with learning disabilities has been limited to the oral modality. Analysis of both oral and written narrative discourse skills of individuals with and without learning disabilities is provided by a study by Montague, Maddux, and Dereshiwsky (1990). Preadolescent and adolescent students with and without learning disabilities heard/read and retold stories in Task 1, and in Task 2 generated their own written stories following the provided opening statement. In accordance with the findings in the above review of story grammar, all students, both with and without learning disabilities, demonstrated an understanding of narrative discourse schema in both modes, although to a more rudimentary degree by students with learning disabilities.

A striking difference between the products of the two groups was the quantity and quality of internal response information. That is, stories retold or self-generated by students with learning disabilities contained significantly fewer internal responses, attesting to their scanty attention to or expression of characters' thoughts, feelings, goals, and motives. Although other deficits were evident, it was observed by the authors that the shorter story length typically produced by subjects with learning disabilities would have been increased in proportion to the inclusion of sufficient information in the internal response category. This pattern may be interpreted as exemplifying Myklebust's (1965) analysis of concreteness in the written stories of

Right Hemidecorticate
(has only left hemisphere)

Effective use of anaphoric pronouns
and linkage to prior referents
Effective use of Given/New
information

Left Hemidecorticate
(has only right hemisphere)

Less effective linking of pronouns
to prior referents; fewer pronouns
Excessive repetition of noun references
Less effective use of Given/New
information

Figure 1.   Cohesion in narratives by left and right hemidecorticates. (From Newman, J.E., Lovett, M.W., & Dennis, M. [1986]. The use of discourse analysis in neurolinguistics: Some findings from the narratives of hemidecorticate adolescents. *Topics in Language Disorders, 7,* 31–44, reprinted by permission.)

children with learning disabilities; that is, ideation that is bound to the observable, with a lesser tendency toward abstract expressions (D.J. Johnson & Myklebust, 1967).

Among other findings, written stories of students with learning disabilities through 11th grade continued to be inferior to those of normally achieving students in organization, cohesion, and episodic structure. The aforementioned limitations in ability to process affective information showed no appreciable gain across grade levels (Montague et al., 1990).

The findings of deficits in narrative discourse skills reported above take on added significance in light of their possible relations to more general academic achievement. In a longitudinal study of language subtypes in 6- and 7-year-old children with learning disabilities, Feagans and Appelbaum (1986) found that children whose narrative abilities exceeded their syntactic and semantic skills were less likely to experience academic failure than children whose narrative abilities were poorer than their measured abilities in syntax and semantics. "Narrative ability was shown to be relatively important in predicting academic outcomes" (p. 363). (See Chapter 6 for discussion of subtyping research.)

Writing Problems

As was stated at the beginning of this chapter, the severity of language deficits varies widely across reports by different authors about different populations. This variation is no less true in the area of written language than oral language. The writing performance of individuals with learning disabilities has been studied across many dimensions by a number of investigators (Gajar, 1989; Graham, 1990; Houck & Billingsley, 1989; D.J. Johnson & Myklebust, 1967; Moran, 1988; Newcomer, Barenbaum, & Nodine, 1988), whose findings and interpretations are summarized.

Expository Prose   Most of the foregoing discussion of deficits in discourse processing, oral and written, has been devoted to the narrative mode. It is important at this point to consider the difference between written narrative and expository prose with reference to the demands these genres place on the writer. As Westby (1989) pointed out in her discussion of reading comprehension, processing of expository prose is more demanding than processing of narratives. "The relative independence of content facts, content schemata, and text grammar marks a major difference between expository prose and stories" (p. 203). In other words, comprehension of expository prose requires construction of meaning without the support of familiar story grammar structure, plus the intake of factual information based more on bottom-up than top-down processing. The distinction between the two forms of written discourse applies equally to the expressive process of composition.

Students with learning disabilities are less likely to compose text that conforms to expectations for writing in the expository genre. They have exhibited problems in generating and organizing content of acceptable quality and quantity (Graham, 1990). These limitations have been attributed, in part, to a disruption of the writing process resulting from difficulties with and concerns about the mechanics of writing described above (Graham, 1990; Moran, 1987). It is presumed that slow, effortful composition may interfere with the development of and memory for ideas and their coherent associations.

Graham (1990) studied the effects of three conditions on the composition of expository prose by fourth- and sixth-grade students with learning disabilities: 1) traditional writing procedure, 2) dictation of oral texts onto audiotape at a normal rate of sentence generation, and 3) dictation to an adult scribe, requiring a slowed rate of composition in order to allow time for the scribe to finish writing each sentence before producing the next sentence in the composition. The effects of an additional procedure, production signaling (i.e., prompts to write/say more about the topic) were examined in each of the three composition conditions. Results are reported in the appropriate sections below. Overall, under the condition of slowed dictation, compositions were significantly longer than those produced under other conditions and were judged to be of higher essay quality than written compositions.

Productivity/Fluency   Writers with learning disabilities tend to be more limited in their amount of written output than writers without such disabilities in terms of number of words and sentences produced. They have been observed to be more fluent in the oral than the written modality. The subjects in Graham's (1990) study produced significantly longer essays in the condition of slowed oral dictation than in writing. It has been suggested by a number of authors that this restriction in written output may be related to difficulties with the mechanics of spelling and punctuation, to be discussed below. The superior results secured under conditions of slowed oral dictation were attributed by Graham (1990) to elimination of the disruptive demands of attention to the mechanics of writing. This difference in fluency between the oral and written modalities is illustrated by the sample presented in Figure 2 of oral and written production by the same 10-year-old boy with specific learning disabilities (provided by D.J. Johnson & Myklebust, 1967).

The positive response of subjects in Graham's (1990) study to production signaling led to significant increases in quantity of content. This outcome was interpreted to signify that students with learning disabilities tend to terminate the composing process too soon, possibly because "producing expository text may be particularly difficult for [learning disabled] students" (Graham, 1990, p. 790). The degree of effort may be an important factor in reducing motivation for composition.

Syntactic Maturity   One aspect of reduced syntactic maturity in the writing of students with learning disabilities is a tendency to use limited variations in sentence types (Moran, 1988). These constraints are contrasted with the greater variation observed in oral communication. Another issue, that of structural complexity in the writing of individuals with learning disabilities, is still unresolved. Studies of different age groups yield conflicting results and interpretations.

No significant between-group differences were found in number of morphemes per T-unit produced by fourth-, eighth-, and 11th-grade students with and without learning disabilities (Houck & Billingsley, 1989). Normally achieving secondary school students exceeded students with learning disabilities in mean morphemes per T-unit (Moran, 1988). College students with learning disabilities achieved higher scores on mean words per T-unit than students without such disabilities (Gajar, 1989). Furthermore, while Moran (1988) found no between-group difference in percentage of complex T-units produced by secondary school students, T-units produced by fourth- and eighth-grade students with learning disabilities were less complex than those of normally achieving peers (Houck & Billingsley, 1989). Of course, it is recognized that length of T-unit is not an unequivocal measure of clausal complexity, since length may be an effect of the addition of adjectives and prepositional phrases, which do not determine syntactic complexity at the sentence structure level (Gajar, 1989).

Analysis of other indicators of syntactic maturity has revealed that children and adolescents with learning disabilities use less elaborated noun and verb phrases and less frequent optional modifiers such as adjectives, adverbs, prepositional phrases, and clausal comple-

A short time ago the United States Navy sent up a moon. This moon is traveling around our earth extremely fast. Sometimes it is less than 400 miles from the earth. At other times it is more than 2,500 miles away. The Vanguard has had many failures, but one morning the pencil-shaped rocket was sent into space. The transmitters inside the moon are run by two different sources of electricity. One is powered by the sun. This is called a solar battery. The other is just an ordinary battery. The Museum of Science and Industry has put up a few new exhibits on the Vanguard. Now we may trace its flight.

A

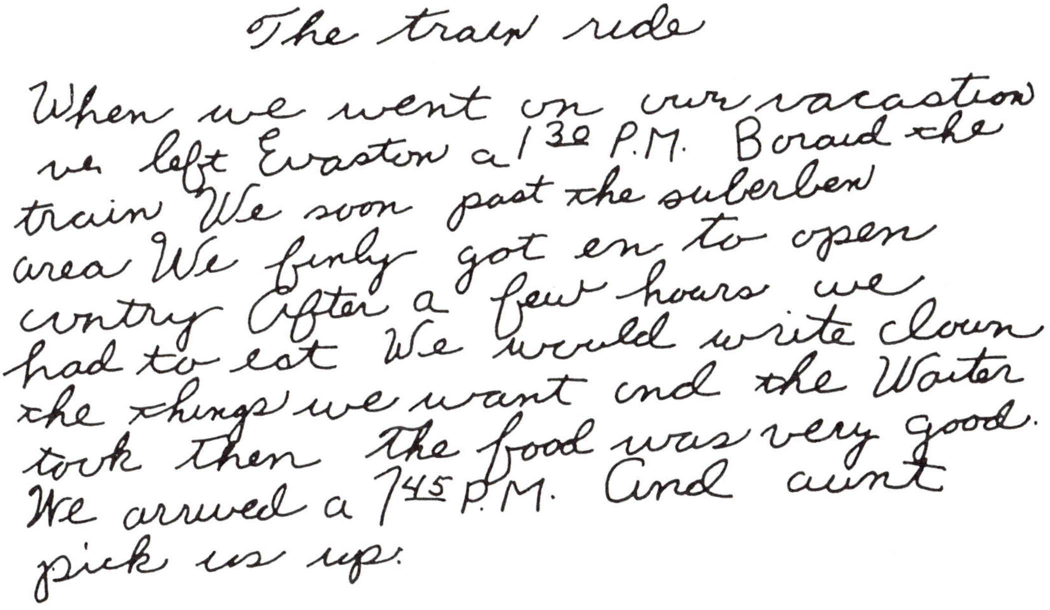
The train ride

When we went on our vacation we left Evaston a 1 30 P.M. Boraid the train We soon past the suberben area We finly got en to open contry After a few hours we had to eat We would write down the things we want and the Waiter took then the food was very good. We arrived a 7 45 P.M. And aunt pick us up.

B

Figure 2. Samples of oral (A) and written (B) language production by a 10-year-old boy with learning disabilities. (From Johnson, D.J., & Myklebust, H.R. [1967]. *Learning disabilities: Educational principles and practices.* New York: Grune & Stratton; reprinted by permission.)

ments (Moran, 1988). In addition to the possible constraints imposed by difficulty with the mechanics of writing mentioned above, it is speculated that some limitations in verbal memory may impede the construction of more elaborated sentences (D.J. Johnson & Myklebust, 1967).

Quality of Content Narrative or personalized style is frequently used when expository prose is appropriate for academic tasks. However, even the quality of narration in the stories of children with learning disabilities has been found to reflect a delay in the internalization of story schema (Newcomer et al., 1988). In response to picture stimuli, 8- to 11-year-old children with learning disabilities wrote fewer narratives that met the criteria for stories (i.e., beginning, middle, and end plus some conflict and resolution) and more descriptions of the pictures without any sequencing of events than were produced by normally achieving peers. In his early study using the Picture Story Language Test, Myklebust (1965) found that children with learning disabilities were less imaginative, less elaborated, and more concrete in expression of ideas in their written stories than were controls.

There is a possibility that the use of picture stimuli may tend to elicit more concrete descriptive than narrative responses in the written output of some children with learning disabilities. There is some lack of agreement about the impact of modality on composition. Newcomer et al. (1988) reported that, even in the oral modality, their subjects with learning disabilities generated fewer stories reflecting narrative schema than did normally achieving peers. However, Moran (1988) reported that, in her own study and other studies surveyed, adolescents with learning disabilities performed at a level equivalent to achieving students on oral composition with respect to ideation and organization, as well as linguistic complexity and productivity. The oral modality was found more favorable for the retelling of stories by students with learning disabilities than was the written modality, in terms of responsiveness to the thematic importance of the material and the amount recalled (Fuchs & Maxwell, 1988).

In Graham's (1990) study of expository composition, the slowed condition of oral dictation resulted in higher essay quality than did written composition in terms of the use of almost twice as many textual units such as premises, reasons, elaborations, and conclusions. However, some incidence of nonfunctional units (e.g., repetitions or irrelevant content) were noted in both conditions in reaction to productive signaling.

Vocabulary   Students with learning disabilities in grades 4, 8, and 11 were found to use significantly fewer words with seven or more letters (a measure of vocabulary maturation) than did normally achieving students (Houck & Billingsley, 1989). College students with learning disabilities used fewer different words than did peers without such disabilities in their written compositions. This measure has been found to be the best predictor of composition ratings at the unversity level (Gajar, 1989).

Errors and Omissions   Omissions of words and word endings along with errors of agreement and tense occur with a higher frequency in the writing of individuals with learning disabilities than in the writing of those without such disabilities. This pattern has been observed at all age and grade levels (Houck & Billingsley, 1989; D.J. Johnson & Myklebust, 1967; Moran, 1988). These omissions and occasional substitutions of words are considered to be a probable manifestation of attention lapses and less efficient proofreading skills.

Punctuation and Capitalization   Moran (1988) observed that apparent difficulty with sentence structure in the writing of students with learning disabilities reflected failure to master the mechanics of punctuation of sentence boundaries, not basic syntactic immaturity. Thus, the high frequency of sentence fragments and run-on sentences is attributed to this failure. Associated with sentence punctuation is the use of capitalization. Houck and Billingsley (1989) reported that, in this skill, "11th graders with learning disabilities still have not achieved the level of accuracy obtained by [normally achieving] fourth graders" (p. 567).

Spelling   Spelling disability is a widely recognized characteristic of dyslexia (Boder, 1971; Bradley, 1983; M.M. Gerber, 1986; D.J. Johnson & Myklebust, 1967; Siegel & Ryan, 1984). Moran (1988) reported that students with learning disabilities, when questioned about their relatively unelaborated writing style, have said that they do not try to write more extensively because they are unable to spell many words. In her comparison of the writing of students with learning disabilities and that of low-achieving students without learning disabilities and high-achieving students, Moran (1988) found that only lower spelling accuracy distinguished students classified as having learning disabilities from low-achieving students in regular education classes.

Houck and Billingsley (1989) found more spelling errors by students with learning disabilities than their normally achieving peers across grades 4, 8, and 11. They did note some improvement from grades 4 to 8 by both groups but no significant improvement by either group between 8th and 11th grade. D.J. Johnson and Myklebust (1967) provided a sample of a severe spelling disorder in an adolescent (Fig. 3).

Research on Spelling Problems Ehri (1989) and M.M. Gerber (1986) have analyzed patterns of dysfunctional spelling in terms of categories of errors observed in normally developing young children in stages of emergent literacy. The classifications by these two authors are similar, but terminology differs slightly. Descriptions and examples of error categories are as follows:

> *Precommunicative* (Ehri)/*Preliterate* (Gerber): Scribbles or assortments of letters and nonletters demonstrating no knowledge of correspondences between phonemes and graphemes (e.g., *KO/muffin*; *8T/eighty*).
> *Semiphonetic* (Ehri)/*Prephonetic* (Gerber): Alphabetic representations of some but not all sounds in words (e.g., *PL/pickle*; *UM/human*).
> *Phonetic* (Ehri and Gerber): Representations of sounds heard in words, even when such representations are inaccurate (e.g., *DOKTDR/doctor*; *HIKT/hiked*).
> *Transitional* (Gerber): Recognizable approximations of conventional spellings with legal letter sequences, but some incorrect letter combinations (e.g., *PEAKED/peeked*).
> *Correct* (Gerber): Conventional spellings produced at times with variable speeds and self-corrections.

The following examples of spellings generated by a 22-year-old man with dyslexia were reported by Ehri (1989):

> *THRUT/truck*   *CHREAT/chicken*   *GERAT/drinking* (p. 363)

Increasing incidence of spellings approximating accuracy were observed with maturation. However, "the preponderance of errors produced by [learning-disabled] students were similar to those expected of normally achieving children who were 3–5 years younger" (M.M. Gerber, 1986, p. 531).

A number of other researchers have found some correlation between specific aspects of reading and spelling skills. Table 8 summarizes some of the characterizations of types of spelling difficulties identified and described in these studies.

Differences in the ability to adopt appropriate strategies in different conditions were demonstrated in Bradley's (1983) study of spelling and reading problems. She found that 55% of young normally achieving readers/spellers who were not successful on a visual memory task were successful on various auditory organization tasks (the ability to group words on the basis of sound patterns, segment speech sounds, and generalize from a known word, *fight*, to an unknown word, *light*), but only 4.9% of readers/spellers experiencing deficiencies were successful on an auditory organization task. Bradley (1983) concluded that, although the two groups were equivalent in visual memory, normally achieving readers/spellers were able to shift to an auditory strategy when appropriate to task demands, whereas readers/spellers with deficiencies were apparently unable to use an alternate auditory strategy when the task requires such a shift. It is suggested that, beyond visual memory and/or auditory analysis, some more general ability to reason or develop rules for the processing of information may be involved in the inferior performance of the reader/speller with deficiencies.

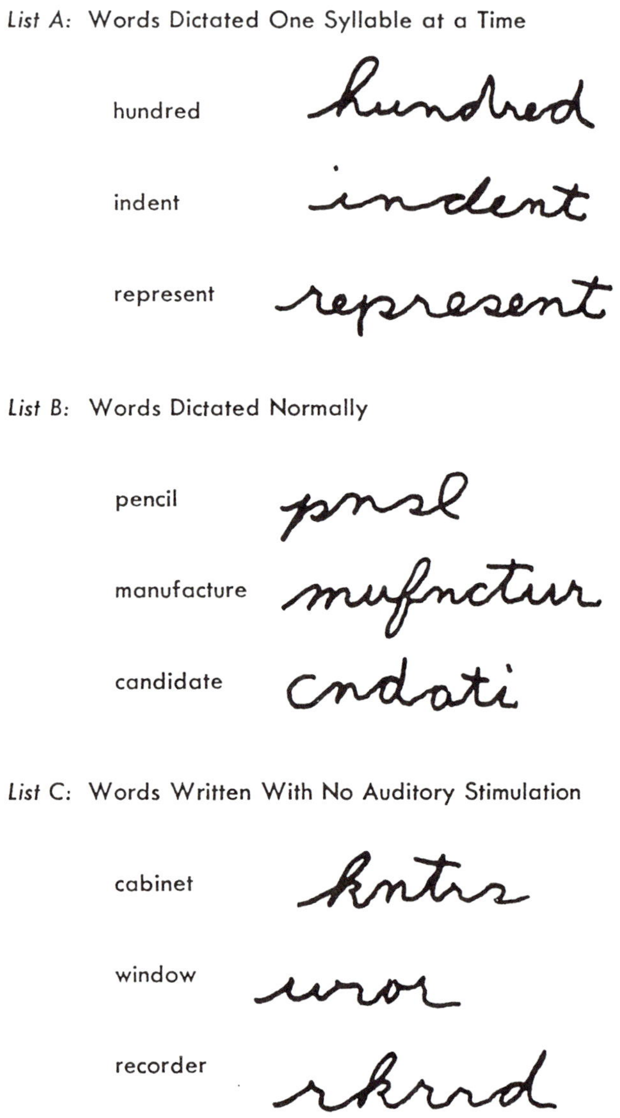

List A: Words Dictated One Syllable at a Time

hundred   *hundred*

indent   *indent*

represent   *represent*

List B: Words Dictated Normally

pencil   *pnsl*

manufacture   *mufnctur*

candidate   *cndati*

List C: Words Written With No Auditory Stimulation

cabinet   *kntr*

window   *wror*

recorder   *rkrrd*

Figure 3. Samples of production by a 15-year-old boy with severe spelling disorder. (From Johnson, D.J., & Myklebust, H.R. [1967]. *Learning disabilities: Educational principles and practices.* New York: Grune & Stratton; reprinted by permission.)

Viewing spelling problems from a different perspective, Jimenez and Rumeau (1989) attribute spelling deficiencies to instructional method. Spelling errors were identified in written passages and classified as follows:

Omissions (e.g., *frenship/friendship*)
Additions (e.g., *raydio/radio*)

Table 8. Classes of spelling problems in patterns of disability

Investigators	Spelling types	Characteristics
Treiman and Baron (1983)	"Phoenicians" rely heavily on sound/spelling rules	Good at spelling regular words Poorer at spelling exceptional words
	"Chinese" rely heavily on word-specific visual images	Good at recognizing familiar sight words Poorer with unfamiliar words requiring analysis of sound–letter correspondences
Rourke (1983)	Phonetically accurate (PA) excessive reliance on phonemic analysis	Difficulty going beyond phonemic information in order to use visual gestalts (visual memory not believed to be a factor)
	Phonetically inaccurate (PI) linguistic deficits	Difficulty with phonemic segmentation, retrieval, and synthesis Visual memory deficits

Mixing of letters and/or syllables to the point of illegibility
Vertical reversal (e.g., *mau/man*)
Corruption by dividing a word and attaching a final syllable to the next word
Letter-order errors (e.g., *sopt/stop*)
Similar looking letters (e.g., *jellow/yellow*)
Similar sounding letters (e.g., *freguent/frequent*)
Static letter reversals (e.g., *dib/did*)
Unions of words that should be written separately (p. 197)

Different patterns of spelling errors were associated with either a phonics or sight-word approach to reading, with certain types assumed to result from an undue emphasis on rote learning of grapheme-phoneme relations in early reading and writing instruction. Since many normally achieving students have become good spellers under both instructional methods and many students with learning disabilities have failed to master spelling under either condition, it is difficult to generalize from these findings and their interpretation to an understanding of the marked and persistent spelling disorders frequently manifested by individuals with learning disabilities throughout their life span.

M.M. Gerber (1986) and M.M. Gerber and Hall (1987) have speculated about factors that may be disruptive to spelling acquisition in students with learning disabilities. It was observed that spelling performance did improve as a result of an intensive training approach consisting of adult imitation of student errors and modeling of correct spellings. Instances of failure to generalize from successful training to spontaneous use were thought to result from possible information processing deficits, such as poor attention control, inadequate content and organization of spelling knowledge, memory overload, slow rate of mastery, and inadequate integration of new spellings with preexisting knowledge. "If the dynamic interdependency among these processes is disturbed at early stages of acquisition, initial difficulties are severely compounded over time" (M.M. Gerber, 1986).

Writing and Reading Expository Prose

The results of a study of students' skills in writing and reading expository text serve as a fitting conclusion to this section on discourse processing problems. Englert, Raphael, Anderson, Gregg, & Anthony, 1989) examined the writing and reading performance of fourth- and fifth-grade students classified into three groups: 1) those with learning disabilities, 2) high achievers, and 3) low achievers without learning disabilities. Students with learning disabilities demonstrated markedly deficient skills in comparison with the other groups on the following measures:

> Written expository texts and written summaries of two passages were significantly less well organized and contained significantly fewer ideas.
>
> Comprehension and recall of expository prose passages were characterized by significantly fewer of the passage ideas and significantly poorer organization of ideas recalled.

The authors concluded that, in reading, subjects with learning disabilities were relatively insensitive to the text structure of expository prose. Regarding writing skills, Englert et al. (1989) concluded that the students with learning disabilities "had yet to acquire a working knowledge of the organizational framework that would help them retrieve systematically relevant ideas from background knowledge and organize their ideas to produce well-organized and coherent prose" (p. 13).

Summary

Repeatedly throughout the foregoing discussion of various aspects of language reported to be problematic for individuals with learning disabilities, patterns have emerged that raise questions about the nature of the deficits that apparently have a negative impact on academic performance. Certain questions relate to the possible interaction between language and cognitive deficits in the processing of information. This issue is addressed throughout much of Chapter 8. Another issue that must be considered is a distinction between the relative roles in learning disability of deficits in the development of the primary language systems (phonology, syntax, and semantics) and deficits in metalinguistic skills. In a similar vein, a third question concerns a possible distinction between deficiencies in primary linguistic abilities and deficiencies in the *ability to use* linguistic knowledge (or pragmatics) for skilled verbal communication in the performance of academic tasks. Both of these latter issues are considered below.

METALINGUISTIC DEFICIENCIES

The role of primary versus metalinguistic deficiency in reading and writing failure is not yet clear. While deficits in metalinguistic skills have been viewed by many as causal to reading disability, Van Kleeck (1984b) advanced the notion that they may indeed be *fostered* by reading. It is not unlikely that early reading failure may have a profound circular effect on the later development of both primary language and metalinguistic abilities.

Although there is little doubt that many students with learning disabilities have experienced delays in language development through preschool and, in some cases, into the early school period, numerous reports cited above seem to attest to gains in the acquisition of primary linguistic systems through later school years into adolescence. It is, of course, acknowledged that certain deficits continue to be overtly observable in some adolescents and young adults with learning disabilities, but these and other less overt deficiencies may not generally be of an order of severity that would justify classifying many of these individuals as having a language impairment. From their research, Wiig and Semel (1984) could not conclude that deficits in auditory processing and oral production were necessarily coexistent. Rather, they supposed that a deficit in one aspect of language may, in all likelihood, be counterbalanced by assets or adequate performance in other areas.

In accordance with the tentative conclusion reached by Kamhi and Catts (1986), it may be the case that the language abilities and disabilities of individuals with learning disabilities range along a continuum:

> At one end of the continuum would be the language-impaired child who has had a severe expressive and/or receptive language delay in the preschool years. At the other end would be the poor reader who has had no history of language problems but is reading significantly below grade level. (p. 345)

The point is made, however, that within this continuum there are discontinuities reflected in the lack of correspondence in degree of severity between the two types of disorder. One of the characteristics distinguishing individuals with reading impairments and writing deficiencies from those without such deficits appears to be degree of metalinguistic awareness.

In retrospect, many of the research tasks on which selected aspects of syntax and semantics have been tested involve examination of metalinguistic rather than primary linguistic abilities. This author holds a view similar to that expressed by Van Kleeck (1984b), that tasks requiring subjects to give word definitions, synonyms, antonyms, analogies, and the like, or to recognize and correct grammatical or morphological anomalies in sentences are tapping into heightened language awareness rather than tacit linguistic knowledge. It is not maintained that such skills are not pertinent to the performance of many educational tasks, but it is necessary to differentiate between abilities and disabilities in these domains.

Metalinguistic Deficits and Reading Disability

That metalinguistic deficits do affect academic language performance is most evident at a functional, rather than contrived, level in written language skills, both receptive and expressive. The reader will recall the extensive research presenting evidence of a relationship between heightened phonological awareness and early reading acquisition. At the skilled level, it is maintained that the differences between speech and reading can be explained "only if we regard reading as a deliberately acquired, language-based skill, dependent upon the speaker-hearer's awareness of certain primary linguistic activity" (Mattingly, 1972, p. 145). It may therefore be the more limited ability of the individual with learning disabilities to bring to a level of heightened awareness his or her primary linguistic knowledge that lies at the heart of the reading problem in many cases.

Metalinguistic Deficits and Writing Disability

Metalinguistic deficits are readily observed in the writing process. According to the above descriptions of the discrepancy observed between the oral language structure of adolescents with learning disabilities and the structure realized in their written output, reduced awareness of sentence form and of the mechanics used for marking sentence boundaries must account for at least part of the inferior quality of their writing. Spelling may be viewed as a special case of metalinguistic deficit. Since spelling requires heightened awareness of sound-letter correspondences and of other aspects of word structure, the prevalence of markedly severe spelling problems among individuals with learning disabilities would seem to attest to a prounced deficiency in this particular area of metalinguistic abilities. Failure to detect errors of omission and/or additions of words, which is not observed in the spoken language of these individuals, is characteristic of ineffective proofreading, implicating a lower level of linguistic awareness.

Beyond these structural aberrations signifying inferior monitoring of written language, reports of the content of both oral and written discourse lead to the assumption that speakers and writers with learning disabilities tend to construct messages that fail to communicate with clarity, completeness of information, or appropriateness of style. In this area, the boundary between metalinguistics and pragmatics becomes blurred.

Metalinguistics and Pragmatics

Two types of pragmatic deficits have been inferred. One type has been categorized as inadequate awareness of the stylistic appropriateness of written composition for particular functions. That is, the rambling narrative or personalized style frequently observed in these students' writing is generally inappropriate for the academic functions requiring objective, logically organized expository prose. Admittedly, this deficiency may be the result of factors other than lack of pragmatic knowledge. Restricted experience with written language, insufficient or inadequate instruction, and reduced motivation may all contribute to failure to develop control of expository written prose (Shaughnessy, 1977). The other type of metalinguistic-pragmatic deficit most frequently inferred about the discourse deficiencies of the individual with learning disabilities is the failure to adequately take the perspective of the listener-reader.

Taking the Perspective of Readers/Listeners Insufficient awareness of information possessed or required by the message receiver may be a factor influencing the reported sparsity and lack of specificity of verbal output. This phenomenon has been investigated in a number of studies of referential communication abilities of children with and without learning disabilities.

The dyadic barrier game format has been used to study both expressive communication and receptive processing skills in a situation requiring explicit verbal encoding and decoding of oral directions without visual support. Children with learning disabilities, compared to normally achieving peers, have been observed to provide less specific, task-relevant information in terms of spatial relations and pronoun reference (Bryen, 1981) and more contradictory or repetitious information (Bunce, 1989). Listeners with learning disabilities appear to be as capable as their normally achieving counterparts in following directions but less efficient in the use of questions to gain additional necessary information (Bunce, 1989; Spekman, 1981).

The research provides evidence supporting the notion of a production deficit in the communication of subjects with learning disabilities. For example, Bunce (1989) reported no significant difference between the performance of subjects with and without learning disabilities after five 25-minute training sessions for subjects with learning disabilities over a period of 2 weeks. These beneficial effects were found to persist in a follow-up testing situation 6–8 months later.

It should be noted that subjects in the cited studies had not been identified as having an overt language impairment. Also, although the communication skills required for the experimental task have been roughly equated with those required for classroom demands, there is a recognized need to examine performance in the educational versus experimental setting (Spekman, 1981). From the present author's perspective, this is judged advisable because of a difference between the context-supported experimental task in which concrete objects are used and the decontextualized receptive and expressive language processing demands of education.

The foregoing information contains some degree of overlap between metalinguistic and pragmatic factors. Other research has investigated the use of language for specific functions by children with language-related learning disabilities.

PRAGMATIC CORRELATES OF LEARNING DISABILITIES

The nature of pragmatic deficits in people with learning disabilities defies simplistic description or attribution. Studies of pragmatic abilities/disabilities in individuals having learning disabilities led a number of investigators to implicate cognitive and social competence (Brinton & Fujiki, 1982; Brinton, Fujiki, & Sonnenberg, 1988; Bryan, Donahue, & Pearl, 1981; Bryan & Bryan, 1978; Donahue, 1981, 1986; Donahue & Bryan, 1983; Meline & Brackin, 1987; Spekman, 1981). Students with learning disabilities have been reported by these researchers:

To be more hostile than normally achieving peers in communication

To be more likely to ignore interpersonal initiation from peers

To be less assertive, less tactful, and less persuasive in conversation

To be less likely to seek more information in the presence of message inadequacy

To be less likely to request clarification in the absence of comprehension

To provide significantly less information necessary for task completion

To be less proficient in monitoring message adequacy

Most investigators report that, under particular controlled conditions such as modeling, instruction, and reward, these children have demonstrated the requisite linguistic and social skills for performing appropriate speech acts. "The fact that these skills were immediately acquired without laborious remediation suggests that modelling intervention was not teaching children new behaviors, but rather demonstrating when to mobilize existing ones" (Donahue & Bryan, 1983, p. 271).

Repair of Communication Breakdown

One area that has had a specific impact on academic performance has been the failure of many students with learning disabilities to initiate repairs of communicative breakdown, particularly in requesting clarification in the absence of comprehension. It is suggested that their history of communication and social difficulty "may have led them to doubt their own comprehension skill and overestimate their partner's ability to provide adequate messages" (Donahue, 1986). Another interpretation attributes the passivity of the child with learning disabilities in communication breakdown to a "failure of the learning disabled to understand the social obligations required of listeners in such circumstances" (Spekman, 1981).

More recent investigations of these issues have examined the ability and inclination of children with language deficits to respond to repeated requests for clarification, designated as "stacked clarification requests" (Brinton et al., 1988). In their comparison of subjects who had a language impairment with children without impairment matched for chronological age and language age (younger children), Brinton et al. found that some differences existed in response to different types of requests for clarification under repeated conditions:

> Children without impairment of the same chronological age complied more frequently than the other groups by supplying additional and/or background information.
>
> Children with language impairment and younger children matched for language age complied more frequently by revising the *form* of response.
>
> Children with language impairment produced more inappropriate responses than other subjects.
>
> Children with language impairment ignored repeated requests for clarification more frequently than other subjects.

It was observed by the investigators that the children with language impairment seemed to find the task of stacked repairs more taxing than did the other groups. They concluded that the discrepancy between the group with language impairment and other groups was not completely explained in terms of limited ability with language form and content. "It was not the case that the impaired subjects lacked repair strategies, but rather that they lacked persistence in applying them" (Brinton et al., 1988, p. 390). This lack of persistence was interpreted as a possible reaction of these children to their deficit, in terms of retreat for fear of making errors. This suggestion is in accordance with a characterization of students with learning disabilities as those whose sensed inadequacy inhibits motivation for sustained effort. Thus, it is not always easy to determine whether certain performance problems stem from psychosocial or pragmatic factors.

Functional Communicative Competence

Questions have been raised regarding the generalizability of the results of these and other studies of selected aspects of communication on small samples of children with learning disabilities. In his review of 19 studies of pragmatic competence of students having learning disabilities, Dudley-Marling (1985) found a lack of unified support for the assumption that these students as a group have pragmatic deficits. Furthermore, the fact that some samples were identified as having language impairment and others as being free of identifiable language impairment confounds the issue of linguistic versus social or cognitive inadequacies as possible causal factors.

McCord and Haynes (1988) studied the naturalistic conversations of subjects with and without learning disabilities (8–11 years old), none of whom were identifiable as having language impairment. Damico's (1980) nine measures of discourse (adapted here) served as the basis of analysis:

> Failure to provide necessary amount or type of information
> Use of nonspecific vocabulary without clarifying antecedents
> Need for multiple repetitions before improvement in comprehension
> Poor topic maintenance: inappropriate shifts without transitional cues
> Inappropriate responses, suggestive of inattention or unresponsiveness to prompts or probes of others
> Linguistic nonfluency in the form of frequent disruptions, hesitations, and so on
> Revision behavior in terms of false starts and self-corrections

Delays of inordinant length before responding

Turn-taking difficulty manifested by not allowing others to comment on previous information or to add/request further information

Results revealed significant group differences on failure to provide necessary information, need for repetition, and poor topic maintenance. No significant differences were found between subjects with and without learning disabilities on the other six categories of discourse errors analyzed. While quantitatively there was no significant difference between groups on discourse errors, qualitatively it was observed that the two groups of subjects tended to make different kinds of errors. Therefore, it was noted that "based on Damico's (1980) guidelines for making problem/no problem decisions, this study suggests that some [learning-disabled] subjects as well as the [non–learning-disabled] subjects exhibited mild pragmatic deficits" (McCord & Haynes, 1988, p. 241).

In conclusion, it would appear that students with language-related learning disabilities are more likely to experience pragmatic deficits as a result of a sensed inadequacy in verbal communication and social interaction. However, even students with learning disabilities not identified as having language impairment are apparently at greater risk than normally achieving peers for less adequate use of language for social and academic functions. It is recommended that speech-language pathologists and classroom teachers be alert to the pragmatic problems of students with learning disabilities in assessment and referral for special services (McCord & Haynes, 1988).

SUMMARY AND CONCLUSIONS

All of the foregoing evidence attests to a relationship between learning and language disabilities. Ceci (1987) has expressed his preference for the term *language/learning disability* instead of *reading disability*. However, the diversity of the population with learning disabilities precludes generalizations about the nature of the relationship. Groups studied have varied from those overtly delayed or deficient in oral language to those exhibiting problems only in the decontextualized language of education, written and/or oral. Subjects in studies of language-reading relationships have also covered a range of ages, with, at times, resulting discrepant findings. For example, the oral language skills found related to reading comprehension in young children with reading disability differed from those relationships observed in older subjects, with younger children appearing to place greater reliance on syntactic and lexical information and older students relying more heavily on the use of narrative discourse processes (Snyder & Downey, 1991).

The following tentative conclusions about the nature of language-related learning disabilities are regarded as plausible:

Slower, less efficient processing of verbal information in working memory may interfere with optimal integration of words and propositions for comprehension of the written and oral language of education.

Impaired comprehension may result from reduced available capacity for accessing relevant stored schematic knowledge.

Bottom-up deficiencies in perceptual pickup of verbal information may contribute to the formulation of incomplete or inaccurate phonological representations.

An impoverished semantic knowledge base may negatively affect verbal information
   processing as a result of reduced top-down effects and may contribute to retrieval
   difficulties.
Individuals with language-related learning disabilities may vary in their ability to construct or sustain internal representations of linguistically encoded information in the
   absence of contextual support.
Deficient sensitivity to organization of verbal information may interfere with optimal
   comprehension and/or composition of extended passages of written discourse.

Some students who possess basic linguistic competence may process the decontextualized language of literacy only by expending a degree of effort that is stressful to an extent that
limits motivation to maintain performance at the level required for academic success. Thus,
there is reason to believe that in these individuals there is a lesser inclination to engage in
extended verbal processing, whether in the form of expressive elaboration or of the decoding,
storage, and retrieval of higher levels of linguistically encoded information. The degree to
which such limitations have an impact on communicative effectiveness, both academic and
social, continues to be the subject of research.

We may characterize students with language-related learning disabilities as individuals
with low versus high verbal abilities, required to function in an educational process that, by its
very nature, places high verbal demands on them. Low verbal abilities may be determined by
either genetic diversity or neurological malfunction, with probable variation in causality
among members of this population.

Scholars of language disorders hold different views about causality of specific language
impairment—that is, delayed or deficient language development in the absence of documented sensory, intellectual, or emotional disorder. In view of the scanty evidence of neuropathology in most of these children, some investigators have inclined toward the genetic diversity explanation of limitations in language proficiency (Dale & Cole, 1991; Leonard, 1991;
Tomblin, 1991).

It has been reasoned that, in the area of language, there is likely to be a range of proficiency analogous to that observed in such domains as musical ability or physical prowess in the
population at large, and that some individuals fall at the lower end of a normal continuum
(Leonard, 1991). Support for the genetic diversity hypothesis may be drawn from studies revealing familial patterns of limited language proficiency (Olson et al., 1989; Tomblin, 1991)
and of reading disability (B.A. Lewis, 1990; B.A. Lewis et al., 1989).

Although receptive to the genetic diversity position, which tends to deemphasize the relevance of attempts at neurological explanations, some scholars argue that research aimed at
identification of the mechanisms underlying language development continues to be of value.
That is, the neurological substrates of language performance, whether normal or impaired,
merit efforts directed at increased understanding and explanation (J.R. Johnston, 1991).

This debate about causality of specific language impairment is not dissimilar to the one
that has engaged scholars in the field of learning disabilities at large. The shift in definitional
terminology from "minimal brain damage" to the more ambiguous clause "presumed to be due
to central nervous system dysfunction" appears to reflect the absence of a solid consensus
about the issue (see Chapters 1 and 6).

It has been repeatedly emphasized that the classification "learning disabilities" encompasses heterogeneity in type and degree of impairment, therefore probably reflecting variations

in etiology. Aram (1991) has pointed out that, in the category of "specific language impairment," descriptions and implied causality may stem from research on different populations. That is, while the larger, less severe population of school-referred cases may reflect the low end of a genetically determined normal distribution, more severe problems of clinical cases may be attributed to abnormality. Therefore, in the overlapping population of language-related learning disabilities, ruling out some types of neurological impairment in all cases may not be justified.

In addition to the language deficiencies described above, the academic difficulties experienced by students with learning disabilities may involve, to different degrees, cognitive deficits and psychosocial problems. These topics are discussed in Chapter 8.

8 / Cognitive and Psychosocial Correlates of Learning Disabilities

A language-related learning disability is obviously not an isolated phenomenon. Chapter 7 has examined learning disabilities in relation to their linguistic correlates. The present chapter focuses on correlates in two other areas: cognition and psychosocial variables. First, the tightly bound relationship between language and cognition, already identified in the review of cognitive information processing theory and research, is examined from the perspective of disability. Second, psychosocial correlates are addressed because of the not uncommon view that low achievement in academic language-related learning exacts a cost in personal and social adjustment.

COGNITIVE CORRELATES OF LEARNING DISABILITIES

Both research and theory on cognitive deficits associated with learning disabilities have increased significantly over the last decade. An examination of the cognitive correlates of learning disabilities requires discussion of the separate areas of perception, attention, and memory and the interaction among them. In each of these areas theoretical developments and research have undergone some shifts in perspective.

Perception

Views on the role of perception in the field of learning disabilities have shifted over time. Different emphases have been placed on the relationship of perception to reading and to other aspects of learning. In this section, the hypothesized relation between visual-perceptual impairment and reading disability is examined first. Then, research on other aspects of auditory and visual perceptual deficits in learning disabilities is summarized.

Visual Perception and Reading Disability   In the area of reading disability, early views that visual-perceptual deficits were a cause of reading disability have not been supported by subsequent research. (This body of literature was reviewed in Chapter 1.) Because of the failure of early research to establish the value of perceptual and perceptual-motor assessment and training, the Board of Trustees of the Council for Learning Disabilities issued a position paper (1986) opposing such practices as part of learning disability services.

During the 1970s, some alternative notions about perceptual processing were advanced that differed from the early conceptualizations of learning and reading disability alluded to above. For example, it was demonstrated that poor readers performed as well as skilled readers in the initial phase of visual information processing, during which perception occurs—that is, during the 0- to 300-millisecond interval following stimulus presentation. However, poor readers were significantly inferior to skilled readers in processing information during the interval of 300–2000 milliseconds, when coding of information for memory occurs (Morrison, Giordano, & Nagy, 1977). This led to the conclusion that poor readers were deficient not in perception but, rather, in the higher order encoding of perceived information for organization and retrieval.

Indeed, results of another study pointed to an *overadherence* to visual-perceptual information by poor readers (Klees & LeBrun, 1972). That is, poor readers tended to focus unduly on perceptually present letters and words rather than on the elaboration of relationships among words necessary to comprehension. Thus, in relation to reading disability, the assumed visual-perceptual deficits were not empirically demonstrated as a causal factor.

From a different perspective, the theories about perception discussed in Chapter 3 are pertinent to attempts to explain apparent perceptual problems observed in children with reading disabilities. Specifically, the proposed interaction between top-down, knowledge-based processing and bottom-up, data-based processing is relevant to this issue.

Reading Errors Caused by Linguistic Versus Visual Deficits   One of the more persistent myths about learning disabilities is the claim that people with dyslexia see letters or sequences of letters backward, thereby implicating a visual-perceptual impairment. However, empirically it has been found that, among the reading errors made by the poorest readers in a group of third-grade subjects, only 15% were due to letter sequence reversal (e.g., *was* for *saw*), and only 10% reflected letter orientation confusions (e.g., *b* for *d*). Confusion between such reversible letters as *b* and *d* occurred much more frequently when presented in words than when presented singly (Shankweiler & Liberman, 1972).

Furthermore, poor readers who may make such reversal errors have demonstrated intact visual perception by accurately copying letters and short words, even though they tended to make more errors than good readers in naming the words they have accurately copied (Vellutino, 1979). The greater difficulty experienced by poor readers in copying longer letter strings forming words, and their less accurate naming of these words, has been attributed to poorer verbal memory and deficient verbal knowledge. In other words, without adequate top-down verbal knowledge (of both oral and orthographic patterns), the visual processing system may become overloaded, leading to inaccuracies (Vellutino, 1979; Vellutino & Scanlon, 1986). The benefits of top-down processing reflect the notion of a trade-off between the amount of information "behind the eyeball" (stored in the brain) and the demands imposed upon the perceptual processing of information "in front of the eyeball" (Smith, 1973). The reversal and naming errors of poor readers have been interpreted, then, as evidence of a linguistic versus a perceptual deficit.

A striking example drawn from Vellutino's investigations is the finding that good young readers and poor young readers were equally inaccurate in processing the stimulus word *loin* as *lion*. That is, both groups identified an unfamiliar word as a familiar word, exemplifying the tendency to perceive information in the light of present knowledge. It is therefore surmised that children with language deficiencies are likely to bring less linguistic knowledge to bear during the processing of letter configurations that form words. Thus, the difficulties manifested by children with language-related learning disabilities in integrating the visual information of print with their verbal correspondences lie in the verbal, not the visual-perceptual, area (I.Y. Liberman & Shankweiler, 1979; I.Y. Liberman et al., 1982; Shankweiler & Liberman, 1979; Vellutino, 1979; Vellutino & Scanlon, 1986).

Perception and Information Processing Deficits   Although the belief that visual-perceptual impairment is causal to reading disability has been refuted, inefficient auditory- and visual-perceptual skills may, indeed, have a negative effect on learning. In contrast to individuals without learning disabilities, subjects with learning disabilities have demonstrated a tendency to process information in a more global, diffused, less differentiated perceptual style (E.K. Brown, 1974; Guyer & Friedman, 1975; Keogh & Donlon, 1972). In these studies, conducted during the 1970s, higher error rates and slower response time (longer latencies) were more prevalent in the verbal than the visual-perceptual mode by these children. However, more recently, there have been reports of inefficient and imprecise scanning of visual information as well as of lapses in auditory verbal pickup in the following of instructions and directions by individuals with learning disabilities with and without hyperactivity (Cotugno, 1987; Swanson, 1985).

Interpretation of research findings by such investigators as Kamhi and Catts (1986) and Brady and coworkers (1983; 1987), discussed in Chapter 7, and Ceci and Baker (1989), to be discussed below, along with the work of Tallal and her colleagues (Tallal & Piercy, 1973, 1974, 1978; Tallal, Stark, Kallman, & Mellits, 1981) provides support for the possibility that some problems experienced by individuals with learning disabilities may reflect auditory-perceptual deficits. However, a distinction should probably be made between what may be a primary perceptual problem in speech sound discrimination, possibly related to articulation disorders (and other phonologically related aspects of language development), and a deficit in phonological awareness widely assumed to be related to reading disability. That is, these are, in all probability, perceptual skills of a different order. Furthermore, what remains unclear in the area of reported perceptual deficits is the degree to which other phenomena such as attention and memory are implicated.

Attention

Attention deficits in children with learning disabilities have been legendary, yet there has been some lack of clarity about the nature and prevalence of the various aspects of the problem. The characteristics of distractibility, hyperactivity, and impulsivity are presented in conjunction with related issues in learning disabilities that require resolution. Investigations of and contrasting viewpoints about these different aspects of attention disorder are reviewed. Research on physiological measures and selective attention deficits will be described, along with consideration of the interaction between attention disorder and reading disability and a possible ca-pacity deficit that may limit attention under certain conditions.

Attention Deficit Disorder   The term *attention-deficit disorder* (ADD) in the *Diagnostic and Statistical Manual of Mental Disorders* (third edition) (*DSM–III*) of the American Psychi-atric Asociation (1980) is used to describe a variety of maladaptive behavior patterns. The *DSM–III* differentiated between ADD with and without hyperactivity as separate clinical en-tities. In the 1987 revision (*DSM–III–R*) (American Psychiatric Association, 1987), the dual category was collapsed into a single category—attention-deficit hyperactivity disorder (ADHD)—with the addition of another category, undifferentiated attention-deficit disorder. Shaywitz and Shaywitz (1991) have reported opinions among authorities that "ADD without hyperactivity represents a clinically meaningful entity and should be included in *DSM IV*" (p. 70). They also have noted that the term ADD is frequently used in the literature to signify both ADD and ADHD, resulting in confusion among these entities.

The following criteria for attention-deficit disorder with hyperactivity are listed in the *DSM–III*:

A.   Inattention (at least three of the following):

   (1)   often fails to finish things he or she starts
   (2)   often doesn't seem to listen
   (3)   easily distracted
   (4)   has difficulty concentrating on schoolwork or other tasks requiring sustained attention
   (5)   has difficulty sticking to a play activity

B.   Impulsivity (at least three of the following):

   (1)   often acts before thinking
   (2)   shifts excessively from one activity to another
   (3)   has difficulty organizing work (this not being due to cognitive impairment)
   (4)   needs a lot of supervision
   (5)   frequently calls out in class
   (6)   has difficulty awaiting turn in games or group situations

C.   Hyperactivity (at least two of the following):

   (1)   runs about or climbs on things excessively
   (2)   has difficulty sitting still or fidgets excessively
   (3)   has difficulty staying seated
   (4)   moves about excessively during sleep
   (5)   is always "on the go" or acts as if "driven by a motor" (*DSM–III–R*, pp. 43–44)

Questions have been raised about the diagnostic efficacy of both categorical classification models (as in the *DSM–III*), which are usually based on specific criteria, and dimensional classifications (such as rating scales), which specify attributes and cutoff points for inclusion (Fletcher, Morris, & Francis, 1991). These authors stated that existing methods result in lack of precision in definition of the disorder and controversy about identification of children with or without attention disorder. These problems have a negative impact on decisions about inclu-sion of children in special service delivery programs (Epstein et al., 1991).

Shaywitz and Shaywitz (1988) have observed that, in the absence of adequate diagnostic guidelines, there may be a confounding of behavior disabilities (hyperactivity/impulsivity) with learning disabilities. In their comprehensive review and analysis of the literature on ADD, they stated: "The implications of these findings are that hyperactivity or ADD and learning disabilities are two separate disorders and that one does not necessarily predict the other" (p. 402). Nevertheless, the two conditions are frequently associated with each other. Cantwell and Baker (1991) considered the possibility that the relationship between them may be reflexive in nature. That is, attention deficits may contribute to learning failure, and learning failure may result in hyperactive behavior. They do point out, however, that there is scant evidence that ADHD leads directly to learning disability; many children with ADHD do not manifest learning disabilities. The distinctions or interactions between these disorders continue to require further consideration (Doris, 1993).

Learning Disabilities and ADD

Distractibility   Many children who have ADD along with a learning disability seem to have a short attention span; that is, their ability to concentrate is limited in duration. A reduced ability to focus on external task-relevant stimuli or to flexibly shift between internal and external processing is viewed as devastating to concentration and learning (Rudel, 1988).

While it has been widely believed that distractibility is due to the child's inability to inhibit reaction to competing environmental stimuli, laboratory research has demonstrated that subjects with ADD do have the ability to filter out such distractions. However, many of these laboratory experiments fail to make demands for performance of a duration that would equal the demands of real-life educational tasks. Therefore, they may not present conditions analogous to those situations that may make the child vulnerable to external distraction (Rudel, 1988).

A second point requiring consideration is that distraction may be generated *internally* through intrusion of feeling, fantasies, and thoughts unrelated to the task at hand. The child with ADD may not have the attentional controls needed to filter out these internal intrusions. Whether externally or internally caused, an impaired ability to maintain attention in task performance frequently leads to impulsive responding.

Impulsivity   Impulsivity is a pattern of overly quick response in the absence of adequate information processing or monitoring of appropriateness or accuracy. Impulsive children often respond before directions for task performance are completed, engage in inadequate planning prior to taking action, and exhibit ineffective organization of material.

Kinsbourne and Caplan (1979) provided a neurological hypothesis for this phenomenon of impulsivity. They discussed the counteracting operations of two mechanisms. The first component programs rough-and-ready decisions almost as soon as a task attracts attention. The second component imposes checks that defer response until decisions have been monitored for appropriateness. In children who are impulsive, however, the second component appears to be underactivated. Based on Kinsbourne and Caplan's model, it appears that, once children with attention problems are primed to respond, it is more difficult for them to inhibit premature response.

A relationship between impulsivity and learning problems is assumed: "children who have cognitive and behavioral impulsivity would be expected to have academic problems because they make decisions too rapidly based on inadequate data" (Cantwell & Baker, 1991, p. 92). Under some experimental conditions, however, the reaction time of impulsive children with learning disabilities has been observed to be slower, rather than always faster, than that of children without such disabilities. Rudel (1988) suggested that such variability may be an indicator of shifts from underarousal to overarousal, reflecting poor *modulation* of the attention system instead of an actual *deficiency.*

Hyperactivity   The nature and etiology of attention disorders, and more specifically hyperactivity, have been the subject of debate over the past two to three decades. From the medical perspective, hyperactivity has been viewed as a symptom of neurological impairment (Denckla, 1972). However, Ross (1976), after extensive review of research on attention disorders, including hyperactivity, questioned the neurological assumption:

> We don't know why some children are "difficult" [hyperactive] children, they seem to be born that way; they may have a constitutionally determined behavioral style, a temperament, that sets them apart from other children who are reported to be "easy" to raise. Nothing in their history suggests that these "difficult" children are neurologically damaged children. (p. 89)

Research Findings   Recent research has continued to study the phenomena of learning disabilities and ADD and their possible interactions or distinctions. Because of the multifaceted nature of attention and its interaction with other confounding variables, research into attention disorders has employed a variety of methods and focused on different aspects of the phenomenon. A substantial body of the literature is devoted to the phenomenon of hyperactivity.

Studies of Hyperactivity and Learning Disabilities   A number of studies have compared and contrasted hyperactivity and learning disabilities (Cotugno, 1987; Dykman, Ackerman, & Holcomb, 1985; Richards, Samuels, Turnure, & Ysseldyke, 1990; Schworm & Birnbaum, 1989). Results of these studies are synthesized in Table 1. In general:

> While both groups [hyperactive and nonhyperactive learning disabled] show severe impairment in selective attention when compared to control groups, [hyperactive learning-disabled] children appear more compromised as performance requires increasingly complex integrated cognitive functioning (e.g. pacing *and* scanning; pacing, *scanning and* attending. (Cotugno, 1987, p. 566)

It is inferred by Richards et al. (1990), in agreement with Shaywitz and Shaywitz (1988), that these patterns of inattention ascribed by numerous investigators to individuals with learning disabilities may reflect diagnostically mixed samples with an overrepresentation of subjects with ADD combined with hyperactivity.

Types of Attention Problems in Learning Disability   To present another perspective, Douglas and Peters (1979) suggested that the attention problems observed in children with

Table 1.   Attentional characteristics of children with learning disabilities and hyperactivity

	Attentional characteristics
Learning disability	Apprehension about difficult tasks Susceptibility to distraction in relation to task avoidance Deficient in selective attention Not deficient in sustained attention
Hyperactivity	Deficient in sustained attention Excessive activity during task performance Impulsive Unsystematic or incomplete in informational search
Learning disability and hyperactivity	Slow in selective attending Distractible Poor regulation of motor tempo Less active visual scanning Difficulty holding information in memory

Based on Cotugno (1987), Dykman, Ackerman, and Holcomb (1985), Richards, Samuels, Turnure, and Ysseldyke (1990), and Schworm and Birnbaum (1989).

learning disabilities are likely to be the result, not the cause, of their academic failure. Moreover, important distinctions have also been drawn between pervasive and situational attention disorders. For example, Douglas (1983) argued that attention deficits manifested in a child's behavior on particular tasks (versus pervasive distractibility and/or hyperactivity) may reflect the characteristics of the task itself rather than reaction to a distractor. In other words, children with learning disabilities may respond differently to tasks that are or are not important and rewarding to them both in the laboratory and in their real world. Some of the patterns observed in children with attention deficit and learning disabilities (Kinsbourne & Caplan, 1979; Rudel, 1988; Shaywitz & Shaywitz, 1988) are:

> Increased error rate with increased task duration, suggesting deficient attentional *vigilance*
>
> High error rate attributable, possibly, to unsystematic and/or inefficient search strategies involving a reduced tendency to decenter attention from a single salient cue to other relevant or critical stimuli
>
> High error rate resulting from predominant use of random trial and error, rather than logically based problem-solving behavior
>
> Failure, at times, to make any response to task stimuli after a preparatory signal

Attention-Deficit Disorder and Reading Disability   The relations between attention, reading ability, and aspects of language deficit were explored in a series of studies by Felton and Wood (1989). Among the many findings was a relationship between certain cognitive deficits, ADD, and reading disability subtype. The reader will recall from Chapter 6 the following subtypes of reading disability:

> *Dysphonetic:* Difficulty with phonological analysis and sound/letter correspondences leading to problems decoding unfamiliar words
>
> *Dyseidetic:* Difficulty with acquiring and retaining recognition of sight words, with adequate phonological processing skills
>
> *Mixed:* Difficulty with both phonological and visual word attack skills (Boder, 1971)

A clear-cut distinction was observed by Felton and Wood (1989) wherein the majority of subjects in the subtype groups other than dysphonetic were classified as having ADD (i.e., dyseidetic, 80%; mixed, 69%; and nonspecific, 80%). However, only 31% of the dysphonetic group were classified as having ADD.

In a longitudinal study, follow-up assessment of a proportion of the original subject sample produced some rather surprising results. Of the 27 subjects with reading disability available for a second assessment 1–2 years later, 16 (59%) were reclassified according to subtype. Of the reclassified group, 13 (81%) had been identified as having ADD in the original classification. The authors speculated that: "Given the high number of ADD children who changed subtype, it is at least plausible that some of the changes from test to test were due to attentional factors" (p. 7).

Dysphonetic readers, with a relatively low incidence of ADD, appear to manifest major phonological processing problems primarily responsible for the reading difficulty independent of attention problems. It is interesting to note that dyseidetic readers, who seem to have adequate phonological processing skills, demonstrate word retrieval and rapid naming problems that may interfere with the acquisition of sight words. Failure to acquire sight words at a level of automaticity is considered a detriment to fluent reading. Felton and Wood (1989) suggested that attention problems may exacerbate such deficits.

Further findings derived from study of a sample of first-grade children from the general, nonreferred population revealed that attention disorders, deficits in phonemic awareness, and deficits in rapid naming were all identifiable at this early stage. Each pattern was observed to be detrimental to early reading achievement but *not necessarily in the same children*. Felton and Wood (1989) reasoned from their findings that all children with reading disabilities may not be deficient in the skills critical to reading. Some may have an attention deficit disorder that, if diagnosed early, may lead to appropriate pharmacological or instructional treatment, thereby preventing the establishment of a persistently disabling condition. Dykman and Dykman (1991) have endorsed the administration of psychostimulant medication for children with ADD and reading disability because of the observed benefit in tasks that require sustained and/or effortful performance.

Effortful Versus Automatized Attention   While it is generally recognized that attention is necessary to learning, it is not considered sufficient. A variety of other variables, including working memory, stored knowledge, and processing strategies, are believed to interact with attention and are implicated in learning and reading failure. From one viewpoint, failure to master certain critical skills to the point of automaticity is seen as a cause of inefficient and ineffective allocation of attentional resources. R.J. Sternberg and Wagner (1982) asserted that individuals with learning disabilities present evidence of slower and less complete mastery of tasks that others have acquired to the point of automaticity. Therefore, children with learning disabilities continue to allocate inordinate amounts of attentional resources to those tasks that the individual with normal function performs with little or no attentional demand or conscious effort. Children with learning disabilities have been reported to benefit from the use of psychostimulant drugs to increase their tolerance for the intensive overlearning needed for their achievement of skills at the automatic rather than effortful level (Dykman et al., 1985).

The degree of effort required to perform certain attention-demanding tasks was investigated by Swanson (1984b). Based on the findings, it was assumed that individuals with learning disabilities may exert effortful attention in encoding processes that are automatic or effortless for individuals without learning disabilities, particularly in language-related academic skills.

This point has been made a number of times in the previous chapter with reference to the more effortful, less automatized phonological decoding and encoding skills of poor readers/spellers/writers, along with the deficits in their rapid word or meaning retrieval. All of these less mastered, more effortful skills divert attentional resources from the processing of meaning in reading and writing (J. Kagan, 1983; LaBerge & Samuels, 1974; Shankweiler & Liberman, 1972).

Physiological Studies   A group of studies using such physiological measures of attending as heart rate deceleration, alpha wave rate reduction (i.e., slowed rate, or idling speed, of the alpha waves in brain activity detected by electroencephalograms), and reaction time were conducted during the 1970s (Czudner & Rourke, 1972; Fuller, 1978; Rourke & Czudner, 1972; Sroufe, Sonies, West, & Wright, 1973). Results during task performance revealed that, in contrast to controls, subjects with learning disabilities manifested significantly less cardiac deceleration, less attenuation of alpha waves, and slower reaction time to signals. All of these findings appear to indicate some reductions in the allocation of attentional resources under experimental task performance conditions by individuals with learning disabilities. More recently, research using electroencephalography (EEG) and brain electrical activity mapping (BEAM) techniques has yielded findings of greater amounts of alpha waves, representing decreased cortical activity, in subjects with learning disabilities (from research reviewed by Haynes et al., 1989) and underactivation of the frontal lobe in subjects with dyslexia (Duffy, Denckla, Bartels, & Sandini, 1980). These phenomena were viewed as suggestive of ADD by the investigators.

Selective Attention Studies   During the 1970s, a series of studies employed the Central-Incidental Learning Task (Hagen & Hale, 1973; Hagen & Kail, 1975) to study children's ability to attend to task-central versus task-incidental information. In this study, children were shown a series of cards, each containing two pictures (e.g., an animal and an object). Subjects were instructed to attend to only one of the items (e.g., the animals) for future recall. Subsequently the children were tested first on their ability to recall only the central items (i.e., animals) and then on their ability to match objects with the animals originally paired with them (incidental recall). Children with learning disabilities were reported to perform significantly more poorly than children in control groups on central, but not incidental, recall (Hallahan, Gajar, Cohen, & Tarver, 1978; Hallahan, Tarver, Kaufman, & Graybeal, 1978; Tarver, Hallahan, Kaufman, & Ball, 1976). Results of these earlier studies were interpreted as evidence of a delay in the development of selective attention in children with learning disabilities.

Reid and Hresko (1981) viewed these early results differently, pointing out that, in every case reporting inferior recall for subjects with learning disabilities in contrast to controls, the central recall scores of the subjects with learning disabilities exceeded their own incidental recall scores. This is regarded as evidence that the subjects *with learning disabilities* were selectively attending and that lower scores on incidental recall were more likely due to inefficient processing than inattention.

This viewpoint received some support from the findings that, although students with learning disabilities scored lower and demonstrated greater distractibility than controls on experimental tasks of selective attention, they were also observed to be slower in processing information (Richards et al., 1990). On the basis of their own research and analysis of other studies, Richards et al. (1990) interpreted recent evidence as suggestive of the view that slower pickup of information by the central processing system "is likely to be the root of selective attention problems for children with [learning disabilities]. Rapidly presented information may be attended to, but likely is lost or disordered before it is processed" (p. 135).

This effect may have been evident in studies employing a speeded sorting task that eliminated the memory component but required attention to critical features (Copeland & Reiner, 1984; Copeland & Wisniewski, 1981). These studies produced the following results:

Subjects with learning disabilities took longer to sort than subjects without learning disabilities.

Across repeated trials, subjects without learning disabilities reduced their error rate while the error rate of subjects with learning disabilities *increased* with repeated trials.

On stimuli containing more critical features, subjects with learning disabilities made more errors than controls.

Thus, on a task designed to examine attention to central information with less confounding effects from memory processing, children with learning disabilities manifested less efficient and effective performance than age-mates without disabilities. A subsequent study using the same speeded sorting method included training in verbalization of critical features concurrent with sorting as a potential enhancer of selective attention. This activity proved to be more interfering than facilitative for the group with learning disabilities; they made more errors under this condition than did controls (Copeland & Reiner, 1984).

It has been pointed out above and elsewhere (Reid & Hresko, 1981; Ross, 1976) that verbal labeling, while facilitative to some groups and in some tasks, is not always an appropriate strategy and may actually hinder performance. This detrimental effect may be due either to the fact that covert labeling does occur at the automatic level or to deficient language ability that is unequal to the verbalization task without cost to performance of the primary task.

Interactive effects of verbal ability with selective attention in dichotic listening tasks were examined in a study by Swanson and Obrzut (1985) comparing children with and without learning disabilities. Summarized, it was found that children without learning disabilities had higher selective attention scores under all orienting conditions, demonstrating their superior ability to flexibly access different features from their word knowledge store. Swanson and Obrzut (1985) concluded that "disabled children are less able to attend selectively to distinctive word features because of word knowledge deficits" (p. 416). One may conjecture with reasonable confidence that, in the face of inferior verbal knowledge, language-related tasks would, indeed, tend to be more effortful, placing heavier demands on resources available for selective attention.

Information Processing Issues: Capacity or Strategy Deficit?

Bridging the functions of attention and memory in language-related learning disabilities are the overarching theories about the nature of the deficits from current information processing perspectives. The controversy about capacity versus strategy deficit was prominent in the literature throughout the 1980s. On the one hand, a considerable body of research throughout the 1970s had provided support for the hypothesis that the student with learning disabilities was a passive learner whose academic failure was attributable to inadequate development and/or use of facilitative strategies. On the other hand, the possibility has been considered that constraints may reside in the "architectural" features of the information processing system, including the capacity of short-term memory, the durability of the memory trace, and the speed of various processing operations (Torgeson & Greenstein, 1982). Such features are viewed as relatively impervious to change through training or volitional control. It is, perhaps, relevant to these issues that children with attention disorders have been observed to improve under stimulant drug therapy in their concentration, attention maintenance, planning for problem solution and selective attention (Pelham, 1988), thus implicating some neurologically based constraints on performance.

A more recent research review has led to the hypothesis that improved academic performance associated with stimulant drug therapy may be due to beneficial changes in attitude and motivation instead of changes in basic cognitive processes (Henker & Whalen, 1989). It is still unclear whether increased willingness to comply with the demands of tasks that are challenging and not particularly enjoyable is attributable to positive effects of medication on neurological or psychological causal factors.

The dilemma about the nature of the deficits was expressed by Swanson (1982):

> One is plagued with persisting questions as to what limitations, if any, remain constant in learning disabled children's performance: what constraints are there on cognitive structures; and, more importantly, how do these constraints interact with the kinds of strategies these children can use?" (p. x)

More recently, attention has focused on the determining influence of the knowledge base, including level of language proficiency, on the basic components of information processing and on the potential for strategy development and use. In the discussion that follows, research on memory deficits in learning disabilities is considered from these vantage points, with particular emphasis on interactions between aspects of memory and aspects of language.

While it has not been maintained here or demonstrated in the literature that all reading disabilities are language-deficiency based, an impressively large proportion of the population studied has presented evidence of such a relationship, as was demonstrated in Chapter 7. Therefore, since much of the recent research on reading disability has focused on relevant aspects of language, reading disability and language-related learning disability will be regarded as virtually synonymous in the following consideration of the research and theory in this area.

Memory

Research and theory about memory in the field of learning disabilities has paralleled current models of memory as a normal cognitive process, as discussed in Chapter 3. Memory is central to learning, that is, the storage and retrieval of information. As discussed in Chapter 4, the processing of discourse, both written and oral, involves aspects of memory. Memory deficits have been widely reported in people with learning disabilities. In this section, the nature of those deficits is explored.

Various investigators have studied different components of memory in an attempt to understand a student's failure to store, retain, and/or retrieve information. Some have focused on sensory storage and short-term memory capacity, whereas others have studied the strategic components of working memory whereby information is transferred from short- to long-term memory through rehearsal, organization, and/or elaboration. This reflects the debate over whether capacity or strategy is the more important component in memory deficits in learning disabilities. Semantic orientation, semantic knowledge, and accessibility of knowledge have been the subjects of both empirical research and theoretical speculation. The amount and diversity of the literature is increasingly daunting. The following sections sample research and theory in each of the areas identified above.

Short-Term Memory Deficits in Learning Disabilities

Echoic Storage   One area of research in short-term memory concerns the actual capacity for storage of input. The reader will recall from Chapter 3 descriptions of *echoic storage* as auditory sensory memory and *digit span* as a measure of the number of information chunks held in short-term memory. A study of the echoic storage capacity of poor and good readers demonstrated shorter digit span for poor readers (four to five digits versus five to seven digits for good readers) and a greater decrease in recall of this auditory information by poor readers following delay or interference (Sipes & Engle, 1986). Further evidence supported the likelihood that this difference in echoic memory entails the activation of auditory phonetic features rather than the duration of sensory information per se. This conclusion is in accordance with the findings of numerous investigators, cited in Chapter 7, that short-term memory deficits in children with language-related learning disabilities appear to reflect inadequate or inefficient activation of phonetic codes in the storage of information for transfer to working memory.

In their review of research, Spear and Sternberg (1986) noted: "There is considerable evidence that the short-term memory difficulties of disabled readers are restricted to memory for materials that can be coded verbally, such as letters, words, pictures, and numbers" (p. 19). The precise nature of this deficient ability to process verbally codable information in short-term memory has been open to various interpretations within the capacity-strategy debate. Some evidence has been provided supporting the hypothesis of short-term memory capacity deficit in certain individuals with learning disabilities. Other investigations have led to conclusions about maladaptive visual/verbal encoding. The following section discusses relevant research on these issues.

Differences in Short-Term Memory Span   While a substantial body of research points to a maladaptive mode of information processing as more probable than span capacity limitation as a causal factor in the memory deficits of individuals with learning disabilities, it is not possible to rule out limitations on short-term memory span in all cases. A subgroup of children with learning disabilities (approximately 15%–20%) have been found to have severe memory span difficulties (Torgeson, 1988b), manifested in deficient memory for sequential verbal material such as digits and sentences presented aurally or visually. These children have not demonstrated deficits in the recall of the gist of meaningfully organized information or in comprehension of oral language of relatively limited complexity. Difficulty has been reported only in comprehension of specific types of complex prose that place heavy demands on storage processes in working memory. Thus, Torgeson (1988b) inferred that, "Since phonological codes are particularly well adapted for storage of information about the order of items as well as their identity . . . performance on a wide variety of *verbatim* recall tasks is affected (p. 609) [italics added for emphasis].

Extreme difficulties on span tasks and complex naming tasks are attributed to a deficit in the ability to efficiently extract and operate on certain phonemically coded information over brief time periods. Torgeson (1988b) identified some of the tasks adversely affected by such a deficit as:

> Difficulty in early reading and spelling acquisition
> Difficulty with rapid and accurate pronunciation of words
> Difficulty following strings of oral directions

Torgeson (1988b) left open the question about whether the phonological coding deficits of this group of children should be regarded as necessary but not sufficient to account for reading disability.

Restricted Use of the Verbal Code   There is general agreement that children with language-related learning disabilities fail to benefit from the use of their own linguistic code to enhance storage and retrieval of information, both visual and verbal (Spear & Sternberg, 1986; Swanson, 1983; Vellutino & Scanlon, 1986). It appears that, whereas skilled readers utilize two intact routes for the storage and retrieval of information (the visual and the verbal), poor readers seem to rely predominantly on the visual route (Swanson, 1984a). Evidence exists suggesting that the combined processing in the visual and verbal codes places heavy demands on those individuals with reading/learning disabilities (Swanson, 1986). This phenomenon is the subject of speculation. For example, Perfetti and McCutchen (1982) have questioned whether it is the degree of effort required in the activation of phonetic codes in the performance of verbal tasks that has negative consequences on such processes as reading.

Effort and Performance of Verbal Tasks   Results of Swanson's (1984a) study were suggestive of capacity deficits in children with learning disabilities. They were found to be penalized by time pressure in tasks requiring the manipulation and recall of verbal material at different levels of difficulty. It is thought posible that, for children without such disabilities, certain verbal encoding processes (e.g., word recognition or phonic decoding) are sufficiently automatic to free up capacity for performing higher level processes, such as reorganization of material for recall. Conversely, poor recall by children with learning disabilities has been attributed to less tolerable attentional demands imposed by high-effort verbal tasks that limit available capacity for the function of executive control processes in working memory (Swanson, 1984b).

Working Memory and Learning Disabilities   In a recent study of the components of working memory in different groups of children, Swanson and his colleagues (Swanson, Cochran, & Ewers, 1990) investigated performance on tasks designed to reflect: the executive control component, a peripheral visual-spatial storage component, and a peripheral verbal storage component. Peripheral systems are those that store information processed through perceptual and motor mechanisms (e.g., an "articulatory loop" for storage of verbal input and a "visual-spatial scratch pad" for storage of images and spatial information). The central executive system controls higher level processes such as organization of information and retrieval of relevant information from long-term memory.

Through factor analysis of results, six subtypes of subjects were derived, one of which was clearly identifiable as having learning disability, "exhibiting distinct deficiencies in working memory components" (Swanson et al., 1990, p. 65). Although the subjects with learning disabilities were inferior in functions of both peripheral (verbal and visual) and central executive processing, it is suggested that "the memory problems of children with [learning disabilities] may be more functionally related to higher order processes, such as central processing ability" (p. 61). What has remained unclear to these authors is whether the deficit in working memory reflects a limited capacity or some specific language processing limitation.

Differences in Semantic Knowledge, Semantic Coding, and Mnemonic Performance It will be recalled from Chapter 3 that encoding information at a meaningful level enhances recall. A body of literature cited in that chapter reported on the memory benefits of semantic (deep) coding (i.e., the assignment of meaning) in contrast to processing information at the more superficial level of physical features, whether visual (e.g., features of orthography) or verbal (e.g., sounds that rhyme).

The literature reviewed and summarized here on studies of semantic coding by individuals with and without learning disabilities resists clear-cut generalization of results and their implications (Ceci, 1982, 1984; Ceci & Baker, 1989; Cermak & Moliotis, 1987; Howell & Manis, 1986; Swanson, 1983, 1984a, 1986; Swanson & Obrzut, 1985; Swanson & Rathgeber, 1986). Methods for experimentally examining and analyzing the relationship between semantic coding and memory have varied widely, as the following examples of procedures illustrate:

Memory for named versus nonnamed pictures
Response to semantically related words such as synonyms/antonyms at automatic and
    purposive levels of attending

Recall of material according to superordinate classification

Sorting and recall of words on the basis of shared semantic versus phonemic versus orthographic features

Unscrambling anagrams to match target words (e.g., natir/train) for recall, in lists of
semantically related and unrelated words

Pairing superordinate terms with true or false exemplars (e.g., "This is an animal" while
displaying a picture of a dog or a pumpkin)

Results of such studies present evidence of basically intact knowledge of semantic associations and categorization in subjects with learning disabilities. That is, no differences were
found between groups with and without learning disabilities on recognition of associations
between words that are synonyms or antonyms, and on knowledge of items belonging to the
same category.

However, differences between groups have been observed in other dimensions of semantic processing. Subjects with learning disabilities have shown:

1. A lesser tendency to employ semantic coding in the recall of visual material (Ceci, 1982;
    Swanson, 1983, 1984b)
2. A lesser tendency to activate superordinate knowledge in response to presented verbal
    stimuli (Ceci & Baker, 1989)
3. Slower retrieval of superordinate knowledge from semantic memory in processing both
    written and pictured words (Cermak & Moliotis, 1987; Howell & Manis, 1986)
4. Lack of complete correspondence, in some cases, of categorical clustering during encod-
    ing and recall of the clustered information, suggesting a qualitative difference in semantic
    processing (Swanson & Rathgeber, 1986)
5. A greater tendency to engage in phonemic rather than semantic processing of words for
    recall (Ceci & Baker, 1989)
6. Less benefit from being primed by a highly related word in speed of naming target words
    (Ceci, 1982)

Swanson and his colleagues (1990) have proposed that at least some important differences
between reading ability groups are reflected in their varying ability to conceptualize information in semantic codes. It is conceivable that encoding of words by children with language-
related learning disabilities may *fail to fully and effectively activate relevant features* and/or
that these individuals are *less proficient in the elaboration of semantic codes*. It will be recalled
from Chapter 7 that many individuals with language-related learning disabilities have demonstrated limitations in their semantic knowledge, suggestive of fewer and weaker links in the
semantic network. It is also evident from the results presented here that, although *basic* semantic knowledge may be intact, individuals with learning disabilities are less inclined to access it
as readily or rapidly as individuals without such disabilities in the performance of demanding
tasks requiring memory for visual and verbal material.

The tendency of children with learning disabilities to fail to process information at the
deeper semantic level and the relation of this tendency to memory was explored by Ceci, Ringstrom, and Lea (1981) in a study that is sufficiently illuminating on this issue to warrant some
descriptive detail. Subjects were classified on the basis of their performance on auditory and
visual memory tests as: 1) impaired in auditory but not visual memory, 2) impaired in visual

but not auditory memory, 3) impaired in both auditory and visual memory, or 4) having no impairments in auditory and visual memory.

The experimental tasks consisted of the presentation of prepared lists of words in the auditory modality and pictures in the visual modality with instructions to remember as many as possible. Subjects first performed a free recall task. Then recall was cued by either semantic or nonsemantic cues. The semantic cues consisted of category names. The nonsemantic cues in the auditory modality were phonetic (rhyme) or gender of speaker's voice. In the visual modality, nonsemantic cues were color or location of items in the pictures.

Results revealed that a memory impairment in a specific modality was associated with a relative reduction in semantic processing in that modality, in contrast to evidence of semantic processing in the unimpaired modality. Controls responded successfully to an overwhelmingly large proportion of semantic cues in both auditory and visual modalities.

For purposes of further clarification, the following modality-specific results are provided. For those with auditory memory deficits, on the auditory cueing task the proportion of words recalled in response to semantic cues was 36%, while nonsemantic cues produced successful recall of 44%. In contrast, performance on the auditory cueing task by those with visually but not auditorally impaired memories was highly successful in response to semantic cueing, approximating performance of controls.

In the visual cueing condition, subjects with only auditory memory impairment responded with significantly superior recall in response to semantic rather than nonsemantic cues. For those with visual memory impairment, the semantic cue superiority effect in the visual modality disappeared. Impairment in both visual and auditory memory was associated with poor response to all cues. *These results strongly suggest that reduced memory in either modality was related to diminished semantic processing in that particular modality.*

Strategic Use of Semantic Knowledge   Account is increasingly taken in the literature of the distinction between existing knowledge, whether declarative or procedural, and the tendency to use such knowledge strategically to enhance learning. Swanson (1988a) designed a study aimed at determining subtypes of memory deficiencies among individuals with learning disabilities. Results revealed eight memory subtypes with some overlap between groups. A common factor across all subtypes of subjects with learning disabilities, as compared to controls, was inferior use of structural aspects of semantic knowledge, such as organization, categorization, association, or elaboration, on demanding learning tasks. Such deficiencies in higher level central processing operations have been regarded as characteristic of the passive learner.

Research and Theory About Strategy Deficits and Learning Disabilities   The characterization of the individual with a learning disability as a passive learner (Torgeson, 1977, 1979) received widespread acceptance for more than a decade. Such a description has been based largely on research reporting deficient use of active strategies for storage and recall of information. A suggested revision of this view has been advanced by Swanson (1989), whose investigations have led him to argue "that a more accurate characterization of [learning-disabled] children is that they are *actively inefficient* learners" (p. 10). From this perspective, children with learning disabilities have been reported to employ active strategic thought processes, but appear limited in their ability to use more effective strategies with flexibility. Both of the above views implicate deficiencies in the use of strategies for enhancement of memory and learning.

From her review of the literature, Worden (1986) observed that "there is much evidence that voluntary control processes for strategic encoding may be deficient in the learning disabled" (p. 243). Such deficiencies have been described as a disinclination to generate active elaboration of information and to engage in planful, organized activity for employing structure as a mnemonic strategy (Torgeson & Greenstein, 1982).

Rehearsal and Categorization Deficits   Two of the most frequently cited strategic processes involved in the enhancement of short-term memory capacity have been rehearsal and elaboration through categorical clustering. In Chapter 7, it was noted in some early studies that, although many children with learning disabilities demonstrated the ability to use categorical clustering at some levels of complexity, they did not tend to employ this strategy spontaneously to facilitate memory as frequently and effectively as achieving peers (Bartel, Grill, & Bartel, 1973; Ring, 1976; Suiter & Potter, 1978). It has also been reported that children with learning disabilities evidenced poorer rehearsal strategies than children without such disabilities (Bauer 1977, 1979; Tarver et al., 1976; Torgeson & Houck, 1980). Categorical clustering is one type of elaborated rehearsal that has received attention in memory research with populations both with and without disabilities. Research in this area has continued throughout the past decade with increasing refinements in methodology and interpretation of results.

A number of studies have reported poorer recall by subjects with learning disabilities of material requiring spontaneous clustering of stimulus items as a form of elaborative rehearsal (Bauer, 1977, 1979; Wong, Wong, & Foth, 1977). Analysis of performance patterns has revealed that when rehearsal has been used, subjects with learning disabilities tended to use a less sophisticated strategy than subjects without disabilities, with their performance resembling a pattern characteristic of younger children without disabilities (Ornstein, 1978). That is, they rehearsed single items repetitively rather than groups of items concurrently.

> This must have placed them at a distinct disadvantage when it came time to remember the words, since they could draw only from a disjointed series of episodes rather than from a well-organized network of responses in which one word recall might possibly evoke others. (Ornstein, 1978, p. 117)

The more mature cumulative rehearsal strategy tended to be used by subjects without learning disabilities.

Further analysis has demonstrated that skilled readers'/learners' superordinate clustering reflected a higher level of abstraction in semantic organization than the more conceptually superficial organizational patterns observed in the recall of subjects with learning disabilities (Swanson, 1984b). The quality of information organization into categorical networks is apparently a developmental phenomenon differentiating skilled readers according to age. It is noteworthy that this developmental difference in the ability to impose organization on material for improved recall was observed even in older versus younger subjects with learning disabilities (Cermak & Moliotis, 1987).

Interesting effects have been found by Wong and her associates (1977) under varied conditions of organizational cueing and task time, as shown in Table 2. In this study, poor readers rehearsed less actively and, when given unlimited time, did not seem to use the opportunity to generate organization facilitative to recall to the extent manifested by readers without disabilities. However, both the children in this study and adults with learning disabilities (Sandman & Wilhardt, 1988) performed almost as well as control subjects on free and cued recall tasks when they were provided with organizational structure by the investigators. It was concluded

Table 2. Benefits in recall of organizational cueing and task time for readers with (LD) and without (NLD) learning disabilities

	Untimed condition	Timed condition
+ Cueing	LD inferior to NLD	NLD and LD equal
− Cueing	LD inferior to NLD	LD inferior to NLD

Adapted from Wong, Wong, and Foth (1977).

that basic processes related to storage and access of information from long-term memory did not differentiate adults with and without learning disabilities, since under conditions that did not require active initiation of a mnemonic strategy, adults with learning disabilities performed as well as controls (Sandman & Wilhardt, 1988). It has been suggested that individuals with learning disabilities may have the capability of abstracting categories from *presented* material, but may not be as able as counterparts without disabilities in chunking material for later *retrieval* (Cermak & Moliotis, 1987).

Questions about this strategy deficiency require attempts at explanation. Why do individuals with learning disabilities but without intellectual impairment fail to develop and use strategies that facilitate voluntary memory? Why do they demonstrate the ability to effectively use such strategies when externally guided to do so but fail to employ them spontaneously with flexibility and appropriateness?

One possible answer may be drawn from the literature on normal child development. A study by Guttentag (1984) examined the effects of mental effort on the use of cumulative rehearsal by children at different age levels. Younger children who did not spontaneously engage in cumulative rehearsal were instructed in its use. However, it was demonstrated that the use of a cumulative rehearsal strategy by children who were developmentally unready to employ it spontaneously required the investment of measurably greater effort than was required by those who were developmentally ready. It was suggested that there may be a tendency to avoid use of a strategy that requires a high level of effort. Children with learning disabilities have been found to perform more poorly under conditions of high effort (Swanson, 1984a). There is ample evidence, cited in Chapter 7, that many cognitive-linguistic educational tasks are effortful for those with language-related learning disabilities, to a degree that may indeed reduce motivation to engage in active, strategic processing of information for the enhancement of memory.

While this account of persistent strategic deficits is plausible and possibly accurate, it is not regarded as fully explanatory by scholars who take cognizance of the importance of knowledge stored in long-term memory, both declarative and procedural, in determining task performance. A prevalent current view maintains that there is an inseparable relationship between strategic enhancement of memory and an adequate knowledge base, with particular emphasis on the quality and use of verbal knowledge.

Interaction Between Knowledge and Strategy Deficits   There does appear to be a relationship between the tendency to employ elaborative strategies (e.g., categorical clustering) and the developmental status of existing knowledge. To illustrate, Rabinowitz and Chi (1987) asked: "Why would the learner choose to use a categorization strategy if the categorical relations among the items were never noticed?" (p. 92). From this viewpoint, deficits in the strategic use of certain levels of organization of material for memorization may be attributed either to less enrichment of associational links in the structure of semantic memory or to lower levels of activation, with resultant deficits in accessibility.

Readers will recall from Chapter 7 that word-finding problems have been attributed to deficient quality of word knowledge in long-term memory (Kail & Leonard, 1986). Analysis of discourse processing results led to the conclusion that this subgroup of children with learning disabilities (those with word-finding problems) did not appear to have more limited short-term memory capacity or inferior syntactic coding abilities. Rather, these results suggest that the poorer recall for discourse was attributable to problems in identifying individual words and their syntactic roles in clauses and sentences, thus implicating limitations on the depth and breadth of word knowledge.

It is maintained that an insufficient knowledge base (in both semantic and general world knowledge) may account for strategic and nonstrategic learning deficits in individuals with learning disabilities (Kolligian & Sternberg, 1987). Poor performance on many memory tasks may be due to the disadvantage imposed by requirements to process new information in the context of insufficient old information. Furthermore, information that should ideally have been automatized may still require effortful allocation of resources, thereby slowing speed of processing to the extent that time constraints cannot be met. Under these conditions, working memory cannot function optimally.

Results of a study of vocabulary learning by adolescents with learning disabilities underscore the validity of the above contention (Griswold, Gelzheiser, & Shepherd, 1987). Comparing eighth graders with and without learning disabilities on study patterns and results, Griswold et al. (1987) observed that, although scores of subjects with learning disabilities on the vocabulary learning task were inferior to scores of controls, no differences were observed in the use of study strategies by the two groups. That is, both groups appeared to similarly employ rehearsal, self-testing, note taking, and study time. The best predictor of performance was prior tested vocabulary knowledge and reading comprehension. It is not unlikely that a generalized verbal proficiency may contribute more than memorization strategies to vocabulary acquisition. It is also possible that richer semantic knowledge may facilitate less observable, self-generated covert strategies drawing on that knowledge that may interact in memory for verbal material.

Knowledge × Process × Context View of Learning Disabilities   In a searching review and reevaluation of previous research and underlying assumptions, Ceci and Baker (1989) called into question widely held premises about qualitative differences in children with learning disabilities. They argued that, under varying conditions requiring the use of different knowledge domains, these children have demonstrated cognitive processes similar to those in children without disabilities. Results of his earlier research had convinced Ceci that children with learning disabilities went through the same cognitive steps as children without disabilities but did so more slowly and less efficiently.

A major disparity between these groups appears to reside in the linguistic domain, with language deficits constituting the most prevalent characteristic among children with learning disabilities. As a result of the language deficit and its associated cognitive correlates, it is reasoned that the knowledge base in these children may be less well developed than that of achieving peers, "and this lack of development could set limits on how effectively they encode, retrieve, abstract and infer in these domains" (Ceci & Baker, 1989, p. 94).

Among many interesting findings in Ceci and Baker's review was evidence leading to the conclusion that the children with learning disabilities in their sample processed more at the phonemic level than the semantic level on the experimental dichotic listening tasks. This finding may be interpreted as one more bit of evidence of a tendency in children with language-related learning disabilities to engage in shallow rather than deep processing of information in certain demanding tasks requiring verbal encoding. Further general conclusions attributed learning disabilities to impoverished semantic knowledge. Ceci and Baker argued that:

> the manner in which linguistic stimuli are represented in long-term memory constrains how effectively one can attend, remember, and discriminate them. The more dimensions that cross-cut these stimuli and the more attributes and node structures that connect them and get cross-activated in their presence, the better they can be processed. Even something as basic as the speed with which a stimulus can be recognized has been shown to depend on how elaborately it is represented in long term memory. (1989, p. 98)

On the basis of their observations of skilled performance by children with learning disabilities on problem solving in particular contexts (e.g., video games) in contrast to their less than adequate performance on decontextualized tasks requiring similar cognitive information processing skills, Ceci and Baker (1989) contested the prevailing conceptualization of learning disabilities as a reflection of a basic underlying processing deficit. Rather, they are persuaded that "limited knowledge base in a particular domain may account for ineffective processing in that domain" (p. 99), and they proposed that learning disability be examined from an individual difference perspective that encompasses an interaction between processing capabilities and knowledge base. With particular reference to reading disability, individual differences in degrees of deficit in phonological processing, word knowledge, and schematic knowledge may serve as causes of problems with decoding and/or comprehension.

Regarding learning in general, it may be inferred that, if the knowledge representations in the linguistic domain are suboptimal for processing information in those language-related tasks requiring elaboration through activation of internodal connections, reduced depth and breadth of processing would be an inevitable result, adversely affecting information storage and recall. Such a conclusion, regarding memory problems associated with language-related learning disabilities in particular, is congruent with all of the foregoing reports of linguistic/cognitive deficits in the literature reviewed.

Deficits in Memory for Prose   Research in memory has predominantly used word and picture stimuli rather than connected discourse. Memory for prose is inextricably involved in the vast body of research and theory devoted to reading comprehension, an area whose dimensions preclude inclusion within the confines of this chapter. Examination of research in this section is limited to a sample whose major focus is on memory for prose by individuals with learning disabilities.

In Chapter 7, a substantial body of research on narratives was reviewed. However, the emphasis in those studies was essentially, although not exclusively, on the organization and quantity of linguistically encoded information generated or retold by subjects with and without learning disabilities. Worden (1986) has reviewed and reported on research investigating the performance of these groups on the comprehension and recall of prose. Some of the findings from studies of the performance of both adult (community college) and school-age and adolescent students with learning disabilities (P.A. Weaver & Dickinson, 1982; Worden, 1986; Worden, Malmgren, & Gabourie, 1982; Worden & Nakamura, 1983) are:

Recall of fewer propositions from prose text than students without learning disabilities
More erroneous information in recalled text
Reduced sensitivity to information order in paragraph organization
Less accurate answers to comprehension questions
Recall of fewer superordinate, but not subordinate, ideas
Less proficiency in distinguishing levels of importance among ideas

Despite the above deficiencies, repeated opportunities to study text led to an improvement in performance by students with learning disabilities to a degree that approximated the improvement of students without such disabilities. Thus, Worden (1986) concluded that, although students with learning disabilities do not appear to process textual material for effective recall as readily as students without such disabilities, they do not have a permanent deficit in this area. General maturation, coupled with further linguistic development, is believed to foster improved performance under facilitating conditions.

> Taken as a whole, these results suggest that ability-group differences in the use of text structure to aid recall will be greatest for younger subjects under less-than-optimal conditions. Adults and/or subjects who have been trained to recognize the structural features in question show minimal differences. (Worden, 1986, p. 253)

Implicated in the disparity between characteristic performance by many students with learning disabilities and their demonstrated potential under more facilitating conditions is the phenomenon of metacognition.

Metacognitive Deficits   Metacognition was described and discussed earlier in Chapter 3 as the knowledge about and regulation of one's cognition (A.L. Brown & Palinscar, 1982). "The distinction between cognitive and metacognitive aspects of performance refers to the distinction between knowledge and understanding of that knowledge in terms of awareness and appropriate use" (Wong, 1980, p. 29). More specifically, metacognition includes awareness of what strategies, skills, and resources are necessary for task performance and self-regulatory abilities to foster successful task completion. These include planning stepwise activities, evaluating their effectiveness, and revising procedures in the face of encountered difficulties (L. Baker, 1982).

From their own research and extensive review of the literature, Borkowski, Estrada, Milstead, and Hale (1989) concluded that children with learning disabilities appear to demonstrate metacognitive deficits in a wide variety of tasks. Metacognitive deficits may be classified into two areas: metamemory and metacomprehension.

Metamemory   Metamemory, including awareness of strategies facilitative to learning, is one component of metacognition that has been previously reported to be delayed or deficient in students with learning disabilities (Borkowsi, Johnston, & Reid, 1987). As noted above, individuals with learning disabilities have been described as passive learners whose inferior performance on memory tasks may be attributed in large measure to inadequacies in goal-directed behavior (Torgeson, 1977), with possible negative effect on the deliberate selection and use of strategies that enhance performance.

Borkowski et al. (1987) have argued that failure to use facilitative strategies spontaneously may be due to metamemory deficits; that is, inadequate development in some children with learning disabilities of knowledge about and understanding of the behaviors that contribute to success on memory and learning tasks. They have been found to be less informed about internal (e.g., rehearsal) versus external (e.g., making a list) storage strategies.

Inefficient learners have been found less likely to employ facilitative strategies for more complex academic learning (Pressley & Levin, 1987), such as

Underlining and note taking

Selection of helpful retrieval cues from text

Making meaningful integrations of materials that require association

Going beyond given information to elaborate relations among elements in order to achieve more meaningful (hence, memorable) representations

The all-too-prevalent failure of students with learning disabilities to generalize trained strategies to new but similar tasks has been characterized by Borkowski et al. (1987) as a metacognitive deficit. The transfer of strategies to other relevant tasks was believed to require sufficient motivation to engage in "deliberate, conscious, goal-directed activity" (p. 150).

Worden (1987) has called attention to some problems with the metamemory model in accounting for the inactive learner's failure to generalize trained strategies for memory and learning tasks. She noted that, whereas Borkowski et al. (1987) mentioned deficits in auto-matic processing as one possible contributory factor, it received but passing attention in their discussion, in contrast to their focus on poor strategy choice and execution and the lesser motivation of the passive learner to engage in active strategy use. Worden (1987) has reasoned that:

contrary to the view expressed by Borkowsi, Johnston and Reid, these students may well under-stand the role of effort in learning, but it is precisely because learning is so much more effortful for them than for their nondisabled classmates that they try to avoid using strategic behaviors. (p. 222)

This issue of the possible interaction between cognitive and motivational factors in learning disabilities is discussed below.

Metacomprehension   Individuals with learning/reading disabilities have been reported to manifest deficits in the metacognitive functions of planning, monitoring, and checking com-prehension (A.L. Brown, Bransford, Ferrara, & Campione, 1983). The following descriptions of metacognitive deficits oberved in this population have been reported by a number of authors (L. Baker, 1982; Bos & Filip, 1982; Forrest-Pressley & Waller, 1984; Garner & Reis, 1981; Paris & Oka, 1989; Short & Ryan, 1984; Stevens, 1988; Wong, 1987):

Limited awareness of the purpose of reading as a meaning-getting act

Failure to adjust reading activities to meet different goals (e.g., details versus general impression)

Deficiencies in recognition of factors contributing to difficulty in text comprehension (e.g., level of organization or logical relations)

Failure to detect or react constructively to incongruities between new information and present knowledge

Reduced tendency to perceive syntactic or semantic ambiguities and to detect errors

Failure to recognize flawed comprehension

Reduced resources for coping with comprehension difficulties

Failure to use strategies flexibly to meet task demands in reading and studying

In a different but related vein, students with reading disability have been found to attribute their failure to low ability or luck instead of to such controllable factors as effort. "The affective consequences of causal attribution become antecedents to future action such as persistence or goal selection" (Paris & Oka, 1989, p. 36). Negative causal attribution has been regarded as a factor contributing to deficient metacomprehension (Borkowski, Weyhing, & Carr, 1988).

Wong and Wilson (1984) asserted that empirical research should be aimed not only at identifying metacognitive deficits but at programmatic intervention studies that provide both information and benefits. It may be reasoned that observed benefits of training metacognitive skills would provide some support for the assumption that corresponding metacognitive deficits are causally related to comprehension difficulties.

A number of studies have examined the effects of instruction in metacognitive skills that may be classed into the following categories:

> Stimulating goal-oriented behavior through preposed and/or self-generated questions, and predictions and verification of anticipated content
> Developing awareness of specific purposes of reading through search for main ideas, inferencing, and summarization
> Monitoring comprehension by detection of inconsistencies or errors
> Evaluating task performance by checking candidate responses against models

Another related, but separate, instructional research focus has been on the explicit restructuring of students' long-standing attitudes about attributions for failure and success believed to have an impact on the investment of effort in metacognitive activities.

A summary of condensed descriptions of experimental procedures for metacomprehension instruction and major findings from a sample of research are presented in Table 3.

Issues About Metacognitive Deficits and Learning/Reading Disabilities Reported benefits from research on cognitive and metacognitive instruction for students with learning/reading disabilities are believed to further illuminate understanding of the nature of these students' academic failure (Wong, 1985a). "In short, [learning-disabled] children's strategic deficits reflect their lack of metacognitive skills" (p. 159).

Some caveats have been sounded about the assumed role of metacognitive skills in all aspects of performance. L. Baker (1982) observed that *awareness* of memory strategies may be neither necessary nor sufficient for appropriate use of such strategies. She also called into question the validity of verbal report as an index of metacomprehension activity, commenting on the observed nonverbal behavioral evidence of comprehension monitoring in the absence of verbal report. Furthermore, she cautioned about assigning too large a weight to metacognitive factors in reading failure, to the detriment of attention to such decoding factors as deficient phonemic awareness and processing speed. These aspects of reading have frequently made excessive attentional demands on students with reading disability, and attention deficits may place limitations on the amount of resources available for metacognitive reflection (Loper, 1982).

Wong (1987) has taken note of the interaction among such factors and the development of metacognitive abilities apparently possessed to a degree by students with learning disabilities: "because decoding consumes LD readers' attention and efforts, they are unable to develop higher order metacognitive skills such as awareness of organizational factors in a passage and how these facilitate studying" (p. 193).

Table 3. Instructional research in metacomprehension: Procedures and major findings

Study	Subjects	Procedures	Results
Pflaum and Pascarella (1980)	Middle school, learning disabilities	Detection and correction of errors disruptive to comprehension, transfer of responsibility from teacher to students for monitoring and evaluation	Increased comprehension for subjects with at least 3rd-grade decoding skills
Bos and Filip (1982)	7th grade, skilled and unskilled readers	Advance cueing for detection of an inconsistency disruptive of comprehension	85% of unskilled and skilled readers detected the inconsistency, demonstrating effective comprehension monitoring
Schumaker, Deshler, Alley, Warner, and Denton (1982)	Junior high, learning disabilities, 4th-grade reading level	Multipass; scanning, self-questioning, search for main ideas, search for detail, comprehension monitoring, and self-evaluation	Marked improvement on test grades for textbook material; increased motivation in face of improvement
Wong and Jones (1982)	Junior high, learning disabilities	Search for main ideas, self-questioning, prediction of important information for comprehension testing, study and evaluation	Improved identification of main ideas; better than controls on comprehension and recall of content
Hansen and Pearson (1983)	4th grade, poor readers	Preposed questions to direct attention to key ideas, elaboration questions to stimulate inferencing, predictions about anticipated information	Trained subjects superior in recall of inferential material
Short and Ryan (1984)	4th grade, poor and good readers	Preposed *Wh-* questions to stimulate self-instruction in location of important story components for comprehension, plus attribution training Attribution training alone	Improved awareness of purposes of reading, improved reading comprehension in terms of error detection No significant gains
Holmes (1985)	4th and 5th grade, poor readers	Combined use of key word cues, self-questioning, checking candidate inferential responses against yes/no questions; controlled level of passage difficulty	Experimental subjects superior to controls on posttest inferential questions and on a standardized reading achievement test
Palinscar and Brown (1986)	Junior high, remedial readers	Self-generated questions, summarization, clarification, and prediction of subsequent content plus reciprocal teaching	Improved comprehension generalized to classroom performance
G.E. Miller, Giovenco, and Rentiers (1987)	4th and 5th grade, below- and above-average readers	Self-instruction, self-questions and/or self-statements to guide effective identification of purposely embedded errors	Below-average readers performed as well as above-average readers on comprehension questions and on detection of one out of two types of errors

(continued)

Table 3. (continued)

Study	Subjects	Procedures	Results
Stevens (1988)	6th–11th grade, remedial readers	Search for main ideas, evaluation of adequacy of identification and summaries via computer tutorial models and feedback	Generalization of identification of main ideas in expository text
Borkowski, Weyhing, and Carr (1988)	10- to 14-year-olds, poor readers	Summarization of paragraphs plus strategy training plus attribution training	Combined summarization, strategy, and attribution training produced 50% improvement in comprehension
		Attribution training alone	No significant improvement

Another issue concerns the efficacy of explicit attributional training in increasing motivation for engaging in metacognitive activity. Attribution training combined with strategy and metacomprehension training in the studies in Table 3 has been reported beneficial, but attribution training alone resulted in no significant gains. In other words, verbal instruction directed toward heightening awareness of benefits of effort on successful performance appear to have limited efficacy in stimulating enhanced motivation to engage in metacomprehension activities. In contrast, control of the difficulty level of the verbal material in the passages to be read was observed to have beneficial effects. "The apparent better performance by the Strategy Plus Material group and the Material Only group points out the importance of letting students work with materials that give success" (Holmes, 1985, p. 546).

In light of present concerns with the language deficits of many individuals with learning disabilities, some, but not all, of these metacognitive ineptitudes may be regarded as related to primary linguistic and metalinguistic deficiencies. These issues are addressed in greater detail in subsequent chapters on intervention.

Summary of Cognitive Correlates of Learning Disabilities

Perception The claim that visual-perceptual impairment is a major cause of reading disabilities has been largely discredited. Auditory-perceptual deficits at the metalinguistic level have been implicated in the problems with phonological awareness associated with failure in reading acquisition. However, there is only inconclusive evidence that, as a generality, individuals with learning disabilities exhibit the primary auditory-perceptual deficits that may contribute to language impairment. Although deficiencies in auditory and/or visual perception may, in some cases, reduce the effectiveness and efficiency of information processing, the relative role of bottom-up data processing deficits and top-down knowledge deficits remains the subject of debate, requiring further research. Some ostensible perceptual deficiencies may be attributed to attentional factors, since it is difficult to clearly disentangle effects of these two mechanisms.

Furthermore, although on certain tasks children with learning disabilities may demonstrate inadequacies in perceptual information processing, on other tasks they appear to adhere unduly to perceptual information, to the detriment of higher level processing. In accordance with the assumption that the proficient user of the tool of language is more capable of achieving mental distance from perception, in order to process information at more abstract levels

(Oleron, 1977), the frequent reports of concreteness manifested by individuals with language-related learning disabilities may indeed reflect a reduced propensity for using language to free thought from the influence of perception.

Attention   Review of relevant research has led Cooney and Swanson (1987) to suggest that the attentional *resources* of persons with learning disabilities are adequate for performance of most learning and memory tasks. Such a generalization would seem to require a qualification with regard to persons with language-related learning disabilities; it is reasonable to conjecture that, in the verbal domain, demands for attention allocation under certain conditions may stress available resources. It will be recalled that Swanson and his colleagues (1990) left unanswered the question about whether problems observed in children with learning disabilities were due to limited capacity or to some specific language processing limitations.

Referring briefly to previously cited neuropsychological theory, available research evidence points to a reduced tendency of children with language impairment to activate a verbal mental set and maintain such a set for verbal effort over time in the presence of competing attentional demands. Assuming some possible neuropsychological difference between language-deficient and language-proficient individuals in this regard, it seems plausible to assume that the greater effort required to engage in demanding verbal activity would implicate a *functional* difference in available attention capacity. That is, while attentional resources may be *structurally* intact and adequate at a global level, by virtue of the greater effort required to sustain a verbal mental set, these resources may be functionally more limited for language-related information processing by individuals with some degree of language impairment. Since degrees of language deficiency vary widely in the population with learning disabilities, the above assumptions would probably apply to different extents commensurate with severity of impairment.

Memory   There is compelling evidence that voluntary memory performance in academically related tasks is closely tied to linguistic knowledge and its use in the encoding and storage of information. Regarding the memory deficits of individuals with language-related learning disabilities, limitations in linguistic activity are implicated in:

> Phonetic encoding in short-term memory
>
> Slower access to verbally coded information
>
> A generalized disinclination to supplement visually coded with verbally coded information
>
> An apparent relative impoverishment of the semantic knowledge base, with an accompanying deficit in the activation of semantic knowledge in elaborative strategies for enhancement of storage and retrieval of information in purposive memory tasks

It is acknowledged that the issue of the relationship between elaborative organization and recall continues to require additional clarification. A number of investigators have reported that children with learning disabilities have demonstrated the ability to employ semantic organization when induced to do so to facilitate recall. However, such reports are at times qualified. For example, it has been reported that the organizational processing deficits in children with learning disabilities became more apparent at higher levels of linguistic and conceptual complexity (Ring, 1976). Subtle limitations in their semantic knowledge base may contribute to reductions in the quality of conceptual elaborations that may have a detrimental effect on spontaneously generated organization for the storage and recall of information (Ceci & Baker, 1989).

Although research and theory in memory make a strong case for the relationship between organization and memory, some important unanswered questions remain, particularly with reference to the function of persons with language-related learning disabilities in this respect. Two such questions would address the extent to which quantity and quality of knowledge affect the efficacy of organization for memory, and the extent to which heightened effort and slowed speed of verbal information processing might have a negative impact on the active use of elaborative strategies and the depth of semantic processing in learning and memory tasks with time constraints.

Beyond the ineffective encoding strategies for information storage, deficient retrieval of information from semantic memory to working memory, along with deficits in selective attention, have been posited as characteristics of memory problems in people with learning disabilities (Brainerd, Kingman, & Howe, 1986; Fletcher, 1985; Swanson, 1988b). Furthermore, it is not unlikely that failure to engage in facilitative active processing strategies reflects some metacognitive deficit, possibly attributable in part to a learned helplessness. Such metacognitive deficiencies may stem from the persistence of reading and learning disabilities perceived by the individual as evidence of an inability to succeed (Paris & Oka, 1989), thereby reducing motivation and intentions to learn (Hagen, Barclay, & Newman, 1982). "After experiencing failure, the 'helpless' child engages primarily in one sort of metacognitive activity, namely, nonproductive thoughts about his or her lack of ability" (p. 22).

The Failure Cycle

The effect of all the above variables appears to be a vicious spiral with cumulative negative impact on the individual with learning disabilities. Whether deficits are attributed to some genetically programmed difference or delay in the areas of language and cognition or they reflect some neurological malfunction is not fully understood. What is apparent from the research on linguistic/cognitive deficits is the likelihood that children with language-related learning disabilities enter the educational experience ill-equipped to meet the language and learning demands of the classroom.

Failure to achieve academic success has debilitating consequences for the student. A complex cyclic interaction among a number of factors occurs, as schematized in Figure 1.

1. Linguistic deficits are important determinants of reading disability and auditory verbal learning problems in education.
2. Difficulties in processing the linguistically encoded information transmitted in education are major causes of academic failure.
3. Academic failure reflects and contributes to a reduced knowledge base in both semantic and general information.
4. Academic failure results in low self-esteem and fear of further failure.
5. An impoverished knowledge base, possible constraints on information processing capacity, and a sensed inadequacy, individually or in combination, interfere with the development and efficient use of effective learning strategies. The inactive or inefficient learner is more subject to distractibility and response impulsivity.
6. Failure to actively employ effective information processing strategies reduces the probability of academic success.
7. Repeated experiences of academic failure and persistent reading disability are attributed by the student to an intrinsic inability to succeed.

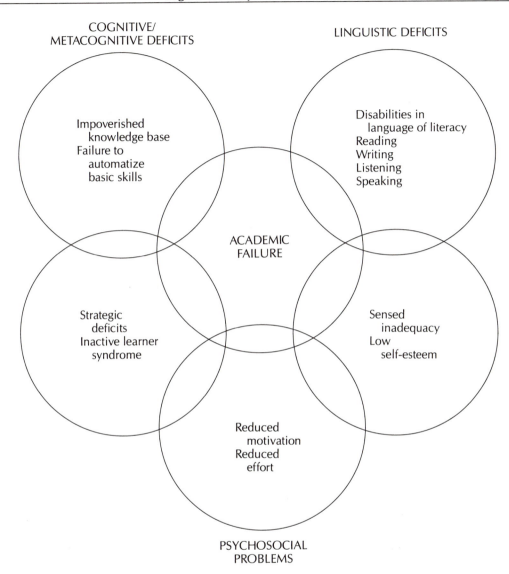

COGNITIVE/
METACOGNITIVE DEFICITS

LINGUISTIC DEFICITS

Impoverished
knowledge base
Failure to
automatize
basic skills

Disabilities in
language of literacy
Reading
Writing
Listening
Speaking

ACADEMIC
FAILURE

Strategic
deficits
Inactive learner
syndrome

Sensed
inadequacy
Low
self-esteem

Reduced
motivation
Reduced
effort

PSYCHOSOCIAL
PROBLEMS

Figure 1.   The failure cycle of language-related learning disabilities.

8.   Learned helplessness reduces motivation and effort, with a resultant decreased probability of present and future academic success, continued impoverishment of the knowledge base, and failure to master basic skills.

Thus, in cyclic fashion, academic failure associated with language-related learning disabilities is reflexive and self-perpetuating. The accompanying emotional problems experienced by many individuals having learning disabilities require further consideration and exploration in order to understand their nature and the role they may play in the disability.

PSYCHOSOCIAL CORRELATES OF LEARNING DISABILITIES

While many individuals with learning disabilities reportedly have personal and/or social mal-adjustment problems, these problems are not, apparently, universal in this population. In one laboratory examining children with learning disabilities, approximately one half of those studied exhibited "completely normal personality functioning" as measured by Rourke and Fisk (1981, p. 2). Of the 93 adults in a learning disabilities clinic population, 36% had received counseling or psychotherapy; however, others not in therapy expressed a need for some therapeutic support (D.J. Johnson & Blalock, 1987). Reports from other clinicians and researchers indicate that many of these individuals are at risk for secondary emotional problems, including "low self-esteem, poor self-concepts, social isolation, withdrawal, anxiety, depression and frustration" (D.J. Johnson & Blalock, 1987, p. 288). Some of the research investigating these problems and the theoretical issues that continue to be debated are reviewed.

M. Sanders (1979), while acknowledging the existence of neurogenic learning disabilities as a clinical entity, also took cognizance of a popular preference for the label "learning disabled" rather than "emotionally disturbed" by many parents and teachers.

> The development of the learning disabilities field is thus a mixed blessing, for while it has contributed greatly to the understanding and remediation of children's learning problems, it has also provided a new distraction for parents unable to acknowledge psychogenic emotional problems in their children or in themselves. (p. 5)

She noted, in addition, that educators who previously felt impotent to remedy emotional disturbance welcome the justification to treat learning problems from an active educational orientation.

Problems with Differential Diagnosis

A major issue that continues to defy clear-cut resolution is the distinction between primary and secondary emotional disorder. That is, while emotional problems related to learning disabilities are widely recognized, there is lack of complete agreement about whether they are causal to or resultant from the learning problems. Notwithstanding the clause in the official definitions of learning disabilities that excludes primary emotional disturbance as a criterial handicapping condition, psychologists frequently find it difficult to clearly discriminate between those emotional problems that are a secondary overlay to academic failure and those that are determinants of such failure.

One of the problems in differential diagnosis has been identified (Lufi & Cohen, 1988; Mokros, Poznanski, & Merrick, 1989) as undue reliance on the WISC–R (Wechsler, 1974). It has been assumed that individuals with emotional disturbance may be distinguished from individuals with learning disabilities by the absence of a discrepancy between Performance and Verbal IQ scores falling within the normal range. However, the WISC–R results alone have been found to produce excessive overlap between these groups and normally achieving populations. It is recommended that the WISC–R be used in conjunction with other procedures, such as personality tests (Lufi & Cohen, 1988).

Analysis of performance on a number of cognitive measures, along with selected WISC–R subtests, revealed no quantitative differences between children diagnosed as having an auditory learning disability and those diagnosed as being emotionally disturbed (Reeves, 1980). Qualitative analysis did reveal that children with emotional disturbance responded to tasks more readily than did those with learning disabilities and had less difficulty shifting to higher, more symbolic levels of meaning. However, their responses more frequently manifested bizarre and idiosyncratic interpretations. On certain tasks, children with learning disabilities tended to respond more concretely and descriptively, whereas the responses of subjects with emotional disturbance were more frequently tangential.

M. Sanders (1979) provided descriptions of types of emotional disturbance that might appear clinically to reflect auditory learning problems or generalized reductions in academic performance:

> *Withdrawal*—This behavior pattern may range from temporary or periodic to total withdrawal from the school situation. When this pattern is chronic and severe, it is usually indicative of childhood schizophrenia. In this case both the demands and the gratifications of the educational experience are ignored. These children are not stubborn, angry, discouraged, or conditioned to fear of failure. However, for reasons of their own, they have no interest in the world of school. They tune it out completely. Less severe, transitory withdrawal may be a reaction to temporary serious disruptions, such as illness or death.
>
> *Weak ego control*—In the presence of positive motivation and the ability to establish peer relationships, children with weak ego control seem to lack the emotional stamina to sustain attention to school tasks. They repeatedly need diversion and teacher attention and tend to have temper tantrums or to resort to tears when things do not go well. These children may give the impression, at times, of lack of comprehension of questions or tasks by virtue of apparently unrelated responses. It is suggested that these distortions may reflect over-preoccupation with their own concerns and a tendency to overpersonalize information or events to the point that objectivity is lacking. In a one-to-one exploration, it is possible to determine that the apparent auditory processing or expressive communication disability may, in fact, be attributable to interference by an emotional problem.
>
> *School phobia*—Some children may not have been ready to leave the security of the home and enter into competition with other children. These children may be generally immature, resembling younger children emotionally, cognitively, and, at times, linquistically.
>
> *Encapsulated school-related problems*—In some cases difficulty is experienced only in specific aspects of the school situation that may impinge on a particular emotional problem. For example, a child may have a neurotic conflict in dealing with authority in general, manifesting itself in situations in which teacher-imposed demands must be met.

Although it is considered important for those dealing with students with learning problems to be aware of the existence of such emotional problems, it is not here maintained that their incidence is necessarily frequent nor primarily causal among those students classified as having learning disabilities. Research within recent years tends to indicate heterogeneity in the population with learning disabilities regarding primary and secondary personal and social adjustment problems, with the evidence favoring the predominance of a secondary emotional overlay rather than serious psychogenic disorders.

Research on Psychological Problems in Learning Disabilities

Research reviewed by Bruck (1986) led to the conclusion that many of the emotional problems of persons with learning disabilities reflect adjustment problems resulting from labeling or academic failure. There was a higher than normal rate of anxiety, withdrawal, poor self-esteem, and depression, but the severity in most cases was not judged to be of clinical significance. Encouragingly, most of the earlier adjustment problems appear not to persist past compulsory school age. Follow-up study revealed that, while most of the adults manifesting adjustment problems had documented histories of such problems as children, a sizeable proportion (54%) with childhood problems during school age were well adjusted as young adults.

Externalizing and Internalizing Problems   Some of the emotional problems of children with learning disabilities are described by researchers as externalizing conduct problems, whereas others are classified as internalizing personality problems. An example of externalizing conduct problems is inappropriate behavior stemming from school-related anger. Students with learning disabilities have been found to differ significantly from students without such disabilities in their degree of school-related anger (Heavey, Adelman, Nelson, & Smith, 1989). Beyond the implications of anger for behavior, it was pointed out that "anger has other, less observable deleterious effects, especially as a potential precursor to depression" (p. 50). Thus, there may be some relationship between externalizing conduct problems and internalizing personality problems, such as depression.

Childhood Depression and Learning Disabilities   D. Goldstein and Dundon (1987) have identified a group of children enrolled in a special school for children with learning and emotional difficulties who met the criteria for childhood depression. Although the mean score on the Children's Depression Inventory was significantly higher for children with learning disabilities than the mean score for children without such disabilities from similar ethnic background enrolled in public school classes, it was significantly lower than the mean score of those enrolled in classes for children with emotional disturbance. It was thus found that a subgroup of children with learning disabilities met the criteria for social and emotional disturbance. Follow-up study of the two groups over 1–3 years of remedial education led to the conclusion that those children originally classified as having learning disabilities and social-emotional disturbance were not validly diagnosed as having learning disabilities because of their impressive gains in response to treatment of their emotional problems. In contrast, the inferior educational progress made by children classified as having learning disabilities but not originally classified as having social-emotional disturbance suggested that their learning problems were not attributable to primary emotional problems.

This distinction is supported by Mokros et al. (1989), whose findings led them to assert that children whose cognitive performance does not show gains with improvement in mood may best be classified as having a primary learning disability with superimposed affective disorder. It is, however, acknowledged that many children assumed to have a learning disability may also suffer depression as a primary disorder. For those children suffering from depression or other affective disorders, from an attention-capacity framework it is believed that depression or anxiety may place undue demands on available resources, to the detriment of optimal information processing.

Anxiety in Children with Learning Disabilities   In addition to depression, anxiety is a frequently reported condition accompanying learning disorder. The levels of manifest anxiety in children receiving part-time special services for learning disabilities and those in full-time learning disabilities classes were compared with each other and with those of children without such disabilities (Stein & Hoover, 1989). Even though the severity of the disability differed between the part-time and full-time groups, the level of manifest anxiety was comparable between the two groups and significantly higher than that of the group without disabilities. The authors made no claims for having determined the direction of cause and effect, acknowledging the possibility of a relationship between anxiety and learning disability. However, it is suggested that mainstream class conditions may have increased the opportunity for failure and resultant anxiety in these part-time students with learning disabilities, thus providing some support for the claim that an emotional problem may develop in reaction to the threat or experience of academic failure.

It is not surprising that students with a history of academic failure tend to have a low self-concept. There is evidence, however, that the poorer global self-concept demonstrated by the group with learning disabilities actually reflects a more specific *poorer academic* self-concept (Cooley & Ayers, 1988). "When this academic component was removed [from the results] the self-concept differences disappeared" (p. 177). As discussed briefly above, it has also been found that those students manifesting low self-concept are inclined to attribute their successes to factors external to themselves and to attribute academic failures to factors internal to themselves, such as low ability. These findings about attributional tendencies have been interpreted as causally related to reduced motivation and feelings of helplessness. As conceptualized above, the low self-concept of individuals with learning disabilities in terms of anticipated failure interacts cyclically with reduced incentive to make the effort to succeed, thus virtually guaranteeing continued status as a failure to the self and others within the social milieu (Cooley & Ayers, 1988; Paris & Oka, 1989).

Social Adjustment Problems

Social maladjustment, behavioral problems, and peer rejection have been reported among the wider population of children and adolescents with learning disabilities. Different theoretical assumptions have determined the nature of research methods used to study social adjustment problems in efforts to describe and explain them.

Social Imperception Hypothesis   A theory advanced by Rourke et al. (1989) attributing maladaptive social behavior in children with learning disabilities to social imperception or deficits in the ability to notice and interpret nonverbal cues from the environment has had its adherents throughout the past two or more decades (D.J. Johnson & Myklebust, 1967; Lerner, 1971; Wiig & Semel, 1984). Citing an example of visual imperception in learning disabilities, Wiig and Semel (1984) reported on a visual perception evaluation of an adolescent with learning disabilities, results of which evidenced visual inattention, distractibility, poor visual memory, and problems in perception of orientation and direction of movement. However, it is important to notice that these results include descriptions of deficiencies not limited to perception itself. Nonetheless, the theory postulates that visual imperception may be related to right hemisphere dysfunction, involving impaired perception of important changes in facial expression, gestures, and body postures that signal certain interpersonal messages. A relationship is assumed between such imperceptions and reduced affective sensitivity and limited knowledge of social rules, resulting in poor social skills (Wiig & Semel, 1984). Inappropriate interaction with other people in a manner and to a degree that is disruptive to social relations tends to cause rebuff and rejection, which, in turn, is believed to disturb the development of a positive self-image, frequently causing a reaction of hostility and aggression.

More recently, evidence from a study of patterns of lateralized cognitive deficits in children with learning disabilities "did not support the hypothesis that [learning disabled] children with right hemisphere impaired cognitive profiles would exhibit higher rates of aggression and disregard for social norms" (Glosser & Koppell, 1987). Some other scholars who have reviewed and critiqued extensive bodies of research in this area have called into question the methods and/or the generalizations about the implications of the findings cited as support for a neurologically based social-perceptual deficit (Maheady & Sainato, 1986; Pearl, 1987). For example, it has been observed that experimental situations may be too dissimilar to the range of actual social contexts to permit generalized assumptions about the nature and degree of social imperception in children with learning disabilities (Maheady & Sainato, 1986). From another point of view, it is argued that these children do have the ability to interpret social displays, but are less accurate because they pay less careful attention (Pearl, 1987).

In the absence of data judged sufficiently convincing to justify attributing social problems of children with learning disabilities to primary cognitive deficits, Bruck (1986) favored the position that environmental factors play a significant role in the development of social-emotional difficulties. She postulated that a contributing factor to these problems is the interaction between parent, teacher, and peer reactions to the child with learning disabilities.

With equivocal results and questions about methodological validity, it is advised that efforts to apply the theory of social imperception to remedial training "be reserved until that time when psychometrically sound measures of these skills are developed and when the relationship of these abilities to overall social competence are more clearly delineated" (Maheady & Sainato, 1986, p. 396).

Cognitive Deficit Hypothesis   From a Piagetian cognitive developmental perspective, rather than a neuropsychological view, it has been suggested that poor social skills in children with learning disabilities may reflect delay in the ability to take another's perspective (Pullis & Smith, 1981). Evidence supporting this hypothesis has been interpreted from results of studies showing that children with learning disabilities scored significantly lower than achieving children on role-taking tasks. Such deficiency is believed to be related to delayed development in decentration. These attributes have been the focus of a considerable body of research in the verbal communication patterns of children with learning disabilities (reviewed in Chapter 7 in the section "pragmatic deficits").

Results of other studies of role taking reviewed by Pearl (1987) also suggest reductions of social knowledge and sensitivity to another's perspective among subjects with learning disabilities. However, some inconsistencies in the findings of these studies exist to an extent that warrants further investigation for clarification. For example, lack of correlation has been established between ratings on role taking and other measures of social competence (Bruck & Hebert, 1982; E.C. Horowitz, 1981).

Research on Social Interaction   Regardless of theoretical differences, there is relative unanimity in the literature about the types of patterns observed in the social interaction among children with learning disabilities and significant others, with some variations in reports of degree of severity. For example, Bruck (1986), reporting on studies of peer ratings, found that, while children with learning disabilities were not rated as the most socially valued peers, they were not largely, or predominantly, socially isolated. In fact, some investigations found more between-group similarities (children with versus without learning disabilities) than differences, and the existence of severe problems in only a small segment of the population with learning disabilities.

In contrast to Bruck's (1986) findings, L. Perlmutter's (1986) survey of relevant studies strongly suggests that children with learning disabilities tend to be less well liked than their classmates without such disabilities, and less well regarded by parents and by other adult observers unaware of classification status. Frequently these children have been observed to act as "class clowns" in a compensatory effort to secure attention from peers who are likely to ignore or rebuff them. These observations have been supported by the results of sociometric studies.

In an interesting experimental procedure, children with and without learning disabilities engaged in teacher–learner dyadic interactions. In one condition, the dyad consisted of age peers; in another condition, older children with learning disabilities were teachers of younger children. Naive observers rated social behavior. The children with learning disabilities received higher ratings for socially acceptable behavior when interacting with younger children than in interaction with age-mate children without such disabilities. The ratings of "teachers" with learning disabilities, which were lower than those of subjects without such disabilities in the age-mate condition, actually increased to the level accorded "teachers" without disabilities when interacting with younger children.

These results appear to warrant the conclusion that children with learning disabilities have the *ability* to perform adequately when granted the favorable status generally given by younger to older children. Further investigation of research inclined L. Perlmutter (1986) toward a developmental lag theory, rather than a social-perceptual deficit, to account for the observed social deficiencies. This hypothesis received support from the finding that many adolescents with learning disabilities are likely to seek social interaction with younger children. The impact of the developmental lag was regarded as increasing with age, since the social environment continues to grow in complexity, placing those who are less mature at a greater disadvantage.

One of the acknowledged weaknesses of all research in learning disabilities is the heterogeneity of the population, making it difficult to generalize implications of findings in one group to all individuals with learning disabilities. From the above reports, it may be assumed that some of the inconsistencies reported in describing the social problems of those students with learning disabilities stem from disparities among the characteristics of the groups studied. One dimension on which children with learning disabilities have been reported to differ among themselves is hyperactivity, a characteristic frequently incurring negative social reactions.

Contrast Between Learning Disabilities and Behavioral Disorders   There is a need to distinguish between the social-behavioral characteristics of students with learning disabilities and those of students with behavioral disorders (Margalit, 1989). Comparisons were made between teacher ratings of behavior for boys with learning disabilities in classes for students with learning disability grades 1–4, and those made for boys demonstrating behavior disorders in regular education classes, grades 1–4. Among other findings, children with learning disabilities were rated more dependent, more introverted, and less hostile than the boys with behavioral disorder. Margalit (1989) favored a cognitive deficit hypothesis to explain the inability of children with learning disabilities to learn complex social problem-solving skills.

She viewed these deficits in interpersonal development from an information processing framework, suggesting that difficulties in processing the information of social interaction should be treated as one of the defining characteristics of persons with learning disabilities.

A longitudinal study by J.D. McKinney (1989) provided some information about behavioral subtypes of students with learning disabilities and relations between subtypes and academic progress. Cluster analysis yielded seven subtypes, which were collapsed into four composite groups for statistical and theoretical reasons. Two groups, comprising 34.9% of the students, were characterized as displaying social-emotional behavior within the normal range and one group showed low positive behavior. Other groups were described as follows:

> *Attention Deficit* (28.6%): showing deficiencies in task-oriented behavior and independence but normal personal-social behavior
> *Conduct Problems* (14.3%): displaying mild attention deficits and elevated distractibility and hostility
> *Withdrawn Behavior* (11%): rated as overly dependent and introverted (primarily composed of girls)
> *Global Behavior Problems* (4.8%): significantly impaired in all classroom behaviors

In examining category membership over a 3-year period, one of the most interesting findings was that from year 1 to year 3, it was more likely for children with learning disabilities originally classified as demonstrating adaptive behavior to be reclassified into more maladaptive patterns; that is, 54% were reclassified from the adaptive group into groups predominantly demonstrating attention deficit or problem behaviors. Only 11% moved from original maladaptive to more adaptive patterns. It is also of interest to note that, longitudinally, children with learning disabilities but without significant behavior problems made significant academic gains, although continuing to show subaverage achievement, whereas those children with attentional and behavioral disorders declined in relative progress compared to rate of gain by other subgroups and average learners.

Summary of Psychosocial Problems and Learning Disabilities

Apparently all children with learning disabilities do not demonstrate significant social-emotional problems. However, the psychosocial concomitants of learning disability in this heterogeneous population are of a dimension that warrants continued investigation. Research into the components of the phenomenon of learning disabilities in general, and evaluation of particular cases, requires determination of the primary or secondary nature of the social-emotional problems accompanying academic failure.

CONCLUSIONS

From the foregoing research and its theoretical implications, it is evident that the problems of individuals with language-related learning disabilities are multifaceted, with complex interactions among the linguistic, cognitive, and psychosocial factors. In the intervention process, consisting of both assessment and treatment, all of these aspects of possible deficit require consideration. However, the heterogeneity of the population to be served demands individualized, rather than generalized, approaches.

III

SERVICE DELIVERY TO STUDENTS WITH LANGUAGE-RELATED LEARNING DISABILITIES

9 / Assessing Language Abilities in School-Age Children

Jack S. Damico and Charlann S. Simon

> One's approach to language assessment must reflect a *model* of language that takes into account several considerations, ranging from the purposes of the assessment to one's conceptualization of the very nature of language. (Bryen & Gerber, 1981, p. 115)

This statement stresses the fact that blind use of a "test battery" is not language assessment. To engage in assessment, one must have a model of what language is and how it works. Furthermore, this model should be able to bring one closer to understanding why some children have difficulty both comprehending information and demonstrating this comprehension through oral and written language.

For many years, language models and assessment methodologies reflected the position that standardized tests must be used to determine deviance, to systematically examine particular aspects of language, and to document delay on the basis of comparing performance of the child with that of a sample of his or her peers. Over the past two decades, however, pragmatics research has focused on the dynamic interactions among listener and speaker roles, message content, and the context in which communication occurs. This body of knowledge has provided us with tools to observe language use in natural contexts and has encouraged clinicians to pay more attention to message content that is an integral part of the communication context in which the listener (reader) and speaker (writer) must demonstrate language proficiency. While standardized tests may be necessary to meet legal guidelines for placement in special education and may answer some specific questions about underlying linguistic, cognitive, and metalinguistic skills, these results may not provide the most valuable information for describing language problems or planning intervention programs.

This chapter emphasizes the value of conceptualizing language as a complex behavior that cannot be adequately described by standardized testing. It is suggested that description—followed by explanation of behaviors observed—occupies the premier position in assessment. As noted by Muma (1978), an individual's score on a standardized test is less important than learning how that individual functions in obtaining that score. Based on this conceptualization, clinical practices are presented here that can be used to determine the degree to which an individual's communication is functional relative to the referral context. With school-age children, referral for language evaluation is usually linked to deficits observed in the classroom. Information presented in this chapter reflects the increasing emphasis on descriptive assessment involving criterion-based, communication-based, and curriculum-based assessment.

A POSITION STATEMENT ON THE ASSESSMENT OF LANGUAGE AND COMMUNICATION

Assessment decisions are grounded in one's conceptual/operational model. That is, what we do reflects how we think. The operational model used is based on certain premises about the nature and development of language as well as the purposes of language assessment. These premises are in a constant state of revision as we incorporate new research findings and clinical insights.

The premises underlying assessment suggestions presented in this chapter are:

1. Language is a rule-governed symbol system capable of representing or coding one's understanding of the world.
2. Language is a generative system that permits various combinations of words to code the same thoughts and feelings, and it can be used to produce unlimited novel utterances.
3. Language is a complex ability that requires simultaneous and integrated functioning. Verbal and nonverbal contextual variables must be synthesized during comprehension and formulation of messages.
4. Language is a social code that reflects the community in which a child learns the symbol system, and it may include the use of various dialects.
5. Language functions can describe the communicative purposes for using language.
6. There is a developmental sequence in the emergence of language structures and functions.
7. Language and cognitive development are intertwined in development and use.
8. If there are deviations in an individual's rule knowledge/use (or structure/function), relative to peers within the language community, this may reflect deficits in communicative competence.
9. Assessment of communicative competence must include consideration of structure and function, relative to the cognitive level at which an individual is operating, and the dialectal variation of the community in which language was learned.

Based on these nine premises, the traditional conception of language proficiency as a set of minimally interacting components (i.e., syntax, phonology, semantics, morphology, pragmatics) that are autonomous in nature appears too simplistic (Canale, 1983; Crystal, 1987; Cummins, 1984; Hubbell, 1981; Kirchner & Skarakis-Doyle, 1983; Oller, 1979, 1983; Shuy, 1981; C.S. Simon, 1985, 1987). While providing a convenient format for language assessment and sample analysis, these divisions do not reflect real communication. That is, a division of language into modules does not describe the intricacies and complexities of communication behaviors. In practice, these linguistic dimensions are nondivisible (Carroll, 1961; Crystal, 1987; Oller, 1983).

Increasingly, language proficiency is being conceptualized from a synergistic perspective in which the various dimensions of language are considered complex and integrated. These linguistic dimensions function together to formulate, transmit, and comprehend meaning. In addition, this synergistic perspective implies that language is not a closed system. Rather, it is closely linked with other semiotic and cognitive abilities and is influenced by extraneous intervening variables such as motivation, experience, learning, and anxiety. The practice of assessment, therefore, should reflect this more synergistic focus on communicative ability (Damico, 1988, 1991; C.S. Simon, 1986, 1989).

To observe events systematically and synergistically and analyze products of these events, it is essential to first acquire an understanding of the language system being studied. This would include not only an understanding of the divisions categorized as phonology, morphology, syntax, and semantics, but also how these divisions are integrated to produce communication and how sociocultural factors affect language use. In addition, it is necessary to study the contexts in which an individual is asked to perform in listener/reader and speaker/writer roles.

This chapter highlights this emphasis on the synergistic construct of language assessment. Throughout the chapter there is an integration of various types of assessment procedures that comment on the effectiveness of one's language to formulate, transmit, and comprehend meaning. Evaluators are encouraged to observe events systematically and analyze products of these events. This necessitates not only an understanding of the way that meaning is coded by structure for a particular purpose, but also how contextual and sociocultural factors affect language use.

IMPLEMENTATION OF ASSESSMENT

The synergistic model of assessment leads to questions concerning the purposes of assessment, the context in which assessment occurs, and the techniques and tools utilized during the evaluative process.

Purposes of Assessment

The initial purpose of assessment is to determine whether or not an individual is a competent communicator in academic and social situations regardless of causal factors. That is, it is imperative to determine if communicative problems do exist in the referral context. If communicative problems do exist, then the second purpose of assessment is initiated: to determine the reasons for this lack of communicative success. This is important since our current educational system places speech-language pathology services in special education. It is necessary, therefore, to ensure a differentiation between children who are unsuccessful mainstream communicators because of an intrinsic language-related learning disability and children who are unsuccessful communicators for other reasons (e.g., cultural diversity, dialectal differences, lack of motivation, poor previous instruction). It is not appropriate from pedagogical, fiscal, legal, or ethical perspectives to place a child into special education unless the communication problem is truly due to an intrinsic language-related learning impairment. Consequently, the methods utilized should be specific and comprehensive enough to provide an explanation for difficulties noted. To accomplish this descriptive requirement, Damico (1991) suggested a bilevel analysis paradigm consisting of a descriptive analysis phase and an explanatory analysis phase.

Descriptive Analysis Phase   At the descriptive analysis level, the evaluator utilizes procedures or instruments (detailed below under "Techniques and Tools of Assessment") to comment on the student's relative competence in the context of interest. At this level, the issue of a language-related learning disability is not considered. The essential question is one of success or proficiency as a communicator. To address this question of proficiency, the behaviors utilized in assessment must comment on the functional aspects of language usage through the application of valid criterion-based, communication-based (L. Bloom & Lahey, 1978), and curriculum-based (N.W. Nelson, 1989; Tucker, 1985) indices that serve to comment on specific abilities and behaviors needed to function as a successful communicator in the referral context. For example, a student's ability to find key words in a textbook passage, the ability to use specific and sufficient vocabulary, and the ability to seek clarification through questioning appear to be three essential skills necessary for successful communication in the classroom environment.

The use of these behaviors as indices for effective communication enables the evaluator to *focus on the functional aspects* of language as communication. This is consistent with the current construct of language proficiency. When analyzing true language use, the evaluator asks one specific question: "How proficient a communicator is this child in the context of interest?" By addressing this question, the evaluator seeks to observe and describe the child's ability to fulfill three criteria that operationally define proficiency: the effectiveness of meaning transmission, the fluency of meaning transmission, and the appropriateness of meaning transmission.

Effectiveness of Meaning Transmission   The effectiveness of meaning transmission is the first operational criterion of proficiency. That is, how well can the child use language to formulate, relay, or comprehend a message? This is the primary objective of language as communication. In keeping with the premises discussed previously, this ability to transmit a message effectively is not tied to a specific language structure, register, or mode of transmission. Meaning can be transmitted effectively in many ways (e.g., telegraphic speech, Standard English, a dialectal variety, a gestural system). Regardless of how it is achieved, if the meaning is transmitted then communication is accomplished and the individual is effective.

Fluency of Meaning Transmission   The second criterion, fluency of meaning transmission, involves two considerations. First, the evaluator must determine if the child relays or comprehends the message within an appropriate period of time. For the normal flow of communication to occur, it is necessary that the child adhere to the temporal constraints of conversation. Taking too much time to formulate, relay, or comprehend a message usually interferes with communication. Second, the evaluator must determine if the child is able to repair an interaction if the first attempt to transmit meaning is not successful. Can the child revise an initial utterance that was not sufficiently formulated? How well can the child use context, experience, or expectancy to make sense of something not immediately comprehended? To be proficient communicators, children must not only be effective in meaning transmission, they must also be fluent in this transmission.

Appropriateness of Meaning Transmission   The appropriateness of meaning transmission is the third criterion. Since language and communication are highly influenced by cultural or societal factors and expectancies, it is not enough to transmit meaning effectively and fluently. The child must also transmit meaning by using the codes, registers, and modalities appropriate to the context. Failure to do so typically results in less communicative success in that specific context. For example, an individual using Standard English in an environment in which a dialectal form of Vernacular Black English is the norm will typically fare poorly. Although the individual will be able to get meaning across successfully and fluently, the inappropriate structural form will label the speaker as an outsider and one not culturally and linguistically attuned to the community (Labov, 1972).

Discussion From the functional perspective, then, a proficient communicator is one who can meet all three criteria during conversation. Problems with any of the three will typically result in communicative difficulty and should require further investigation. It must be stressed, however, that failure to meet these criteria in no way indicates that the child has a language-related learning disability. This decision cannot be made at the descriptive analysis level. This level only identifies the problematic behaviors that make the child less proficient than is expected or required.

If the descriptive analysis, with its emphasis on the functional aspects of communication as identified by valid indices of necessary abilities and behaviors, indicates that the child is a successful communicator in the context of interest, then the evaluation is finished. There is no need to conduct any further analysis since few problematic behaviors will have been noted. In this case, the evaluator has a functional description of how the child successfully handled the communicative tasks in the context of interest, and these skills and abilities may be used as evidence of the child's communicative proficiency. However, if the descriptive analysis has identified problematic behaviors that result in the child being an unsuccessful communicator in the context of interest, then it is necessary to conduct the explanatory analysis phase of this bilevel paradigm.

Explanatory Analysis Phase This second phase of the bilevel assessment paradigm attempts to determine the causal factors for the problematic behaviors noted in the descriptive analysis phase. It is in this phase that the question of differentiation between an intrinsic language-related learning disorder and various extrinisic factors is considered. In this phase the evaluator carefully analyzes the problematic behaviors that were documented through the appropriate tools or procedures and attempts to determine if these behaviors can be explained by any extrinsic factors such as cultural diversity, test anxiety, fatigue, poor testing practices, or dialectal diversity. If these extraneous variables do not sufficiently account for the problematic behaviors, then the evaluator conducts a linguistic analysis. To conduct this analysis, the evaluator reviews all of the problematic behaviors noted within the linguistic context and determines whether or not there is a systematicity to the problematic behaviors observed. That is, there is an attempt to link the occurrence of these behaviors with the occurrence of some underlying linguistic variation.

For example, it might be noted that a child is not a proficient communicator because he or she has frequent inappropriate responses to the queries of others. In analyzing this behavior, the evaluator discovers that 85% of the child's inappropriate responses occur when the questions involve higher levels of cognitive and linguistic abstraction. Further analysis might pinpoint that, while the student responds accurately to questions beginning with *what* and *where,* there is a significant deterioration in response to *why* and *how* questions. In this case, the problematic behavior (inappropriate responding) is used to identify the child's actual language difficulty (inability to function at or above a particular level of linguistic abstraction). The problematic behavior, therefore, is only an index to help determine the real underlying linguistic difficulty. There are a number of linguistic analysis procedures that can aid the clinician when conducting an explanatory analysis. Some of these procedures, along with the actual questions to ask in conducting the analysis, are discussed below under "Techniques and Tools of Assessment."

To meet the objectives of communicative assessment within the synergistic perspective, therefore, a descriptive assessment approach is necessary that makes use of functional and realistic language behaviors derived from criterion-based, communication-based, and curriculum-based assessment. In adhering to this approach, the evaluator will be more effective in meeting the objectives of assessment: determining if an intrinsic disorder exists and documenting both the indices of this problem and the underlying causal factors.

Context of Assessment

From a synergistic perspective and within a functional model, language behavior is viewed along with potential distractions and influences rather than apart from them. Oller (1979) stated that language tests are most effective when they are pragmatic; the behaviors analyzed are observed and collected in a situation in which they are affected by the temporal constraints of real interaction, there is intentionality, and the tasks are contextually embedded. The behaviors most relevant to assessment objectives are those that occur when language is functioning holistically to transmit meaning within real contexts. Determining one's "communicative competence," therefore, is dependent on first acknowledging the impact of the communication context. If one wants to find out how proficient a student's classroom communication and metalinguistic skills are, the ideal context for observation is in the classroom.

For school-age children, the classroom becomes a major focus because of the amount of time spent here and the significance of success in this setting to the formulation of a child's self-concept. For example, a teacher might say, "Johnny doesn't understand directions." During observation, an evaluator notices that at the beginning of class, when the assignment is being given, Johnny is fumbling with his notebook and looking for a pencil. The attention needed to comprehend the direction was not present. It is possible to obtain a passing comprehension score in a treatment room for students like Johnny. Environmental distractions and personal disorganization, however, might inhibit a comparable performance in class. It is only when the observation and the performance context are matched that accurate evaluation can occur or generalization of later therapy objectives can be ensured.

Based on the work of Canale (1983), Cummins (1983), Luria (1981), and Westby (1985), Damico (1991) detailed three major manifestations of language-as-communication to observe when conducting naturalistic assessment: oral monologic communication, oral dialogic communication, and contextually constrained communication.

Oral Monologic Communication   During many communication events, individuals have time to prepare or plan or there is some external structuring by another person (Ochs, 1977). For example, a youngster might be asked to think about and create a story or retell a story just heard. Other examples are when someone is given a sequence of pictures or asked to relate an important event that has been discussed many times before. In each of these cases, there is an opportunity to present predetermined content that has logically structured form with transitions and cohesive ties. The individual need not actively attend to changing context and interaction, since they have been placed on hold while "performance" of the preplanned activity occurs. As Westby (1985) noted, this is a necessary academic skill that is exemplified by description, giving directions, telling a story, telling jokes, or delivering speeches.

Oral Dialogic Communication   The second manifestation is one that speech-language clinicians typically conceptualize when talking about language analysis—oral dialogic speech. This involves communicative interaction that is unplanned. The child may formulate a message, but once it is given, the turns of the interactional dyad determine the child's subsequent utterances. The child must be able to adjust to the changing needs and demands of the linguistic and nonlinguistic context to be successful. This type of language is typically seen in true conversational interaction or in responding to the multiple queries of others. Preplanning of the linguistic structure, the content, or even the purposes of the discourse is not possible. This manifestation is particularly important for social effectiveness.

Contextually Constrained Communication   The third type of language that should be targeted for assessment involves meaning transmission in situations in which the context rigidly controls the way that the communication may be structured. Because of contextual, situational, or format constraints, there are specific ways that an interaction may proceed in terms of the language code used, the content expressed, and even the interactional rules that are followed. There is a strict adherence to predetermined rules and expectations not applied in the other two manifestations. For example, a job interview is a situation in which the context rigidly controls the way that communication may be structured.

The classroom is a contextually constrained situation (Mehan, 1979; Ripich & Spinelli, 1985; C.S. Simon, 1979, 1987; Wallach & Miller, 1988). There are distinct interactional patterns between the teacher and student that are very different from normal conversational discourse, and in some situations dialectal forms may be judged unacceptable even when they effectively transmit meaning in a fluent manner. N.W. Nelson (1989) summarized classroom language by saying, "In schools, much emphasis is placed on learning to read and write language, on learning to talk about language, on using language to learn how to do to other things, and on using language to learn about things" (p. 170).

Another important instance of contextually constrained communication involves formal test taking. This situation requires response to questions and performance on tasks that are typically isolated from intentionality and real communicative meaning. Consequently, these activities are more cognitively demanding and have less contextual embeddedness (Cummins, 1983; Oller, 1979). Children perform testing activities not because they want to do so but, rather, because someone with power requires them to do so. Although such test-taking ability is only important in certain situations and not a true reflection of one's overall communicative ability, it is beneficial for the professional to note whether or not the child exhibits difficulty within this delimited situation. Poor test-taking ability can cause the child to be misclassified or may result in a needless reduction of teacher or parent expectations. Such formal test-taking ability is only important because of our society's unbalanced emphasis on such activities (Damico, 1991).

Discussion   When collecting data in natural situations, all three types of language use must be observed to conduct a complete evaluation. While this tripartite division may tend to overlap at times, it does allow for an in-depth description and is consistent with clinical experience. It is possible that a child may experience communicative difficulty with one of these manifestations and not the other two. As discussed by Cummins (1984), each communicative situation varies according to its degree of contextual embeddedness and cognitive complexity.

The child's inability to handle these two dimensions may be reflected in differential performance across these three manifestations, which occurs because the cognitive demands of contexts vary. An individual might be able to display social communicative competence when engaged in informal interactions, but may have a history of academic language difficulties in classroom interactions. This breakdown in language proficiency is an instance of the child reaching a level of incompetence when trying to cope with the more intricate demands of classroom communication. This example of the child reaching a level of incompetence in one or more of the manifestations may be taken to any extreme. For example, a student may display proficiency in explaining how to proceed with a manual arts project—because vocabulary, concepts, sentence patterns, and self-confidence are intact—but be unable to cope with a plot and character analysis in a literature assignment.

Taken together, the issues considered under the purposes of assessment (i.e., the bilevel analysis, a functional focus, and use of communicative referencing) and within the context of assessment (i.e., pragmatic methodology, collection in natural settings) enable the evaluation to be more valid and enable the clinician to accept more performance variation than would the more traditional approach to assessment. It requires, however, a divergence from the traditional. In this approach, the process of assessment involves a different focus and strategy. When the clinician receives a referral, for example, there is no need to select discrete point tests to analyze specific components of the child's linguistic abilities. The clinician should not be concerned with the child's use of receptive syntax or expressive morphology apart from actual communication and should not attempt to assess these isolated skills with a formal norm-referenced test. Rather, the assessment should proceed in the following manner:

1. The clinician receives a referral or district data that direct attention to an at-risk student.
2. Procedures are selected that will answer this question: "How proficient is the individual as a communicator in oral monologic, oral dialogic, and contextually constrained communication situations?"
3. The clinician engages in a descriptive analysis of performance per situation. If the results indicate there are no problems with the effectiveness, fluency, or appropriateness of meaning transmission, evaluation is ended. Selected notations might be shared with those who regularly interact with the individual.
4. If problematic behaviors are noted in any one of the three observational contexts, the clinician moves into the explanatory phase of assessment. Additional procedures—including possible probes—are selected as the clinician attempts to explain the occurrence of communication difficulties. This is the stage in the evaluation process in which the clinician engages in analysis of language structure, metalinguistic awareness, neurological processing, and other related factors.

To conduct assessment through this process, however, requires the availability of a psychometrically strong set of language tests or procedures. Fortunately, there are numerous tools and procedures that fit within this synergistic model. These tools and procedures encompass several assessment formats and come from a variety of disciplines. Each one, however, can be used effectively and productively within the synergistic model. It is to these techniques and tools that the discussion now turns.

TECHNIQUES AND TOOLS OF ASSESSMENT

The techniques and tools discussed in this section are those that match the purposes of assessment and can be used within the appropriate contexts. These tools or procedures tend to assess language holistically and descriptively rather than from a discrete point perspective, focus more on the functionality of language rather than tuning in to superficial structural aspects, and utilize communicative referencing more frequently than normative referencing. Additionally, these tools are more consistent with the pragmatic methodology and may be more easily applied in natural settings than other tools or techniques. The theoretical bias revealed at the first of this chapter, therefore, is maintained in test selection.

Issues of Test Selection

Several issues pertaining to selection of tests and evaluative procedures must be mentioned before discussing the specific tools. This information will aid the clinician in test selection and will demonstrate that many of the testing procedures previously utilized in the assessment of children believed to have language-related learning disorders also fit within this more synergistic assessment process. To select assessment tools properly, tests must be appropriately classified, triangulation of data must be stressed, and there must be an emphasis on psychometric strength.

Classification of Tests   When selecting appropriate testing procedures, there is a wide range of tests from which to choose. These tests have been classified and differentiated in numerous ways over the last several decades (e.g., formal-informal, standardized-nonstandardized, language structure versus language use tests, screening measures versus in-depth tests). Within the traditional model of language assessment these distinctions have some relevance. Within the synergistic model, however, these distinctions are less important. Within this framework it is more beneficial to classify tests according to four dimensions: the level of analysis applied, the language context targeted, the test's placement along the discrete point–pragmatic continuum, and the type of assessment format used.

The classification of language tests as being appropriate to the descriptive analysis phase or the explanatory analysis phase has been discussed. Basically, those tests and procedures that address functional aspects of communication to determine the child's level of proficiency as a communicator are utilized in the descriptive analysis phase. Those that are designed to conduct detailed and in-depth analysis of paradigmatic and syntagmatic aspects of language functioning *after* the descriptive analysis are utilized in the explanatory phase. Similarly, little discussion is needed regarding the classification of tests and procedures according to the three manifestations of communication. These have been detailed, and specific tools that fit under each manifestation are listed later in this section. Some discussion is needed, however, regarding the other two dimensions that act to differentiate language tests.

Discrete Point–Pragmatic Continuum   The major theoretical difference between the traditional approach to language assessment and the emerging approach involves the conception of language as modular versus synergistic. That is, can language be operationally broken down into its components, analyzed, and still be true language behavior (a discrete point methodology), or does this fragmentation of language strip its essentialness and leave the evaluator with something less than language during the evaluation? If language cannot be broken down and maintain its uniqueness, then it must be collected and analyzed as it functions holistically (a pragmatic methodology). In actuality, all language tests can be arranged along a continuum between these two polar extremes. To the extent that a test is designed to analyze specific and discrete units of a particular aspect of language structure (e.g., a receptive morphological marker such as past tense -*ed*), it is closer to the discrete point pole. To the extent that a test is designed to analyze language as it functions to relay an intention or operate at a level of displacement, it is closer to the pragmatic pole. Tools such as the Test of Auditory Comprehension of Language or the Test of Language Development are more discrete point in nature, whereas the Test of Pragmatic Skills, the Porch Index of Communicative Ability in Children, and the Preschool Language Assessment Instrument are more pragmatic in nature. Within the synergistic model, the tools selected should be those closer to the pragmatic rather than the discrete point pole.

Type of Assessment Format Used   Another dimension of language tests involves the actual strategy or format used to obtain and code the behaviors assessed. While there are numerous formats used, most can be classified under four major headings. The first is the largest category, *probes*. This format has been utilized in the design of many of the traditional language tests, and there are many variations within this category. For example, there are picture elicitation probes, question-and-answer probes, probes using puppets, and those using elicited imitation. Additionally, there are both formal and informal probes. That is, many have been carefully researched, subjected to peer review, and made available to the profession (formal probes), whereas others, for various reasons, have been designed and used only in a limited area and typically without much empirical substantiation or peer review. Although these tools vary to some extent, they all focus on certain aspects of language, attempt to reduce extraneous variation by controlling the test environment, and require a high degree of procedural standardization.

Structured probes are useful for systematically and efficiently acquiring information on an individual's ability to cope with those language functions that are emphasized in academic settings. For example, a natural discourse interaction might not provide an opportunity for the individual to demonstrate facility in using language to explain, describe, inquire, or summarize. Specific probes, however, can be administered that permit observation of a youngster's ability to shift rapidly from one of these language functions to another (C.S. Simon, 1984).

Rating scales and protocols make up the second assessment format. This format allows the evaluator to observe the student as a communicator and then rate or describe individual aspects of the child's behavior according to a set of reliable and valid indices of communication. The procedures under this category enable observation in certain types of settings or during specific tasks; then, after the child is no longer present, the evaluator or the informant completes the rating scale or protocol. Two frequent variations of this format are checklists and interview questions. Typically these tools have some sort of evaluation (e.g., a numerical scale, an age range, a semantic differential, a forced judgment of appropriate/inappropriate) for each behavior on the scale or protocol.

The third assessment format involves the use of *language sampling* procedures. The child completes whatever task is required and this performance is audiotaped, transcribed, and then analyzed. Over the past 20 years, this format has continued to gain popularity. There are specific discussions available on how to collect language samples (e.g., Barrie-Blackley, Musselwhite, & Rogister, 1978; J. Miller, 1981; Stickler, 1987), and although the actual data collection procedures are quite uniform under this format, numerous analysis procedures have been designed.

The final general assessment format involves *direct and on-line observation*. This data collection approach is still relatively new in speech-language pathology, but it has been used for many years in other disciplines. In general, procedures under this heading require direct and real-time observation of the targeted child while he or she is engaged in communication. The clinician not only observes the child's performance but also immediately codes the communicative behaviors observed. Typically these procedures utilize communicative referencing to a greater extent than do the other formats, and they also require more training to conduct a successful evaluation.

It should be noted that this assessment format dimension is completely separable from the discrete point–pragmatic dimension. Within each of the four general formats there are both discrete point and pragmatic tests. The methods used to elicit and code behaviors are not necessarily dependent on the way that language proficiency is conceptualized and operationalized. Consequently, selection of the assessment format is typically dependent on the personal preference of the clinician rather than other factors.

Triangulation of Assessment Data   Another important issue to consider during test selection is the concept of triangulation. Advocated extensively in ethnography, this concept ensures that the data collected and analyzed are valid. Based on a loose analogy from navigation, wherein multiple readings are taken to increase the accuracy of fixing one's location on the map, triangulation in language assessment involves the comparison of data relating to the same language manifestation taken at different points in time or through different assessment formats. By collecting and analyzing data in this manner, the evaluator can obtain different perspectives on the targeted behavior.

For example, at the descriptive analysis level a rating scale may show an individual has difficulty detecting absurdities in sentences. This may indicate that "piecing together segments of information" is a problem. By using tools from several formats, a better description can result. A formal probe might be as effective at indicating a problem with absurdities as are informal curriculum-based probe procedures. Overlapping information from several different tools makes it possible to determine the breadth and depth of this type of language difficulty. The examiner can then conduct an explanatory analysis with a formal probe designed to evaluate the child's ability to make inferences as well as an analysis procedure based on levels of abstraction. These help determine if the problem is an intrinsic language difficulty. At times it is helpful to mix assessment techniques that are structured (probes) and those based on the analysis of language behaviors occurring during discourse (rating scales, sampling, observations). The contrast frequently provides insight.

Need for Psychometric Strength   Finally, test selection requires an awareness of the psychometric strengths of the tests considered: the tools of choice must be reliable, valid, and clinically useful. From the standpoint of test design, a language assessment tool is valueless if it cannot provide reliable data across testing instances, contexts, or evaluators. In like fashion, language tests must exhibit construct validity if they are to be effective measures of proficiency. Finally, even reliable and valid tests must be clinically useful. If a test cannot be easily adapted to the public school environment, then it is of little benefit. For example, videotaping and fine-grained analysis of communication is a very powerful way to analyze language data, but it simply will not achieve widespread use in the schools because the time and expense needed to conduct such analysis are prohibitive in that environment.

Determining psychometric adequacy is a very complex task that requires close review of the technical manuals and the studies documenting reliability and validity. Detailed discussion of these issues is outside of the scope of this chapter. The reader is encouraged, however, to carefully consider the psychometric issues when selecting tests and procedures.

After addressing the issues involved in test selection, clinicians must determine which techniques and tools are most appropriate for their purposes. A wide range of available procedures that fit within the synergistic framework are discussed in the following pages.

Assessment Procedures at the Descriptive Analysis Level

Oral Monologic Communication

Evaluating Communicative Competence (C.S. Simon, 1986)   In 1984 Simon introduced an evaluation procedure that was dedicated to helping clinicians who have found most standardized tests to be of little use in gathering descriptive information on the communication skills of school-age children. The administrative "scenario" allows an evaluator to systematically gather descriptive data on language processing and expressive language tasks that probe competence in coping with communication demands found in discourse and classroom interactions. In particular, there is an emphasis placed on offering an opportunity to observe auditory memory, integration, and evaluation abilities and the cognitive planning and linguistic skills students need to apply when they use language for a variety of functions. This data collection method consists of 21 components (Table 1).

The functional-pragmatic model is based on the premise that assessment tasks should simulate everyday communication interactions. While a language sample format sets the stage for collection of this type of data, short answers on standardized tests do not permit observation of higher level expressive language functions required in classroom responses (e.g., inquiry, description, explanation). The selected tasks are an attempt to "rig" an evaluation session so that optimal data are gathered within a limited time frame. Therefore, the functional-pragmatic evaluation procedure has certain limitations that Simon has attempted to rectify in more recent clinical practices. For example, systematic observation and screening of classroom communication performance now precede use of Evaluating Communicative Competence.

The Story Reformulation Analysis Procedure (Chappell, 1980, 1985)   This procedure was designed as a screening tool for the adolescent population, but it may be used with students at the fourth-grade level and above. The child is required to retell or reformulate a prepared story. A set of general and specific scoring criteria are provided in a protocol format. Scoring focuses on four major areas of story reformulation: setting the plot, interrelating events, shifting the plot, and concluding the plot.

Clinical Narrative Analysis   While there are numerous procedures utilizing the language sampling format to analyze narrative abilities, Hedberg and Stoel-Gammon (1986) discussed two that are clinically effective: narrative-level analysis and story grammar analysis. The analysis of narrative levels (Applebee, 1978) allows the clinician to determine how well the child is able to organize and structure narratives. Both developmental and communicative referencing information is used to analyze the child's ability to produce a coherent text by linking concepts to the central theme of the narrative. There are six basic levels of organization: heaps, sequences, primitive narrative, unfocused chain, focused chain, and narrative. This analysis has proven effective in describing poor language users (Hedberg & Stoel-Gammon, 1986; Westby, Van Dongen, & Maggart, 1989). Story grammar analysis is more elaborate. This approach analyzes both the effectiveness and appropriateness of meaning

Table 1.   Content components from Evaluating Communicative Competence

Auditory Tasks
1.   The Interview
2.   Identification of Absurdities in Short Sentences
3.   Identification/Explanation of Absurdities in Statements
4.   Integration of Factors to Solve a Riddle
5.   Comprehension and Memory for Facts
6.   Comprehension of a Paragraph
7.   Comprehension of Directions

Expressive Tasks
8.   Sequential Picture Storytelling
9.   Maintenance of Past Tense in Storytelling
10.   Maintenance of Present Tense in Storytelling
11.   Tense Shifts Based on Introductory Adverbial Phrases
12.   Semantically Appropriate Use of Clausal Connectors
13.   Stating Similarities and Differences between Two Stimuli
14.   Sequential Directions for Using a Pay Telephone
15.   Description of Clothing and a Person
16.   Explanation of the Relationship between Two Items
17.   Barrier Games
18.   Twenty Questions
19.   Creative Storytelling
20.   Situational Analysis and Description
21.   Expression and Justification of an Opinion

Excerpted from Simon (1986).

transmission by focusing on structural and functional relation rules that operate within narrative production. Hedberg and Stoel-Gammon have found this analysis scheme particularly effective with upper elementary and adolescent students.

Other Tests of Oral Monologic Communication   Although only three procedures are detailed here, there are other effective oral monologic procedures available. For example, G. Brown, Anderson, Shillcock, and Yule (1984) developed a set of assessment procedures using the protocol format that reflect on various task-based activities. This procedure allows analysis of the description of static relationships, dynamic relationships, and abstract notions. Also included within the probe format is the story retelling activity in the Verbal Memory II Subtest of the McCarthy Scales of Children's Abilities (D. McCarthy, 1972). Other language sampling techniques have been described by Garnett (1986), Merritt and Liles (1987), and Roth (1986), while Culatta, Page, and Ellis (1983), Norris and Bruning (1988), and Westby et al. (1989) suggested some excellent assessment protocols. J.R. Johnston (1982) summarized four different perspectives on narratives (story grammars, scripts, texts, and communication acts) to create clinically oriented questions applicable within a protocol format.

Oral Dialogic Communication

Clinical Discourse Analysis (Damico, 1985a)   Utilizing a language sampling format, this procedure employs a set of 17 communicatively referenced behaviors and the theoretical work of Grice (1975) to determine conversational proficiency. The behaviors focus directly on the three criteria of proficiency previously discussed. The 17 problematic behaviors are: failure to provide significant information to the listener, the use of nonspecific vocabulary, informational redundancy, the need for repetition, message inaccuracy, poor topic maintenance, inappropriate responding, failure to ask relevant questions, situational inappropriateness, inappropriate speech style, linguistic nonfluency, revision behavior, delays before responding, failure to structure discourse, turn-taking difficulty, gaze inefficiency, and inappropriate intonational contour. This procedure has been used extensively with the school-age population.

Pragmatic Protocol (Prutting & Kirchner, 1983, 1987)   This assessment procedure focuses on verbal, paralinguistic, and nonverbal aspects of communication to derive a judgment of conversational proficiency. In the procedure, the examiner observes the child in conversation and then completes this protocol. The general conversational categories are: speech acts produced, topic manipulation, turn-taking ability, lexical selection and use, lexical specificity, cohesion, stylistic variation, intelligibility and prosodics, kinesics, and proxemics. This tool has demonstrable reliability (Prutting & Kirchner, 1987) and validity (Duncan & Perozzi, 1987).

Informal Assessment Observations   Within the Communication Skills Transfer Report of Evaluating Communicative Competence (C.S. Simon, 1986), there is another assessment tool based on the protocol format. Using a 5-point scale, the examiner comments on the child's proficiency with basic language concepts, language production in terms of form and function, stylistic flexibility, cognitive-linguistic organization, comprehension, and speech parameters. The data employed to make these judgments are typically observations of conversational interactions.

Test of Pragmatic Skills (Shulman, 1985)   This test is designed to comment on the ability to signify conversational intent. Four guided play interactions serve as a medium through which this ability is evaluated. Ten conversational intentions are elicited and a 6-level response rating scale is used for scoring different degrees of appropriateness within the tasks. This tool provides both descriptive data based on communicative referencing and quantitative data based on normative referencing. The design allows an examination of the child's ability to interpret the conversational stimuli needed to maintain dyadic sociocommunicative interaction.

Porch Index of Communicative Ability in Children (Porch, 1979)   The probe format for this test was originally designed to assess neurological deficits in adults. This adaptation for children, however, is effective in describing communicative proficiency from an informational and/or neurological processing perspective. The General Communication Mean score is the most accurate single score for the description of oral dialogic communication. It combines the child's performance on 10 different subtests crossing four modalities (verbal, pantomime, auditory, and visual). The multidimensional scoring system employed within this test allows for both quantitative (normative-referenced) and qualitative description of performance.

Social Interactive Coding System (Rice, Sell, & Hadley, 1990)   This direct observational procedure describes the child's verbal interactive status in conjunction with the setting, the conversational partner, and the activities during which the interaction occurs. Interactive behaviors such as conversational initiation, repetitions, verbal and nonverbal responses, and the language/dialect used are coded. This tool requires a 20-minute observational period during which the examiner observes and codes behavior for 5 minutes and then takes a 5-minute break to fill in any coding gaps. This "5 minutes on, 5 minutes off" cycle is repeated four consecutive times. Developed originally for preschool children, this procedure does have direct application for description of the school-age population.

Other Tests of Oral Dialogic Communication   There are, of course, many more oral dialogic tools that may be mentioned. In terms of additional procedures within the probe format, The Word Test (Jorgensen, Barrett, Huisingh, & Zachman, 1981), the Interpersonal Language Skill Assessment (Blagden & McConnell, 1985), and the Language Processing Test (Richard & Hanner, 1987) are all effective in focusing on specific aspects of oral dialogic communication. Within the protocol format, Spotting Language Problems (Damico & Oller, 1985), Loban's Oral Language Scale (1976), The Pupil Rating Scale (Myklebust, 1971), Fey's coding scheme for profiling social-conversational participation (1986), and the Adolescent Conversational Analysis (Larson & McKinley, 1987) each fit within the functional-pragmatic model. Schwabe, Olswang, and Kriegsmann (1986) have designed a protocol based on various sampling and observational procedures designed to assess the constituent variables needed for requesting information in true interactional settings. Finally, several other functional language sampling procedures have been discussed by J. Miller (1981) and by Stickler (1987), and both Calvert and Murray (1985) and Damico (1985b) have developed direct observational procedures focusing on speech acts, contextual factors, and problematic behaviors that differentiate good from weak communicators in real conversational activities.

Contextually Constrained Communication

Classroom Communication Screening Procedure for Early Adolescents (C.S. Simon, 1989)   This procedure is designed within the probe format to identify students with potential classroom communication difficulties. Although a criterion-referenced tool aimed at students in transition from elementary school to junior high school, it is effective for most adolescents experiencing academic difficulty. This procedure focuses on the wide range of communicative behaviors needed to understand and complete assignments, to comprehend the language of the classroom, and to formulate and reason during classroom discussions and assignments. It may be used as a group screening procedure or administered to only one student at a time. The manual for this procedure provides an in-depth discussion of various analysis procedures that may extend the findings of this specific tool.

Curriculum Analysis Form (Larson & McKinley, 1987)   This protocol comments on the student's ability to communicate within the structured classroom context. Through a series of questions and checklists, there is an evaluation of the child's ability to handle textbook language and organization, classroom interactions, test-taking ability, and the child's attitudes toward the classroom communicative tasks. Although most effective with adolescents, it can be adapted for elementary school students.

Classroom Pragmatic Skills (Creaghead & Tattershall, 1985)   These authors have compiled a set of diagnostic questions and communicative skills needed to be successful in the classroom. By organizing these behaviors into a protocol, a rich description of the child's ability to use language within this context is possible. The major areas of analysis are knowledge about the school routine, knowledge about communicative routines, the ability to use written language formats, giving and following oral directions, giving and following written directions, and the comprehension and use of figurative language.

Analysis Checklist for Classroom Interactions (N.W. Nelson, 1985)   This informal assessment protocol is designed to comment on the communicative interactions of both the teacher and the child in the classroom environment. Through a detailed set of 20 questions, the examiner is able to determine whether the teacher–child dyad is a successful one. If not, then the mismatch between teacher talk and student comprehension is identified. This tool may be used effectively in conjunction with curriculum-based assessment strategies.

Test of Written Language–2 (Hammill & Larsen, 1988)   This battery assesses written language by using probes, protocols, and the language sampling format. Ten aspects of the written language are analyzed: vocabulary use, spelling, style, recognizing and correcting illogical sentences, sentence combining, thematic maturity, contextual vocabulary, syntactic maturity, contextual spelling, and contextual style. This test employs both criterion referencing and normative referencing to comment on the child's communicative performance.

Curriculum-Based Assessment   A long-standing classroom assessment technique that has been recently touted is curriculum-based assessment (N.W. Nelson, 1989; Tucker, 1985). This set of assessment strategies typically employs probes, protocols, and direct observation to determine the language demands of the curriculum and how well the child can handle those demands. Tucker (1985) described this procedure as reliance on the curriculum content to assess an individuals' performance capabilities. This is logical since the focus of interest is the child's success within this contextually constrained environment. The use of curriculum-based language immediately ties general assessment findings to the reality of language interactions in the classroom and the educational tasks at hand.

Through data gathering and direct observation, the examiner describes the actual curriculum in the child's specific classroom, the potential environmental factors at work (e.g., scheduling), the task expectations placed on the child, and the linguistic and communicative demands of selected aspects of the curriculum. Once this is determined, the examiner observes and works with the child within the actual curriculum to determine when and how the child experiences difficulty. For example, during math class the child might experience difficulty with particular problems because of their requirement that weight comparisons be made. By actively participating with the child while the classwork is done, it is recognized that the child has a poor comprehension of comparatives that results in difficulty. Furthermore, the child lacks the communicative ability to ask for clarification or assistance from the teacher. The specific problem is identified not only within the curriculum but also within the interactional abilities of the child. Many of the protocols discussed in this section can be effectively applied to curriculum-based assessment.

Careful observation is a valuable component of curriculum-based assessment. It is important to become aware of how information is presented—in texts and by teachers—as well as how it is received (Gruenewald & Pollak, 1990; Samuels, 1987). Since speech-language pathologists have been exposed primarily to remediation contexts rather than mainstream educational contexts, much can be learned by:

1.   Observing classrooms in action
2.   Reviewing texts and worksheets that caseload students use
3.   Interviewing students during independent work time
4.   Taking achievement tests and/or taking lecture notes

By "getting on the other side of the desk," one gets a more realistic perspective of communication roles a student is expected to take and the coping mechanisms students use. Initial observational notations on difficulties are relative to the context where they occur rather than an artificial setting. In this situation, the speech-language pathologist can record patterns of unproductive learning behaviors that impede comprehension or expression of a child's understanding of curriculum content. For example, some students might have difficulty pronouncing key words (e.g., *specific, transoceanic*). This inhibits willingness to participate. Linking careful analysis with observation enables effective curriculum-based assessment.

Other Tests of Contextually Constrained Communication   As with the other two manifestations of communication, there are numerous other assessment tools and techniques that are appropriate within this manifestation. For example, excellent protocols may be derived from the work of Archer and Edward (1982), Bassett, Whittington, and Staton-Spicer (1978), Vetter (1982), and Calfee and Sutter-Baldwin (1982). There are also other probes available. There are informal probes such as written and oral cloze procedures (Laesch & van Kleeck, 1987; Oller, 1979), probes of figurative language (Seidenberg & Bernstein, 1986), language learning tasks (Connell, 1986), and assessments of writing (Isaacson, 1985), as well as formal probes such as the Detroit Tests of Learning Aptitude–2 (Hammill, 1985), the Formal Reading Inventory (Wiederholt, 1985), and the Kaufman Assessment Battery for Children (A. Kaufman & Kaufman, 1983).

Assessment Procedures at the Explanatory Analysis Level

If the child is found to have communication difficulties in the descriptive analysis phase of assessment, the explanatory analysis phase is initiated. The question of interest at this point is, "*Why* do we see the problematic behaviors that identified the child as a poor communicator during descriptive analysis?" This question allows us to determine whether the occurrence of the problematic behaviors is due to factors extrinsic to the student or due to an intrinsic language-related learning impairment.

To conduct an explanatory analysis of the child and the child's problematic behaviors, the evaluator must be able to answer a set of questions pertaining to the child's communicative performance during the descriptive analysis phase. This involves two components. First, the evaluator must have sufficient information regarding the child to answer the explanatory analysis questions. This requires additional information on the child's history, environment, and current social, familial, and academic circumstances. Second, the evaluator must know what questions to ask in order to conduct the explanatory analysis.

In addition to the data collected using the triangulation strategy during the descriptive analysis phase, there are several other procedures that can help provide additional relevant information on the child being assessed. Gallagher (1983) provided an effective list of prereferral questions that may assist in obtaining additional linguistic and nonlinguistic data pertaining to the child's communicative performance during collection of a language sample. Similarly, Peck (1989) designed a procedure for obtaining additional information on a child's interactional environments at the dyadic level, the situational level, and the contextual level. This protocol focuses on responsiveness to the child's attempts to communicate, the dyadic partner's communicative abilities and strategies, the social climate experienced by the child, and the child's access to and familiarity with the communicative setting within which he/she was observed. Each of these factors plays an important role in explanatory analysis. Within the classroom environment, Ortiz (1988) provided a protocol collecting data on the academic environment's orientation toward the students (empowering versus disabling), and Larson and McKinley (1987) and Ripich and Spinelli (1985) suggested various tools to collect academically relevant data within the school environment. Finally, R.L. Sinclair and Ghory (1987) provided an excellent discussion on what occurs when children experience academic difficulty as a result of a host of factors and how these difficulties may result in a process of disabling that produces "marginal students." Broken into stages and levels of marginality, this material is invaluable in determining the child's reactions to the academic environment.

In conducting explanatory analysis, the evaluator should apply a set of questions that will help structure the explanatory analysis phase (Damico, 1991). The questions (asked in the following sequence) will guide this analysis phase:

1. Are there any overt variables that immediately explain the communicative difficulties? Among the potential considerations:
    a. Are the documented problematic behaviors occurring at a frequency level that would be considered within normal limits, or are they occurring in random variation?
    b. Were there any procedural mistakes in the descriptive analysis phase that account for the problematic behaviors?
    c. Was there an indication of extreme test anxiety during the descriptive assessment in one context or format but not in subsequent ones?
    d. Is the student a monolingual speaker of another language?
    e. Was there significant performance inconsistency between different contexts or formats within the targeted manifestations?
2. Is there evidence that the problematic behaviors noted can be explained according to normal second language acquisition, cross-cultural, or dialectal phenomena? (See Damico [1991] for further discussion.)
3. Is there any evidence that the problematic behaviors noted can be explained according to any bias effect that was in operation before, during, or after the descriptive analysis phase?

These three general questions address the possibility that the problematic behaviors are due to extraneous variables. If there are no extrinsic explanations for the data obtained in the descriptive analysis phase, then there must be a greater suspicion that the child does have an intrinsic language-related learning impairment. If this is the case, then the child should exhibit some underlying linguistic systematicity that accounts for the majority of the problematic behaviors noted. The final question in the explanatory analysis should therefore be asked, and the analyses needed to answer this question should be performed.

4. Is there any underlying linguistic systematicity to the problematic behaviors noted during the descriptive analysis phase?

It is within this question that the real *linguistic* analyses occur. This question reflects directly on the possibility that there are underlying intrinsic factors linked to language-related learning impairments.

To answer this question, the evaluator conducts a modified co-occurring structure analysis (Muma, 1978). This analysis typically requires the collection of communicative data in a form that lends itself to analysis (e.g., transcription of responses from probes, language samples, narrative transcriptions, detailed written observations). The evaluator takes only the data that contain problematic behaviors and tries to determine if these problematic behaviors are the result of some type of difficulty with the syntagmatic and paradigmatic dimensions of language. That is, since the problematic behaviors are only manifestations of a potential language-related learning impairment, the evaluator attempts to determine the underlying linguistic causes. This is an important point. Linguistic analyses will only reveal the systematicity of impairment when the actual instances of difficulty (the problematic behaviors) are analyzed. As with the descriptive analysis phase, there are a number of techniques and procedures that may be used to conduct explanatory linguistic analysis. Some of these procedures will be discussed according to a division along syntagmatic and paradigmatic lines.

Syntagmatic Analysis Procedures The syntagmatic dimension of language refers to the characterization of meaning transmission according to linear and sequential ordering of linguistic units (i.e., phonemes, morphemes, and propositions). What we commonly refer to as morphology, syntax, and phonology are actually aspects of this syntagmatic dimension. Several systematic analysis procedures and some probe activities have been found to be very effective when conducting syntagmatic analysis.

Language Assessment, Remediation, and Screening Procedure (LARSP) (Crystal, 1979, 1982; Crystal, Fletcher, & Garman, 1976) This grammatical profiling system enables the evaluator to determine if the problematic behaviors are due to an increase in grammatical complexity at the phrasal, clausal, or discourse levels. The most extensive grammatical analysis system currently available, Crystal's procedure is arranged according to three primary dimensions: the main types of organization in sentence structure and function, the main stages of grammatical acquisition, and the main patterns of grammatical interaction used between the interactants. Although the procedure requires training, the time needed to learn the system is worthwhile. Additionally, since only those utterances with problematic behaviors are analyzed, the time requirements for this analysis procedure are less demanding than might be suspected.

Systematic Analysis of Language Transcripts (SALT) (J. Miller & Chapman, 1983) This computer-aided procedure performs morphemic and other structural and functional analyses that enable the evaluator to conduct effective syntagmatic (and some paradigmatic) assessments. In addition to an optional feature that allows the evaluator to configure specific analyses, this procedure codes utterance types, specific words and morphemes, verbal and nonverbal data of interest, and bound morphemes in obligatory contexts. Given the range of this procedure to code structural, lexical, and functional aspects of communication, it is an effective explanatory analysis tool.

The Temple University Short Syntax Inventory–Revised (A. Gerber, Goehl, & Heuer, 1988) This formal probe is designed to describe the child's ability to use basic functional syntactic and morphological forms during interaction. The test employs a lotto game strategy to enlist children's willing participation, and it provides descriptive and developmental data. The paired elicitation-imitation responses of the same structures is intended to allow comparison of language knowledge and language use.

Other Syntagmatic Analysis Procedures Several other syntagmatic procedures worthy of mention are the grammatical analyses described by L. Bloom and Lahey (1978), Kamhi and Johnston (1982), Muma (1978), and Stickler (1987), and the coherence and cohesion analysis by Halliday and Hasan (1976). Each may be employed to effectively conduct syntagmatic analysis.

Paradigmatic Analysis Procedures The paradigmatic dimension of language refers to the characterization of meaning transmission according to ordered categorization, classification, and usage of sets of semantically related terms that can occur within the same linear position. Classifications of semantic categories, parts of speech, levels of linguistic displacement, and abstraction are aspects of this dimension. As with syntagmatics, tools and procedures are available to analyze problematic behaviors within this dimension.

Profile in Semantics (PRISM) (Crystal, 1982) This semantic profiling procedure enables the evaluator to determine if an increase in semantic complexity at the lexical (PRISM-L) or grammatical (PRISM-G) levels can account for the problematic behaviors. Divided into these two major sections, both lexeme and morpheme strategies for coding meaning are addressed (some syntagmatic information is included). The focus is on paradigmatic relations such as synonymy, hyponymy, and incompatibility, and the tool does code some types of developmental errors. The lexical analysis is very comprehensive and frequently quite enlightening.

Preschool Language Assessment Instrument (Blank et al., 1978) This probe technique is designed to analyze language according to increasing levels of linguistic displacement. Four levels of perceptual language distancing are used to organize the test stimuli and determine the child's ability to function with increasing levels of linguistic abstraction. By virtue of its content, progressing through levels of increasing abstraction, and its complex scoring procedures, the test is well designed to provide explanatory analysis information. Subsequent to the publication of this formal probe, Blank and Franklin (1980) modified the procedure for use within the language sampling and protocol formats.

Analysis of Metalinguistic Awareness Another important aspect of the paradigmatic dimension focuses on the child's level of metalinguistic awareness. As discussed by Van Kleeck (1984a) and Van Kleeck and Schuele (1987), this ability to consciously reflect on various components and properties of language is an indication of higher level linguistic skills. This may be particularly important in academic settings and may provide an explanation for many of the contextually constrained problematic behaviors noted in the descriptive analysis phase. For example, many classroom tasks are dependent on metalinguistic and metacognitive skills (Torgesen, 1982; Wong, 1982). This is exemplified by the need to observe the child's ability to exhibit the task persistence required to accurately complete rather mundane assignments, as well as engage in tedious analysis and sequencing of segments in a multipart written direction. This type of information can contribute to our understanding of why a student "doesn't understand directions" (Tunmer & Cole, 1985). There are several tools that can analyze this paradigmatic ability.

The Test of Language Competence–Expanded Edition (Wiig & Secord, 1988) describes metalinguistic awareness from ages 5;0 to 8;11 (Level 1) and 9;0 to 18;11 (Level 2). Both forms of the tool focus on recognition of ambiguous sentences, making inferences to achieve comprehension, re-creating speech acts or sentences, and comprehending and explaining figurative language to tap metalinguistic awareness. This tool also employs specific behavioral observations that are very helpful in describing the child's use of language strategies.

Other Paradigmatic Analysis Procedures There are additional procedures that are effective when conducting paradigmatic analysis. Schuele and Van Kleeck (1987) have provided a protocol for analysis of metalinguistic ability; additional probes of metalinguistic ability are Assessing Semantic Skills through Everyday Themes (ASSET) (Barrett, Zachman, & Huisingh, 1989) and the Analysis of Language of Learning (Blodgett & Cooper, 1987). Each of these measures is quite effective. Tough (1981) and Wallach and Miller (1988) discuss important aspects of intelligence and thinking skills that may be adopted for successful analysis. Finally, the Test of Problem Solving (Zachman, Barrett, Huisingh, & Jorgensen, 1984) provides another probe that focuses on the paradigmatic dimension from the perspective of critical thinking skills.

SUMMARY

When assessing the language and communicative abilities of children suspected of exhibiting language-related learning impairments, there is a trend toward a functional-pragmatic model of assessment. This model presents several clinical and practical implications regarding descriptive analysis that focus on the functional aspects of communication, employing a pragmatic methodology within naturalistic settings. Although this approach may be unfamiliar, it presents several advantages over the traditional assessment approach. With this assessment model, speech-language pathologists are able to conduct effective and valid language assessment as befitting their school-based role as "language specialists."

10 / Interdisciplinary Language Intervention in Education

TRENDS IN SERVICE DELIVERY

It has become increasingly evident that the problems of students with language-related learning disabilities require services that overlap the boundaries of allied but separate disciplines. Professionals in the fields of education and speech-language pathology have been called on to interact in ways that have contributed to alterations in models of service delivery. This chapter provides an account of some of the changes that have been taking place in the roles and functions of speech-language pathologists in the educational setting and some of the issues related to interdisciplinary collaboration between educators and language specialists.

Historically, service delivery for schoolchildren with language problems adhered to the clinical model of one-to-one or small group therapy by the speech-language pathologist in extraclassroom settings. While this pull-out model has been an appropriate approach for the treatment of a variety of communication disorders, such as stuttering, defective articulation, or voice problems, its use for remediation of language disabilities in the schools has been found wanting.

In a number of states, there has been a trend toward in-class intervention by speech-language pathologists. In part, this alternative has been preferred because of concern about the negative effects of withdrawing children from the site of educational instruction (Christensen & Luckett, 1990). Furthermore, viewing language from pragmatic and semantic perspectives, treatment of language disabilities by speech-language pathologists in sterile isolation from real-life situations and functions has been judged counterproductive (L. Miller, 1989). More specifically, growing awareness of the interrelationship between language deficits and aca-

---

A portion of the material in this chapter appeared in Gerber, A. (1987). Collaboration between SLPs and educators: A continuing education process. *Journal of Childhood Communication Disorders, 11,* 107–123; reprinted by permission.

demic failure has underscored the need to integrate language intervention with educational processes (N.W. Nelson, 1981, 1989; Wallach & Miller, 1988). From the perspective of an educator and authority in reading instruction, Palinscar (1989) has advocated the use of school communication contexts as a primary setting for service delivery to children referred for speech and language problems.

For all of these reasons, efforts have been made more recently by speech-language pathologists to design education-based models of service delivery. Frequently this kind of intervention has entailed ongoing interaction with classroom teachers and, in many cases, participation in the educational process on a collaborative basis. This interdisciplinary approach permits consideration of the numerous factors that are involved in learning and learning failure, including knowledge and analysis of classroom language demands and expectations, attitudes and belief systems of teachers, and individual learning styles of students (L. Miller, 1989; N.W. Nelson, 1986a).

Throughout the past decade, five major types of classroom-based intervention programs have been developed, all of which are, to varying degrees, interdisciplinary in nature:

1. The language specialist teaches a self-contained language classroom;
2. The language specialist team teaches with the regular classroom teacher, special education classroom teacher or resource teacher;
3. The language specialist provides one-to-one classroom based intervention with selected students;
4. The language specialist consults with the classroom teacher or special service providers (regular and special education teachers, reading specialist, learning disability teacher, psychologist, social worker, nurse, etc.); and
5. The language specialist provides staff development, curricular development, or program development to the school or district. (L. Miller, 1989, p. 156)

The remainder of this chapter provides descriptions of some classroom-based approaches exemplifying the above types of intervention and discussion of some of the issues involved in their implementation. It will be noted that certain examples of the five formats listed above overlap in some of their components, thereby resisting completely clear-cut classification.

The Self-Contained Classroom

When language remediation is considered to be a primary need and when the stimulation of language development and accompanying cognitive growth are judged prerequisite to successful academic learning, self-contained classrooms have often been conducted by speech-language pathologists. Such classes have been established for preschool children, early school-age children at a preacademic level, and for primary-grade children at a beginning academic level. Variations in format and function have been designed for middle and secondary school students with language-related learning disabilities.

A Language Acquisition Preschool Classroom (Bunce, 1990)   The Language Acquisition Preschool (LAP) is a classroom-based program for 3- to 5-year-old children with language impairment, children learning English as a second language, and children developing normally, who serve as peer models. The Educational Coordinator of the program has an interdisciplinary background of training, certification, and extensive experience in elementary education and speech-language pathology.

In the daily schedule of activities, a whole language approach (see discussion below) is employed in conjunction with specific intervention procedures for individual children's needs. Goals and procedures focus on language, cognitive, motor, and personal/social skills within the context of a typical preschool program:

> *Circle Time,* during which children are encouraged to participate in verbal turn taking, asking questions, listening, and deciding in what activities they will engage
>
> *Free Play,* during which four centers provide opportunities for art, block building, labeling objects/pictures, and either solitary play or interaction with peers or adults in child-centered activities
>
> *Dramatic Play,* during which children discuss setting up roles and enacting scripts, engage in turn taking, and develop vocabulary and grammatical competencies needed for enacting the scripts
>
> *Story Time,* during which children are exposed to literature books, puppets, and/or flannel board stories; stories may be read, told, or made up by children
>
> *Music and/or Finger Play,* during which children learn rhymes, follow directions, and enjoy rhythms and patterns
>
> *Outside Playtime*
>
> *Snack Time,* during which conversation is fostered and requests are made for juice and crackers
>
> *Small Group Time,* during which children engage in a variety of activities (e.g., cooking, experiments) and compose summaries of their experiences for written recording by the adult
>
> *Sharing Time,* during which children display items they have brought from home and engage in speaking to the group, asking and answering questions about the objects

The program employs a thematic approach to provide consistency of content in many of the verbal activities. It also fosters early literacy development in a naturalistic educational environment.

An Early School-Age Preacademic Class for Children with Communication Disorders (Feinberg, 1981)   This class was conducted in a school for children with neurological problems and various types of learning disabilities. The children enrolled in this class lacked "the prerequisite skills to succeed in a nursery school, a typical kindergarten or a regular learning disabilities classroom" (Feinberg, 1981, p. 249). For these children with varying degrees of expressive and/or receptive language impairment, the group setting was judged ideal for language stimulation in naturalistic, educationally oriented contexts.

The teacher, a speech-language pathologist, and her assistant, who had a training background in early education, served as group facilitators, promoting the process of peer modeling. "Older or more skilled children can provide models for target performance for younger or less skilled children in both language behaviors and general social behavior" (Feinberg, 1981, p. 253). Choral responses in certain language tasks provided support for children who were reluctant to respond individually because of sensed inadequacy.

Goals included development not only of more mature language form but also of the language related to curriculum subjects. For example, readiness for math and science was developed by teaching quantitative, spatial, and temporal concepts and terminology, and readiness for social studies was developed by developing awareness of the nature of family structure and of the community, and teaching relevant vocabulary. The program also aimed at the development of cognitive and social skills related to classroom performance, such as: "attending behavior, listening behavior, appropriate classroom behavior, self-help skill, seeking and accepting assistance when needed, complying with group and game rules, etc." (Feinberg, 1981, p. 258). Parents were informed about the nature of their children's problems and the ways they could help to further their progress both in school and "beyond the realm of classroom into the very texture of the child's life experience" (Feinberg, 1981, p. 265).

A Special School Classroom-Based Program (Parish, 1989)	A private school was established to provide language stimulation in self-contained classrooms for children ranging in age from 18 months to 9 years who were considered at risk for failure in public school. Speech-language pathologists were teachers of preschool classes, and experienced teachers conducted classes from kindergarten through first, second, and transitional grades beyond.

The teachers in this program have the responsibility of understanding language development and of guiding children through developmental stages. In their classes they provide individually designed instruction based on evaluation of each child's level of language development and learning style. Extensive experiences in the outdoors on the school's campus are used as bases for language stimulation and problem solving, along with fostering social and motor skills. In addition, art lessons are used to help children learn about organization, symbols, sequencing, and other relationships. Children are guided in the development of strategies that help them compensate for their areas of difficulty; they are also encouraged to let teachers know what ways they think they learn best. The goals and intervention approaches throughout the school are the result of interdisciplinary interaction.

An Early Academic Public School Classroom for Children with Communication Disorders (McBride & Levy, 1981)	A self-contained classroom in a regular public school was established for 5- to 6-year-old children whose language delay or deficit, in the presence of normal intelligence, placed them at risk for academic learning disabilities. The teacher was a speech-language pathologist who had taken coursework in early childhood education and learning disabilities. Thus, her professional preparation for this assignment was interdisciplinary.

The classroom environment was rich in its stimulation of verbal communication throughout all its activities. Information about each child's communication abilities was derived from evaluations performed jointly by the classroom teacher and the school speech-language pathologist. A regular kindergarten curriculum guide was modified to provide content suitable for the linguistic/cognitive level of the children and was adjusted in an ongoing fashion to meet changing needs and competencies. Teacher-child discourse in the implementation of the curriculum was also adjusted to ensure successful communication at the children's level of language development.

Within this global program for stimulation of oral language growth, there was also a central emphasis on fostering emergent literacy through an experiential unit approach to beginning reading. The concepts and the language contained in a book selected for beginning reading were analyzed. The material derived from this analysis served as the basis for the construction of a theme-based, ongoing project of rich, first-hand experience for the children, the goal of which was to make the linguistic and conceptual contents encountered in the book meaningful.

The theme of the book was centered on a park. In collaboration with the teacher, the children constructed a representation of a park in a section of the classroom. Throughout the semester, as aspects of the park and its contents were made and added, the objects and activities formed the basis of formal and informal instruction in such areas as vocabulary, spatial relations (comparative size and distance), body parts of animals in the park, one-to-one correspondence in counting, and so forth. In the course of many of these activities, accompanied by verbal discourse, the teacher took advantage of opportunities to use sentence patterns to be encountered in the beginning reader, thus preparing the children for success in their initial reading experience. Throughout the program, efforts were directed at developing both the language of social discourse and the literate language of education in both its written and oral forms.

A Middle School Program for Development of Classroom Communication Skills (Despain & Simon, 1987)   The ACCESS program (Accent on Classroom Communication and Study Skills) described here qualifies to a limited extent for inclusion in the category of self-contained classrooms. While the use of L. Miller's (1989) classification system necessitates placement of this program within this category (in the absence of another available slot), it would be more accurate to characterize it as an alternative classroom approach (N.W. Nelson, 1989).

In a middle school with departmental instruction in separate classrooms, some of the seventh- and eighth-grade students had been enrolled in remedial reading classes conducted by reading specialists. The speech-language pathologist had been asked by the principal to administer a language screening of all seventh-grade students who had scored below the 40th percentile on a reading achievement test. Results revealed a 53% failure rate on the language screening by these students with reading disabilities.

The speech-language pathologist was asked to visit the remedial reading classes to observe students' performance, assist in analysis of areas of language deficit, and develop, as a result of this diagnostic teaching, a language-based remedial reading program in conjunction with the reading specialist. (This aspect of the program would qualify it for inclusion under the consultation/collaboration category of classroom-based intervention discussed below.) However, the speech-language pathologist developed a communicative skills curriculum for the students with demonstrable language deficiencies and implemented this curriculum in the classroom.

A comprehensive program was developed that encompassed all faculty in the ACCESS program who taught subject matter courses. Education focused upon the development of strategies for fostering the requisite linguistic and cognitive skills within the contexts of science, social studies, and English. The speech-language pathologist served as a guest teacher in the English classes once a week for each seventh- and eighth-grade section, providing instruction in classroom communication skills within the context of the classroom. (Students with the most severe problems were included in the traditional pull-out case load for individual or small group therapy as well.)

The following list includes a sampling of the goals for the communication skills class:

> *Developing comprehension skills* by promoting such abilities as: 1) focusing attention on all critical details of oral and written directions, 2) increasing awareness of multiple meanings of words by attention to context, 3) learning to block out competing background noise and movement, and 4) monitoring comprehension and seeking clarification when confused
> *Developing expressive language skills* to serve such functions as: 1) relating a well-sequenced, detailed account of an experience; 2) sharing and justifying opinions;

3) summarizing lesson content or directions; and 4) formulating questions asking for clarification

Developing meta-skills, such as analyzing and manipulating complex sentences and using cognitive monitoring questions to improve academic task performance:

(1) What is the task?
(2) Am I doing it?
(3) How well have I done it? (C.S. Simon, 1987, p. 115)

Developing classroom pragmatic skills through: 1) increasing awareness of classroom formats, 2) developing appropriate student-teacher interaction, 3) adopting effective learning habits, and 4) developing test-taking skills

Throughout the total curriculum of the ACCESS program, interdisciplinary interaction contributed to the evolution of an alternative approach to education, one whose primary intent was not to cover content but, rather, to use content for the development of school language and thinking skills. Posttests of ACCESS students on classroom communication skills, curriculum-based vocabulary, informal reading inventory, and standardized reading subtests revealed measurable gains on mean scores.

A Secondary School Program   A Language/Study Skills Class (Buttrill, Niizawa, Biemer, Takahashi, & Hearn, 1989) was designed for secondary school students enrolled in the general education program. Thus, it was one of the classes in the departmentalized curriculum that included social studies, English, mathematics, business education, and physical education. The teacher of the Language/Study Skills class served as a resource to students with language-related learning problems and as a resource for general education teachers; therefore, this model combines features of the self-contained classroom approach and the consultation/collaboration approach.

The speech-language pathologist performs the traditional function of assessment, placement, and review of students with communication problems. In the role of teacher, the language specialist has designed and implemented a classroom-based curriculum aimed at fostering strategies for successful, language-related academic performance; that is, teaching students with language-related learning disabilities "how to learn" (Buttrill et al., 1989, p. 190). The following areas are covered in the program (Buttrill et al., 1989, pp. 190, 191, 194):

1. Academic organization, including time management, recording of assignments, and breaking tasks into smaller steps
2. Study skills, including text analysis, study strategies, note-taking methods, test-taking strategies, and reference skills
3. Critical thinking, including
    a. general thinking behavior involving observation and description, comparison and contrast, hypothesis formation, generalization, and prediction
    b. problem solving involving identification and definition of the problem, analysis of the problem, and development of options
    c. higher thinking skills involving inductive reasoning and deductive reasoning
4. Listening skills, including tuning in, recognition of organizational cues, and relating new to old information
5. Oral language production, including developing expanded word knowledge (synonyms,

figurative language, analogies, etc.), and expanding syntactic complexity for interesting verbal style

6. Written language development, including small group discussion for prewriting stimulation of ideas, use of outlines for organization, and development of proofreading skills

The classroom approach as an alternative to the pull-out model has been judged more efficient with regard to secondary school students' schedules and more effective in meeting curriculum demands. It is also more acceptable to these adolescents because academic credit is awarded for this class assignment.

Team Teaching

The demarcation between types of classroom-based service delivery is frequently blurred because of the multifaceted nature of their design and implementation. This overlap is apparent in the three examples offered in this section. Each of the programs described exemplifies as at least part of its structure a self-contained classroom intervention context. However, to one degree or another, the design and implementation of the curriculum are the result of teamwork between the speech-language pathologist and the special or general education teacher.

A County-Wide Eclectic Language Intervention Program for Preschool and School-Age Children (N.W. Nelson, 1981)   In a county school system, self-contained language classes were established for children at the preschool level and upward to 9- to 12-year-old students. Some classes, mainly at the preschool level, were taught by speech-language pathologists; others were taught by special education or learning disability teachers. However, throughout the program, teamwork between these professionals produced a format that alternated between "structured activities that focus on the form of language and more naturalistic activities that focus on its content and use" (N.W. Nelson, 1981, p. 14).

Taking cognizance of the interactional nature of language systems and the resulting interrelatedness of deficits and relative strengths in areas of children's language, this program was designed to provide language stimulation across all modalities and to integrate language stimulation with academic studies. One underlying assumption has been that not only may listening and speaking serve as a basis for reading and writing, but oral language development may also benefit from processing language in the written modality. For example, in some instances, written forms may enhance perception of phonological sequences in words that present perceptual difficulty in the oral modality.

The team teaching character of the program was implemented by assigning "varying time commitments by teachers of the speech and language impaired and teachers of the learning disabled" (N.W. Nelson, 1981, p. 14). It was acknowledged that, for many children whose language had not developed to age-appropriate levels under normal naturalistic stimulation, some intensification of input structure was required to foster growth. "The provision of consultative and classroom models of language generally do not eliminate the need for some direct service" (N.W. Nelson, 1989, p. 181). However, to overcome the negative effects of such focus on structure in isolation from naturalistic situations and to enhance the integration of gains in language knowledge and use into real-life functions, the program provided daily oscillations between the learning experiences in form and function. Thus, each day in this program, at a specific time in a designated space in the classroom, individuals or small groups worked on aspects of language form with content and use controlled. Work on meaningful language use in experiential and subject matter learning contexts took place in other parts of the room, providing "a shift between individual or group activities and whole group interaction" (N.W. Nelson, 1981, p. 14).

A substantial part of the activities was directed at writing and reading about children's experiences, construction of a classroom newsbook, and development of individual students' personal newsbooks. These books were, at different times, dictated by children and written by teachers. This process provided opportunities for teacher-modeled expansion of linguistic form. Furthermore, teacher-written material on topics of interest encouraged the pragmatic function of reading to learn.

Pretesting and posttesting provided evidence of positive gains in verbal IQ scores and on other language and achievement tests. The interdisciplinary approach to intervention resulted in a high rate of placement into mainstream classes.

A Program for Bicultural Children with Language-Related Learning Disabilities
(Westby, 1987; Westby & Rouse, 1985)   In a predominantly Hispanic public school in the southwest, children from families who spoke New Mexican Spanish or Chicano English and who demonstrated limited competence in both languages were enrolled in a special class. The language-related program for this class was designed by a team consisting of an Hispanic speech-language pathologist and an Anglo teacher. The goals were to increase communicative competence in informal social language and in literate school language.

The instructional approach consisted of two levels: high-context activities and low-context activities. High-context activities were essentially nonacademic experiences, such as field trips, art projects, cooking, and pretend play. The emphasis in these situations was predominantly the teacher's verbal input, without any pressure on the children to comply with verbal responses. The level of language used by the teacher in accompaniment with these experiences was easily comprehended by the children and slightly in advance of their developmental stage. "Language was context dependent. Thus a student could say 'Give me that thing there' and be understood" (Westby & Rouse, 1985, p. 20).

Pretend Play situations required more verbalization by the children. The teacher set the situational framework and, in early stages, participated in the action, thereby providing models for the verbal interaction. In later stages of the process, the adult shifted to the role of stage manager, directing children to speak as one of the characters, but with no pressure for correctness of utterances.

Low-context activities fell into two classes: familiar and unfamiliar topics. In low-context familiar activities, adults modeled informal discussions about topics related to the children's experiences. Children were encouraged to emulate the model in talking about an experience of their own. They were free to refrain from responding, but the adult dialogue was aimed at guiding the children toward the use of more explicit language when they were motivated to speak.

Low-context unfamiliar activities were similar to those encountered in a traditional classroom: for example, calendar time, book reports, and so forth. Material was written on the blackboard and attention was directed toward words, sentence patterns, and punctuation. "Language was not used to communicate a need-meeting message or share personal information, but was used to talk explicitly about language" (Westby & Rouse, 1985, p. 21). Responses were judged for correctness.

The speech-language pathologist and the classroom teacher worked jointly as a team for certain parts of the day. At other times each professional worked with half of the class simultaneously. Both of them worked together to design curricular activities for half of each school day. The overall purpose of this team-taught classroom was to help the children progress through a continuum of high-context to low-context language-related activities. This process was accomplished by using a variety of teacher strategies to enable, support, encourage, and sustain children's verbal performance without making them feel threatened or inadequate in their communicative efforts.

A Transdisciplinary Program for the Development of Literacy (L.P. Hoffman, 1990) In view of a recognized need to integrate instruction in all areas of language and communication (reading, writing, listening, speaking, spelling, and handwriting) with each other and in content learning experiences, this program for school-age children with severe communications problems is designed to actively engage all members of a transdisciplinary team in the efforts to promote linguistic, cognitive, and social growth. The team may consist of special educators, speech-language pathologists, social workers, career educators, and so forth. While each team member performs specialized professional functions independently (e.g., assessment) and/or jointly (e.g., in individualized education program conferences), all these diverse professionals participate in classroom-based intervention procedures designed to achieve communication goals.

The language goals are identified by the speech-language pathologist. All team members are informed about the students' targeted needs and direct attention to them during academic and social activities. Evaluation of program effectiveness has revealed measurable gains in language comprehension, reading, and mathematics on average each year at all levels, from elementary school through middle and high school. This program has been operating for more than 15 years. Further evidence of its effectiveness is a zero dropout rate for high school students enrolled in the program. Its effectiveness is, in large measure, due to the provision of quality in-service training of program staff to assist them in "performing the expanded roles" (L.P. Hoffman, 1990, p. 83). This issue is discussed in greater detail below.

One-to-One Classroom-Based Intervention

The traditional pull-out method of direct service delivery continues to be advocated and used in numerous instances in conjunction with classroom intervention (L. Miller, 1989; N.W. Nelson, 1989). In some instances, students with more severe problems or attentional deficits are enrolled in the caseload of the speech-language pathologist who may conduct intervention in a more controlled environment, focusing on individual needs and eliminating distracting elements from the learning situation (A. Gerber & Mastriano, 1991; C.S. Simon, 1987). In the one-to-one situation, the opportunity is available for ongoing diagnostic teaching or therapy combined with the warmth of interpersonal supportiveness so often needed by children with sensed inadequacies.

The classroom-based model of pull-out intervention is most effective when it is integrated with the curricular content and educational tasks. Continual consultation with the classroom teacher and/or observation in the classroom are indispensable for securing information about the nature of the material being studied, the language demands of the classroom, and the level of the student's performance. In a more highly structured approach, N.W. Nelson's (1989) curricular-based assessment, described in Chapter 9, provides the language specialist with the information necessary for decision making about selection of language behaviors to be targeted for remediation or development.

Materials to be used in the individual or small group direct service sessions may be drawn from actual classroom texts or task assignments. The advantage of using such materials in individual sessions is that they may be modified to a level of difficulty appropriate to the students' current level of proficiency or need. Furthermore, the likelihood of integrating enhanced skills and knowledge into classroom performance is increased if materials and tasks are common to both situations.

Consultation and Collaboration

"In the collaborative format, the language specialist acts as an information provider for other professionals and for students, as a co-planner, an observer and ethnographer of the student's process, and as an occasional co-teacher" (L. Miller, 1989, p. 158). The collaborator/consultant does not usually serve as the deliverer of primary direct services, but the employment of this model has far-reaching effects in terms of efficiency and effectiveness of service delivery. That is, as a result of interacting with educators instead of limiting services to those who can be served directly, shared specialized information is likely to have a broader influence on more students in the educational environment itself (Damico, 1987; L. Miller, 1989). Consultation and collaboration, however, are demanding professional functions that require skills in both content and the process of interaction among professionals (Russell, 1981). This topic is addressed below in the section "The Challenge of Interdisciplinary Collaboration."

One effective bridge between members of allied professions may be established through the use of questionnaires about students' performance. These may take many forms and may be derived from a variety of sources, such as:

> Commercially published rating scales (e.g., The Pupil Rating Scale: Screening for Learning Disabilities [Myklebust, 1971])
>
> Checklists published in the literature (e.g., A School Readiness Language Checklist [Weiner & Creighton, 1987]) (This instrument is discussed below and the relevant part of it is included in the Appendix to this chapter.)
>
> A pool of questions published in the literature from which relevant items may be drawn (e.g., Factors that Influence Learning to Read and Text Comprehension [Samuels, 1987]; see the Appendix to this chapter)

This section provides examples of programs employing the consultative/collaborative format.

Philadelphia Get Set Screening and Stimulation Program (C.C. Towne & R. Fink, personal communication, 1986)   This program was devised as a creative solution for the problem of screening a large population of preschool children in the Philadelphia Get Set Day Care Centers for the purpose of early detection of speech-language problems. Teachers were trained by a speech-language pathologist to administer the Communication Screen (Striffler & Willig, 1981), an instrument designed for use by a variety of professionals who work with young children. The speech-language pathologist monitored early attempts by the teachers and performed reliability checks on their scoring until reliability was established. She subsequently consulted with the teachers for interpretation of results and recommendations for evaluations of children who failed the screen. This approach fostered early detection of children at risk for language-related learning problems by involving the teachers in one phase of the process.

During the second phase of the program, teachers were trained by speech-language pathologists in a core of techniques aimed at stimulating development in selected aspects of language. The selection was based on certain common patterns of deficit revealed on the screening test. Videotaped demonstrations of a small sample of intervention procedures were followed by a discussion session, in which opportunities were provided for teachers to explore the possibilities of using toys and other play materials as topics for expanded verbalization. Subsequently, speech-language pathologists demonstrated the use of language stimulation activities in the classrooms for teacher observation.

One clearly observable benefit of the complete program was the marked increase in the number of teacher referrals for language evaluation and early professional intervention. This effect was apparently due to the teachers' heightened awareness about child language and its relationship to learning and child development.

Documenting and Facilitating "School Readiness Language" in the Kindergarten Classroom (Weiner & Creighton, 1987)   The heading for this section is actually the title of a paper describing an approach to interdisciplinary consultation/collaboration between speech-language pathologists and kindergarten teachers. The rationale for the proposed methods is based on a recognition of the relationship between the level of language development at school entry and early academic performance. Whereas this recognition is fairly widespread, the means of documenting such levels are generally beyond the professional competence of the kindergarten teacher. Therefore, Weiner and Creighton (1987) asserted that the speech-language pathologist is the professional best qualified to provide the kindergarten teacher with information well founded in developmental psycholinguistic research.

The approach consists of two components. The first is a language behavior checklist organized into four developmental stages, the latter three of which are most pertinent to kindergarten-age children (see Appendix). Each stage of the checklist includes not only specific behaviors but also a description of general characteristics of children's communicative and learning capabilities at that stage.

The language behavior checklist is used by the kindergarten teacher as a structured instrument for observation of individual children in the classroom. Information gathered from this observation serves as the data base for teaching strategies adjusted to each child's current level and for those aimed at fostering needed language growth. In this second phase of consultation/collaboration, the speech-language pathologist and the teacher jointly construct groupings of children on the basis of their language skills and devise ways of altering the language-learning environment to optimize language growth.

Program in a School for Students with Learning Disabilities (Cohen & Schiller, 1981) The model described here was developed to serve the needs of upper elementary- and middle school–age students with learning disabilities who were performing below teacher expectancy in programs designed to remediate reading and learning deficiencies. The classroom teachers in this school were well-trained special educators; however, they were somewhat frustrated because a number of their students did not improve significantly in response to individualized reading instruction. They were also concerned about deficits manifested by some of these students in processing the oral language of instruction. In view of the growing recognition of the relationship between aspects of oral language and reading abilities, the expertise and insights of speech-language pathologists were therefore welcomed by these educators.

The speech-language pathologists analyzed the needs of these children from their own professional perspective. As clinicians, they recognized the need for a therapeutic style of intervention to provide the support required to foster self-esteem and expectations of success in these failure-prone children. In addition to the psychodynamics of the clinician-client interaction in small group sessions, the program provided sound awareness training to foster improved word analysis skills, and stimulation of improved listening, attention to, and memory for information transmitted through oral language. Emphasis was placed on enriching the semantic network underlying vocabulary expansion as a related aspect of receptive language processing.

Teachers observed and eventually participated in each phase of the intervention program. They became increasingly capable of including such procedures in their class curriculum on an ongoing basis and demonstrated the motivation for doing so. Interdisciplinary consultations extended the process of individualizing instruction for the children on the basis of shared information and enhanced understanding among professionals. This proved feasible because of a staff development program that is described briefly in the next section.

Staff Development, Curriculum Development, and Program Development

Efforts at collaboration between educators and language specialists are likely to be enhanced when members of both professions share a body of knowledge about child language and the processes that tend to foster growth in its knowledge and use. Some collaborative programs have contained continuing education components to further such mutual understanding. Following are examples of one program described above and two others not included in the above categories that exemplify three different modes of continuing education for teachers in aspects of language relevant to the goals of interdisciplinary intervention.

A Head Start Continuing Education Program   For 3 years Head Start administrators and teachers had been engaged in observation of and consultation about a small group language intervention program for Head Start children with communication disorders at Temple University (A. Gerber & Mastriano, 1991). At the end of this period, Head Start administrators proposed a continuing education program for teachers in their program to enhance their knowledge about language and its development and disorders, and their awareness of delays or deficits in their children. It was also anticipated that the teachers would gain some new insights into how they might focus more intensively on language stimulation in their classrooms.

Funding was secured for enrolling 60 Head Start teachers in a 1-credit course in Language and the Preschool Child, offered by the Department of Speech (now the Department of Speech, Language, and Hearing) at Temple University. The teachers attended four 3-hour sessions, once a week for a month, conducted by two speech-language pathologists. Classroom lectures were supplemented by assigned readings and videotaped demonstrations of procedures selected from the small group language intervention program.

Each of the four sessions included presentation of some theoretical information on a selected topic about language, followed by a discussion about the application of this theory to principles of intervention and pertinent demonstrations. Teacher participation was fostered to generate creative suggestions about adaptation of the demonstrated small group activities to their classrooms. This kind of exchange heightened the awareness of the speech-language pathologists to the nature of classroom conditions and possible problems encountered by educators, thus exemplifying the bidirectional information sharing necessary to successful collaboration.

Formal evaluation of teacher reactions to this staff development program revealed that the majority of those enrolled found the subject matter very appropriate for their present responsibilities and judged the material immediately useful. They also expressed a desire for demonstrations of language stimulation activities in the classroom itself rather than in the small group clinical setting.

Informal feedback about the benefits of the continuing education project was provided by the chief Head Start speech-language pathologist and staff psychologist, both of whom reported that the nature of teacher referral had changed dramatically. Whereas, prior to participation in the staff development course, children were referred to the speech-language pathologist almost exclusively for "speech" problems, following the course, teachers were much more likely to refer children for language problems. Thus, while there were no available data that this collaboration was effective in changing educators' classroom practices after an all-too-brief exposure to the complex content and skills of a different discipline, there was evidence of valuable consciousness raising as an outcome of such exposure.

The School for Learning Disabilities Program (Cohen & Schiller, 1981)   The results of teacher observation and participation in the small group sessions for learning disabled children with severe reading problems and deficits in processing the oral language of instruction in this program were reported in the previous section. This favorable outcome, however, was made possible by providing intensive teacher education by the speech-language pathologists. Seminars were offered to present the theoretical framework and objectives of both the sound awareness training and the program for improving the processing of oral language in the classroom. Training in the use of the methods and materials was provided in workshops. As a result of this interdisciplinary staff development program, the teachers and the speech-language pathologists developed a productive working relationship to the benefit of the children.

A Classroom Program in the Inner City Schools (A.J. Gerber, 1970)   A request for assistance in improving students' communication skills was received by the Department of Speech (now Speech, Language, and Hearing) at Temple University from the administrators of parochial schools in the neighboring diocese. The department responded with a proposal for providing services to children by assignment of graduate students for supervised practicum experience in the schools in conjunction with a staff development program for the classroom teachers.

Ten parochial school teachers were enrolled in one 3-credit course taught by university faculty. Content included selected aspects of the following areas: communication processes; the relation of language to thought, speech, and language development; phonetics; and sociolinguistics. Principles underlying procedures for expanding speech and language competencies were explored.

As a result of their training in the continuing education course, teachers were increasingly able to observe, analyze, and record patterns of speech and language occurring in their classrooms. This information was shared with the language specialists (graduate students and supervisors) and, to a degree, formed the basis for design of classroom goals and procedures. The language specialists demonstrated procedures in the classrooms on a weekly schedule, and teachers followed through on related procedures during the remainder of the week.

Following one semester of implementation, the effectiveness of this interdisciplinary project was evaluated by having a naive judge observe classes conducted by teachers in the staff development program and others who were not participants. Teachers were rated for the quality of communicative climate they established and for the incidence of the methods employed in the program to foster the development of communication skills. Ratings for communicative climate were more than twice as high for classes conducted by teachers in the staff development program. There were 135 instances of the use of the program's innovative methods by trained teachers, in contrast to 26 instances observed in classes of untrained teachers. Subjective evaluation by the nine teachers who continued in the program revealed six to be enthusiastic and three who were negative about its goals and procedures.

THE CHALLENGE OF INTERDISCIPLINARY COLLABORATION

As an educator, Palinscar (1989) has recognized that the concerns of the disciplines of special education, remedial reading, and speech-language pathology intersect to a degree suggesting "that the time is ripe for collaboration among school specialists" (p. 11). While such interaction among members of these allied but different fields is believed by many scholars and practitioners to hold the promise of enriching repertoires of intervention strategies, it also has the possibility of encountering obstacles and conflicts.

On the one hand, it has been observed that few teachers have had the academic background and practical experience that foster confidence in addressing language-related issues. Therefore, many educators evidence an uneasiness when they are expected to engage in consultation about or collaboration in the area of language (Damico, 1987). On the other hand, many speech-language pathologists, whose training and experience have not included knowledge of or function within the education process, are somewhat at a loss initially when called upon to consult about or collaborate in this milieu (Weiner & Creighton, 1987). Therefore, the challenge of interdisciplinary collaboration entails internal motivation or external pressures to depart from time-honored functions in the exploration of untrodden paths outside their own professional territories.

Two programs exemplifying interaction between speech-language pathologists and classroom teachers report different degrees of collaborative effectiveness. Although the information available in the descriptions of these programs is not isomorphic in scope or level of detail, comparison and contrast of common dimensions should prove illuminating in analyzing factors that may influence the outcomes of interdisciplinary ventures.

Program I (Christensen & Luckett, 1990) provided whole-class language lessons throughout an entire school district in regular education classes from kindergarten to sixth grade. Program II (Iglesias, Pena, & Quinn, 1991) provided language-related services in preschool Rainbow Head Start classes composed of Hispanic and African-American children. Table 1 presents a comparison of these two programs and their outcomes. It is apparent from the descriptions in Table 1 that these two situations differed dramatically in the conditions that initiated the collaborative efforts and affected their outcomes. The following discussion examines principles and processes of collaboration, with further use of illustrations from the two contrasted programs to highlight critical elements.

Damico (1987) stated that an indispensable ingredient for success is acceptance of the need of an interdisciplinary approach and recognition of the benefits to be gained from its design and implementation. This acceptance and accompanying motivation are needed both at

Table 1. Comparison of two programs involving interdisciplinary collaboration

Program I (Christensen & Luckett, 1990)	Program II (Iglesias, Pena, & Quinn, 1991)

Participating Professionals

SLPs and regular classroom teachers in a public school district	SLPs, three classroom teachers, and three aides in a Rainbow Head Start school

Participating Students

Children enrolled in caseload of SLPs and all regular education students in their classrooms	Three classes of 20 children each, consisting of 4-year-old Hispanic and African-American children

Administrative Authorization

State-wide curricular requirement for oral language instruction in regular education Directives from State Dept. of Education and Special Education Policy resulting in extension of SLP's functions to include the regular education classroom	Administrators of the local Rainbow Head Start program sought services of a bilingual SLP to help meet needs of Hispanic-speaking children

Goals

To conduct speech-language enrichment lessons for all students in a class containing any student with a valid IEP for speech-language problems	To aid teachers in the use of communicative strategies that facilitate general verbal development and the development of classroom language and behavior for children at marginal academic risk

Extent and Nature of In-Classroom Intervention

SLPs taught one 20- to 30-minute lesson/week for each participating classroom. For K–2, lessons targeted basic language skills of vocabulary, grammar, reasoning, and oral expression. For Grades 4–6, lessons were aimed at enrichment of the regular curriculum	SLPs spent approximately 2 hours/day, 2 days/week: —Modeling for teachers appropriate level and style of questions and comments in interaction with children with language deficits —Fostering active involvement of children in storybook time —Demonstrating use of sorting activities appropriate to children's developmental levels

Extent and Nature of Consultation/Collaboration

SLPs demonstrated procedures for teachers and consulted with teachers to involve them in observation, monitoring children's responses, and team teaching	SLPS: —Conferred with teachers about interactional patterns they had modeled —Conferred about children's performance and teacher–child interactions —Attempted to guide teachers toward understanding children's level of language development and their needs —Emphasized need for receptive stimulation in advance of expressive demands

Effectiveness of Interdisciplinary Collaboration

Generally positive response because of classroom teachers' concern about directive to teach oral language. Some teachers initially resistant to innovations in their classroom by other professionals. Word-of-mouth recommendations from supportive teachers influenced those less flexible in accepting change	Negative response by teachers because of: —Imposition of program by administration —Threat to existing order —Resentment of instrusion of outsiders —Anxiety and loss of self-esteem because of need to receive outside help —Drain on time and effort when already overburdened —Minimal training, low pay, and low motivation —Resentment at having to cope with children with special needs —Cultural differences in adult–child interactional style and concepts about educational goals and methods —Suspicion about motives of SLPs —SLPs unrealistic, idealistic expectations —Devaluation of teachers by SLPs because of their lack of knowledge about child language

SLP, speech-language pathologist; IEP, individualized education program.

315

the administrative level and by all personnel having direct instructional contact with students. Without *both* the authoritative endorsement of those in high levels of policy making and the active, willing participation of instructional personnel, efforts at introducing change will probably encounter formidable obstacles. The results of differential application of these principles are evident in the two examples offered.

In Program I, a mandate from the highest level of state administration had provided the incentive for teachers to secure interaction with a specialist in an area of expertise outside of their own professional experience. Although there may have been some resistance and even resentment, the mandate was clearly enunciated and compliance was required.

In Program II it became clear that administrators had failed to communicate to teachers the goals of the program and roles of its personnel. Therefore, there was not only resistance to change and resentment of intrusion of other professionals into their territory on the part of the teachers; there was also a misinterpretation of the functions of the speech-language pathologists by teachers who felt they were being observed and criticized. During a confrontational crisis, teachers excluded speech-language pathologists from their classrooms and insisted on a pull-out model of services to children with special speech/language needs. The speech-language pathologists refused to comply with this demand.

From this point onward, a process of conflict resolution was instituted. Differences in perspective were shared. Some of the issues addressed were: 1) the contrast between adult–child interactional styles in the classroom of teachers and those of speech-language pathologists; and 2) the purpose of classroom language intervention—to provide help to these children in a way that went beyond the traditional services of the speech-language pathologist. Subsequently, in later stages of this collaborative process, teachers began to acknowledge benefits from the collaboration, started to ask about problems that frustrated them, and began to share information about the children with the speech-language pathologists. The speech-language pathologists shifted from "telling teachers what to do" to stating problems and drawing information from teachers.

Eventually, teachers developed a greater understanding and acceptance of the methods used for observation and analysis of classroom language-related events and problems. Specialists and teachers adopted more interactive roles, offering suggestions and alternative solutions to problems, with options to accept, reject, or modify recommendations. By adopting principles of conflict resolution (Briggs & Chan, 1987; Day, 1985; G.M. Parker, 1990), collaboration was viewed as an evolving process rather than an imposed product (Iglesias et al., 1991).

Damico (1987) and C.S. Simon (1987) have offered the following suggestions for avoiding such conflicts and resistance by teachers to classroom language intervention by speech-language pathologists:

> Discussion between the speech-language pathologist and the teacher about students receiving services for speech-language problems
>
> Requests by the speech-language pathologist for permission to observe the child under discussion during performance within the classroom
>
> Sharing with the teacher the speech-language pathologist's interpretation of observed performance from a language perspective and making concrete suggestions for remedial or facilitative procedures in the classroom
>
> Offering to give a demonstration of such procedures in the classroom

In summary, a problem-solving mode of interaction in which information flows bidirectionally between the educator and the language specialist is likely to promote collaboration to the mutual benefit and satisfaction of professional participants across disciplinary boundaries. All too often, these boundaries are perpetuated by "terminology barriers" that discourage communicative efforts between specialists and generalists (Garnett, 1986).

Probability of success is enhanced by some type of continuing education that would result in informed practice based on shared knowledge about both language and educational processes. Motivation to engage in such in-service continuing education may emerge in gradual stages through growing awareness of the value of the information made apparent through demonstrations, informal consultations, and sharing accounts about experimentation with innovative approaches. The patient building of a mutually trusting working relationship may prove more effective than premature attempts to impose an intensive study program on resistant professionals (Damico, 1987; C.S. Simon, 1987).

THE WHOLE LANGUAGE APPROACH TO LITERACY AND LANGUAGE INTERVENTION: PROS AND CONS

As one result of the increasing advocacy and implementation of classroom-based language intervention, the whole language philosophy, currently endorsed by many educators as the most viable foundation for literacy acquisition, has had an impact on service delivery to students with language deficits. The whole language approach reflects a reform movement in language arts education in reaction to unduly widespread failure in reading and writing achievement (Schory, 1990).

A major premise of whole language philosophy is that the development of all aspects of language, written as well as oral, results from immersion in a variety of meaningful language experiences at a holistic level (Goodman, 1986). Furthermore, the development of skills in each language modality may foster growth in other modalities. For example, increasing mastery of the writing process may contribute to reading improvement in emergent literacy (Teale & Sulzby, 1986), and acquisition of reading and spelling skills may stimulate growth in oral phonological development (P.R. Hoffman, 1990; N.W. Nelson, 1981; Westby, 1990).

It is also maintained that, because of the inseparable interaction among all linguistic domains (phonology, syntax, semantics, and pragmatics), attempts to teach subskills in discrete areas fly in the face of the actual nature of language processing (Altwerger et al., 1987). From this point of view, fractionating language into subsystems that serve as targets for skill building (e.g., sound-symbol associations, sound blending, and visual word recognition) are eschewed because they are believed to violate the natural processes of language development and use (Altwerger et al., 1987; Chaney, 1990).

However, not all scholars and practitioners subscribe to the premise that equates oral language acquisition with the acquisition of literacy. In some developing countries, while all inhabitants talk, many may not read or write (Chall, 1989). Palinscar (1989) has made the point that "language skills achieved naturally by children in the course of social interaction are highly contextualized skills of communication. This stands in contrast to the decontextualized uses of language present in numerous school literacy experiences" (p. 1). She further asserted that "directed practice plays a more significant role in the acquisition of literacy skills than in the acquisition of language" (p. 2).

In accordance with this view, Chaney (1990) argued that the predominant use of a whole language approach would tend to inhibit the development of the metalinguistic skills demonstrated by research to be related to literacy. With particular reference to those phonological competencies regarded as "a fundamental aspect of learning to read an alphabetic language" (p. 5), Chall (1989) judged a global approach to be less effective in fostering the acquisition of decoding and word recognition skills. Thus, there continues to be support from certain sources for a need to extract and practice to the level of automaticity those subskills that coalesce into fluent, competent reading and writing (Chaney, 1990). It has been reported that numerous practitioners who subscribe in principle to a whole language approach do indeed resort to the extraction of specific aspects requiring the focus of intensified instruction (Pomerance, 1991).

There is also lack of universal agreement among language specialists about the appropriateness of the whole language approach for intervention with children who have language deficits. "Whole language programs assume that children have a certain degree of oral language proficiency. For language-learning disabled students, such assumptions may be incorrect" (Westby, 1990, p. 228).

The whole language philosophy has engendered debate in the field of language intervention as well as in the domain of written literacy. Some language specialists who are proponents of a strong pragmatic theory have claimed that principles of whole language theory are equally relevant for intervention with children who have language impairments (Norris & Damico, 1990; Norris & Hoffman, 1990). These authors take the position that fragmenting language into its components for the systematic teaching of superficial forms (e.g., phonemes, syntactic patterns, or vocabulary items out of context) violates the principles of natural language learning.

They advocate providing a rich linguistic environment and abundant opportunities for talking about things that are intrinsically interesting and meaningful to children. Rather than correcting "errors," which they regard as instances of the natural progression in language acquisition, they propose that intervention consist of high-frequency use of selected aspects of language in repeatable contexts built around themes. These themes are intended to provide the unifying context for a wide variety of meaningful language-related activities. Across time, it is expected that this ongoing language experience immersion would spur gains in conceptual complexity that would impel the development of more advanced language for expression of the experience.

Nonetheless, there are those who continue to believe, despite the influence of the pragmatics revolution, that work on the structure of language has value (N.W. Nelson, 1988b; Wallach & Miller, 1988). "As we have moved further and further away from structural concerns, we have lost some evenness of focus. The study of syntactic competence has become somewhat obscured as our interest in conversational and narrative discourse has advanced" (Wallach & Miller, 1988, p. 145).

The present author has espoused an approach to intervention with students who have language-related learning disabilities that integrates aspects of both approaches as appropriate for different linguistic and metalinguistic goals. In agreement with N.W. Nelson's (1981) eclectic model, discourse skills are fostered through intensified experience with naturalistic language functions; metalinguistic abilities and areas of individual developmental needs are accorded more structured focus. Chapter 11 contains procedures that apply these principles to intervention.

Appendix:
Questionnaires About Student Performance

A SCHOOL READINESS LANGUAGE CHECKLIST[1]

We can now define school readiness language as a list of language behaviors intersecting with curricular requirements and developmental expectations. Depending on the expectations created by the curriculum, any developmental language level can be considered appropriate or inappropriate. The [speech-language pathologist] can help teachers create a match between curricular expectations and the child's level of language ability. Use of the checklist provided below may help to identify abilities of individual children. It is designed to go to the classroom teacher.

To: _____ From: _____
        (child's teacher)   (consultant)

On the basis of

☐ classroom observation
☐ interview with you
☐ screening results
☐ testing results, I have rated _____'s language level at
☐ Stage II
☐ Stage III
☐ Stage IV

The following information is provided to assist you in designing a maximum language/learning environment for this student.

Stage II Language Behavior Checklist

a. ☐ Speaks in 3–4 word "sentences" lacking small function words.
b. ☐ Describes pictures by naming objects in them.
c. ☐ Fidgets and/or looks around during group activity time.
d. ☐ Vocabulary for body parts, colors, etc., is incomplete.
e. ☐ Is more successful at playing alone or near others than with others.
f. ☐ Tested language age is at 2½ to 3½ year level.
g. ☐ Responds to definition request ("What's a horse?") by shrugging or pointing to the appropriate picture or object.

Summary of Stage II. Not yet capable of focusing attention in response to outside direction, these children learn best from an object or experience that attracts their full attention

[1]From Weiner, C. and Creighton, J. (1987). Documenting and facilitating "School Readiness Language" in the kindergarten classroom. *Journal of Childhood Communication Disorders, 11,* 125–137; reprinted by permission.

(e.g., measuring sand, rolling balls, feeling textures). They require much one-to-one attention from an adult or older child who can talk with them about what they are doing or experiencing. Attention to a task can be extended by verbalizing as the child works. Stage II children rely heavily on the environment for understanding directions and making thoughts and wishes known. They may appear to understand requests more than they do by assuming that the expected thing is requested and that any verbalization is a request to do something. Selected suggestions for working with Stage II children are included later under "Strategies for Helping Children Develop School Readiness Language." (Materials and specific activities for working with both Stage II and Stage III kindergarteners are available in K-TALK [Kindergarten-Teacher Administered Language Kit], available through Communication Skill Builders, Inc., Tucson, AZ.)

Stage III Language Behavior Checklist

a. ☐ Uses well-formed simple sentences.
b. ☐ Connects sentences with *and*.
c. ☐ Tells stories with simple sentences connected by *and* and *and then*.
d. ☐ Uses *-s* for plurals, third-person singular, and possession.
e. ☐ Has some vocabulary for body parts, numbers, colors.
f. ☐ Uses social terms like *please, thank you,* and *excuse me*.
g. ☐ Talks with other children about ongoing activity.
h. ☐ Responds to definition request ("What's a horse?") by giving perceptual and functional attributes organized through experience ("You ride it." "My brother has one.").
i. ☐ Follows group instruction if visual cues are present.
j. ☐ Processes complex sentences as though they were simple sentences (answers the question, "The dog that bit the cat ran. What ran?" with "The cat.").
k. ☐ Responds to requests for clarification by repeating utterance.
l. ☐ During group discussion, makes off-topic comments.
m. ☐ Indicates need for clarification by doing the wrong thing.
n. ☐ Tested language age is at 3½ to 4½ year level.

Summary of Stage III.   These children learn best when working in small groups as the teacher moves among them, discussing what they are doing. Capable of attending in a group for only short periods of time, they require frequent opportunities for one-to-one dialogues with teachers as well as for spontaneous conversation with other students. Their primary method of learning is through manipulation of objects, exploration, and experience.

Stage IV Language Behavior Checklist

a. ☐ Relates events about which the listener knows nothing in a way that allows the listener to understand what happened.
b. ☐ Connects information sequentially with words like *because, since, until, while*.
c. ☐ Responds to requests for clarification by providing additional information.
d. ☐ Requests clarification.
e. ☐ During group discussion, makes comments on topic.

f.   □ Has sufficient private speech to work independently.

g.   □ Expresses doubt or speaks about hypothetical situations.

h.   □ Derives meaning from a string of sentences.

i.   □ Can understand and answer questions about a story without looking at pictures.

j.   □ Responds to definition requests ("What's a horse?") with concepts based on experience.("It's an animal that has four legs, a mane, and a tail, and you ride it with a saddle.")

k.   □ Has conversations with other children about what happened or will happen.

l.   □ Tested language age is 5–7 years.

Summary of Stage IV.   Ready for academic tasks, this child can learn from group interaction and from quiet study or interaction with work sheets. Activities that rely heavily on listening skills, such as listening to stories with few pictures shown, or to audiotapes, are appropriate for short periods of time. These children are ready to recall verbal information that will help them formulate hypotheses about concrete objects, events, and processes. Many of them have learned to separate printed words into their component letter parts and to recognize that words symbolize something.

FACTORS THAT INFLUENCE LEARNING TO READ AND TEXT COMPREHENSION

Inside-the-head	Outside-the-head

Inside-the-head

1. Intelligence: Does the student have the intelligence to learn to read?
2. Language of instruction: Does the student understand technical terms used during instruction, such as "word," "sentence," "paragraph"?
3. Decoding ability
   Is the student accurate at word recognition?
   Is the student automatic at word recognition?
   Can the student read orally with expression?
4. Background knowledge and schema
   Does the student have the necessary background knowledge to understand the text topic?
   Can the student make appropriate inferences?
5. Text structure: Is the student aware of text structure used in scientific articles, expository text, narratives, fairy tales, etc.?
6. Anaphoric terms: Can the student find the referent for anaphoric terms?
7. Metacognitive strategies
   Is the student aware of when there is a breakdown in understanding the text?
   Can the student identify the major points and details in a text?
   Can the student synthesize, summarize, and construct a conceptual map of a text?
8. Language facility
   Vocabulary: Does the student have an extensive vocabulary? Does the student know the variety of ways in which a word can be used?
   Syntax: Is the student aware of how various propositions may be embedded in a sentence to make it complex?
9. Graphic literacy: Can the student interpret a variety of graphs and figures?
10. Motivation, attention: Is the student sufficiently interested to focus attention on learning and on the text topic?

Outside-the-head

1. Quality of instruction
   Is the teaching style task and human relations oriented?
   Is there direct teaching of decoding and comprehension skills?
   Is sufficient practice time given so that skills can develop beyond accuracy to automaticity stage?
   Is there quality control over the progress of each student?
   Is the classroom program carefully structured?
   Is the teacher explicit about the goals for each lesson, and does the teacher explain why the goals are important?
   Does the teacher clarify how to do the task?
   If a student cannot answer a question, does the teacher help the student arrive at the correct answer?
2. Text topic: Is the topic one that the student has sufficient background to understand?
3. Conventions of print: Does the student understand the meaning of print conventions, such as quotation marks, exclamation marks, question marks, side heads, capital letters, etc.?
4. Clarity of writing style
   Has the writer correctly judged the audience?
   Is there an appropriate match between information in the text and the reader's background knowledge?
   Do the sentences contain too much information?
   Are there too many anaphoric terms?
   Does the text lack cohesive ties and causal links?
5. Text readability
   Is the vocabulary appropriate for the student?
   Is the sentence structure too complex for the student?
6. Format design and structural text elements
   Does the text have titles, chapter heads, and side heads?
   Does the text use abstracts, statements of objectives, questions at the beginning, middle and end of text, marginal gloss?
   Is the text easy on the eyes?
7. Time: Is enough time given for the student to read and comprehend the text?

From Samuels, S.J. (1987). Factors that influence listening and reading comprehension. In R. Horowitz and S.J. Samuels (Eds.), *Comprehending oral and written language* (p. 310). San Diego: Academic Press, Inc.; reprinted by permission.

11 / Intervention: Preventing or Reversing the Failure Cycle

PRINCIPLES FOR FACILITATING SUCCESSFUL PERFORMANCE

This chapter approaches intervention from the perspective of research on the linguistic, cognitive, and psychodynamic aspects of language-related learning disabilities. It is divided into three parts: 1) enhancing language knowledge, skills, and functions; 2) developing strategies for improved performance of language-based academic tasks; and 3) maximizing classroom success through compensatory adjustments. Throughout all three sections, the psychodynamic factors conceptualized in the failure cycle (see Chapter 8) assume a preeminence in intervention. Thus, a primary tenet of the approach herein proposed is to design goals and select procedures that maximize the probability of students' experience with success. In conjunction with this philosophy is the assumption that responsibility for creation of conditions favorable to successful performance by students with language-related learning disabilities rests with a clinician-educator who is sufficiently informed about language, its processing demands in different functions, and the current level and nature of the students' abilities and disabilities to minimize the experience of failure during students' progress from deficient to more proficient performance on language-related tasks (A. Gerber, 1981).

This approach to remediation of learning deficiencies finds its counterpart in Feuerstein's (1980) construct: *mediated learning experience*. "By mediated learning experience (MLE) we refer to ways in which stimuli emitted by the environment are transformed by a 'mediating agent.' . . . The mediator selects stimuli that are most appropriate and then frames, filters, and schedules them" (p. 15). Mediation of various aspects of intervention may be achieved by different forms of scaffolding.

Scaffolding

As the term implies, scaffolding supports performance in ways that enhance the probability of success. It is provided intensively during early phases of instruction or training and is gradually withdrawn on evidence of increased task or skill mastery. Scaffolding may take a number of forms, among which are creation of optimal task conditions, cognitive modeling, guidance of selective attention, and provision of external support.

Creation of Optimal Task Conditions   The use of curriculum-based materials and tasks during intervention has been advocated for its efficacy in integrating gains in competencies into naturalistic classroom performance (A. Gerber, 1981; N.W. Nelson, 1981, 1989; Wallach & Miller, 1988). However, because many students with language-related learning disabilities have demonstrated the inability to cope successfully with some of this material, and because they tend to associate academic tasks with failure, modifications of such material to levels that reduce demands is frequently necessary to enlist active and successful student participation. In some cases it may be advisable to defer introduction of academic subject matter until some level of competence in related skills has been achieved in high-interest, low-complexity activities. Gradually, progress may be made from early levels of simplification toward age- and grade-appropriate material while retaining motivation and active student involvement (A. Gerber, 1981).

Facilitation of success frequently requires both reduction of the amount of material presented to smaller units and provision of increased time for task performance (Lasky & Chapandy, 1976; Perfetti & Lesgold, 1977; Rees, 1981). Research reported in earlier chapters strongly suggests the deleterious effects of excessive effort on the processing capacity of students with learning disabilities (Swanson, 1984a). Therefore, minimizing factors contributing to undue effort and stress in task performance is regarded as essential in preventing or reversing the failure cycle.

Cognitive Modeling   Philosophically, the view of cognitive modeling advanced here diverges somewhat from the early conceptualization of cognitive behavior modification. Meichenbam and Goodman (1971) reported on their attempts to train impulsive children to control their behavior by the strategy of verbal self-direction. Adults modeled overt verbalization of the processes used in task performance, then had the child verbalize overtly, and finally had the child verbalize covertly. The authors characterized the verbalization during task performance as verbal rehearsal. They found that cognitive modeling plus self-instruction tended to lengthen response latency and reduce errors in impulsive children.

While equivocal generalization of behavioral training was subsequently reported (Meichenbaum, 1980), it was observed that changes in the child's cognitive reactions are central to behavioral change. Cognitive modeling is here viewed as a means of making overt, for the student to observe, a set of executive cognitive strategies usually employed covertly by the successful information processor.

Following modeling by the clinician-educator, the student is given the opportunity to engage in the same task performance, emulating the modeled strategies. In clinical-educational interactions within one-to-one or small group situations, the present author has found the modeling procedure to virtually ensure successful performance if the task is within the student's potential level of ability. Psychologically, it appears that *demonstrating efficacy of enabling procedures* is more potent in enlisting active attempts from students than *telling them what they should do to succeed.* The experience of success under these facilitating conditions has been observed to initiate alterations in students' self-concepts; it is inferred that changes in cognitive structures regarding not only the self, but also alternative options in task performance, are fostered under these conditions.

Guidance of Selective Attention   Training impulsive children to scan and attend to all relevant features of stimuli, to note similarities and differences, and to examine alternatives was found to improve selective attention 5 months after completion of training (Egeland, 1974). Highlighting important information visually, intonationally, and verbally provides priming cues during or in advance of task performance. Specific examples of such techniques are provided below.

The benefits of self-instruction on focusing and maintaining attention have been discussed in earlier chapters. A brief reference to one source (Schunk, 1986) will suffice here: "verbalization can direct children's attention to important task features, assist strategy encoding and retention" (p. 352). Having the child emulate modeled verbalization of critical information is an effective self-instructional technique for fostering task-relevant selective attention.

Provision of External Support   By means of interpersonal interaction as well as the structuring of material, early stages of intervention may scaffold the students' efforts with cooperative execution of tasks along with helpful cues for successful performance. In other words, wherever appropriate and feasible, the failure-associated isolated, unaided struggle to perform may be eliminated, while dyadic or group participation provides assistance and psychological support. As with other variables discussed above, independent performance may be expected only when anticipation of success is realistically based on demonstrated growth in students' skills. The above principles may be applied differentially to the goals and procedures presented in the remainder of this chapter. Many of the procedures have been drawn from the literature and are so documented. Other undocumented procedures are the contributions of the present author.

ENHANCING LANGUAGE KNOWLEDGE, SKILLS, AND FUNCTIONS

The contents of this section have been determined by convergences between those areas of language judged pertinent to academic function and aspects of language deficits identified by research as correlates of academic learning disabilities. As noted in Chapter 9, information about curricular language demands is indispensable to analysis of possible mismatches between educational expectations and student competencies. Whereas material included in this section on intervention goals and procedures covers a broad range of potential problems, selection of particular goals and procedures is dependent on the results of individual assessment through: observation of student performance in educational contexts, formal testing, and consultation with teachers and educational specialists. The remainder of this section is divided into three major areas: 1) oral and written discourse processing: expressive and receptive; 2) word knowledge and word retrieval; and 3) metalinguistic skills.

Oral and Written Discourse Processing: Expressive and Receptive

This section provides procedures and their rationales aimed at developing and/or increasing students' proficiency in processing the language of literacy (oral and written) throughout a range of age and ability levels. The first section addresses the establishment of early concepts about and attitudes toward literacy through exposure and immersion. The next section, "The Oral-Written Connection," presents procedures aimed at developing literacy competencies through integration of language across modalities. Subsequent sections focus on fostering skills in specific functions that tend to involve predominantly, although not exclusively, the use of a particular modality:

> Oral instructional discourse: listening, asking/answering questions, and following directions
> Narrative discourse: nonfictional and fictional
> Reading comprehension
> Writing

A later section on metalinguistics is devoted to the skills that operate at a heightened level of conscious control in the processes of reading and writing.

Most of the procedures presented in this section are appropriate for classroom use, some for total group participation; others may be more effectively implemented in small groups or dyads either within the classroom or in a sequestered environment.

Exposure to Literacy in the Environment

Developing Print Awareness   Immersion in the artifacts of literacy has been regarded as a critical precursor to early reading (Heath, 1983; Van Kleeck & Schuele, 1987). Young children exposed to literate activities in the home also have demonstrated active attempts to engage in early writing (Teale & Sulzby, 1989). The natural environment provides massive amounts of such stimulation through television, advertising, and signs and signals in the external world. The early educational setting may purposively saturate young children with such material in the form of labels and signs placed around the classroom.

GOAL: To foster awareness of print and its functions.

Procedure: Use of labels, signs, and charts to develop awareness of print.

Name cards can be placed on children's cubbies. Labels can indicate where items belong. Children's jobs in the daily schedule can be printed on charts. "At first the teacher will have to interpret and model the use of these printed materials, but the children will soon use them in their everyday activities" (Teale & Sulzby, 1989, p. 8).

After relatively protracted periods of exposure to children's name cards and item labels, games may be played with them:

1. Take all name cards from a group of children, mix them up, and have children reclaim their own or distribute them to their rightful owners.
2. Take labels of classroom items and have children take turns replacing them in their correct locations.

The Morning Message and News (Teale & Sulzby, 1989)   In kindergarten and early elementary grades, children can observe the use of print for other functions such as announcing or recording information.

GOAL: To expand awareness of the functions of print.

Procedure: The adult writes about activities planned for the day while children watch and listen. The morning message may be presented at the beginning of the school day. For example, the adult may write:

"Good Morning. It's Tuesday, February 16. We will be going on our trash walk today. Also, we have a special book about a mystery for our story time today" (Teale & Sulzby, 1989, p. 8). After the message is written, children read it along with the adult. They are also given the opportunity to write the message at whatever level of competence they have developed, with complete acceptance of their product by the adult (Sulzby, Teale, & Kamberlis, 1989). Thus, they have the first-hand opportunity of participating in a literacy event.

Storybook Reading in School and at Home   "Reading aloud to young children *teaches* them about reading" (Teale & Sulzby, 1989, p. 7). Research has shown that early readers tend to come from homes in which literacy permeates daily functions (Glazer, 1989).

GOALS: To develop the concept of reading as a mode of meaningful communication.
To promote a positive attitude toward reading as a source of pleasure.
To foster the development of the language of literacy.

Procedures: Reading to children using pictures, repetition, and dramatization. Reading aloud to children may be done in large or small groups. However, for some "unready children" who have difficulty following a story line (de Hirsch, 1981), a one-to-one situation is more likely to reduce distraction and focus attention. Accompanying story reading with picture illustrations may be effective in making the verbal material more interesting and meaningful for children with receptive language problems.

For young children and particularly those manifesting language delay, "Participation stories, poetry and rhymes, and song books help immerse children into language. The language is repetitive and predictable. Because children are able to anticipate the language, they join the reader and become part of the storybook activity" (Glazer, 1989, p. 23). For example:

The Three Bears: "Who's been sitting in my chair?"
Billy Goats Gruff: "Who is walking over my bridge?"
Gingerbread Man: "I've run away from a little old woman and a little old man, and I can run away from you too, I can, I can."

The frequent utterance of these refrains, preferably in chorus, helps children to become actively familiar with patterns of literate language characterized by a syntactic style that often differs from that of social discourse. This rationale applies equally to the exposure of children to classic nursery rhymes. A study found that knowledge of nursery rhymes by 3-year-olds was a significant predictor of prereading skills (Maclean, Bryant, & Bradley, 1987).

Dramatization of stories that have become highly familiar provides repeated experience in the use of the language of narrative dialogue and a sense of narrative structure, experienced at the sensorimotor level, of the sequence of goals, events, and outcomes.

The Oral-Written Connection   In collaborative approaches to enhancing success in language-related academic tasks, both the teacher and the speech-language pathologist can facilitate the development of written as well as oral language skills (N.W. Nelson, 1988a). From a whole language perspective, development of skills in one aspect of language is believed to foster growth in other aspects. For example, it is maintained that increasing mastery of the writing process can contribute to improvement of reading ability, and both of these academic language skills interact with the oral language processes of speaking and listening (Schory, 1990).

Procedures in this section are designed to stimulate development of literacy by integrating oral and written language, thereby heightening awareness of the nature and functions of print as talk written down.

GOALS: To foster awareness of the relationship between spoken and written discourses
To provide early success in meaningful reading

Procedure: Using the Language Experience approach (Hall, 1976; D.M. Lee & Allen, 1961), have children construct and dictate an oral account of an experience for the adult to record in print.

A major tenet of the Language Experience approach is that meaningfulness is prerequisite to reading comprehension and that meaning for children is based on their experiences. "Thus, by providing opportunity for each child to build his own reading materials until he develops skill and confidence in handling other materials, an adequate background of experiences is made implicit" (D.M. Lee & Allen, 1961, p. v). That is, the child experiences early success in comprehending a written story, because its meaningfulness stems from knowledge the child already possesses and therefore readily constructs.

The following example illustrates a format for writing a language experience story based on a shared experience. Each sentence is written on a separate line in stories for beginning readers, thus increasing salience of segments of the discourse and reducing processing demands:

> Yesterday we went to Sesame Street Alive.
> First we saw Bert and Ernie.
> Then we saw Cookie Monster.
> Next we saw Big Bird.
> After that we had ice cream.
> We had a wonderful time.

After the children dictate each sentence and the adult writes it on a chalkboard or on large sheets of paper on an easel, the children and the adult "read" the sentence in unison as the adult's hand moves in a connected left-to-right manner under the sentence. The smooth, un-broken sweep of the hand encourages production of the natural prosody of oral language in-stead of disjointed word-by-word utterance. Subsequently, individual children may play "teacher" and emulate the adult's hand movement as they lead the group in rereading the story line by line.

These stories may be accumulated in large classroom books, to be read and reread over time. They may be copied by children at whatever level of writing they have developed (in-structed by the adult to "do it your own way"). They may then be illustrated and compiled into children's own individual story books, which they are encouraged to reread at home and in school. The difference in writing proficiency between children's emergent skills and the adult model may be explained as "another way of writing" (Sulzby et al., 1989).

The experience stories may serve to instill a sense of the temporal sequencing characteris-tic of narrative discourse and help children become conversant with terms that signal the ordering of events (e.g., *first*, *next*, *later*, *after that*). They may also be used as material for developing word recognition skills that are contextually based. For example:

1. The adult prints individual words selected from the stories on cards and places the cards in a container. Adult and children take turns drawing a word card from the container and asking another player to find the story in which this word appeared, match the word card to the word in the text, and say the word.
2. Children may be asked to find a word that has a certain meaning or starts with a certain sound. After the word is identified it is read in its context.

Repeated encounters with the material in gamelike activities tend to foster word recognition and rudimentary word analysis with comfort and confidence.

Intensive use of the Language Experience approach increases the likelihood of preventing the failure cycle. That is, by creating optimal task conditions, early reading success may be fostered. The approach is also suitable for attempts to reverse the failure cycle by providing older children with reading disabilities an alternative route to literacy.

GOAL: To integrate language and literacy intervention with curricular tasks and material.

Procedure: Sensory reporting and narrative recording.

The following procedure applies Moffett's (1968) approach to discourse analysis in terms of levels of abstraction. That is, discourse may report on current events simultaneously with their sensory perception or may provide narratives of past events selectively abstracted from all sensory information on the basis of their relevance to a topic-centered account. (Further detail about the different level of abstraction in discourse is reserved for the section on writing.)

For example, a modified Language Experience approach may be applied to discourse about a simple science experiment on the relationship of oxygen to fire. Materials include a candle affixed to a surface, matches, a glass tumbler, and a tape recorder. As the experiment is conducted, using the tape recorder, a child reports on ongoing events and observations as they occur.

> A candle is standing on a board.
> The teacher is lighting the candle with a match.
> The candle is burning with a bright flame.
> The teacher is turning a glass upside down and putting it over the candle.
> The candle is still burning.
> Now the flame is getting smaller.
> The fire is going out.
> All the oxygen has been used up.
> Fire needs oxygen to burn.

At the conclusion of the experiment, students participate in the conversion of the oral sensory reporting to a written narrative record. To reduce demands on children with writing disabilities, the narrative may be dictated by the children to the adult, who writes the report on the chalkboard. Using a replay of the tape-recorded material, children are asked to convert the form of the information from the present tense of *what is happening* to the past tense of *what happened* (Moffett, 1968, p. 35).

> A candle was placed on a board. The teacher lit the candle. After it burned brightly for a short time, the teacher turned a glass upside down over the candle. The flame stayed bright for a while. Then it started to get smaller and dimmer. After a while the fire went out. It had used up all the oxygen in the glass. We saw proof that fire needs oxygen to burn.

Children read aloud the report they have dictated. Because the material was constructed orally by the children, its content is familiar and meaningful, thereby ensuring a successful reading experience. Procedures described above for analyzing segments of the text in context and out of context may be employed with this kind of material, thus fostering word recognition along with the use of context for prediction.

Science reports of this nature may then be copied by children into their notebooks and reviewed periodically. In this manner, receiving maximal external support under optimal conditions, they may experience success in speaking, listening, reading, and writing in meaningful subject matter context.

Advancing Reading Proficiency and Fluency   It is not uncommon for nonproficient readers to plateau at a level characterized by passive, halting word recognition in the absence of fluency and motivation. C. Chomsky (1976) recognized the need for an approach that would shift focus from individual word decoding to connected discourse and that would "capture their attention and make large amounts of textual material available" (p. 288).

GOAL: To enhance reading fluency through intensive, protracted exposure to simultaneously presented oral and written high-interest-level text.

Procedures: Children are presented with storybooks to read repeatedly as they listen to accompanying audiotaped versions of high dramatic quality.

The process in early stages is conceptualized as a combination of memorization and reading of the textual display. This procedure is continued until the children are able to read the text without the auditory input. Children are encouraged to tape record their own oral reading of the stories either with or without the support of the master tapes. Thus, the procedure exemplifies the principle of scaffolding with external support until mastery permits its withdrawal. The process is then repeated with other storybooks.

Chomsky (1976) also employed gamelike activities for sentence analysis and the analysis and synthesis of words drawn from the story contexts. Some of the procedures used were:

> Making flash card collections for each child's individual needs
> Reading words from flash cards either in isolation form or in context of text
> Timing their own reading of flash cards in their collections
> Finding words in the story that rhyme with a stimulus word
> Finding words in the story that begin or end with targeted sounds or letter configurations

The third-grade children in Chomsky's (1976) study dramatically increased both reading and writing skills over a 3-month period. They took off on their own in spontaneously choosing new storybooks to read. Their success was attributed to added motivation emanating from their experience of success. The process consisted of "radically increased inputs and concentrated attentiveness" (Chomsky, 1976, p. 293).

Echo reading and choral reading are other means of fostering successful reading of more advanced material for older students performing below age/grade level. In echo reading, the adult reads aloud one or two sentences from the text at which the student is looking. The student immediately echoes what the adult has read while pointing to the printed material. In choral reading the adult and the student read aloud in unison. The adult's voice leads the student's decoding and models fluent reading of the text with normal prosody, thereby enhancing the student's comprehension and appreciation of the content. It is recommended that echo reading precede choral reading because it is the less demanding of the two procedures (Gillet & Temple, 1986).

The oral-written connection used in this approach exemplifies an effective means of preventing/reversing the failure cycle by scaffolding performance through the provision of models and external support.

Processing Oral Instructional Discourse "Children whose individual processing strategies do not include linguistic decoding and encoding options for complex syntactic structures and semantic relationships experience difficulty as classroom language demands become more complex and nonverbal support becomes more meager" (N.W. Nelson, 1986a, p. 17). Research reviewed in Chapter 7 indicates that many students with language-related learning disabilities may be unduly taxed by oral instructional discourse because of possible attentional problems and slower, less efficient verbal information processing abilities. Such limitations present difficulties in maintaining a sustained listening set (Wiig & Semel, 1984). Because of a history of such problems in understanding and retaining auditory verbal information, students' motivation to remain actively attuned to extended oral discourse is frequently diminished. The following goals and procedures are aimed at improving listening skills and enhancing success in processing the oral language of instruction.

GOAL: To foster concentration on a topic and exclusion of distractions.

Procedure: Prelistening "warm-up." Buttrill et al. (1989) have suggested a daily prelistening warm-up activity to provide practice in tuning in and tuning out. The adult announces a topic of the day. Students then close their eyes and imagine themselves engaged in some activity related to the topic. They may be encouraged to monitor the degree to which they maintain focus and inhibit intrusion of distractors and may make an oral report to the group in some self-rating procedure.

GOAL: To establish a listening set through the use of active auditory skills.

Procedure: "Whole body" listening. Truesdale (1990) has devised a "whole body" approach for teaching children how to listen. Children are told to use their *ears* to listen with exaggerated stillness to sounds outside their room. They are trained to keep *hands* and *feet* inactive during listening. They are informed that their *brains* think actively but their *mouths* remain inactive to permit effective listening. Finally, they are told to use their *eyes* to look at a speaker when listening.

GOAL: To motivate active listening to oral discourse with the support of visual information.

Procedure: Identifying errors in narratives.

The adult tells a story while displaying pictures illustrating events. The story is tape recorded as it is being told. Students are informed that mistakes may be made in the narration wherein what they hear will not match what they see in the pictures. By detecting and signaling such errors, students win a point. On replay of the taped story, the adult wins a point for each undetected error. This procedure may be repeated with different material over successive sessions, with cumulative score keeping to promote ongoing motivation for spirited engagement in listening activities.

GOAL: To motivate active listening without the support of visual cues.

Procedure: The barrier game.

The barrier game has been demonstrated to stimulate improved referential communication in children with learning disabilities (Bunce, 1989). It may also provide opportunities for students to monitor their listening comprehension. By placing a barrier between the speaker, who describes the construction of a configuration of objects, and the listener, who attempts to replicate the configuration without visual access to its construction, the listener is compelled to acutely attend to the verbal message. Removal of the barrier after completion of the task allows for confrontation between speaker and listener as to the accuracy of message communication. Taping and replaying the speaker's message permits evaluation of the adequacy of information sent and received and provides powerful evidence of inadequacies in either referential communication, message reception, or both. Repeated trials give impetus to increased efforts at careful encoding and decoding of verbal information.

GOAL: To enhance comprehension of the semantic content of instructional oral discourse.

Procedure: Present students with lists of unfamiliar components in forthcoming oral discourse.

Wiig and Semel (1984) have proposed that, in advance of oral instruction, unfamiliar words, concepts, and relationships be clarified by presenting students with a list of definitions or illustrations to increase their meaningfulness. "The students can use the list for reference during the presentation and later questioning" (p. 655). They have also recommended the use of visual aids (e.g., flash cards, slides, photographs, and films) to enhance the meaning of the verbal messages.

GOAL: To facilitate students' ability to detect cues to organization of orally presented verbal information.

Procedure: Outlining.

For older students, the adult may preview a skeletal outline of material to be presented (Alley & Deshler, 1979). For example, students may be informed in advance "Our topic will be discussed under three major headings" (p. 294). Students may be alerted to organizational verbal cues such as "the first point," "a key point," and "in summary" (Buttrill et al., 1989, p. 196).

To help students identify main and supporting ideas, Alley and Deshler (1979) have proposed the following activities:

1. Have students listen to a short selection and suggest a title.
2. Tell a short story and have students summarize it in one sentence.
3. Give three statements, one containing a main idea and two containing subordinate ideas. Have students identify each statement.
4. Have students listen to a class presentation on videotape and identify the main ideas. In the beginning, students should be presented with a worksheet from which they can choose the main idea. Students should discuss why each of the other choices is *not* a main idea (too general, too specific, irrelevant, or inaccurate). (p. 295)

Processing the structure and the content of lecture material may be further scaffolded by following outlines with the support of the instructor (Alley & Deshler, 1979; Wiig & Semel, 1984). That is, the adult (either in actual classroom instruction or in small group remedial sessions) gives a preview of what is coming by reading aloud major headings in the outline. Students then listen to the oral material within the context of the structural written guide. If appropriate to their developmental level, they may be encouraged to write down important cue words and phrases under relevant headings. The adult may model efficient listening and note taking by condensing units of spoken text into stripped down content words that abstract the gist (Graves, 1991).

GOAL: To direct attention to critical factual details.

Procedures: Preposed *wh-* questions, summarization.

Students may be alerted to upcoming factual information by preposed *Wh-* questions (Buttrill et al., 1989). Following segments of lectures on key points, the adult may model the construction of minisummaries of factual content. Subsequently, students may emulate this procedure.

Further support for the processing of oral instructional discourse may be provided by creating optimal listening conditions. These procedures are to be discussed in the final section of this chapter.

Assessment of Discourse Ability   Curricular content and pedagogical methods remain the responsibility of the classroom teacher. However, for students with language-related learning disabilities, benefits may accrue through collaboration between the speech-language pathologist and the teacher in two areas of oral classroom discourse: following directions and response to and use of questions. A number of factors that may have an impact on the ability of children with language-related learning disabilities to process directions and questions have been identified:

> Linguistic complexity and length of teacher utterance (N.W. Nelson, 1988b; Wiig & Semel, 1984)
>
> Rate of presentation (N.W. Nelson, 1984; Wiig & Semel, 1984)
>
> Level of abstraction (Blank, et al., 1978)
>
> Emotional state (N.W. Nelson, 1988b)
>
> Certain classes of terms referring to logical, spatial, or temporal relations (Amidon & Carey, 1972; Wiig & Semel, 1984)

It has been stated in earlier chapters and elsewhere in the literature (L. Miller, 1990; Wallach, 1990) that some young children may enter the educational experience unready to meet some of the language demands placed on them, with resultant early failure to comprehend or respond appropriately to comments, directions, or questions spoken by the teacher. This mismatch between teacher language and child language/cognitive abilities frequently causes the child to withdraw from active listening or to engage in impulsive responding accompanied by a high rate of error in task performance. Therefore, a critical goal of early intervention is to ensure *successful* participation in classroom activities that involve the child's verbal comprehension and expression. Prerequisite to the achievement of this goal is the adult's accurate assessment of the level of discourse at which the child can currently function and understanding of the processes by which growth to more advanced levels may be fostered.

Some guidelines to stages of readiness in young children, or children of any age who have language-related learning disabilities, are provided by Weiner and Creighton (1987), among which are the following:

> Attentional capacity
>
> The ability to work alone

The need to associate verbal information with manipulation of concrete material
The ability to listen to verbal information divorced from immediate contextual support

One assessment approach, designed by Blank et al. (1978), provides teachers and language specialists with a system both for assessing the child's present level of discourse processing ability and for facilitating growth in discourse processing skills under optimally supportive conditions. Although the levels of language-perception distance have been delineated in previous chapters, they are reiterated here with examples of intervention procedures for convenience of reference. Intervention procedures may be administered by a teacher or speech-language pathologist.

Level I—Matching Language to Perception
Procedure: Scanning for a matching object.
Adult presents an object (e.g., a knife, a crayon) and a card containing an array of many common objects. The child is instructed to look at the object held up by the adult and then to point to one like it on the picture card.

Level II—Selective Analysis of Perception
Procedure: Scanning for an object defined by its function.
Adult presents a card containing an array of common objects, including a knife, and instructs the child to "find something we could cut with."

Level III—Reordering Perception
Procedure: Following a set of directions.
Adult presents a doll wearing clothes, an empty box, and a doll's hat. The child is instructed to: "First, take the socks off the doll, then put the hat in the box, and then put the box on the floor" (Blank et al., 1978, p. 123).

Level IV—Reasoning About Perception
Procedure: Predicting changes in structure.
Adult stacks four blocks in a vertical column. Pointing to the bottom block, he/she asks the child what would happen if the bottom block were taken away.

The reader is referred to Blank et al. (1978) for a complete description of items used for testing that may be employed as items in a hierarchy of training. This material is recommended as a guide for stages of development at which children may be expected to engage successfully in educational discourse. Moreover, since higher level discourse skills are increasingly required to meet educational demands, progress toward such advances without undue frustration for the child is fostered through a suggested approach using simplification procedures (Blank & White, 1986).

Simplification Procedures   The simplification procedures are far from simplistic and require a thoroughgoing understanding of the system of discourse levels and sensitivity to the child's responses to discourse demands. The principle of simplification is based on the concept of progression through a continuum of abstraction. "Specifically, when children fail because questions are beyond their level of information or skill, the teaching adult should reformulate the following dialogue at a simpler level" (Blank & White, 1986, p. 5).

The following example has been excerpted from Blank and White (1986, p. 5):

Adult: Why do we use tape for hanging pictures?
Child: 'Cause it's shiny.
Adult: Here's a shiny piece of paper and here's a shiny piece of tape.
   Let's try them both. Try hanging the picture with the shiny paper.
Child: (does it)
Adult: Does it work?
Child: No, its falling.
Adult: Now try the tape.
Child: (does it)
Adult: Does it work?
Child: Yeah, it's not falling.
Adult: So, why do we use the tape for hanging pictures?
Child: It won't fall.

It can be seen that, when the child demonstrated an inability to reason about perception in the absence of first-hand sensorimotor experience, the level of demand was reduced to the point at which the language was matched to perception. From this simplification procedure, the child was able both to experience success and to be guided to a higher level of function in response to questions and commands.

From a somewhat different perspective, Wiig and Semel (1984) reported on linguistic/ cognitive components that may cause difficulty in direction following by children with language-related learning disabilities. "They may find it hard to execute commands that contain adjective sequences, prepositional phrases, right-left directions, number facts, or linguistic concepts of time or condition" (p. 484). For intervention, Wiig and Semel proposed a sequence of difficulty in tasks and the use of materials that are designed to foster improvements in processing of oral directions, among which are:

Following oral commands for gross motor actions (e.g., "Run to the closet and get your coat and put it on.")

Following oral commands for fine motor actions (e.g., "Draw a blue bird." [pause] "Take a green crayon." [pause] "Draw a tree.")

Following oral commands that contain adjective sequences (e.g., "Touch the big red circle and the small blue circle.")

Following oral commands that contain prepositions (e.g., "Pick up a red crayon and put it next to the book.")

Following oral commands that contain number facts (e.g., "In a deck of cards, find two aces. Find a nine of hearts. Find a seven of spades.")

Following oral commands that contain linguistic concepts (e.g., "After I write my name, you write yours.")

In research on normal language acquisition, temporal terms such as *before* and *after* have been found to present difficulty for kindergarten children in carrying out commands embedded in subordinate clauses (Amidon & Carey, 1972). Young children were found to do better with directions using *first* and *last* to indicate order. It was suggested that *first* and *last* are easier to process because they occur in main clauses, whereas *before* and *after* are more difficult to process because they occur in subordinate clauses. It has also been reported that temporal information is more readily processed when order of mention parallels order of occurrence (H. H. Clark & Clark, 1968).

He fixed the car before he went swimming.

After he fixed the car he went swimming.

GOAL: To create conditions that will foster improvement in children's ability to process oral directions in the classroom.

For children who have difficulty attending to, comprehending, and/or retaining auditory verbal information, it may be preferable to initiate intervention procedures in a one-to-one or small group situation free from distracting background stimuli. Directions of a nonacademic, gross motor nature may precede the fine motor or symbolic activities "that are not related to their drives" (de Hirsch, 1981, p. 62).

Procedure: Following oral directions.

The following examples reflect principles discussed in several sources (Amidon & Carey, 1972; Blank et al., 1978; Blank & White, 1986; M.H. Clark & Clark, 1968; de Hirsch, 1981; Wiig & Sewel, 1984). Selection of the type and level of procedures must be based on a determination of the present capabilities and needs of individual children.

> To Child 1: "First touch Mark. Then touch Amy."
>   "Right! You touched Mark before you touched Amy."
> To Child 2: "First touch Amy. Then touch Mark."
>   "Right! After you touched Amy, you touched Mark."
>   (Adult presents a bell and a drum)
> To Child 1: "Ring the bell before you hit the drum."
> To Child 2: "After you hit the drum, ring the bell."
> To Child 3: "Ring the bell after you hit the drum."
> To Child 4: "Before you hit the drum, ring the bell."

The above progression may require repeated trials over time accompanied by the simplification process described above. That is, while attempting to move children along in their ability to process the more advanced forms, it may be necessary to revert to the simpler form (e.g., "First ring the bell. Then hit the drum.") followed by adult expression of the more advanced form, as demonstrated in the first illustration.

Procedure: Visualization of oral directions.

Visualization has been found to result in gains on memory tasks (Levin & Allen, 1976). It has been used as an aid in children's processing of oral directions (N.W. Nelson, 1988b). Visualization of oral directions may be taught by drawing simple designs with crayons, incorporating pauses for visualization of each part of the direction:

> "I will draw something, and I will tell you how to draw the same thing. After I tell you what to draw, close your eyes and make a picture inside your head. Then open your eyes and draw it. Let's see if our drawings are the same."
> Two-part direction: "Draw a circle." (pause) "Draw an X in the circle."
> Three-part direction: "Draw a square." (pause) "Draw a circle under the square." (pause) "Put a dot in the middle of the circle."

Designs are compared after completion. A similar procedure may be used with verbal rehearsal after each element:

In stage 1, rehearsal can be done aloud ("Let me hear it.")
In stage 2, rehearsal can be whispered ("Keep it a secret.")
In stage 3, rehearsal can be covert ("Talk inside your head.")

Any of the above processes may be transferred to more "academic" tasks for children who are engaged in the use of written language. For example, visualization may be taught to an individual child or a group in a classroom-like setting using paper, pencils, and a blackboard or easel paper.

"First fold your paper down the middle like this."
"After you have folded your paper, write your name at the top."
"After you have written your name, copy these letters."
"Say the name of each letter before you write it."
"I will tell you again."
"Before you write the letter, say its name."
"After you finish copying the letters, you may draw a picture."
"I will tell you again."
"You may draw a picture after you finish copying the letters."

These directions may initially be given individually with pauses between the sequenced items to permit processing and completion of each step before proceeding to the next item. When children demonstrate successful processing under these facilitating conditions, the attempt can be made to combine two steps in a sequence.

It is, of course, necessary to observe the performance of the children under these more demanding conditions to determine if there are signs of overloading. If such signs are detected, the simplification process should be instituted without punitive penalty. Thus, continually operating on the scaffolding principles stated at the beginning of this chapter, the adult assumes responsibility for the child's success *and failure*, with the accompanying obligation to alter conditions to facilitate success and minimize failure without imposing blame or a sense of inadequacy upon the child.

GOALS: To focus attention on critical elements in oral directions for the accurate location of targeted information.

A fairly common problem for students with language-related learning disabilities is difficulty attending to all critical elements in directions for performing academic tasks.

Procedure: Cue cards for attending to critical elements.

Display a red card on which is printed the word *where*. Display a yellow card on which is printed the word *what*. Students have reading books or textbooks whose readability is well within a comfortable level. The adult gives directions for finding specified information in a designated location. Before saying the location, the adult holds up the *where* card. Before saying the targeted information the adult holds up the *what* card. For example:

(Holding up the *where* card) "On page 250 in the first paragraph (holding up the *what* card) find the name of the explorer."

Students compare their findings and may engage in playful competition to see who finds the answer first. With success achieved in locating material that is perceptually present, directions may subsequently be aimed at location of information requiring higher order processing (e.g., "Find a word that means *strong*" "Find three words that tell you how long ago this happened"). Scaffolding with the cue cards may be discontinued when students give evidence of having internalized the attending strategy.

Processing Questions: Answering and Asking   The prominent role of question asking and question answering in education has been noted by numerous authors (Blank & White, 1986; Klein & Harris, 1986; N.W. Nelson, 1984; Silliman, 1984). Difficulties experienced by students with language-related learning disabilities in responding to questions and asking questions to secure needed information or request clarification have been reported in the literature reviewed in Chapter 7. Problems vary according to age, grade, and curricular demands. Therefore, suggested intervention procedures address different types and levels of question asking and question answering.

Wh- Questions   An early study by Ervin-Tripp (1970) led to the conclusion that some of the difficulties experienced by immature listeners may be attributed to their inattention to the nature of the particular *Wh-* word and the information it seeks. Rather, the responses of these listeners appear to indicate that they attend to the nature of the verb, using a strategy that requires supplying a part of the sentence that seems to be missing:

> *Q:* "Why was the boy sleeping?"
> *A:* "In bed."
> *Q:* "When did you eat?"
> *A:* "A sandwich."

Some older children with language-related learning disabilities have been observed to respond in a similar manner:

> *Q:* "When will you be going away?"
> *A:* "I'm going to my grandmom's."

Another factor found to influence the ability to comprehend and respond to Wh- questions is the reference to information not present in the immediate environment. Parnell et al. (1986) reported that, while all subjects, with or without language disorders, had greater difficulty responding appropriately and accurately to questions about things not perceptually present, the children with impaired language manifested a more profound deficiency under these conditions. *Why* and *when* questions were most difficult, and even *where* questions, usually mastered early, presented problems for the children with language disorders "when the question concerned nonimmediate referential sources" (p. 105).

Wiig and Semel (1984) suggested the following order of difficulty of *Wh-* questions for children with learning disabilities: *What–who–which–where–when–why–how–whose*. Taking all the above information into account, intervention designed to foster growth while ensuring a high success rate might apply the principle: *Whenever possible, ask children questions that they are likely to be able to answer*. This would entail following an order of question type and provision of information through either experience, modeling, or supportive prompts.

GOAL: To develop the ability to answer *Wh-* questions about phenomena not present in the immediate environment.

Procedures: Adult modeling; storytelling with classes of *wh-* material.

The adult may engage in modeling and turn taking:

"I get up at 7:00. When do you get up?"
"I go away on vacation in July. When do you go on vacation?"
"I go to Ocean City every summer. Where do you go?"
"I come to school on the train. How do you come to school?"

Subsequently children may engage in asking similar questions of peers using color-coded cards for the various *Wh-* words (i.e., *When* cards are blue, *Where* cards are green).

Another procedure designed to foster processing *Wh-* question words in the decontextualized language of literacy accompanies storytelling with color-coded *Wh-* questions. For example, the adult writes headings of *Wh-* words on a chalkboard or easel in different colored chalk or magic markers. Items that would be appropriate answers to questions containing each *Wh-* word are listed in the appropriate column. For the story "The Three Billy Goats Gruff," the color-coded lists might consist of the following:

Who	What	Where	When	Why
Billy Goats Gruff	Green grass	On a hillside	One day in summer	To eat grass
Troll		Across the river	All morning	
		Under the bridge		

The adult asks questions, using the various *Wh-* words. Using a team-game format, members of each team are given turns responding. They earn a point for their team if they correctly name the color of the *Wh-* word and another point if they select the correct item from the appropriate list of responses. This procedure is suitable for children who have some minimal reading skill (A. Gerber, 1981, p. 194).

Other Questions   All too frequently, efforts to stimulate growth in asking and answering questions are limited to relatively simple form and content in contrived activities. To assist the student with learning disabilities in meeting the language demands of education, intervention needs to address the wide variety of questions that are asked about subject matter and or content-related processes by teachers and by textbooks and workbooks. A number of systems for describing and categorizing academic questions are found in the literature. N.M. Sanders (1973) grouped academic questions into three major categories:

1. Memory questions, involving recognition or recall of information given in a passage
2. Translations, involving the expression of ideas in different form
3. Interpretation, involving higher order cognitive operations

(See Chapter 5 for detailed descriptions.) Another taxonomy of question types has value for both teachers and older students in terms of emphasizing the purposes the questions serve (Alley & Deshler, 1979):

1. Recall or recognition questions assessing acquisition of information
2. Descriptive or comparative questions for organization of data
3. Synthesizing or summarizing questions requiring formation and/or identification of relationships and conclusions
4. Judgmental questions requiring evaluation of conclusions or relations
5. Open-ended questions stimulating divergent thinking

Reflecting a pragmatic perspective, the terms *requestive* (N.W. Nelson, 1984) and *elicitation* (Silliman, 1984) have been used more recently. Requestives require a factually accurate response product, whereas elicitations evoke the process of mental activity in the course of problem solution. Item 1 in the above listing of Alley and Deshler's taxonomy is an example of a requestive, while other items in the list may be classified as elicitations.

Much attention has been directed at children's ability to answer questions in instructional discourse. Wiig (1989) stressed the equally important ability to ask questions as a strategy for self-directed learning or for seeking clarification. Purposes of gathering information, organizing information, isolating significant features, verification of information, and proving or disproving hypotheses are served by active questioning behavior (p. 87).

GOAL: To develop the ability to progress from asking hypothetical "potshotting" questions to asking constraint questions.

Procedures: Twenty Questions.

Twenty Questions is a game that can be structured to foster development of question asking and answering skills in a nonthreatening activity. The use of a nonacademic activity is considered preferable for early stimulation of targeted skills, followed in gradual stages by the introduction and modification of classroom material. C.S. Simon (1980) recommended the use of category cards for focusing questions and answers. For example, a category card on which is printed the word *animal*, *vegetable*, or *mineral* is selected, under which pictures of objects that are exemplars of that category are placed face down.

Questioning may be modeled initially or scaffolded by the adult to channel questions in order to increase effectiveness. This might take the form of constraint questions eliciting categorical information that would tend to narrow the field of inquiry, rather than the inefficient, impulsive potshotting characteristic of the immature information seeker (Wiig, 1989). For example, the adult might overtly verbalize the thinking process related to this kind of information seeking: "Is it found inside a building? No? Well, now I know it can't be furniture or kitchen utensils." A turntaking version might be employed wherein the adult and a child alternate asking the questions as a partnership, thus juxtaposing mature questioning with that of a less mature questioner.

GOAL: To promote the ability to formulate and respond to questions in a naturalistic communicative interaction.

Procedure: Role reversal in questioning about nonacademic activities.

The process of modeling is used in a turn-taking format. First the adult asks for information the child possesses as an "expert," such as the playing of a game (e.g., baseball). Questions might include:

"Who are the players?"
"Where are they placed?"
"What does the shortstop do?"
"What are the rules for calling a 'strike' and a 'ball'?"
"When is a fly ball an out?"
"How many foul balls is a batter permitted?"

Next, the child asks the adult questions about an activity in which the adult is "expert" (e.g., baking a cake).

Asking directions offers another opportunity for modeling questions in a turn-taking format (A. Gerber, 1981). For example, the adult might begin by asking:

"How far is it to your house?"
"Which way do you turn when you leave the schoolyard?"
"How long does it take you to walk there?"
"How many streets do you have to cross?"

The roles may again be reversed, with the child asking directions to the adult's home or some other place of interest.

GOAL: To apply improved processing of questions to academic tasks and situations.

Procedure: Questioning about academic material.

Following nonacademic activities, procedures may shift to material of a more academic nature, but still involving information well within the students' knowledge and skill level. For older students, curriculum-based subject matter and tasks may form the content of questions asked by an adult and, in turn, by students:

Arithmetic: "How do I cancel fractions?"
Language Arts: "Where do I find the vowel markings in the dictionary?"
Social Studies: "How do I find out the distance between two points on the map?"
    (A. Gerber, 1981, p. 195)

Wiig (1989) provided a variety of activities designed to foster asking and answering of questions in social and academic contexts (e.g., interviewing and role playing). Two examples are appropriate for older students. In a small group, students develop plans for doing their homework assignments. After listing assignments and other activities that require allotments of their time, students question each other about how much time they estimate each assignment will take and how they plan to fit these tasks into available time slots.

In the classroom after a unit on a theme has been completed, a "TV Quiz" game may be played using either an audiotape recorder or video recording equipment if available. The adult may first play game-show host by preparing a number of questions on the topic (e.g., "Where do polar bears live?" "How do they travel from place to place?" "How do they hunt for their food?"). Following the adult model, different children take turns playing host and contestant. Contestants may play in partnerships, which permit support and joint effort to reduce the likelihood of failing to answer a question. At the completion of the game, the recording is replayed so that students may watch or listen to it.

Simplification of Academic Questions   Some of the foregoing examples of questions asked of students have been relatively simple in their form and in the responses required. Yet even relatively simple questions may be excessively demanding for young children with language-related learning disabilities. The simplification process advocated by Blank and White (1986) is appropriate for modifying task demands in order to increase children's effective responses. In conjunction with simplification of questions, it is recommended that an optimal balance be maintained between teacher questions and teacher comments in order to avoid placing undue demands on children not ready to respond at a particular level of instructional discourse. Comments may be formulated at a higher level of complexity, to stimulate linguistic and cognitive development, while questions may be posed at a simpler level (Blank & Marquis, 1987).

GOAL: To foster children's ability to answer questions by reducing processing demands in order to promote success.

Procedure: Simplification of questions.

Questions encountered in textbooks and workbooks are often of a level of complexity that taxes the processing abilities of the student with language-related learning disabilities. These processing abilities may be improved through the use of exercises that train children to analyze and reason using a simplified questioning process. For example, in a demonstration for young children of the relationship of particle size and aperture size, a mixture of barley and salt is poured through a sieve over a bowl.

> Adult comment: "The salt went through because it is smaller than the holes." (reasoning about perception)
> Adult question: "What stayed in the sieve?" (matching language to perception)
> Adult question: "Is the barley bigger than the holes?" (analyzing perception)
> Adult comment: "The barley didn't go through because it is bigger than the holes." (reasoning about perception)

The simplification process described above, which facilitates successful discourse processing by the younger child, may be applied at a more advanced level in a similar but not identical fashion.

Questions at the conclusion of textual passages that may exceed in complexity the student's language processing ability may be reduced to a simpler level to facilitate compliance with task requirements. For example, following a passage in which a character in a book gives an account of a trip to a logging camp, the question is asked: "What suggestions could you give Bob that would help him make his talk more lively and more informative?" This question, which involves identification and evaluation of multiple items, may be broken down to the following series of simpler questions, each requiring focus on a single aspect of the material. Subsequently, the more complex original question may be posed on a second trial with increased probability of a successful response:

> "Was Bob's talk interesting to read about (or listen to)?"
> "What parts of it were not interesting?"
> "How could he have made it more interesting?"
> "What parts could he have left out?"
> "What other things would you have wanted to know more about?"
> "O.K. You have some good ideas about how to make Bob's talk better. Let's read the question as it was written in the book. What suggestions could you give Bob that would help him make his talk more lively and more informative?"

Other sources of difficulty may be the unfamiliarity or abstractness of the terms and/or concepts they represent, which may require interpretation. On occasion, such terms and/or concepts may co-occur with a high degree of information compression. For example, in a language arts textbook, 12 short sentences are listed on which the student is asked to perform an analysis about noun phrases. The following series of questions requires both metalinguistic knowledge and primary linguistic skill to process information of a challenging degree of density for the child with a language-related during disability:

In which six sentences is the subject a noun by itself?
In which five sentences is the subject a noun with its marker?
In which sentence is the subject a noun with two noun markers?

The following simplification is suggested:

"Find a sentence that has a subject that is a noun all by itself. Look at all the other sentences. How many can you find with that kind of subject noun?"

"Find a sentence with a subject that has a noun with its marker. How many more can you find with that kind of noun phrase?"

"Can you find a sentence with two noun markers?"

"Now go back to the book and read the questions the way they are written. Read the first question. You know the answer. Now you can answer that kind of question" (and so forth).

This kind of tutorial support is feasible in a one-to-one or small group interaction. If it is provided intensively over a period of time, the likelihood of the students' acquisition of coping strategies in the classroom is increased but not guaranteed. The classroom teacher's understanding of possible sources of difficulty with academic questions is indispensable to facilitation of success and reduction of failure and frustration by the student with language-related learning disabilities. This issue is discussed at the end of this chapter.

Narrative Discourse: Nonfictional and Fictional Research reported in Chapter 7 presents evidence of deficits in the narrative abilities of children with language-related learning disabilities. Narrative skills are important to classroom success in the performance of both oral and written academic tasks that may range from descriptions of personal experiences to curriculum-based explanations and reports of processes and events (N.W. Nelson, 1988b). "At the broadest level, *narratives* are verbalized memories of past or ongoing events" (Heath, 1986b, p. 84). They may be fictional or nonfictional. Goals and procedures for developing nonfictional narrative skills are presented first.

Nonfictional Narratives Heath (1986a) described three types of nonfictional narratives:

Recounts: verbalization of past experiences on request by a listener
Accounts: spontaneous sharing of experiences and internal reactions
Eventcasts: verbal explanations of ongoing or planned activities

Engaging children in the production of recounts, accounts, and eventcasts as mediated learning experiences (Feuerstein, 1980) is aimed at furthering conceptual, linguistic, and pragmatic growth (McBride & Levy, 1981). With adult scaffolding, children may be led from contextualized to decontextualized language use (Heath, 1983, 1986b) and to the construction of coherent discourse characterized by topic maintenance (Blank & Marquis, 1987).

GOAL: To foster the ability to verbalize descriptions of attributes of objects and to recount events related to object acquisition and use.

Procedure: Show and Tell.

Show and Tell is a well-known and widely used format of oral discourse in early education. McBride and Levy (1981) have developed some guidelines for promoting discourse skills that progress from reference to the here-and-now (matching language to perception) to higher levels of abstraction. The approach consists of three major phases or components:

1. The adult scaffolds the child's description of concrete attributes and/or functions of an object the child has brought to school by questions that guide observation, labeling, and synthesis of information. Skillful questioning may require the use of simplification processes discussed above. For example:

    Adult: "What color is it?"
    Child: "I don't know."
    Adult: "Is it red, yellow, or blue?"
    Child: (no answer)
    Adult: "Can you find something else in the room that is the same color?"

2. The adult scaffolds responses to requests for information that goes beyond the here-and-now. For example:

    "Who gave it to you?"
    "Where do you keep it at home?"
    "Who else plays with it?"

3. Children in the group are guided to become questioners, following the adult's model.

Following elicitation of information by the use of the above methods, it is here suggested that the child be given the opportunity to synthesize a narrative about the acquisition and use of the object in a dictated story that the adult records in written form. Thus, the oral activity of Show and Tell may provide the substance for language experience writing and reading activities.

Show and Tell is not limited to showing. An important component is giving accounts of interesting events that the child has experienced away from the school. This aspect of show and tell provides bona fide opportunities for decontextualized narration.

GOAL: To promote the ability to give a sequentially ordered, topic-focused narrative of events without the support of present context.

Procedures: Event descriptions using monologues, sharing time, and prompts.

A child tells the group about something that happened at home, on a trip, or at a special occasion. The adult scaffolds elaboration of information and logical ordering by questions and/or prompts that elicit a coherent narrative that takes into account listener needs. For example:

"Where did this happen?"
"Who was with you?"
"What happened first?"
"Just tell us about the surprise party now."

A somewhat different approach to the monologic format of Show and Tell is the discussion of topics in Sharing Time. "Sharing Time can be modified to ease the transition into literate monologues by beginning with a group discussion of a topic familiar to all students" (Westby, 1989, p. 230). The adult writes a number of topics on cards (e.g., "What would happen if you didn't get something you had wanted for Christmas?"). Students draw cards from a pile and engage in interaction with other children and the adult by telling personal narratives about the topic. If instances of wandering from the topic occur, members of the group remind the speaker about the topic of discussion to maintain topic focus.

A variation of the use of verbal prompts is the use of written prompts. For example, the card with the topic question may be displayed to the speaker to direct the narrative back to the topic. Also, color-coded cards similar to those described above in the section on "Processing Questions" may may be used to elicit necessary information. That is, if a child has neglected to provide information about the setting for an event, the adult or another child may hold up the card that says *where*.

Narrations of events may also provide content for language experience stories, thus once again integrating the development of oral and written language competencies within functional contexts.

GOAL: To foster the production of logically sequenced, topic-focused descriptions of steps in a process.

Procedure: Eventcasts.

The extensive variety of activities suggested by Blank and Marquis (1987) as vehicles for naturalistic discourse that fosters the development of ideas through language are ideal material for young children's nonfictional narratives. These may take the form of eventcasts. For example, children in one group create a game out of colored paper shapes large enough to be stepped on and a diagram for a pathway of shapes to be stepped on. They discuss rules for play of the game (Blank & Marquis, 1987, p. 159). Following this stage of creative interactive discourse, which may take the form of an eventcast, the children may narrate procedures for play of the game for other groups of children to follow. This may take the form of a tape-recorded narration or of a written narration of the sequenced directions.

Another version of eventcasting employs the activity of sand painting (Blank & Marquis, 1987, p. 133). Sand painting consists of drawing an abstract design with glue on a paper, then pouring sand of different colors over the paper through a funnel, and finally shaking off the sand and leaving the residue adhering to the glue design. One child who has performed the task may provide an eventcast as other children follow the directions. The eventcast would include exposition of the reasons for each procedure as well as the narration of the sequenced procedures.

For older children, narratives of science experiments may follow sensory reporting (Moffett, 1968). An example of this procedure has been provided above in the section on "The Oral-Written Connection." Social studies content is highly suitable for the creation of temporal sequences of events and cause-effect relationships. The adult may scaffold the task performance by presenting time lines of historical events. External support may be provided by having different small groups of students work together to construct narratives in response to the following questions: "What happened?", "When did it happen?", and "Why did it happen?" Groups may then compare and evaluate their historical narratives.

Following the reading aloud of a narrative account of an historical event by the adult, students may be asked to summarize the narrative, prompted by the unfinished statement written on the chalkboard: This story was about _____. As students offer their comments, those comments are written on the chalkboard. The adult then models a summarization of all information given, thus scaffolding the process (C.S. Simon, 1987, p. 119).

Fictional Narrative Discourse In stories generated or retold by students with language-related learning disabilities, research has demonstrated the following deficiencies: less information, fewer complete episodes, reduced usage of some of the categories of story grammar, less connection of episodes in terms of causality, difficulty staying on topic, and failure to express relationships between events and feelings (Garnett, 1986; Roth, 1986). In comparison to normally achieving peers, these students performed like younger children. Narrative skills reportedly develop from less to more mature forms along the following dimensions:

> Description of objects, people, or actions related to an event ("heaps") (Applebee, 1978)
> Chaining of events linked temporarily or causally (Applebee, 1978)
> Linking of logically chained elements to a central theme (Applebee, 1978; Norris & Hoffman, 1990) and maintenance of topic focus (Garnett, 1986; Westby, 1985)
> Expansion of story grammar components to include more episodic detail of action, consequences, and descriptions of internal reactions in terms of feelings and motives (Norris & Hoffman, 1990); Peterson & McCabe, 1983; Stein & Glenn, 1979)

Therefore, intervention is aimed at fostering development in a number of aspects of storytelling.

GOALS: To stimulate progression from more primitive narrative forms (Applebee, 1978) to more advanced narratives that coordinate actions among characters and ascribe causes and motives for actions and emotional reactions to events.

Westby (1989) suggested the following criteria for judging the level of story structure:

1.   Is the narrative merely a descriptive sequence or does it have a temporally based sequence?
2.   Is the narrative merely an action sequence or does it have causally related events?
3.   Is the narrative merely a sequence of reactions or does it imply goal-directed behavior?
4.   Does the narrative consist of abbreviated episodes or is it elaborated?
5.   Does the narrative consist of multiple complete episodes that are embedded and interactive?

It has been recommended that a story structure simpler than those used for analytical research be employed for educational purposes (Page & Stewart, 1985; Thomas, Englert, & Morsinck, 1984):

> *Setting*: introduction of main character(s), time, and place
> *Problem*: predicament the main character attempts to resolve in order to achieve a goal
> *Response*: internal response by main character(s) to the problem and attempts to achieve the goal
> *Outcome*: results of actions and evaluative response by main character(s)

Further simplification may be used as a starting point for early narratives by young children or those older students with more severe language disabilities (N.W. Nelson, 1988b):

> Initiating events
> Attempts (including motivations)
> Consequences (including emotional reactions of character(s))

Procedures: Reading, storytelling/retelling, instruction on story grammar components, book reports.

The following intervention strategies range from simple to more advanced levels of performance. Procedures may be selected on the basis of their suitability to the present level of students' abilities and determined needs for progress.

1.   Engage in frequent reading/telling of stories at a scheduled story time in a designated part of a room (Garnett, 1986). Familiar stories with cumulative, circular, or progressive nar-

rative structures or repetitive refrains foster young children's awareness of the chaining of episodes. Encourage children to "join in the chant as they capture the rhythm and repetition of the language" (Van Dongen & Westby, 1986, p. 78).

2. Present pictures of episodes from well-known stories and have children retell the stories using the pictures as cues to events and their temporal order. A variation is employed by having children select those pictures from a mixed group that best represent the story sequence (Page & Stewart, 1985). Prompts may be given verbally or in written form for expressing a beginning; temporal relationships among episodes (e.g., *then* relations); causality; expression of relationships among characters, their traits, and their feelings; and an ending to the sequence of events (N.W. Nelson, 1988b). After using a sequence of picture cards that illustrate events in a story, pictures may be turned face down. Children may take turns relating episodes they remember, in response to adult prompts for producing temporal connectives (e.g., *after that, finally*) (C.S. Simon, 1980).

3. Using a wordless picture-story book, the adult asks the child to tell a story as it would appear in a book: "Pretend you're the teacher reading a story to the class. You can see the book, but the children cannot. Read it in a way that will make the class understand the story." (Westby, 1989). The adult scaffolds extended narrative production beyond the descriptive level by prompting with any of the following categories of question:

a. Reporting: What happened here?
b. Projecting: How does the boy feel?
c. Reasoning: Why does the boy feel angry?
d. Predicting: What will happen next? (Westby, 1989, p. 214)

During or following storytelling by adult or child, group discussion may further explore predicted outcomes, feelings and motivations, and other possible courses of action (Garnett, 1986).

4. In a story corner, display a chart that lists story grammar components that serve as a guide for storytelling and discussion:

setting—Who? Where? When?
event—What happened to the main characters?
goals—What are the main characters trying to do?
attempts—What happens when they try to do it?
reactions—What are their feelings? What are their plans?
end—How does it turn out? (Garnett, 1986, p. 54)

An alternate approach for children with limited reading ability would employ oral comments by the adult storyteller that enhance awareness of the content and the structures of the narrative by making explicit:

who was performing the actions
what the actions were
how the characters felt
where the events took place
how the story turned out (Wallach & Miller, 1988, p. 102)

5. The adult may read or tell a story, stopping before the end to allow different children to create alternative endings, providing explanations in terms of characters' reactions.

6. Storybooks are assigned for home reading with parents' help when needed. Westby (1989) provided suggested formats for book reports at different levels of complexity to be com-

pleted with parental assistance. The following examples are selected from the sequence of seven levels:

Book Report 1

1. Identify title either by naming or pointing to it on cover.
2. Identify author either by naming or pointing to it on cover.
3. Draw a picture of a favorite part of the story.
4. Describe the pictures in the book.

Book Report 3

1. Identify title either by naming or pointing to it on cover.
2. Identify author either by naming or pointing to it on cover.
3. Name the major characters.
4. Relate three things, in sequence, that happened in the story.
5. Retell the story using the pictures.

Book Report 5

1. Identify title by naming.
2. Identify author either by naming or pointing to it on cover.
3. Identify a feeling exhibited by one of the main characters.
4. Explain how you know a character is experiencing a particular feeling.
5. Retell the story using the pictures. (Westby, 1989, p. 234)

The reader is referred to Van Dongen and Westby (1986) and Westby (1989) for suggested stories and books of different levels of complexity that exemplify particular aspects of narrative.

Reading Comprehension   In Chapter 4, information was presented about the interaction between top-down and bottom-up processing involved in comprehension of extended units of written as well as oral discourse. From the top-down cognitive processing perspective, comprehension necessitates creation of relevant contexts for interpretation of textual material by activation of schematic knowledge possessed by the reader/listener (Jenkins & Heliotis, 1981).

From the material reported in Chapters 7 and 8, there is evidence that poor readers are less inclined than good readers to achieve an optimal balance between bottom-up and top-down processing, thereby rendering the act of reading laborious, meaningless, and frustrating. Among other difficulties, poor readers are reportedly less apt to detect and use higher level organizational structure (Kamhi, 1989; N.W. Nelson, 1988b), apparently regarding the nature of reading as the sounding out of words, not as the construction of meaning (Westby, 1989). Westby (1989) identified three components necessary for comprehension: content facts, content schemata, and text grammar (or organizational structure).

The following goals and procedures are designed to stimulate active processing of textual information in order to facilitate comprehension.

GOAL: To activate schematic knowledge in advance of reading stories or expository text.

Procedure: Prereading topic discussion.

In accordance with the principles stated at the beginning of this chapter, it is recommended that, in early stages of intervention with students who either are at risk for reading failure or have a history of reading failure, reading material should be both familiar in content and readily comprehensible. Class discussions in advance of reading about a topic are helpful in activating knowledge currently possessed by the students. For example, before reading a story about a birthday party, have young children share their own experiences and ideas about birthdays (Kawakami & Hu-Pei-Au, 1986).

For older students, high-interest material about sports, contemporary music figures, movies, television, and current events is likely to invoke schematic knowledge and motivation. Group discussion prior to reading develops a pool of information drawn from students' own knowledge to which new textual information may be meaningfully related. Excellent sources for material appropriate in terms of content level, passage length, and reading difficulty are periodicals for school-age students. Two examples are *News for You* and *Current Science* (Table 1).

GOAL: To enable comprehension of written text by controlling the level of linguistic difficulty.

Procedure: Modify passages from classroom textbooks to reduce semantic and syntactic complexity while retaining age-appropriate content.

Abrahamsen and Shelton (1989) improved the comprehension and retention of textual information by students with language-related learning disabilities by making the following changes in reading passages: passive to active voice, perfect tense to simple past tense, clarification of anaphoric reference, elimination of relative clauses, and reduction of multimeaning words. (The original and altered passages may be found in the appendix to the chapter.

GOAL: To scaffold comprehension for children with language-related learning disabilities by providing all necessary external support.

Procedure: Scaffolding during reading aloud.

Norris (1989) described a bidirectional approach to reading and language intervention whereby the language of a text may serve as material for stimulating linguistic growth and the same procedures scaffold reading for meaning. In brief summary the procedures are as follows:

1. A passage of text is selected or prepared consisting of language students are capable of decoding but that presents comprehension problems because of syntactic or semantic content.
2. As the child reads the passage aloud, the speech-language pathologist listens for indications that the student is experiencing difficulty with some aspects of the language.
3. Feedback is provided to the child by either the adult or other students:
   Prompting inference by questions referring to prior text
   Pointing to a unit of text and providing a conceptual framework
   Providing a concrete interpretation of an abstract statement

Table 1.   Sources of periodicals for school-age students

Current Science
  Subscriber Services
  P.O. Box 16673
  Columbus, OH 43216

News for You
  New Readers Press
  Laubach Literacy Int.
  Box 131
  Syracuse, NY 13210

Providing a familiar synonym for an unfamiliar word

Summarizing information at a conceptual versus a factual level

The reader is referred to the paper by Norris (1989) for a detailed description illustrated by a sample transcript of the process.

GOALS: To stimulate active semantic and syntactic processing through use of contextual cues in the construction of sentence meanings.

Procedures: The Cloze procedure.

The Cloze procedure is useful in activating the linguistic knowledge possessed tacitly by all competent language users. Sentences are presented from which selected words are deleted (either every nth word, or content words, or function words). The adult or students in the group may read the sentences aloud, inserting a click or a tap to signal word deletion. Students fill in the gaps with candidate words (either from a multiple choice list or by free choice) and discuss reasons for word choices, invoking prior or subsequent textual context or world knowledge (A. Gerber, 1981; N.W. Nelson, 1988b).

It is here suggested that sentences used in initial stages of instruction contain everyday familiar material. After a measure of skill has been mastered, sentences may be drawn from curricular material (N.W. Nelson, 1988b). Scaffolding provided by group interaction may be gradually withdrawn, first by having pairs of children collaborate on filling in the blanks, and, subsequently, by having children work alone and compare their results after completion of a number of sentences.

GOAL: To foster top-down processing of expository prose by directing attention to organizational guides and words that signal structure.

Procedure: Text organizers.

Wallach and Miller (1988) have proposed the use of text organizers to heighten students' awareness of the macrostructure of the discourse before actually reading (or listening to) the text.

> Primary level organizers, such as title and major headings, are used as cues for making guesses about what the passage will be about.
>
> Secondary level organizers, such as major boldface headings, are used to confirm predictions about the gist of the passage.
>
> Tertiary level organizers, such as topic paragraphs, are used to update guesses or predictions at a level of more specific detail (p. 106)

Westby (1989) has suggested that students be made aware of key words that signal types of expository text organizations serving different functions. The following examples (p. 249) illustrate the process:

Type	Function	Key words
Sequence	How to do something	first, next, following
Cause-effect	Reasons for something happening	because, since, therefore, consequently
Comparison/contrast	How two things are the same or different	same, alike, however, on the other hand

Key words that signal organizational structure also function as one class of linguistic devices that establish cohesion among discourse elements (Halliday & Hassan, 1976; van Dijk, 1985). Children with language-related learning disabilities have been reported to be less proficient than normally achieving peers in processing cohesive devices (Liles, 1985, 1987).

GOAL: To foster understanding and effective processing of conjunctions.

The crucial role of various types of conjunctions in the processing of discourse meaning was stressed in Chapter 4. These terms must be understood if relations between the propositions they connect are to be comprehended.

Procedures: Paraphrasing, construction of conjoined sentences, conjunction identification.

1.   Present multiple instances of the occurrence of each of the selected conjunctions in spoken sentences. Model paraphrasing the sentences:

> A: Although he was uncomfortable, he fell asleep anyway.
> B: He was uncomfortable, but he fell asleep anyway.
> A: The votes were counted and subsequently the result were announced.
> B: The votes were counted, and afterward the results were announced.

2.   Follow procedure 1, but have students paraphrase.

3.   Present lists of conjunctions on which students have worked. Present lists of short sentences or clauses to be connected by the appropriate conjunctions. These may be written on cards or as sentence strips for students who would be more motivated by physical manipulation of the material, or on duplicated sheets for more mature students who are capable of performing the manipulation mentally. Examples of material are:

> Conjunctions: therefore, nevertheless, furthermore, in spite of, although, on the contrary, subsequently, accordingly, in addition
> Sentences:
> She read the instructions carefully./The dress fit perfectly.
> They studied all night./They failed the exam.
> Pay raises were deferred./Work hours were increased.
> We never took a penny./We actually contributed to the cause.
> He entered the campaign late./He was limited in funds.
> Students may say the conjoined sentences they have constructed, recording them on tape. On listening to their sentences on replay, students may evaluate the acceptability of their utterances and those of their peers.

4.   A speech may be written by the adult in which cohesive conjunctions occur with a reasonably high frequency. Copies of the speech are distributed to students. As the adult delivers the speech orally, students may follow the text and circle instances of the cohesive conjunctions, thus experiencing their use in connected discourse without demands for effortful decoding of printed text while engaged in processing meaning.

GOAL: To promote the students' active processing of textual meaning by establishing associations between pro-forms and referents.

Another type of cohesive device is anaphora—that is, reference to a previous element in a text by pronouns or pro-verbs. The most frequently encountered type of reference is the pronoun, which refers to a prior noun or noun phrase. At times there are multiple referents (e.g.,

"The Indians often brought the settlers food during the first year of colonization. *They* gave it to *them* throughout the long hard winter.") In some cases the referent for a pronoun is an entire proposition (e.g., "Immigrants to this country initially came predominantly from northern and western Europe. After that, there was a rapid influx from other areas.") (A. Gerber, 1981).

Procedures: Train students to actively identify referents for proforms through a succession of levels of difficulty.

One system for controlling levels of difficulty is as follows:

> Initially pronoun and referent are contained within the same clause:
> e.g., *Kangaroos* carry *their* babies in pouches.
> Next, the referent may be in one clause and the pronoun in another clause in the same sentence:
> e.g., *Mammals* produce milk with which *they* nurse *their* young.
> Subsequently, the pronoun and referent may occur in separate sentences:
> e.g., With *weasels and hares*, nature performs a minor miracle. By the time the first snow falls, *they* have replaced brown fur with winter white.
> Ultimately, the referent in a previous sentence may be an entire clause:
> e.g., It is estimated that *Europe lost over sixty million of its people by emigration* from 1815 to 1914. *This* was due to economic conditions and persecution. (A. Gerber, 1981, p. 189)

Pro-verbs, frequently encountered in the anaphoric use of *do* or *have*, can present problems for the student with language-related learning disabilities:

> A flower dies. When it *does*, the petals fall off. (A. Gerber, 1981, p. 190)
> He promised to mow the lawn. If he *doesn't* he gets no allowance.
> She said she would come by noon. If she *hasn't*, go alone.
> They planned to win. Because they *hadn't* there was no award.

Students may work in dyads, with one underlining an anaphoric pronoun or pro-verb and the other hunting for its referent and underlining it, drawing a connection between the two items. They may then substitute the referent for the proform in a paraphrase, thereby increasing their activity in comprehension of the meaning of the sentence or larger unit of discourse.

GOAL: To stimulate active, purposeful search of text for information in response to preposed questions.

Procedures: Preposing questions on material to be read.

Priming textual processing by preposed questions in advance of reading has been reported to be effective in fostering comprehension (Hoskins, 1990; Wallach & Miller, 1988; Wong, 1980, 1985; Wong & Jones, 1982).

Using a brief passage containing material that is high in interest and familiar in content, the adult may ask students to locate specified factual information. For example, in an article about Alfred Hitchcock in *News for You*, students may be asked to find out how many pictures he had made, what his first and last films were, and which one was his most famous movie, all in separate trials to avoid overload. After students report individual facts in response to preposed questions, the adult may model a paraphrased minisummary of the information. Following success at the factual level, students may be directed to locate information that requires some inferencing based on the text but drawing on knowledge outside the text (e.g., "When you read the next paragraph, think about what made Hitchcock's movies so popular.").

Students with language-related learning disabilities have been observed to be less inclined to "read between the lines" for complete comprehension—that is to "perceive and discern the causes, conditions, and consequences that are implied but not stated" (Wiig & Semel, 1984, p. 256). Preposing inferential questions has been reported to result in increased comprehension and learning from text (Hansen & Pearson, 1983).

GOAL: To promote textual elaboration through inferencing

Procedure: Development of an inferential set.

C.S. Simon (1980) has provided examples of nonacademic material for early stages of training in drawing inferences on the basis of perceptual information, logic, and evidence.

> Perceptual inference: "You notice as you drive by a church that a group of people are dressed in long gowns and tuxedos and that there is rice lying on the ground. Therefore, you infer _____."
>
> Logical inference: "California is bigger that Pennsylvania. Pennsylvania is bigger than Rhode Island. Therefore you infer _____."
>
> Inference from evidence: "Joe worked as a janitor at the bank. There was a bank robbery. Joe suddenly started flashing a lot of money. Therefore, you infer _____."

Another activity that may be fruitful in furthering the process of inferential thinking is the interpretation of cartoons. Although the given information is pictorial, the interpretation of accompanying verbal material frequently requires the drawing of inferences. The humor and the nonacademic nature of the material is likely to elicit ready participation in an activity not perceived as threatening. For example: "Dennis the Menace sneezed from putting too much pepper on his food. His mother heard him and made him go to bed. Why did she do that?" (A. Gerber, 1981, p. 207).

Wallach and Miller (1988) propose the following procedures for developing an inferential set:

> The adult reads part of a story aloud to the group. Students discuss aspects of the story that relate to their own personal experiences as a basis for making predictions about a character's behavior or reactions. Questions are then posed that stimulate inferencing about aspects of the story. Students write on strips of paper or discuss orally what they infer about actions and reactions of characters. The adult engages students in an effort to weave together their inferences into a unified text. Students then read or listen to the entire story and discuss ways in which their ideas were similar to or different from those in the text. If there are inferential questions at the end of the story, students may engage in discussion of the answers. (p. 127)

Thus, the process of inferencing is scaffolded by external support and optimal conditions for success.

Children's poetry that requires inference for interpretation may be read aloud by the adult and discussed by the group of students.

> The Acrobats
> I'll swing
> By my ankles
> She'll cling
> To your knees
> As you hang
> By your nose
> From a high-up
> Trapeze

> But just one thing please
> As we float through the breeze—Don't sneeze
> (Silverstein, 1974, p. 10)

After students have achieved success in group interaction, they may work independently on material appropriate for their reading level.

In Summary   Reading comprehension involves the active construction of meaning through complex interactions among top-down and bottom-up processes. Reading comprehension is further enhanced by the use of the metacognitive strategies of planning and monitoring, discussion of which is reserved for a subsequent section on strategy development.

Written Expression   According to Scinto (1986), written language not only entails higher cognitive functions, it fosters them. "If oral language forms the initial ground for the formation of mind and self, written language brings that initial development to a further plane of development" (p. 172). Vygotsky (1962) stated that the written monologue is the most elaborate and demanding form of speech, requiring deliberate thought and complex exact expression since "tone of voice and knowledge of subject are excluded" (p. 144).

It is not surprising, therefore, that written expression poses problems for students with language-related learning disabilities. The nature of these problems was reported in Chapter 7 and is here summarized as follows:

> Limited productivity, with less fluency in written than oral language.
> Limited stylistic repertoire, with tendency to use personalized narrative when expository prose is task appropriate.
> Limited options in syntactic variation, with limited elaboration of noun and verb phrases.
> Restricted vocabulary.
> Frequent errors in spelling, punctuation, and word omissions.

Goals and procedures in this section are directed at the first two problem areas; the latter three are addressed in sections devoted to word knowledge and metalinguistic skills.

The oral-written connection is particularly relevant to the development of productivity. As has been noted above, fluency and spontaneity are more characteristic of oral than written expression. Therefore, in accordance with principles recommended for application throughout intervention procedures, creation of optimal conditions for goal achievement with a high probability of success entails guiding students in a gradual progression from present levels of relative proficiency in the oral modality to levels in need of further development in the written modality.

GOAL: To effect a transition from oral discourse to written discourse while creating a positive attitude toward the act of writing.

Procedure: From an emergent literacy perspective, young children's natural inclination to communicate through some form of written expression is encouraged.

Children may write their own stories in their own way, using illustrations and inventive spellings, thus allowing for spontaneity free of concern for correctness by adult standards. Giving them ample opportunity to read their stories aloud grants them respect as authors.

The adult can write messages or dictate stories modeling mature language form. Children may be told that this is another way of writing. Those who are motivated to emulate more mature forms may be helped to construct words by scaffolding sound awareness and representation of sounds by letters. In this way, immature writers may be guided but not pushed toward the acquisition of more advanced levels (Scott, 1989; Sulzby et al., 1989)

It is suggested that attention may be drawn incidentally to conventions of writing in the adult's written messages—for example: *"it's* means *it is"* (Scott, 1989, p. 326). The adult may model use of such conventions as elementary punctuation: "I put a period here to show that this is the end of my first sentence." The period may be written in a different color in order to highlight it.

GOAL: To promote students' ability to take the perspective of the reader by providing all necessary information for message clarity.

Procedure: Modified barrier game.

The barrier game format may be modified to transmit messages in written rather than oral form. Students may be assigned partners. Each member of the pair draws a configuration of shapes on a concealed paper and then writes instructions for replicating the design. The instructional messages are exchanged. Each student reads the partner's message and follows the directions for replicating the design described. After executing the designs, members of the partnership compare designs and evaluate the written messages for clarity of instruction.

GOAL: To foster creative writing of narratives.

Procedures: The generation of written stories by older children may be supported by carrying over those procedures described above that are used to aid in oral narration.

Stewart (1985) recommended that story components, such as setting, problem, response, and outcome, be modeled by the use of examples from familiar stories. Nonexamples are presented as contrasts. Examples and nonexamples may be written on cards and given to students for sorting. For example, when the focus is on *setting*, a nonexample story part would not include information about a major character, place, or time.

The following steps for the development of story-writing skills provide support through the oral-written connection:

1. Adult reads a story aloud
2. Children discuss the story
3. Children dictate their own stories, either re-told or generated
4. Group composes lists of attributes of characters in a story heard or read
5. They may add or subtract attributes and create new characters
6. Children engage in sensory writing about settings, either in the present situation or other places at other times
7. Children discuss a story plot and suggest creative changes in events, characters, time and setting (Stewig, 1990)

Group discussions on topics of current interest or controversy among older students may foster a transition from oral to written expository prose:

1. The discussion may be tape recorded.
2. On replay of the recording, students may be guided to identify main points, which are written on the chalkboard.
3. Further analysis of the replay leads to organization of information subordinate to the main points. The adult and students jointly engage in constructing an outline of the discussion content.

4. From the outline, statements are generated by members of the group expressing ideas that
    cohere into paragraphs.
5. Alternate phrasing and/or terminology may be elicited by the adult or volunteered by mem-
    bers of the group for refining effectiveness of expression.
6. Upon completion of the group composition on chalkboard or easel, students may make their
    own individual copies.

Thus, applying the principle of scaffolding through provision of external support, the student
group and the adult engage jointly in what may also be viewed as a modeling of processes
leading to the construction of written composition under conditions that optimize success at a
stage of minimal competence.

Wallach (1990) has described procedures for capitalizing on adolescents' interest in and
knowledge about sports to motivate a transition from fluent oral discourse to written productivity:

1. Students engage in a conversation about a sporting event.
2. They then simulate a telecast reporting monologically, assuming viewer access to visual infor-
    mation that supplements commentary.
3. Subsequently they may give a radio sportscast of the event wherein information must be made
    explicit verbally without visual support.
4. Finally students may engage in sportswriting, making the transition from the oral to the writ-
    ten form.

GOAL: To effect transition from narrative to expository text composition.

Procedure: Guidance for producing written text at higher levels of abstraction.

The first two levels of discourse composition proposed by Moffett (1968) were employed
in the transition from sensory reporting to narration, described above in the example of the
science experiment with the candle and the inverted glass tumbler. This system of increasing
levels of abstraction progresses from *narration* to *generalization* and finally to *theorizing*. Extending the above example beyond the level of narrating how the effects of placing an inverted
tumbler over a lighted candle resulted in the extinguishing of the flame, guidance may be
provided to help students construct text at the higher levels of abstraction:

> *Generalization*—"From this demonstration it may be concluded that oxygen is needed
> for fires to burn."
>
> *Theorizing*—"In order to prevent fires from breaking out when oxygen is being used,
> smoking is prohibited in the vicinity."

A different classification of modes of discourse ranks them in the following order of increasing
processing demands: narration, description, exposition, and persuasion (Phelps-Terasaki,
Phelps-Gunn, & Stetson, 1983). Part of a suggested procedure for progress through these levels is as follows:

> Topic: loneliness
> Narration: Recount your loneliest moment to a friend
> Description: Describe a lonely person
> Exposition: Describe causes of loneliness
> Persuasion: Persuade your classmates that it is/is not worse to be a lonely teenager than a lonely old
>   person or a lonely young adult (Phelps-Terasaki et al., 1983, p. 378)

GOAL: To further development of skills in planning and generating content for written
composition.

Procedures: Construction of frameworks of discourse types, study of examples in selected passages.

For generating narrative content, a number of the procedures described above for character and plot generation may be useful. Planning for expository prose may be assisted by construction of frameworks for different types of discourse. Stewart (1985) has suggested four types of expository text most frequently encountered in children's textbooks and the kinds of guides that may be constructed during the planning of content:

> *Description* that focuses on characteristics or features of the main topic. Guides may be constructed with spaces to fill in attributes of shape, size, color, texture, etc. After relevant details are recorded the adult may model the use of the guide as a framework for constructing text.
>
> *Comparison-Contrast* that focuses on likenesses and differences among objects, events, and/or processes. Guides may be constructed to assemble lists of contrasting features. The adult may model construction of separate paragraphs for the discussion of the different dimensions.
>
> *Sequence* that presents steps or serialized ideas in a progression. Guides may be constructed that list the steps and the key words indicating serial order. The adult may initially model how this information may be expressed in composition form. In the composition process, students may consult their sequence guides for ordering of content.
>
> *Enumeration* relates a series of points to a specific topic. Outlines are useful guides for constructing and organizing ideas and their relationships. A variation of an organizing scheme is the construction of a "statement pie" consisting of a topic and "all the pieces of the pie" that support the main ideas. (Stewart, 1985, p. 356)

Other sources of support for the process of composition may be drawn from selected passages exemplifying identified patterns of rhetorical organization: statement of a problem and discussion of solutions, generalization followed by specific examples, and so forth. Students read the passages and prepare outlines of contents. Subsequently they give brief oral presentations from their outlines to either small groups or an entire class, receiving feedback from peers about the communicative effectiveness of the speech. An alternative to "public speaking" is individual tape recording of speeches, which may be listened to for self-evaluation and possible revision. Students may then write a transcription of the taped composition.

The need to integrate skills developed in remedial instruction to curricular material has been increasingly advocated (N.W. Nelson, 1981, 1986a, 1988b; C.S. Simon, 1987; Stewart, 1985).

GOAL: To apply compositional skills to academic functions such as report writing.

Procedure: Information charts.

As a class project, charts may be constructed containing all necessary material: on one axis categories of information and on the other axis sources of information. The adult supplies the topic and categories of information. Students provide information for the slots in the grid. When the chart is completed the students write a report using the category headings as topic sentences and subordinate data as supportive detail. Gradually, the adult supplies less of the information and students are responsible for providing increasing amounts (Stewart, 1985).

Summary   Following the scaffolding of adult modeling and group support, the above procedures may be used by individual students for independent construction of compositions. The foregoing goals and procedures have been designed to foster acquisition of basic composition skills for students with language-related learning disabilities. They have not addressed the refinements of style characteristic of more advanced writing competence. One aspect of such development is expanded word knowledge and flexible vocabulary usage. This is covered in the following section.

One final issue requires at least brief mention. The use of word processors or computers has been viewed with optimism as a facilitator of writing skills for students with learning disabilities. Bridwell-Bowles (1987) reported that preliminary evidence provides some tentative support for such a claim. Whether this is due to the use of a novel medium or whether the computer makes the act of writing and revising easier is not as yet clear. However, it does seem to allow students to write more, and this is judged as potentially beneficial (Bridwell-Bowles, 1987).

Word Knowledge and Word Retrieval

The literature reviewed in prior chapters provides substantial evidence of a relationship between the qualitative and quantitative dimensions of semantic knowledge and reading/writing proficiency and strategic learning. The following goals and procedures are aimed at fostering enrichment of semantic knowledge and enhancing its organization.

Word Meanings and Their Relationships   Traditionally, development in children's organization of word knowledge was characterized as a syntagmatic to paradigmatic shift (Crais, 1990). That is, given the stimulus word *dog*, children of kindergarten age tended to make an association such as *dog-bite*, where 8- to 10-year-olds would be more likely to make an associative response such as *dog-cat*. This phenomenon has been reinterpreted as a shift from event-based or episodic association to semantic organization (K. Nelson, 1977; Petry, 1977). This trend in conceptual and vocabulary development is believed to reflect decreased reliance on physical context (Petry, 1977). It has further been noted that introduction to educational activities such as categorizing, listing, and associating words fosters continued reorganization of the lexicon (Crais, 1990).

GOALS: To foster elaboration of word meanings and enrich associative pathways among word relationships.

Numerous activities have been recommended to foster categorization of words along a variety of dimensions, such as perceptual attributes, function, composition, location, and superordinate class (Wiig & Becker-Caplan, 1984).

Procedure: Sorting activities.

Training in the grouping of items on the basis of some underlying commonality may take a number of different forms at different levels. At the early level, the concept of item grouping and the understanding of the classification process may be more readily fostered by physical manipulation of familiar objects in sorting activities. These activities may consist of selecting out of a mixed array:

1. All items of the same identity (e.g., "Put all the blocks in the box.")
2. All items serving the same function (e.g., "Put all the things you eat with over here.")
3. All items sharing the same attribute (e.g., "Put all the blue blocks over here.")
4. All items found in a similar location (e.g., "Put all the things that belong in the kitchen over here.")

At more advanced levels, a category may be named, with students asked to supply instances of category membership (e.g., *transportation-train*) (Wiig, 1989). Instances of a class may be named, with students asked to supply the superordinate category label (e.g., a drawer, a cup, a box—containers) (A. Gerber, 1981). Material from magazine and catalogue advertisements may be grouped according to substance or function. Curricular texts may provide material for classification (e.g., illustrations of body parts in a biology text may be grouped according to function) (Wiig, 1989).

Another activity fostering categorization skills in the absence of perceptual support is a guessing game. The adult says:

"I am thinking of something that is clothing you wear in winter."
"I am thinking of something you cut with."
"I am thinking of something that grows in the ground."

Procedure: Semantic organizers.

A number of practitioners have developed procedures for the systematic organization of concepts and the language that represents relationships among concepts. Pehrsson and Robinson (1985) have provided an extensive range of materials that progress from levels appropriate for the young preschool child to those designed to enhance writing and reading skills in upper elementary and junior high school. Their semantic organizer approach directs its efforts at the acquisition of schematic knowledge in conjunction with increasing awareness of form that represents content. In describing the process of readying children for later performance with language in its written form, Pehrsson and Robinson (1985) stated:

> Activities involving the sequencing of activities and real experiences, as well as story telling and reading, are important readiness activities and bases for the future development of episodic organizers. However, long before the introduction of such organizers . . . children need to learn to categorize actions and things in relation to a given topic—categorization of subordinate comments or subtopics under a superordinate (major topic or idea). (p. 38)

It is worth noting that this approach, leading to eventual application of categorization of ideas, takes the process well beyond the all-too-frequent practice of limiting categorization to objects. Basing the methodology on the recognized need of young children to comprehend at the concrete level of real-life experience, the first stage in this approach engages preschool up to first-grade children in what the authors term *realia organizers*.

This procedure employs a large picture of a familiar real-life *activity*, such as a family eating a meal at a table. The adult presents a number of real objects, some of which are related to the pictured activity and at least one of which is not (e.g., a dish, a cup, a glass, a knife, and a car). Pieces of twine are available to connect the items related to the pictured activity. However, for the unrelated item (e.g., the car), the twine connecting it to the picture is overlaid with a cross-out piece that signifies negation or exclusion. This activity is first constructed by the adult; children direct and confirm the connections. Following the joint construction of the realia organizer, it is dismantled and reconstructed by the children without adult intervention.

Another phase of this approach is the collection of pictures of actions that are referents for verbs. Pehrsson and Robinson (1985) recommended both magazine pictures and the use of stick figure drawings (labeled Lollypop) performing various actions. Introduction to printed words is accomplished by the use of cartoon-like balloons in which are written single words depicting the pictured action (e.g., *Stand, Sit*). Verb organizers are constructed by connecting with pieces of twine pictures of people, animals, or objects that can perform the pictured action and an instance of exclusion (e.g., *run*) (boys, dogs, mice, but not fish).

A more advanced procedure for elaborating relations among words involves having children draw diagrams similar to those illustrated concretely above for representing elaborated meaning relationships for words and concepts. For example,

> *Toads*—written in a central rectangle to which lines are drawn connecting features such as *dry skin*, *live in water*, etc. with other features that are not characteristic (e.g., *jump far*) crossed out. (Pehrsson & Robinson, 1985, p. 83)

Other examples are weather, connected to a webbing of related words such as signs of change, types of storms, prediction, names of instruments for measuring and prediction (Baldwin & Henry, 1985), and guitar, printed in a concept ladder that represents features and other related words such as Kind of?—instrument, Parts of?—strings, and Made of?—wood, metal, plastic (Blanchowicz, 1986). Additional procedures include having students compare words on the basis of shared or contrasting features, such as "In what ways are a car and a boat alike? In what ways are they different?" (Wiig, 1989), and:

> Having students construct a grid composed of a list of related words on one axis (car, bike, motor cycle) and a list of attributes on the other axis (2-wheeled, motorized). Columns of + and − marks are entered to indicate presence or absence of attributes. (Crais, 1990, p. 57)

Extending Breadth and Depth of Vocabulary Knowledge   Expanding word knowledge and extending such knowledge from concrete to more abstract meanings is a concomitant of the language of literacy. Vellutino and Scanlon (1985) have called attention to the relationship between words with common derivations but at different levels of complexity or abstraction.

GOAL: To deepen understanding of word meanings by developing awareness of relationships between root words and derivations.

Procedure: Matching cards with root words and derivations.

For upper elementary grade or secondary school students, a small group activity may be conducted as follows. Cards are prepared on which words are written that share a common root, one word on a card:

mystery	mysterious
able	disability
know	knowledge
crime	criminal
spirit	inspire
mine	mineral
decide	decision
literature	illiterate
society	sociology
revere	reverent

The adult keeps the cards with the words in the left-hand column, and the other words are dealt to the students in the group. The adult turns up one of the words, reads it aloud, uses it in a sentence, and then asks who has a word that may be paired with the target word (e.g., "Able. I am able to walk, run, and jump"). The student who has the word "disability" places the card on the table and uses the word in a sentence. If the word match is acceptable, the student wins the pair. If the student is unable to use the word in a sentence, a model is provided by either the adult or another member of the group. After a model is provided, other members of the group may volunteer other sentences using the target word.

Multiple Meaning Words   Restricted word meanings may be one factor contributing to comprehension difficulty. While it is not possible to familiarize students with all words that have more than one meaning, exposure to the phenomenon of multimeaning words is a step toward the development of awareness that some words may look or sound alike but mean different things in different contexts.

GOAL: To attune students to the existence of multiple meaning words in order to facilitate flexibility in comprehension and production.

Procedure: Generating sentences for a designated number of meanings for a given word.

A set of cards is prepared on each of which is written a word with a number next to it that indicates the number of different meanings the word may have:

> bridge—4   (a span, a card game, a dental prosthesis, the verb "to close a gap")
> run—4   (move quickly, be a candidate in an election, a tear in a stocking, excreting moisture from the nose)
> bank—4   (place to keep money, border of a river, slope at a curve in a road, dependability ["you can bank on it"])
> fly—3   (moving through air, insect, a baseball hit)
> spring—4   (a season, a flow of water, an energetic leap, a tightly coiled wire)

A dyadic or group activity may be conducted in which a card is displayed and participants try to generate sentences using the word in different meanings until the designated number has been reached. If students are unable to generate sentences exemplifying all meanings, the adult may model a sentence for that meaning. Then group members may volunteer other examples.

Quantifiers and Qualifiers   Quantifying and qualifying terms convey important shadings of meaning in reading comprehension, understanding of test questions, and written expression. Students with language deficits may either fail to process these terms or process them imprecisely.

GOAL: To develop an awareness and understanding of subtle nuances in meaning through the use of quantifiers (Wiig, 1989) and adverbs of magnitude (Nippold, 1988a).

Procedures: Sorting objects using quantifiers, ranking by magnitude.

Using words such as *all, none, many, few, some, any, something, anything,* and *several,* younger children may be asked to first sort objects into groups. The adult may ask students to use the appropriate terms in stating which objects share or do not share common features (e.g., all of these are hard, some of these are round, a few of these have points) (Wiig, 1989).

Lists of adverbs may be presented to preadolescents and adolescents in conjunction with a rating scale. The list may contain words such as *slightly, somewhat, rather, pretty, quite, decidedly, unusually, very,* and *extremely* (Nippold, 1988a, p. 34). The adult reads aloud a brief passage, the last sentence of which contains a combination of an adverb of magnitude and an adjective it modifies. Three versions of the last sentence may be prepared (e.g., The weather in this part of the country seems to be changing. Last winter was extremely mild. Last winter was unusually mild. Last winter was quite mild.) Students assign a rating of 1 to 3 to judge relative degrees of magnitude among the adverbs. After each rating task is completed, students compare ratings and discuss agreements or disagreements among their judgments.

A somewhat different version of this task would have children arrange a group of related descriptors along a semantic gradient (e.g., from hottest to coldest: *cool, hot, lukewarm, boiling, freezing, tepid, cold*) (Blanchowicz, 1986, p. 647).

Vocabulary Expansion   It has been observed that the acquisition of new vocabulary throughout the school years and beyond tends to occur more readily from contextual abstraction than direct teaching of word meanings (Nippold, 1988a). However, in view of their impoverished world and word knowledge, children with learning disabilities may be at a disadvantage when new learning must be attempted on the basis of the surrounding context (Crais, 1990). In addition, less extensive exposure to the vocabulary input gained by skilled readers further contributes to impoverishment of world and word knowledge. Therefore, children with learning disabilities may require guidance in how to learn new words from context.

GOAL: To scaffold acquisition of new vocabulary in meaningful contexts.

Procedures: Story retelling, direct instruction, assessment of current knowledge, news story analysis.

New words may be presented in a story retelling activity. Crais (1990) found that focus on one novel word per practice story resulted in successful retention and use by the children in their retold stories.

Children may benefit from direct instruction about meaning of unfamiliar words in the context of curricular reading activities. For example, The student reads an unfamiliar word like *buffoon*. The adult may say, "*buffoon* means clown. Your teacher may become angry if you behave like the class buffoon. What does buffoon mean?" Students take turns giving the meaning (Pany, Jenkins, & Schreck, 1982).

Within the context of an announced topic during reading for information, children may be asked what they already know about the vocabulary encountered. The adult may ask, "From the words you know, what will this chapter be about?" (Blanchowicz, 1986, p. 646). Subsequently students may be engaged in *exclusive brainstorming*. The topic (e.g., Tropical Rain Forests) is written on the chalkboard. A group of less familiar words that might be encountered in the text is also written on the board (e.g., *foliage, avalanche, moisture, frigate, undergrowth, highrise*). Students are asked to indicate which words would *not* be likely to appear in a passage on this topic. Reference may be made to a dictionary for definitions of unknown words. For readers with disabilities, the activity would be scaffolded by the adult who assists in location of the word and by reading a clear-cut definition aloud. Students discuss why they would exclude particular words. Current word knowledge is then expanded and enriched from subsequent reading (and/or listening to) the text including the targeted vocabulary.

Material drawn from the newspaper has been used to develop vocabulary for sixth-, seventh-, and eighth-grade students in a remedial reading class (Laffey & Laffey, 1986) using the following procedures:

1.   An article of interest is selected.
2.   Unfamiliar vocabulary words are selected from the article and written on the chalkboard.
3.   The adult pronounces the words; students imitate pronunciation, then the adult explains meanings.
4.   The passage is read either individually (by the adult or a child, depending on reading proficiency) or in unison to provide support for the less proficient children.
5.   The meanings of the words are discussed by the group in the context of the material read.

6. Relations among words are identified and discussed in order to extend and strengthen connections in a semantic network.
7. In a follow-up writing activity, a paraphrase is constructed by the students using as many of the new vocabulary items as possible. For students whose resources may be overtaxed by such a task, the composition may initially be a joint venture between group members and the adult.

Synonyms   The following procedure is suggested to foster vocabulary expansion in terms of less commonly used synonyms, since these less familiar terms appear with increasing frequency in more advanced levels of written text. The example is designed at a level appropriate for preadolescent and adolescent students.

GOAL: To expand vocabulary for comprehension and flexibility of written expression through knowledge about different terms that express similar meanings.

Procedure: Substitution of synonyms for familiar words.

The adult tape records a brief passage of prose at a level well within the students' comprehension ability. After students have listened to the passage, the adult presents cards containing less familiar synonyms that can be substituted for a word in the final sentence (e.g., "Helen had studied hard for her history test. She had no problem answering most of the questions. However, the last question was a *little* tricky." [slightly, rather, somewhat]). A student records a repetition of the final sentence, substituting one of the less familiar terms. The tape is replayed to allow students to hear their own use of the more advanced items.

C.S. Simon (1980) has had children place synonym cards under related base words; for example:

stroll	glance	vacate
amble	peek	abandon
strut	gaze	depart
swagger	stare	desert
plod	glare	renounce

Subsequently, students read a brief passage and revise it by substituting synonyms:

A: The policeman walked around the property. He looked into doors and windows. Then he left.
B: The policeman strolled around the property. He peeked into doors and windows. Then he departed.

Other approaches to vocabulary and concept enhancement are suggested by Yoshinaga-Itano and Downey (1986), who recommended connecting new words to old schematic or scriptal knowledge. For example, a medical script may include the following elements, expanding from the known *doctor* and *nurse* to such terms as *needle/injection, medicine/prescription/ medication, drug store/pharmacy*, and so on. This approach can be helpful in aiding students to acquire the meanings of unfamiliar terms encountered in subject matter.

Figurative Language   Nippold and Fey (1983) found that, although on literal vocabulary tests there was no significant difference between preadolescents with and without histories of language difficulty, those with a history of language difficulty scored significantly lower than normally developing peers on comprehension of figurative language. Errors mostly consisted of assigning literal interpretations to metaphors. Nippold (1985) suggested that intervention in the area of figurative language is likely to be most appropriate for older children with language deficits—that is, those "whose difficulties with literal aspects of language have largely subsided, but who continue to experience difficulty with nonliteral meanings" (p. 3).

Types of figurative language include slang, sarcasm, idioms, metaphors, similes, and proverbs. Idioms express meanings in colorful ways that may reflect localized or obsolete customs (Nippold, 1991; Nippold & Fey, 1983). Metaphors may be predicative, consisting of one topic + one vehicle, or proportional, that is, two topics + two vehicles expressing analogic relations (Nippold, 1985). Similes are a variation of predicative metaphors containing the words *like* or *as* (Nippold, 1985). Proverbs are generally more difficult for younger children to understand (Nippold, 1985); they tend to be successfully interpreted by age 11–12 years (Wiig, 1989).

Some research reviewed by Nippold (1985) reported that similes were easier than metaphors for younger children to comprehend; others found no difference in children's comprehension of the two types of figurative language. Wiig (1989) reported that there is little direct evidence as to the order of acquisition of various types of metaphoric expression, but they have been observed to be produced spontaneously between 8 and 10 years of age. Some data reportedly exist that indicate developmental patterns in children's acquisition of double function terms (i.e., those interpreting physical attributes in psychological terms).

GOAL: To increase understanding of figurative language in a progression from literal to non-literal interpretations.

Procedures: Word selection, riddles, pairing, vignettes, advertisements, literature examples, presentation in context, matching.

A number of the following procedures have been abstracted from research reported by Nippold and Fey (1983) and recommendations by Nippold (1988a, 1991), Roth (1987), and Wiig (1989).

   1.   Children may be encouraged to select familiar words expressing physical attributes that may be used to express psychological attributes (e.g., *hard* for texture of a rock; *hard-hearted* for an uncaring person).

   2.   Examples of similarities between actions of different entities may be solicited from children in the form of riddles (e.g., "Which animal moves like a pogo stick?" Answer: *kangaroo*). Other riddles that incorporate humor along with figurative language may be shared among children (e.g., "How do you catch a squirrel? Climb up a tree and act like a nut.").

   3.   Pictures of objects may be presented that could be paired on either a literal or a metaphorical basis (e.g., *snake-river*. "The river wound like a snake. The river snaked through the valley.").

   4.   Pairs of words may be presented that lend themselves to construction of similes and metaphors (e.g., *eyes-diamonds, mouth-cave, wrestler-gorilla).*

   5.   A brief vignette may be presented with an incomplete ending. Students may select from choices of literal ending, figurative ending, or inappropriate ending. For example, "A gang of tough kids threatened to take Eric's football from him. But he was a track star. They couldn't catch him

   because he ran very fast."
   because he ran like the wind."

because he hung around the schoolyard."

. . . A discussion may be held to consider the relative communicative power of the literal and figurative language.

6. Students may collect similes and metaphors found in advertisements (e.g., Put a tiger in your tank [gasoline]; It's not a shoe. It's a machine [running shoes]).

7. Students and the adult may collect similes and metaphors found in literature. (e.g., "a glittering sleet of broken glass" [Updike, 1986, p. 59]). Adults and students may discuss the features shared between the figurative and literal terms.

8. Idioms are best understood in context. Nippold (1991) suggests reading a story that will contain an idiom at the end. Prior to reading the story the adult announces that it will contain an idiom (e.g., hold your tongues) and that questions will be asked at the end of the story about the meaning of the idiom. The series of questions probes the events and relationships that lead to an interpretation of the idiom. It is further recommended that several different stories that involve the idiom be presented over time in order to generalize the meaning of the idiom.

9. Proverbs may be presented in contexts that facilitate comprehension. For example, a sentence is presented followed by multiple choice interpretations:

A new broom sweeps clean.

a.   The new principal likes to coach the basketball team.
b.   The new principal likes to eat lunch with the students.
c.   The new principal fired all of the old teachers.

Following students' choices, the interpretation may be discussed in terms of the lexical items or relational terms in order to ensure that students have a clear understanding of the terms and their implications. For example:

A broom has fibers. When new, all fibers are of even length.
Therefore, all make contact with the floor, providing the best means of sweeping dirt
    away.
Who was the new broom?
Who was swept away?

After such discussion, the adult may model other applications of the proverb, followed by students' attempts. For example:

Adult: "The new president appointed all new members to his cabinet."
Student: "The new coach threw out all of the old defensive plays."

10. Proverbs may be presented along with literal interpretations in random order. For example:

Don't judge a book by its cover.	Children tend to be like their parents.
Strike while the iron is hot.	Don't delay when the time is right to act.
The leaf doesn't fall far from the tree.	Don't be deceived by outward appearances.

(A. Gerber, 1981, p. 207)

The figurative language is matched to its literal interpretations.

Word Retrieval   In light of the view that word retrieval difficulties in children with language deficits may be attributed to inadequate elaboration of meaning in the semantic network (Kail & Leonard, 1986; Wallach & Miller, 1988), it is recommended that an ongoing project for improving word retrieval accompany the above procedures for enriching word knowledge and expanding vocabulary.

GOAL: To improve speed and accuracy of word retrieval as a result of massed practice in recognizing and producing new vocabulary items.

Procedure: Practicing new vocabulary in spaced and timed trials.

Students may keep a cumulative record of new vocabulary words for each week. They may practice naming words in their list, using free or controlled association (saying all words that describe dwelling places of primitive people, all words associated with plant life in rain forests, etc.). In addition to recording accuracy of retrieval on repeated spaced trials, they may use a stopwatch to time their naming speed on repeated trials of naming pictures representing curriculum-associated terms (e.g., *tepee, lodge, igloo, yurt*). When retrieval is acceptably effortless, a new set of materials may be practiced.

Perceptual Representations and Semantic Knowledge   Although it is surmised that the above procedures designed to enrich semantic knowledge may help to ameliorate word-finding difficulties, it has been recognized that visual- and auditory-perceptual representations of words in the lexicon interact with semantic knowledge in word retrieval (Rubin & Liberman, 1983). On the assumption that such representations may be insufficiently precise or less clearly discriminated in entries of items in long-term storage by some children with word retrieval deficits, training in phonological analysis and visual imagery has been administered in experimental studies with apparent benefit (McGregor & Leonard, 1989; Wing, 1990). On the basis of these preliminary findings, it is here suggested that intervention aimed at fostering semantic enrichment be supplemented with training aimed at increasing the perceptual distinctiveness of items in the lexicon.

GOAL: To strengthen the bonds between perceptual representations and enriched semantic knowledge in order to facilitate word retrieval.

Procedure: Phonological analysis.

Displaying a set of pictures of related objects, the adult provides phonological cues to help children guess the selected target. For example:

> "Here are pictures of five animals (rhinoceros, kangaroo, elephant, hippopotamus, gorilla). I am thinking of one whose name has five syllables."
>
> "Here are some pictures of nine foods (chicken, ice cream, cereal, cheese, hamburger, lettuce, strawberries, watermelon, spaghetti). Find three foods whose names begin with the /s/ sound."
>
> "Here are pictures of a lot of different things. I will say something and you find a word that rhymes with what I have said."

Displayed items	Rhymed cues
clock	rock
chair	hair
kitten	mitten
rocket	pocket
fountain	mountain

Procedure: Visual imagery.

Presenting a stack of printed word cards, each of which represents an object that can be depicted as an image, the adult directs a child to select one card and keep the word concealed from other players. The child is then instructed: "Close your eyes and make a picture in your head of the thing that is written on the card. I will ask you questions about what it looks like. From your answers, we will try to guess what it is." Questions may be asked for eliciting detailed visual-perceptual information—for example:

"Is it long and thin?"
"Does it have a sharp point?"
"Is it made of plastic? (contrasting a ball point pen with a pencil)

"Is it fat?"
"Does it have horns?"
"Does it have a curly tail?" (contrasting a cow with a pig)

Procedure: Semantic cues

Beyond these procedures, research conducted by German (1986) suggests that certain situational contexts and structured task conditions are more facilitative to word retrieval:

It is easier to name a picture than to supply a word in a sentence completion task.
It is easier to retrieve nouns than verbs or superordinate category terms.

Most effective prompts for retrieval, including varied types (perceptual and semantic), are reportedly:

phonetic cues: It starts with a /ka/
semantic cues: It's not a peach, it's a _____.
multiple choice cues: It's either a banana, a cat, or a bowl.

Summary Theoretical foundations for practice in remediating word retrieval difficulties in children remain tenuous. The foregoing suggestions are viewed as exploratory. The principle underlying these procedures is the tentative assumption that such stimulation may foster growth in developing systems even in the presence of some intrinsic weakness.

Metalinguistic Skills

The material included in prior chapters attests to the role of heightened awareness of different aspects of language in the acquisition of literacy. Chapter 7 documents evidence of deficits in metalinguistic skills exhibited by students with language-related learning disabilities. Emerging literacy skills from early to middle childhood fall into three categories: word awareness, phonological awareness, and form awareness (i.e., syntactic and semantic well-formedness) (Tunmer & Cole, 1985).

Word Awareness A useful precursor to early reading is a heightened awareness of a word as a discrete element (Van Kleeck, 1990; Van Kleeck & Schuele, 1987). The development of such an awareness is believed to facilitate the beginning reading task of associating a spoken word with its written correspondent.

GOAL: To develop an awareness of a word as an identifiable entity in a string of words that form an utterance.

Procedures: Word supply and substitution.

> Children may be asked to "just say a little bit of sentence." For example (Fox & Routh, 1975):
> Tommy rode his bike.
> Tommy rode his _____.

Children may be asked to substitute one word for another in a form of word play. For example:

> The dish ran away with the spoon.
> The dish ran away with the fork.
> The dish ran away with the monkey.

Children may be asked to substitute nonsense words for real words. For example:

> A car has four pookies.
> A tree has lots of takas.

Phonological Awareness   "It has now become fairly well accepted that an important part of reading readiness is the development of a metalinguistic perspective that includes awareness of the sound system of a language, and the ability to manipulate it mentally" (N.W. Nelson, 1988b, p. 374). Evidence reported from review of research has provided support for a positive relationship between training in phonological awareness and reading achievement (Blachman, 1989). Although all of the complex processes of reading do not invoke or depend on phonological awareness, slow development in this area is widely believed to disrupt early reading success and to precipitate a host of interrelated deficiencies at higher levels of reading (Catts, 1989; Stanovich, 1986).

Blachman (1989) cited studies that report benefits in word decoding from training in:

1.   Phoneme deletion ("Say *ball*. Now say it again without the /b/.")
2.   Segmentation of a first sound in a syllable from the remaining portion or word ("Say *sss—at.*")
3.   Recognition of beginning and ending sounds in words and sound/symbol relationships, and ability to blend phonetically similar words
4.   Analysis of words into syllables and phoneme segments, followed by training in blending two- and three-phoneme units

Further examination of a number of studies revealed that trained phoneme awareness in conjunction with awareness of associated letters and letter strings produced higher reading and spelling scores than results of training on phoneme awareness alone or of no such training. Based on her review of the literature, Blachman (1989) has recommended the use of procedures to enhance phoneme awareness during the reading readiness stage and in formal beginning reading.

GOAL: To heighten perception of the sound segments in words.

Procedures: Sound identification, ear training procedures, sound/symbol association, rhyming, articulatory cue monitoring.

1.   Young children may be taught to move across a paper the appropriate number of disks to represent the sounds they have heard in words spoken by the adult. A word is modeled

in a drawn out fashion that allows the adult to place a disk for each sound on an arrow on the paper (e.g., *sssaat*). After placing three disks on the arrow to represent the phonemes in the word, the adult sweeps his/her hand across the three disks while repeating the word at natural speed. Children are then instructed to "say it and move it," performing the same task using their own disks. At a later stage, letters are printed on the disks (Blachman, 1989).

2.   The present author has found from teacher report that traditional ear training procedures used in articulation therapy have had beneficial effects on heightened awareness of sound segments in words for phonic decoding. Familiar descriptive labels are assigned to each sound prior to introduction of corresponding letter names. For example, the /m/ is called *the humming sound*; the /r/ is called *the growl sound*, and so forth. After bombarding the children with frequent repetitions of a labeled sound in some introductory story, simple CV or CVC words that start or end with the sound that may be pictorially represented on cards are uttered by the adult. When the adult produces a word starting or ending with the pictured sound, children signal their recognition of the sound by holding up their pictured symbol. After children become acutely attuned to the sounds occurring in words, the letter symbol and letter name may be paired with the pictured symbol.

3.   N.W. Nelson (1988b) recommended the following procedures. Children select a letter from an array to match an associated sound. They write the letter that represents the spoken sound. They say the sound usually indicated by a particular letter. They select written syllables and nonsense words that match a spoken pattern. They write syllables or nonsense words to match spoken sound patterns.

4.   Presented with a group of four pictures, children recognize the "odd man out;" that is, three pictured words rhyme and one does not. By introducing letters along with the sounds, the adult demonstrates that new rhyming words can be made by changing the initial consonant (Bradley & Bryant, 1985).

Included among the methods recommended by Ehri (1989) for support of instruction in phonics and spelling is training in the monitoring of articulatory cues to supplement and enhance auditory perception of sound segments.

GOAL: To intensify awareness of phonemic segmentation of words by heightening awareness of articulatory contacts and postures.

Procedures: Form-A-Sound cards, sensorimotor remediation.

Cohen and Schiller (1981) employed a set of Form-A-Sound[1] cards depicting the articulatory placement of target sounds in conjunction with labels that were descriptive of some aspects of sound production — for example:

p and *b*	lip popper
t and *d*	tip tapper
f and *v*	lip cooler
th	tongue cooler

Emphasis was placed on visual, tactile, and kinesthetic awareness of sound production, using mirrors and pantomiming productions for others to identify. In conjunction with recognition of

---

[1]Form-A-Sound cards are available from Ideal Educational Equipment Company, 20 W. Armat Street, Philadelphia, PA 19144.

sounds through production, corresponding graphemes were paired with the phonemes. In subsequent stages of the program, target sounds and sequences of sounds were represented in series of colored blocks for students to identify word-initial, word-medial, or word-final position of occurrence. These procedures were used with students in upper elementary and middle-school grades.

For the adolescent or adult with persistent dysphonetic problems, the present author has adapted a sensorimotor approach to remediation of articulation disorders (McDonald, 1964). Training is provided in identifying sounds by their articulatory contacts or constrictions of the vocal tract. The student produces designated single sounds and reports on the place and manner of sensed production (e.g., /k/—"the back of my tongue bumped the roof of my mouth"). After proficiency is reached at this level, pairs of consonant-vowel syllables are produced (e.g., *pa-la*) and place of contact is reported (e.g., "My lips touched and my tongue-tip touched the front of the roof of my mouth"). Syllable strings are gradually lengthened and made increasingly complex (e.g., *om-ki-tu, af-tuk*-lib). At first productions are imitated from an auditory model. Subsequently, letters representing the sounds are paired with the modeled configurations. Finally, bisyllabic and multisyllabic real words are analyzed in terms of articulatory contacts and corresponding letters.

Spelling   Although spelling does require phonological analysis skills, the process is not identical with that of reading. A distinction does exist between recognition in reading and recall in spelling. Gibson and Levin (1975) have pointed out that recall of sound-letter correspondence places greater demands in spelling than in reading, because redundancy in reading material allows for prediction and decoding on the basis of only partial processing of the visual display. In contrast, while spelling does require complete recall, it does not rely solely on the ability to encode phoneme/grapheme correspondences.

Most proficient spellers rely on both the auditory and visual channels for processing and recall of letter configurations. Poor spellers have been found to rely heavily on one or the other channel, failing to shift from one to the other as word patterns require (Bradley, 1983; Marcel, 1980). Some poor spellers identified as dyslexic have been found to have a deficit in the ability to store and access visual patterns in the lexical-semantic channel: they have also been found to be slower than proficient spellers in translating graphemes to phonemes (Seymour & Porpodas, 1980).

It is suggested that the visual deficit may reflect inadequate knowledge about the properties of letter configurations. It is also surmised that there may exist a short-term memory problem that causes difficulty maintaining dictated words for a long enough period to allow for encoding the complete phonemic string (M.M. Gerber & Hall, 1987). A possible connection between these two manifestations has been proposed by Seymour and Porpodas (1980): "The formation of visual word recognizers may be facilitated if an efficient phoneme-grapheme channel was available to assist the identification of words and to act as a short-term memory capable of retaining a durable and precise representation" (p. 469).

It has been suggested that the speech-language pathologist may be helpful in stimulating young children's awareness of the sound structure of words to undergird their attempts at graphemic representation in inventive spellings (Hoffman, 1990).

GOAL: To foster rudimentary awareness of sounds and their sequences in words by encouraging their graphemic representations in inventive spellings.

Procedure: Sound encoding using inventive spelling.

Ehri (1989) has recommended that children be encouraged to encode in letters the sounds they perceive in words. These inventive spellings, which may be phonetically accurate although conventionally inaccurate, are accepted by the adult as the children's way of writing at their present stage of development. (See Chapter 10 for discussion of emergent literacy.)

The adult may visually and auditorally model slightly exaggerated production of the sound segments in a word. Children emulate this mode of production and print the letters they believe correspond to sounds they hear, feel, and see (e.g., *BUDR*/butter; *SBUN*/spoon). In this way children use "their letter-name or letter-sound knowledge" (Ehri, 1989, p. 360).

GOAL: To foster the ability to contrast student error patterns with patterns of correct spelling.

It has also been recommended that the adult and the student engage in active analysis of error patterns that interfere with accurate communication between the writer and the intended reader (Hoffman, 1990).

Procedures: Imitation/Modeling.

M.M. Gerber (1986) has reported positive benefits for students with learning disabilities from repeated use of an imitation/modeling approach that provided corrective feedback. The adult first imitated student spelling errors and then modeled correct spelling. Lists were repeated under these conditions until 100% accuracy was achieved on these words. Subsequently other lists were presented consisting of words containing the same spelling patterns in minimally contrastive words. For example:

List 1	List 2
game	name
hide	side
lunch	hunch

(M.M. Gerber, 1986, p. 534).

The adult informed the students that knowledge of spellings in the first list would help their attempts at spelling words in the new list. Over repeated spelling dictation trials, subjects in the study presented evidence of attempts to organize spelling information derived from corrective feedback into more effective strategies for achieving spelling accuracy.

While the major responsibility for spelling instruction has traditionally rested with the classroom teacher, interdisciplinary collaboration between the educator and the speech-language pathologist is likely to produce benefits for children whose phonological awareness is inadequately developed. Furthermore, for children whose speech is phonologically immature or disordered, resort to written representations of words through spelling instruction has the possibility of stimulating development of a more mature phonological system (Hoffman, 1990).

GOAL: To foster awareness of the spelling relationships between root words and their more complex derivations.

Beyond phonology, the teacher and the speech-language pathologist may collaborate in joint efforts to expand word knowledge underlying spelling patterns.

Procedure: Root word highlighting.

A root may be presented at the beginning of a row or list of derived words. Students highlight the root in each member of the list.

medic   *medicine   medical   medicate   medicinal*
photo   *photograph   photographer   photography*

In the first example, children may recognize the vocalic value of the unstressed vowel *i,* spoken as schwa, because of knowledge of the spelling of the root word. The same process holds true for the unstressed *o* in the second example.

Additional Techniques   Through consultation between the teacher and the speech-language pathologist, lists of "demon" words may be accumulated and practiced in game-like activities both in the classroom setting and during small group or individual support sessions. Other remedial devices may include having students keep their own lists of troublesome non-phonetic words that they can consult as needed, thereby compensating to some degree for the visual memory deficit (Moran, 1987).

Development of Increased Awareness and Control of Syntactic Structure   A substantial body of evidence attests to the effectiveness of work on the manipulation and combination of sentence structures of increased complexity on the quality of spontaneous writing (Moran, 1987; N.W. Nelson, 1988a; Scott, 1989). "By increasing the familiarity and fluency of complex sentence patterns, writers are able to generate complex sentences with less burden on working memory; hence there are fewer mistakes" (Scott, 1989, p. 331).

There is also evidence suggesting the beneficial effects on reading comprehension of oral tasks requiring children to detect and monitor semantic and syntactic consistency in presented sentences (Wallach & Miller, 1988). Thus, skills in both reading and writing are apparently strengthened by bringing "implicit syntactic knowledge of the spoken language to bear upon the written language, which again requires the ability to reflect on the structured features of spoken language" (Tunmer & Cole, 1985, p. 302).

Sentence Manipulation   The manipulation of phrasal and clausal units is a strategy designed to intensify awareness of the structure of elaborated and/or complex sentences. By physically operating on written sentences, by motorically assembling, embedding, and permuting the syntactic components, the students' attention is directed to the existence of these structural segments, the relationships among them, and the options for flexible sentence construction.

GOAL: To promote facility in the construction of complex sentences containing relative clauses.

Relative clause constructions have been classified as either self-embedded sentences, wherein the relative clause modifies the subject of the main clause, or right-branching sentences, in which the relative clause modifies the object of the main clause. Wallach (1977) found that, for children 9 years of age or older, nonembedded sentences were easier to process than were embedded sentences. In expressive language, from late childhood through early adolescence, right-branching relative constructions predominate. That is, relative clauses are most frequently postmodifiers of sentence noun objects (Scott, 1988b) (e.g., "The neighbors invited the boy who lived next door to a party."). Less frequently used are center-embedded clauses modifying the subject noun (e.g., "The boy who lives next door invited the neighbors to a party."). Following the developmental pattern, it is recommended that intervention stimulate progress from processing right-branching to center-embedded relative clauses.

Procedure: Construction of sentences with relative clauses.

An enjoyable activity for younger children is the gradual accretion of the right-branching relative clauses in the well-known jingle "The House That Jack Built." Using oaktag strips on which the successive clauses are printed, children carrying the strips may additively construct the complete recursive sentence:

This is the house that Jack built.
This is the dog that lived in the house that Jack built.
(Embedding) That chased the cat.
(Embedding) That chased the rat.

Older children may be made aware of the communicative function of relative clauses; that is, the additional or qualifying information they provide. For example:

In the palace was much treasure.
In the palace was much treasure that the kings had amassed.

This treasure was spent on many things.
This treasure was spent on many things that ornamented the temple. (A. Gerber, 1981, p. 186)

To increase conscious awareness of the structure of relative clause sentences, children in middle to upper elementary school may actively perform the operations involved in their composition by substituting a relative pronoun for the noun that is duplicated in each of two main clause sentences. For maximal attention and active participation, children at the front of the classroom may hold and display word cards for each word in the two sentences to be merged into one. Another child is given a card on which appears a relative pronoun. This child removes a child holding the duplicated noun phrase, substitutes himself/herself in place of the removed noun phrase, and moves children in the second sentence into the first sentence where appropriate. For example:

Sentence 1: The boy brought home a dog.
Sentence 2: The boy had found a dog.
Sentence 3: The boy brought home a dog that he had found.
(right branching)

Sentence 1: The child was lost.
Sentence 2: The child cried for its mother.
Sentence 3: The child who was lost cried for its mother.
(embedded)

Higher level content may be used for older children and/or introduced after easier sentences are successfully manipulated:

Sentence 1: Sound waves strike the ear drum.
Sentence 2: The ear drum sends vibrations to the middle ear.
Sentence 3: Sound waves strike the ear drum which sends vibrations to the middle ear.
(right branching)

Sentence 1: The refugees moved away.
Sentence 2: The community had rejected the refugees.
Sentence 3: The refugees that the community had rejected moved away.
(embedded)

Another activity designed to foster growth in the processing of relative clauses involves shifting right-branching clauses to center-embedded clauses. Using sentence component cards containing a relative clause on a single card and other sentence constituents on individual cards, students physically move the clause strip from a right-branching, object-modifying position to a center-embedded, subject-modifying position. This operation may be performed only on sentences that can tolerate such shifts without resulting in semantic anomaly. For example:

> The audience applauded the performers *who had come from far and near*.
> The audience *who had come from far and near* applauded the performers.

> Astronauts gather information for astronomers *who are interested in outer space*.
> Astronauts *who are interested in outer space* gather information for astronomers.

For older students, word cards or sentence strips may be manipulated at a table or desk in small groups or dyads instead of moving children holding word cards as described above.

Procedure: Breaking relative clause sentences into simple components.

For upper elementary and secondary grade students the following complex sentences may be broken down into simple single-clause sentences by substituting a referent noun or pronoun for the relative pronoun:

> Sentence 1: The Delaware River Basin, which quenches the thirst of about seven million people, usually has an abundant water supply.
> Sentence 2: The Delaware River Basin quenches the thirst of about seven million people.
> Sentence 3: The Delaware River Basin usually has an abundant water supply.

> Sentence 1: Many of the buffalo who had taken refuge in the Yellowstone wilderness were killed by hunters who had followed the railroads west.
> Sentence 2: Many of the buffalo had taken refuge in the Yellowstone wilderness.
> Sentence 3: Many of the buffalo were killed by hunters.
> Sentence 4: Hunters had followed the railroads west.

Students may work in pairs, first performing the task independently and then comparing and discussing their work. It is recommended that the adult model the process before students attempt the task. Material progresses from sentences containing one main and one relative clause to sentences containing multiple clauses. In the latter case, performance may be supported by stipulating in advance the number of single-clause sentences that may be derived.

GOAL: To promote facility in the construction of complex sentences expressing temporal relations.

With regard to temporal relation sentences, the principle of order of mention/order of occurrence in main and subordinate clauses may be invoked in a progression of material from less to more demanding.

Procedure: Composing complex sentences with temporally related clauses.

The process of composing complex sentences from simple sentences may first be modeled along the following dimensions:

> *Two separate simple sentences*: Gold had been valued only for its beauty by the Incas. Gold became an object of greed to the Spaniards.
> Manipulating conjoined main clauses; main clause first and subordinate clause second (M^1S^2); subordinate clause first and main clause second (S^1M^2); order of mention (OM); order of occurrence (OO).

Two conjoined main clauses: First gold had been valued only for its beauty by the Incas, but then it became an object of greed to the Spaniards.

M^1S^2; OM = OO   Gold had been valued only for its beauty by the Incas before it became an object of greed to the Spaniards.

S^1M^2; OM = OO   After gold had been valued only for its beauty by the Incas, it became an object of greed to the Spaniards.

M^1S^2; OM ≠ OO   Gold became an object of greed to the Spaniards after it had been valued for its beauty by the Incas.

S^1M^2; OM ≠ OO   Before gold became an object of greed to the Spaniards, it had been valued only for its beauty by the Incas. (A. Gerber, 1981, p. 183)

The advantage of using preconstructed sentence strips that can be physically manipulated by students is twofold: 1) the activity is attention focusing and motivational, and 2) the unit being manipulated is experienced as a clausal entity rather than as a series of discrete words. This structural perception should have benefit for the word-by-word reader, who appears to process written language with little recourse to the linguistic knowledge applied to oral language structure, including the phonological suprasegmentation of prosodic juncture.

GOAL: To promote facility in the construction of complex sentences expressing disjunction.

Procedure: Composing complex sentences with disjunctive clauses.

Complex sentences encoding disjunctive relationships may undergo manipulation of main and subordinate clauses without the temporal phenomenon of order of occurrence.

Two separate sentences: The size and shape of rocks are changed as a result of mechanical weathering. The mineral content remains the same.

Two main clauses conjoined: The size and shape of rocks are changed as a result of mechanical weathering, but the mineral content remains the same.

M^1S^2 The size and shape of rocks are changed as a result of mechanical weathering, although the mineral content remains the same.

S^1M^2 Although the size and shape of rocks are changed as a result of mechanical weathering, the mineral content remains the same. (A. Gerber, 1981, p. 184)

Clausal manipulation may also be used to heighten sensitivity to subtle but important shifts in meaning nuances, further enhancing processing the decontextualized language of literacy. Activities requiring the transfer of information from main to subordinate clauses, and the reverse, may foster awareness of shifts in emphasis:

Speaker 1. Although much remains to be done, a great deal of progress has been made in the area of race relations.

Speaker 2. Although a great deal of progress has been made in the area of race relations, much remains to be done.

Question: Which speaker feels more strongly about the need to improve race relations?

Speaker 1. In the Middle East, negotiations will take place only if there is withdrawal from occupied territory.

Speaker 2. In the Middle East, withdrawal from occupied territory will take place only if there is negotiation.

Question: Which speaker is more insistent on negotiation? (A. Gerber, 1981, p. 198)

GOAL: To promote facility in the construction of complex sentences expressing conditionality.

Numerous situational and logical relations may be expressed in *if-then* sentences at varying levels of concreteness and abstraction. Material may be constructed with high interest/low complexity for early stages of intervention and progress to more abstract academic content at later stages or with more mature students.

Procedures: Composing complex sentences with conditional clauses, identifying conditional statements.

Pairs of *if-then* clauses may be written on cards and displayed in random order. Dyadic partners take turns, one picking a card from the *if* group and the other picking a suitable clause from the *then* group. For example:

If you play ball near the house	then you may break a window
If you're not at the corner by 8:00	then you will miss your bus
If it rains too hard	then the game will be postponed
If there is a prolonged drought	then salt sea water advances up the river
If taxes are reduced	then there is less money for education
If oxygen is used up	then the flame will go out

Textbooks may be searched for examples of *if-then* statements directly relevant to educational subject matter:

> If resistance of the air were disregarded, then bodies of different weights would fall at the same rate.
> *Questions*: Would bodies of different weights fall at the same rate under all conditions? Underline the condition in which this would be true.

> If Jupiter could hold four moons revolving around it while moving through the heavens, then, it was reasoned, the sun could hold the planets in place as they revolve in their orbits.
> *Question*: Underline the reason for accepting the belief that the sun could be the center of our planetary system.

GOAL: To foster the development of syntactic flexibility.

Procedure: Manipulation of complex sentences.

In the classroom, children holding large cards or oaktag strips on which sentence components are printed may be assembled at the front of the room. Other children holding other sentence components may add themselves to or embed themselves in the original sentence to increase its complexity. Then, in those cases in which elements may be moved, other children move children holding the component cards, creating as many variants of the original sentence as possible while preserving meaning. For example:

> Child 1 displays We are not allowed to watch TV
> Child 2 displays In our house
> Child 3 displays At night
> Child 4 displays Until we have finished our homework

The following versions may be constructed by having children move the movables:

1. We are not allowed to watch TV at night in our house until we have finished our homework.
2. In our house we are not allowed to watch TV at night until we have finished our homework.
3. Until we have finished our homework, we are not allowed to watch TV in our house at night.
4. At night, until we have finished our homework, we are not allowed to watch TV in our house.
5. At night in our house, we are not allowed to watch TV until we have finished our homework.
   (A. Gerber, 1981, p. 197)

An example of sentence components with more mature content suitable for such manipulation by older students is:

Although a cease fire had been declared
The fighting started again
In the Middle East
The day before yesterday

In the interest of conserving space, manipulation of the variant syntactic options of these components is left to the reader.

While initially material is used that controls for semantic and syntactic complexity, in later stages, material may be drawn from subject matter to permit guided experience in the formulation and reading of the types of sentences encountered in textbooks:

> The brown bear on the Alaskan peninsula has so far held his own against the invasion of the white man.
> So far, on the Alaskan peninsula, the brown bear has held his own against the invasion of the white man. (A. Gerber, 1981, p. 197)

After engaging in all of the above manipulation of complex sentences under decontextualized controlled conditions, students may be asked to construct contexts of larger units of discourse in such sentences (Wallach & Miller, 1988). For example, older students may be asked to write a passage on the situation in the Middle East, incorporating some of the sentences practiced.

Detecting and Correcting Errors   Violations of word order or word selection are relatively easy for children to detect and revise. Detection and correction of structural errors are considered more difficult. It is advisable to select patterns of errors requiring correction on the basis of observed students' performance (Wallach & Miller, 1988).

GOALS: To improve students' ability to detect and correct structural errors.

Procedure: Analyzing examples of structural errors.

Sentences taken from students' written work that exemplify omissions of word endings marking tense or plurality may be presented in written form to small groups of children. For example:

> The dog jumped up on the sofa even after I spank him for it.
> Be sure you lock all the door and windows when you leave.

The adult may tell the children that they are to play detective and find all places where a word ending has been omitted and to put it in. After they have finished the task as a joint effort, results are compared among groups. Children then read aloud the corrected versions.

At a more advanced level, sentences may be presented that exemplify types of syntactic errors that frequently occur in compositions by nonproficient writers. For example:

> *Lack of agreement between main subject and verb when separated by an embedded clause*: Most of the jobs that will be available is for stenographers and secretaries.
> *Failure to provide a subject after an introductory clause*: If a person graduated from high school and is going on to college should first know what his chances are for a job.

With the support of the adult, students may be guided to realize the need to monitor and sustain relationships between earlier and later sentence components. Reading such sentences aloud tends to heighten awareness of structural violations.

GOAL: To improve organization of written material by developing awareness and control of paragraph structure.

In writing, control of structure goes beyond the single sentence to the relationship of sentences in paragraphs.

Procedure: Construction of paragraphs from sentences.

Two paragraphs from textual material may be broken down into sentences, each of which is printed on a separate strip of paper. The topic sentence for each paragraph may be printed in a different color to highlight its function. The remaining sentences may be combined in random order and presented along with the topic sentences to pairs of students. For example:

> *Topic sentences*:
> In Colorado, more and more people are colliding with mountain lions.
> There is a problem with elephants in Botswana.
>
> *Sentences to be sequenced in the two paragraphs*:
> Last January, a mountain lion killed a jogger.
> Some people feel that no lions should ever be killed.
> Other people believe that lions should be hunted down wherever there is lion–human contact.
> The elephant population has grown from 40,000 to 67,000 in eight years.
> The elephants damage homes and crops.
> They drink the water needed by other animals and humans. (Sentences from paragraphs in *News for You*, Nov. 6, 1991, p. 21)

The students collaborate on arranging the sentence strips under the appropriate topic sentences in a logical sequence.

As suggested above in other procedures for heightening awareness and control of structure, the motoric manipulation of the components is designed to actively engage students who may be less motivated by traditional paper-and-pencil tasks. After the paragraphs are assembled by use of this highly concrete construction process, the students may write them in paragraph form.

Conclusion

It was stated early on in this chapter and emphasized in the preceding chapter that language intervention, to be effective, must be integrated with academic functions and curricular material. The aspects of language covered in this section represent potential problem areas. The examples of material provided in the suggested procedures have been merely illustrative. Selection of appropriate targets for intervention and appropriate materials must depend on collaboration between the classroom teacher and the language specialist. Only from such a collaborative effort can information be secured about curricular demands and student needs. Under optimal conditions, curricular materials may be modified to serve intervention purposes, and gains from structured intervention may be integrated into classroom performance.

DEVELOPING STRATEGIES FOR IMPROVED
PERFORMANCE IN LANGUAGE-BASED ACADEMIC TASKS

There is ample evidence, cited in Chapters 7 and 8, that students with learning disabilities tend to be passive and/or inefficient learners. Furthermore, the domain of relative inactivity appears to be in the use of language or language-related processes to enhance attention, perception, and memory. That is, students with learning disabilities seem deficient in the spontaneous use of such language-related strategies as verbal self-instruction to focus and maintain attention, verbal rehearsal, categorization, and other organizational methods facilitative to storage and recall of information. They have also been observed to be less inclined to activate schematic knowledge for the elaboration of information that is conducive to comprehension and memory. In this section, principles and examples of language-related strategies are provided that are designed to improve students' academic performance. They are divided into two categories: activating cognitive information processing mechanisms, and development of metacognitive skills.

Activating Cognitive Information Processing Mechanisms

Chapter 3 discussed the facilitative effects of verbally mediated processes on aspects of cognitive information processing. Extensive research on the benefits of strategies employing verbal mediation, clustering, and visual imagery has been conducted by the University of Kansas Institute for Research in Learning Disabilities. Their findings support the efficacy of training adolescents in the use of these learning strategies (Schumaker & Deshler, 1984).

This section presents examples of procedures designed to stimulate activation of verbal mediation strategies for enhancing attention to and memory for information related to academic tasks. Whereas the purpose of intervention in the previous section of this chapter was stimulation of growth in language knowledge, skills, and functions, procedures in this section are aimed at fostering the development of cognitive strategies instead of linguistic knowledge and skills per se. Nonetheless, these strategies are aimed at facilitation of effective *use* of language for enhancing task performance.

In Chapter 8 it was reported that many children with learning disabilities exhibit a tendency to process information in a less differentiated perceptual style. This tendency has been noted both in the inefficient and imprecise scanning of visual information and in lapses in the intake of auditory verbal information. The pattern of impulsivity has been frequently associated with unsystematic or inefficient search strategies and inadequate processing of information prior to responding. Studies by Egeland (1974) and Meichenbaum and Goodman (1971) have demonstrated the beneficial effects of training in self-instruction and in modeled scanning of critical features on the control of impulsive, inaccurate responses.

GOAL: To inhibit response impulsivity by fostering self-directed attention to critical visual and verbal detail.

Procedure: Scanning for critical details.

A series of stick figures containing both similar and differentiating features are drawn in duplicate on separate sheets of paper. The figures may differ along the following dimensions:

> on the head a hat, a bow, or a feather
> arms at the side or raised
> legs together or apart

One sheet is cut into separate figures while the other remains intact for display. The separate figures are arranged in random order, face down in a pile. The adult selects one item from the pile and searches for a match on the display of figures. The adult models verbalization of features to be scanned, touching a finger to relevant features on each figure until a match has been found. For example:

> "I'm looking for the one that has a bow on the head, arms at the side, and legs together. First I'm looking at the heads until I find a bow. I found one."
>
> "Then I'm looking at the arms of that figure. They are not at the sides. I'm looking for another figure with a bow on the head and arms at the sides. I found one."
>
> "Now I'm looking at the legs. They are together. I found a match. Now it's your turn."

Before the child begins the search, the adult may direct attention to critical details on the picture drawn from the pile by ticking off on the child's fingers each relevant feature to be searched (e.g., the head with a hat, arms raised, legs apart). The child is then encouraged to engage in verbal self-instruction in the search for a match.

When the child manifests evidence of employing the combined strategies of self-instruction and systematic search, and demonstrates an appreciation of the benefits of such strategies in successful outcome in a nonacademic activity, the strategies may be applied to an academic task. For example, at a middle-school level, the strategies may be invoked in a map scanning task. In social studies of the state of Pennsylvania, students may be asked to locate its two largest cities, Philadelphia and Pittsburgh, by searching for the convergence of two rivers and three rivers, respectively, while verbally directing the scanning process.

GOAL: To train students in the use of categorization in the storage and recall of information.

Procedure: Developing taxonomic organization strategies.

A study by Gelzheiser (1984) reported positive results from training adolescents to impose taxonomic organization during the study of prose material. Students first applied such categorization strategies in memorization of pictures, single words, and two-word phrases. They were taught the rules for studying taxonomically organized information: 1) sort to study, 2) study by groups, 3) name the group, and 4) cluster to recall.

Following demonstrated improvement in recall of pictures and words, students with learning disabilities applied the strategies to the study of prose passages with subtitles used as organizational cues.

Posttraining results demonstrated that students with learning disabilities performed as well as students without learning disabilities on the use of sorting and studying by the clustering of information. However, the *amount* of information recalled by subjects with learning disabilities was less than that recalled by subjects without such disabilities. It was conjectured that, in light of normal developmental patterns in spontaneous strategy use, the amount of experience individuals have had in using particular strategies may have an effect on the degree of efficacy with which those strategies are employed.

N.W. Nelson (1986b) observed that children with language disorders are less likely than other children to develop taxonomic organization strategies on their own and require many more examples before they are able to generalize the skill (p. 12).

GOAL: To stimulate spontaneous use of categorization as a strategy for organization and recall of information.

Procedure: Sorting or grouping items into categories.

Extensive experience may be given in sorting pictures of items from a mixed array into groups based on selected common properties, such as membership in a superordinate class (e.g., foods, toys), function (e.g., things that cut, things that write), composition (e.g., things made of wood, things made of metal), and so forth. Training may progress to having children supply names of items that belong to a class or supply additional items when the adult has named items without identifying the category. That is, the adult may name hippopotamus, algae, crab, minnow, and crocodile, requiring the child to supply another creature that lives in water (A. Gerber, 1981, p. 172).

Applying the skill of categorization to academic material is exemplified by N. W. Nelson's (1986b) report of a student who constructed a chart organizing information about *deciduous* and *coniferous* trees. The conceptual network was constructed at different levels of sub-classification, such as *broadleaf deciduous*, *broadleaf evergreen*, and *coniferous evergreen* trees (p. 12).

GOAL: To stimulate spontaneous use of the strategy of rehearsal in nonacademic memory tasks.

It will be recalled from Chapter 8 that children with learning disabilities tend to be delayed in their use of the active processing strategy of rehearsal as a mnemonic aid.

Procedure: Developing mnemonic strategies.

In a gamelike activity, series of pictures are displayed and then removed. Children earn points for the number of items they can remember. The adult then models rehearsal of the items before another set of stimuli is removed. Children then emulate the rehearsal process and compare the results with the prior number of points earned (A. Gerber, 1981, p. 170). Buttrill et al. (1989) have also recommended that older students study lists of words first without using the mnemonic strategy and then applying such strategies. "When contrasting the tasks, students quickly perceive how effective such strategies can be" (p. 192).

GOAL: To foster the use of categorization and rehearsal in the processing of textual information.

Procedure: Instruction in categorization and rehearsal of text.

For the elementary school child who is delayed in reading, the following set of procedures has been used to foster active processing of information in a text and to ensure successful reading experience. A first-grade reader is used containing pictured items in conjunction with limited, patterned textual language. The topic of the example presented here is *boxes*. The adult models memorizing material on each page by imposing categories upon the information:

> "The boxes on this page are made of different material."
> (Rehearsing) "Boxes are made of paper, wood, and cardboard.
> (To the child who is looking at the page) "Did I remember them all?"

On subsequent pages the adult models rehearsal and categorization as follows: "On this page there are three boxes that are long and skinny and one that is not." After the adult completes all the pages, the child is given the opportunity to emulate the use of the strategy for processing the information on each page by inspecting, categorizing, and rehearsing the pictured items. Then the child reads the material, which is by now familiar and meaningful.

GOAL: To train the strategies of visualization, organization, and elaborated rehearsal in the processing of text at the instructional level.

Procedure: Instruction in text processing strategies.

Applying the modeling of processing strategies to more advanced text may be facilitated through the coupling of oral tape-recorded passages with the simultaneous presentation of the printed version. While the child inspects the written passage, the tape-recorded passage is played, one sentence at a time. The adult turns off the recorder and models a visualization strategy for rendering the material meaningful. In conjunction with visualization, elaboration of information is modeled through the use of comparison, analogy, and categorical grouping:

> "I'm picturing a baby hedgehog as no bigger than my thumb when it's first born."
> "Now I get a picture of the baby hedgehog being fed by its mother, in just about the same way that other mothers nurse their babies."

In summarized review of content, the adult continues to model how information is stored and retrieved through organizational strategies:

> "First I have to think about how they look, their size, their color, and the feel of their quills." (Child checks accuracy of adult's paraphrased recall by inspecting text.)
> "Now I have to think about how they are fed."
> "Now I have to remember how they change as they grow."
> The adult comments in passing, "See how I'm grouping things that can go together to help me remember."

GOAL: To foster the use of categorization and rehearsal strategies for the study of curricular content.

Procedure: Grouping items by common attributes.

Following segments of subject matter presentation, students are guided to group items on the basis of designated common attributes. For example, in learning the names of the planets, students may be told to classify them according to nearness to or distance from the sun (i.e., those less than 200 million miles or those more than 200 million miles). Thus, in each classification, there are four or five names to remember, versus a total list of nine names (A. Gerber, 1981, p. 172). Students may then be given study time in which to rehearse the list as classified and subsequently perform a recall task to self-assess the efficacy of the use of the strategies. Repeated trials may be permitted in the absence of complete accuracy, with students adopting the active use of cumulative rehearsal to focus on items missed.

The Knowledge Base and Processing Strategies   It has been asserted in Chapter 3 that current theory posits a relationship between a well-developed knowledge base and the effective use of processing strategies. Within the framework of the above sections devoted to fostering both increases in linguistic knowledge and the use of active strategies, it should be acknowledged that "a well-developed knowledge base can completely supplant the necessity to use strategies" (Pressley, Johnson, & Symons, 1987, p. 84) or may contribute to the selection and use of the most appropriate strategies. However, for many individuals with learning disabilities, the knowledge base tends to be impoverished, thereby necessitating intervention to perform both of these complementary functions: expand the knowledge base *and* train the use of facilitating strategies.

Development of Metacognitive Skills

Throughout the past decade there has been a groundswell of theory and practice aimed at the development of metacognitive skills for the student with learning disabilities. Central to the design and implementation of metacognitive intervention are the concepts of *informed training* and *self-control training* (A.L. Brown & Palinscar, 1982). "Informed training involves instruction in the significance of the trained activity" (p. 5). Self-control training induces the student to engage in the executive skills of planning, checking, and monitoring their learning activity. "Self-control training can be regarded as an attempt to emulate more closely the activity of the spontaneous user of the strategy—the trained student is taught to produce *and regulate* the activity" (p. 6).

Running like common threads through most of the intervention aimed at training metacognitive strategies are the following requirements:

1. Explicit and elaborated instruction about the goals of strategies and their task applicability
2. Feedback about efficacy of strategy use in tasks performance
3. Training in monitoring the degree of task achievement resulting from the use of the strategy
4. Identification of the strategies used during task performance along with statements of the reason for their use

(Palinscar & Brown, 1987; Pressley, Borkowski, & O'Sullivan, 1984)

Increasing Text Comprehension   Three components of metacomprehension processes have been identified by Westby (1989): 1) planning what to read and how to read, 2) use of knowledge about cognitive processes, and 3) comprehension monitoring. A.L. Brown (1980) has further enumerated metacognitive processes involved in effective reading comprehension:

1. Understand the specific purpose of reading a particular passage.
2. Identify important ideas.
3. Focus attention on important versus trivial information.
4. Monitor to check on one's own comprehension.
5. Engage in self-questioning to determine whether planned goals are being achieved.
6. Take corrective action to repair failed comprehension.

GOAL: To improve reading comprehension through metacognitive training.

Procedures: Idea location, question prediction, and reciprocal teaching.

Wong and Jones (1982) trained junior high school students with learning disabilities to: 1) locate main ideas, 2) formulate questions about that information, 3) find the answers to their own questions, and 4) review the questions and answers. A prediction component was added to the above procedures. Some subjects were asked to locate and underline material that was considered important enough to be the subject of comprehension test questions. Over a period of four days of metacognitive training of subjects with learning disabilities, those subjects in the prediction condition demonstrated increasing effectiveness in predicting important idea units, recalled more information, and answered more comprehension questions correctly than controls in the nonprediction condition.

A reciprocal teaching approach devised by Palinscar and Brown (1986) has received widespread attention as a demonstrably effective means of activating metacognitive skills in text comprehension. Students and adult take turns assuming the teacher role. The following strategies are trained:

1. *Prediction*, requiring the activation of prior relevant knowledge in anticipation of subsequent information. This provides a purpose for reading, to confirm or disprove predictions. Active use of headings and text-embedded questions is promoted.

2. *Question-generation by students* stimulates more active information seeking than questions posed by teacher or text.

3. *Summarizing* of content within and across paragraphs fosters integration of text information.

4. *Clarifying* teaches students "who can be thought of as making a habit of not understanding" (Palinscar & Brown, 1986, p. 772) to be alert to comprehension barriers such as unfamiliar words, unclear reference, or new or complex concepts, and to reread or ask for help.

After training in the above activities, students and adult engage in a dialogue in which, initially, the adult models the use of the four strategies. Students are encouraged to interact by commenting on the teacher's summaries, adding predictions and clarifications and responding to teacher-generated questions. Gradually, there is a shift of responsibility to students for initiating and sustaining the dialogue, with continued scaffolding by the adult. As students gain proficiency in the use of strategies for comprehension and comprehension monitoring, scaffolding is withdrawn.

Results have been highly effective with adolescents and inner city middle-school children. They have enjoyed assuming the role of teacher. An alternative to adult-child pairing has been the pairing of higher achieving students with lower achieving students in reciprocal teaching. Results have demonstrated benefits for both tutee and tutor. The reciprocal teaching approach is also being applied to young nonreaders by stimulating comprehension of orally presented text. Results are promising in that active processing of oral information is fostered and "reciprocal teaching students are spontaneously engaging in discussion using the four strategies during reading group instruction as well" (Palinscar & Brown, 1986, p. 776).

GOAL: To heighten students' awareness of factors that interfere with comprehension.

Procedure: Detection of contradictions as a comprehension problem.

Children may be presented with a number of short stories in written form along with adult simultaneous oral reading. Each story contains a contradiction toward the end. Children are asked to suggest changes that would make the stories easier to understand (Tunmer & Cole, 1985).

GOAL: To foster self-detection and self-correction of reading errors.

Procedure: Evaluating errors as a comprehension problem.

Pflaum and Pascarella (1980) used a tape recorder to sample oral reading. Initially under adult guidance, students were induced to evaluate the effect of errors on comprehension. Gradually, responsibility for self-monitoring was shifted to the students, who kept a record of their own reading errors and self-corrections.

Monitoring Oral Communicative Effectiveness Research has reported frequent deficiencies in the self-monitoring of message clarity by children with learning disabilities and frequent failure by listeners in this population to recognize lack of precise comprehension (Bunce, 1991).

GOAL: To train speakers and listeners to evaluate the quality of their performance in referential communication.

Procedure: Message quality evaluation in the barrier game.

Bunce (1991) has reported beneficial results from training children with learning disabilities to evaluate the quality of messages spoken and received in the barrier game format. Pairs of children take turns at being speakers and listeners in giving and following directions for constructing configurations, drawing designs, or selecting described pictures from an array. Directions are tape recorded for later reference.

The crucial phase of the activity is the confrontation between speaker and listener when the barrier is removed and patterns are compared. In the event of a mismatch, speaker and listener evaluate the adequacy of the messages sent and received. Replay of the taped directions may be used to resolve disagreement. The outcome of such evaluative procedures is a heightened awareness of the need for and the means of achieving more precision and specificity in message formulation and reception. Subsequent turns allow the participants the opportunity to progressively improve self-monitoring during formulation of and listening to descriptive messages.

Metacognitive Processes in Written Composition   Basic or inexperienced writers "need to develop an awareness of their writing processes and of the dysfunctional strategies and rules that they use" (Greenberg, 1987, p. 36). Four aspects amenable to training for heightened awareness and control are the generation of ideas, organization of content, monitoring message clarity, and editing of the written product. Procedures for teaching organization were presented above and are not addressed here.

GOAL: To heighten students' awareness of the purpose for writing by exploration of ideas about the topic.

Procedure: Developing strategies for generation of ideas.

Greenberg (1987) has proposed that students ask and answer the following questions before initial drafting of a composition:

1.   What do I know about this topic?
2.   How do I feel about it?
3.   What experiences have I had with it and how have these experiences shaped my values and beliefs?
4.   What might I want to explain or show or prove about this topic? (p. 37)

It is apparent that this procedure is appropriate for older students and would need to be modified for use with less mature students. At any level, such activities as talking, reading, and thinking about a topic are conscious, deliberative strategies necessary for the generation of ideas (Greenberg, 1987).

GOAL: To foster awareness of reader perspective and needs for message clarity.

Procedure: Developing strategies for monitoring message clarity.

Following a reading of an initial draft, Moran (1987) has recommended that the adult ask students the following questions:

1.   What do you think your classmates know about your topic (or event)?
2.   What do you want them to know?
3.   Do they need more information or description? Where?
4.   What more do you know (or imagine) about this?
5.   Is there a spot that seems confusing or incomplete? (p. 46)

Peer reactions are also used to provide feedback about where the message is clearly conveyed or where further clarification is needed.

Among other procedures for self-regulation in the composition process, Graham and Harris (1987) reported on a procedure labeled with the acronym SCAN to be used in students' evaluation of sentence adequacy:

1. Does it make *sense*?
2. Is it *connected* to my beliefs?
3. Can I *add* more?
4. *Note* errors. (p. 72)

"Error recognition is an important aspect of writing. To be effective the writer must match conventional usage standards" (Phelps-Terasaki et al., 1983, p. 382).

GOAL: To guide students in the editing of their written compositions for detection and correction of errors.

Procedure: Developing strategies for editing written compositions.

It has been recommended that the students' search for errors be constrained to one designated segment at a time (Hull, 1987). In early stages of training, the focus may be placed on one category of error type at a time (Hull, 1987; Scott, 1989). For example, students may be directed to scan for omission of word endings or for misspellings. At this stage, feedback from the adult is needed to inform students about the degree of success attained in error detection and correction (Hull, 1987).

The use of different colored pens for highlighting specified error types has been suggested (Scott, 1989). This practice may help students to develop the important skill of recognizing characteristic patterns of error (Hull, 1987).

Reading one's own composition aloud slowly is likely to overcome the tendency to read in correct forms where errors actually exist (Scott, 1989). Peer proofreading has been found effective in heightening awareness of the occurrence of errors; it is usually easier to detect errors in other people's work than in one's own. During the process of proofreading a peer's writing, the student's sensitivity to error occurrence is likely to be enhanced to the point of improved self-monitoring for errors during the composition process.

Training Pragmatic Skills for Comprehension Monitoring   It has been observed that many children with comprehension impairments are less likely than normally achieving children to engage in comprehension monitoring (Dollaghan & Kaston, 1986) or in requests for clarification in the absence of comprehension (Brinton & Fujiki, 1982). It has been conjectured that such children are either less aware of the distinction between understanding and not understanding or less likely to take action to repair comprehension failure. These functions have been characterized as metacognitive skills (Dollaghan, 1987).

As discussed in Chapters 7 and 8, another view of these pragmatic and/or metacognitive deficiencies has attributed them to a metacommunication deficit; that is, either individual's doubts about their own ability to understand (Donahue, 1986) or insufficient awareness of message adequacy (Meline & Brackin, 1987). Studies of the failure to monitor comprehension have largely focused on the auditory rather than the written modality.

GOAL: To train students to make requests for clarification

Procedure: Developing ability to request clarification.

Dollaghan and Kaston (1986) exposed young children (age range 5;10–8;2 years) to messages requiring clarification because of any of the following attributes: inadequate acoustic signals, inadequate information, and excessive length and/or complexity. Under carefully controlled conditions, subjects were trained to: 1) identify message deficiencies, and 2) react to them by requests for clarification:

"Could you talk more slowly?"
"What do you mean?"
"Could you tell me in a different way?"
"That was too long for me."
"I don't know that word."

Results indicated that children so trained did learn the request for clarification strategies with relative ease and, according to anecdotal report, tended to generalize the use of requests for clarification to comprehension monitoring in school and at home. Need is acknowledged for further research on diverse groups of subjects with learning disabilities to determine the generalizability of such training to other members of the heterogeneous population of children with language-related learning disabilities.

Fey et al. (1988) have suggested the use of quasi naturalistic play contexts in which communication obstacles may be produced by the adult, followed by the modeling of requests for clarification. For example, in uttering a request for a tool during a construction activity, the adult may insert a cough that obscures the critical words, making the request unintelligible. If the child looks puzzled but does not request communication repair, the adult coaches the child: "You have to ask me, 'Get what?'"

In a modification of the barrier game ("over the shoulder") the adult may deliberately provide insufficient instructional information for the replication of a construction. When the child's performance is thus disrupted, the adult may prompt the child to request more information: "Ask me *which* sticker." Modeling adult responses to ambiguous or inappropriate directions by a puppet provides the opportunity to observe effective requests for clarification without direct first-hand involvement. Following such observation the child may be asked to assign blame for message inadequacy and even to analyze the factors causing comprehension failure.

The ultimate test of the efficacy of all such training is students' ability and willingness to engage in request for clarification behavior in the classroom. The degree of responsiveness of the classroom teacher to such requests is but one factor in the larger process of facilitating success through making compensatory adjustments to instructional and interactional aspects of classroom procedures.

MAXIMIZING CLASSROOM SUCCESS THROUGH COMPENSATORY ADJUSTMENTS

The foregoing intervention procedures have focused mainly on modification of the student's cognitive/linguistic information processing in efforts at promoting growth in areas of relative deficit. It must be recognized, however, that many students with learning disabilities continue to require ongoing modifications of the learning environment in order to minimize the likelihood of academic failure. Such modifications necessitate sensitivity on the part of the classroom teacher to conditions that exacerbate the language/learning problems of these students, leading to adjustments of those conditions in a direction facilitative to the students' ability to cope with performance demands.

Adjustment of Rate and Complexity of Language Processing

It is not this author's intent to equate the auditory language processing difficulties of the student having a language-related learning disability with those of adults with aphasia. Nevertheless, patterns described by Brookshire (1974) from his analysis of adult aphasics' processing of auditory verbal material may be suggestive of types of problems experienced by certain individuals with language-related learning disabilities, possibly similar in kind while vastly dissimilar in degree. Awareness of these patterns may attune the teacher to specific needs for adjustment in instructional style for individual students.

1. *Slow rise time* is demonstrated by individuals who tend to miss the initial part of auditory messages and tend to respond to the last part. Short commands may be missed entirely. It is suggested that this individual's system may require a longer time to shift from a passive to an active processing state, implicating a possible attentional component.
2. *Noise build-up* is inferred to be internal interference with message processing in terms of system overload, anxiety, or fatigue. In this type of problem, beginnings of messages appear to be processed adequately, with successive increments in complexity resulting in processing failure in later portions.
3. A *retention deficit* is apparently related to the length, not the complexity, of the message. It appears that comprehension is not the problem, but increases in the amount of material to be processed do result in poorer performance. A slightly higher incidence of error was found to occur in the middle and final segments of messages compared to those made in initial segments. Here memory span and processing strategies are apparently involved.
4. *Information processing deficit* is the term used to describe the apparent inability to receive and process information at the same time. Individuals with this deficit seem to take longer to process a unit of information than the normal listener. Therefore, while they are engaged in processing an earlier unit they miss the next incoming segment. They tend to respond correctly to first and last elements in a message and miss the middle part.
5. *Intermittent auditory imperception* is described as unexplained shifts between proficient and deficient performance as a result of some undetermined physiological or situational variables.

Information provided in previous chapters and sections underscores the need for teachers to "foster a better match between their talking and their students' listening (N.W. Nelson, 1986a, p. 25). It has also been recommended that students be encouraged to identify the factors contributing to their difficulty in processing of the oral language of instruction. For example, C.S. Simon (1985) identified the following factors:

> Information overload resulting from the density and amount of new material presented.
> Competition between the instructional message and distracting background noise.
> Difficulty processing questions because of excessive demands on memory.
> Unfamiliar vocabulary and concepts.

Lasky (1985) has suggested the use of a system labeled SPERS for analysis of other variables affecting students' comprehension and processing of information in the classroom:

> S—How competent is the student in receiving the language *signal*?
> P—Do variations in *presentation*, such as slowed rate, increased use of examples, or delay before being asked to respond, improve performance?
> E—Do *environmental* factors, such as group versus individual setting, background noise, or speech, adversely affect performance?
> R—Does *response* level determine adequacy of performance? That is, is comprehension

demonstrated under conditions requiring lower level responses, such as pointing, in contrast to higher level responses, such as explaining or comparing, etc.?

S—Does the student employ *strategies* to plan for and monitor comprehension, and for enhancing retention of material?

The frequently reported processing problems of those students with language-related learning disabilities are likely to be ameliorated by such adjustments in instructional style as:

1. Securing attention prior to delivery of messages
2. Slowing speaking rate and inserting pauses at appropriate clausal or phrasal boundaries
3. Reducing the length of instructional messages
4. Reducing the complexity and informational compression of instructional communication
5. Providing repeated opportunities to process the same information in verbatim or paraphrased form
6. Increasing "wait time" for question answering

Butler (1988) reported on a study by Rowe (1987) demonstrating the facilitating effects of extending the interval between questions and expected response from 1 to 3 seconds in terms of retrieval and elaboration of information by both slow and gifted children.

An example of the recommended adjustments that may be made to increase the probability of successful processing of auditory and written language of education is simplification and reduction of directions. In the direction samples below, version 2 is preferable to version 1:

1. "The answer to the question is found on the next-to-the-last line of the fourth paragraph on page 236."
2. "Turn to page 236." (Pause) "Find the fourth paragraph." (Pause) "Find the next-to-the-last line." (Pause). "Look for the answer." (A. Gerber, 1981, p. 162)

Another adjustment might involve simplification and reduction of textual language. For example, the teacher may restate textual passage 1 into version 2:

1. The earth is composed of a central core around which is a section called the blanket, which is then covered by an external crust.
2. "On the inside of the earth is the core, like the core of an apple. The crust is on the outside like the crust of a pie. Between the core and the crust is a layer called the blanket." (A. Gerber, 1981, p. 160)

This example not only includes reduction of length and complexity of sentences, but also contains exemplification of a process aimed at rendering decontextualized abstract language meaningful.

Scaffolding Meaningful Interpretation of Decontextualized Language

A number of sources cited in the foregoing sections of this chapter have attested to the difficulty experienced by many students with learning disabilities in interpreting the abstract or unfamiliar words and/or concepts encountered in the decontextualized language of education. Vygotsky (1962) contrasted what he termed *scientific* concepts with *everyday* concepts, the latter developing from a saturation of rich first-hand experience, whereas the former must be acquired vicariously. He stressed that the process of making scientific processes meaningful required relating these abstract scientific concepts downward to a more elementary, experientially concrete level. There are a number of ways of accomplishing this goal.

Hypostatization is a term used by Davidson (1976) to refer to the process of making high-level information comprehensible through the use of analogy and metaphor. It is maintained that, if explicit information is made sufficiently concrete, the ability to draw inferences is increased. The process may utilize nouns with high image value, found by C.T. James (1972) to be more easily recalled than low-image nouns. An example of hypostatization is:

> *Text* (scientific concept)   With changes in temperature, matter changes its state.

> *Hypostatized version*   When water in the kettle gets hot it turns to steam. The matter (water) has changed to another form. (A. Gerber, 1981, p. 163)

Visual imagery has been found to enhance the integration of information that has been read (Levin, 1976) and to facilitate performance on memory tasks (Levin & Allen, 1976). Pressley, et al. (1987) reported that effects reported by Levin were replicable, in that other research reviewed demonstrated benefits from representational imagery instruction. The following example demonstrates the application of imagery:

> *Text*   Mechanical weathering means that the form and size of rock changes but the chemical composition remains the same.
> *Visual Imagery*   Picture the rocks in a stream. See the big rocks being broken into small rocks. The small pieces are still made of rock. When they are banged against each other and worn by the movement of the water they change their size and shape. But what they are composed of does not change. (A. Gerber, 1981, p. 176)

Encouraging Requests for Clarification

The speech-language pathologist or resource room teacher may recognize the need of students with learning disabilities to seek clarification in instances of communication breakdown and to engage in systematic training of such behavior. However, N.W. Nelson (1986a) takes cognizance of the possibility of specialists inadvertently being at cross-purposes with the classroom teacher, who may expect students to listen and understand without the need for repetition. Interdisciplinary consultation and collaboration, the topic of Chapter 10, is indicated to resolve such potential conflicts. From the present perspective, whose central tenet is the prevention or reversal of the failure cycle, one of the goals of the classroom teacher would be the creation of a classroom atmosphere in which students feel free to ask for more information, request a rephrasing (Dollaghan & Kaston, 1986), buy time (e.g., "Could you come back to me on that?" (C.S. Simon, 1989), and so forth.

Alternative Processing Supports

Assistive devices have been increasingly made available for the older student. Particularly in the demanding task of taking notes on extended classroom lectures, tape recording reduces the requirement for rapid processing of transitory information whose content is usually extremely challenging for students whose verbal processing capacities tend to be overburdened under these decontextualized conditions. Wiig and Semel (1984) pointed out the benefit of such recordings for study and rehearsal of academic material. They also observed that the use of earphones during playback of recorded material may reduce the distraction of extraneous noise.

In addition to tape recorders, some institutions of higher learning maintain libraries of taped textbooks for students with special needs or make available scribes (note takers) and typing services (Blalock & Dixon, 1982). Two national resources for recorded texts are Recordings for the Blind, Inc., and the National Library Service for the Blind and Physically Handicapped (Table 2). To further foster academic success, methods of evaluating achievement may be modified to lessen the negative impact of disabilities on results. For example, some students with reading/writing disabilities may more effectively demonstrate subject mastery in oral rather than written examinations. Others may perform satisfactorily in writing under untimed testing conditions that reduce the stressful effects for performance by students who process verbal information more slowly.

Recordings for the Blind, Inc. maintains an extensive catalogue of textbooks, mainly for secondary school and college students. These are available to individuals certified as having learning disabilities. The National Library Service for the Blind and Physically Handicapped provides both recordings of popular leisure reading material and the equipment for its use. This service is provided to individuals with organically based learning disabilities as certified by a physician.

Analysis of Source(s) of Academic Language Difficulty

Gruenwald and Pollak (1975) have advanced suggestions for teacher analysis of the causes of students' failure in language-based educational tasks. They recommended systematic investigation of the students' possession of concepts involved in instructional language, comprehension of substantive and structural terms, and ability to process extended units of discourse consisting of multiple concepts. They urged interdisciplinary interaction between language specialist and classroom teacher to foster the teacher's ability to analyze not only the student's language processing difficulties, but the possible sources of difficulty in teacher language as well.

CONCLUSION

The introductory chapter presented accounts of historical trends and state-of-the-art descriptions of two separate fields: learning disabilities and language disorders. The topic and contents of this book, however, attest to a significant degree of convergence between specialized areas of these disciplines. It is apparent that, in serving the needs of students with language-related learning disabilities, interdisciplinary collaboration is of paramount importance. Therefore, inevitably, educators and speech-language pathologists share concerns about theory and practice.

The speech-language pathologist is not obligated to possess full knowledge about curriculum and pedagogical methodology, and the educator cannot be expected to be completely informed about the intricacies of language and its disorders. Yet each of these groups of professionals does have the obligation to seek sufficient knowledge in the allied field to permit an understanding of the phenomenon of language-related learning disabilities. It is hoped that this book has made a contribution to such an understanding.

Table 2. Sources of recorded texts

Recording for the Blind, Inc.	National Library Service for the Blind and Physically Handicapped
20 Roszel Road	The Library of Congress
Princeton, NJ 08540	1291 Taylor St. N.W.
(609) 452-0606	Washington, DC 20451
	(202) 882-5500

Appendix:
Reading Passages
of High and Low
Syntactic/Semantic Complexity

The following passages were used in a study by Abrahamsen and Shelton (1989). The material in Passage 1 was originally printed in a text by Eibling, Jackson, and Perrone (1977).

PASSAGE 1: ORIGINAL VERSION

The Gadsen Purchase

In the 1850s many people wanted a transcontinental railroad—one that would connect the East with the West coast. President Pierce wanted the route for such a railroad to run through the South. A survey was made to find the best southern route. The survey showed that this route went across some land in Mexico.

James Gadsen, our minister in Mexico, was asked to try to buy this land. In 1853 the Mexican government agreed to sell it for $10,000,000. The land is known as the Gadsen Purchase. With the Gadsen Purchase, the United States had acquired all the lands—except Alaska—which today make up forty-nine continental states.

The Gadsen Purchase was made with the plan of building the transcontinental railroad along a southern route. But not everyone was happy with this plan. Railroads were fast becoming the key to economic growth—and people knew it. Railroads had already greatly strengthened the economy of the Northeast. It was no surprise when people from different places started pushing to have the transcontinental railroad connect with their region. The strongest push came from Senator Douglas, who wanted the transcontinental railroad to begin in Chicago. (Eibling et al., 1977)

PASSAGE 2: MODIFIED TO REDUCE SYNTACTIC COMPLEXITY

The Gadsen Purchase

In the 1850s many people wanted a transcontinental railroad—one that would connect the East with the West Coast. President Pierce wanted the route for such a railroad to run through the South. President Pierce made a survey to find the best southern route. The survey showed that this route went across some land in Mexico.

The President asked James Gadsen, our minister to Mexico, to try to buy this land. In 1853 the Mexican government agreed to sell it for $10,000,000. The land is known as the Gadsen Purchase. The United States acquired all the lands except Alaska, which today make up forty-nine continental states with the Gadsen Purchase.

The United States made the Gadsen Purchase so the transcontinental railroad travelled along a southern route. But not everyone was happy with this plan. Railroads fast became the key to economic growth—and people knew it. Railroads strengthened the economy of the Northeast. It was no surprise when people from different places started pushing to have the transcontinental railroad connect with their region. The strongest push came from Senator Douglas, who wanted the transcontinental railroad to begin in Chicago. (Abrahamsen & Shelton, 1989, personal communication)

PASSAGE 3: MODIFIED TO REDUCE SEMANTIC COMPLEXITY

The Gadsen Purchase

In the 1850s many people wanted a transcontinental railroad—a railroad that would connect the Eastern part of the United States with the West Coast. President Pierce wanted the route for the transcontinental railroad to run through the South. A survey showed that the best southern route went across some land in Mexico.

James Gadsen, our ambassador to Mexico, was asked to try to buy this land. The Mexican government agreed to sell it for ten million dollars. The land is called the Gadsen Purchase. With the Gadsen Purchase, the United States had acquired all the lands—except Alaska—which today make up forty-nine continental states.

The Gadsen Purchase was made with the plan of building the transcontinental railroad along a southern route. This plan made some people happy and some people unhappy. People knew that railroads had strengthened the economy of the Northeast. People from many different places wanted to be on the route of the transcontinental railroad. Senator Douglas wanted the transcontinental railroad to begin in Chicago. (Abrahamsen & Shelton, 1989, personal communication)

References

Abrahamsen, E.P., & Shelton, K.C. (1989). Reading comprehension in adolescents with learning disabilities: Semantic and syntactic effects. *Journal of Learning Disabilities, 22,* 569–572.

Ackerman, B.P. (1985). Children's use of context and category cues to retrieve episodic information from memory. *Journal of Experimental Child Psychology, 40,* 420–438.

Adelman, H.S., & Taylor, L. (1982). *Learning disabilities in perspective.* Glenview IL: Scott, Foresman & Co.

Adelman, H.S., & Taylor, L. (1985). The future of the LD field: A survey of fundamental concerns. *Journal of Learning Disabilities, 18,* 423–427.

Adelman, H.S., & Taylor, L. (1986a). Moving the LD field ahead: New paths, new paradigms. *Journal of Learning Disabilities, 19,* 602–608.

Adelman, H.S., & Taylor, L. (1986b). Summary of the survey of fundamental concerns confronting the LD field. *Journal of Learning Disabilities, 19,* 391–393.

Adelman, H.S., & Taylor, L. (1986c). The problems of definition and the need for a classification schema. *Journal of Learning Disabilities, 19,* 514–520.

Alba, J.W., & Hasher, L. (1983). Is memory schematic? *Psychological Bulletin, 93,* 203–231.

Algozzine, B., & Ysseldyke, J.E. (1986). The future of the LD field: Screening and diagnosis. *Journal of Learning Disabilities, 19,* 394–398.

Alley, G., & Deshler, D. (1979). *Teaching the learning disabled adolescent: Strategies and methods.* Denver: Love Publishing Co.

Altwerger, B., Edelsky, C., & Flores, B.M. (1987). Whole language: What's new? *The Reading Teacher, 41,* 144–154.

American Psychiatric Association. (1980). *Diagnostic and statistical manual of mental disorders* (3rd ed.). Washington, DC: Author.

American Psychiatric Association. (1987). *Diagnostic and statistical manual of mental disorders* (3rd ed., rev.). Washington, DC: Author.

American Speech-Language-Hearing Association. (1990). Interdisciplinary approaches to brain damage. *Asha, 32* (Suppl. 2), 3.

American Speech-Language-Hearing Association Ad Hoc Committee on Language/Learning Disabilities. (1979). The role of the speech-language pathologist and audiologist in learning disabilities. *Asha, 21,* 1015.

American Speech-Language-Hearing Association Committee on Language Learning Disorders Report. (1989). Issues in determining eligibility for language intervention. *Asha, 31,* 113–118.

American Speech-Language-Hearing Association Task Force on Learning Disabilities. (1976). Position statement of the American Speech-Language-Hearing Association on learning disabilities. *Asha, 18,* 282–290.

Amidon, A., & Carey, P. (1972). Why five-year-olds cannot understand "before" and "after." *Journal of Verbal Learning and Verbal Behavior, 11,* 417–433.

Anderson, J.R. (1976). *Language, memory, and thought.* Hillsdale, NJ: Lawrence Erlbaum Associates.

Anderson, J.R. (1983). *The architecture of cognition.* Hillsdale, NJ: Lawrence Erlbaum Associates.

Anderson, J.R., & Reder, L.M. (1979). An elaborative processing explanation of depth of processing. In L.S. Cermak & F.I.M. Craik (Eds.), *Levels of processing in human memory.* Hillsdale, NJ: Lawrence Erlbaum Associates.

Andolina, C. (1980). Syntactic maturity and vocabulary richness of learning disabled children at four age levels. *Journal of Learning Disabilities, 12,* 372–377.

Andre, T., & Phye, G.D. (1986). Cognition, learning and education. In G.D. Phye & T. Andre (Eds.), *Cognitive classroom learning: Understanding, thinking and problem solving.* Orlando, FL: Academic Press, Inc.

Applebee, A.N. (1978). *The child's concept of story.* Chicago: University of Chicago Press.

Aram, D.M. (1991). Comments on specific language impairment as a clinical category. *Language, Speech, and Hearing Services in Schools, 22,* 84–87.

Aram, D.M., Ekelman, B.L., & Nation, J.E. (1984). Preschoolers with language disorders: 10 years later. *Journal of Speech and Hearing Research, 27,* 232–244.

Aram, D.M., & Nation, J.E. (1980). Preschool language disorders and subsequent language and academic difficulties. *Journal of Communication Disorders, 13,* 159–170.

Archer, P., & Edward, J.R. (1982). Predicting school achievement on data on pupils obtained from teachers: Toward a screening device for the disadvantaged. *Journal of Educational Psychology, 74,* 761–770.

Arffa, S., Fitzhugh-Bell, K., & Black, F.W. (1989). Neuropsychological profiles of children with learning disabilities and children with documented brain damage. *Journal of Learning Disabilities, 22,* 635–640.

Armstrong, S., Gleitman, L.R., & Gleitman, H. (1983). What some concepts might not be. *Cognition, 13,* 263–308.

Arter, J.A., & Jenkins, J.R. (1977). Examining the benefits and prevalence of modality considerations in special education. *Journal of Special Education, 11,* 283–298.

Arter, J.A., & Jenkins, J.R. (1979). Differential diagnosis—prescriptive teaching: A critical appraisal. *Review of Educational Research, 4,* 517–555.

Aslin, R., Pisoni, D., & Jusczyk, K.P. (1983). Auditory development and speech perception in infancy. In M. Haith & J. Campos (Eds.), *Carmichael's handbook of child psychology: Infancy and developmental psychology* (P. Mussen, General Ed.). New York: John Wiley & Sons.

Atkinson, R.C., Herrmann, D.J., & Wescourt, K.T. (1974). Search processes in recognition memory. In R.L. Solso (Ed.), *Theories in cognitive psychology: The Loyola symposium.* Hillsdale, NJ: Lawrence Erlbaum Associates.

Atkinson, R.C., & Shiffrin, R.M. (1971). The control of short term memory. *Scientific American, 225,* 82.

Austin, J.L. (1962). *How to do things with words.* Cambridge, MA: Harvard University Press.

Ayers, J. (1974). *The development of sensory integration theory and practice.* Dubuque, IA: Kendall/Hunt Publ. Co.

Backus, O.L., & Beasley, J.E. (1951). *Speech therapy with children.* Boston: Houghton Mifflin Co.

Baddeley, A.D. (1981). The concept of working memory: A view of its current state and probable future development. *Cognition, 10,* 17–23.

Baddeley, A.D. (1986). *Working memory.* Oxford: Clarendon Press.

Baer, D.M., Wolf, M.M., & Risley, T.R. (1987). Some still current dimensions of applied behavior analysis. *Journal of Applied Behavior Analysis, 20,* 313–327.

Baker, C.L. (1970). Syntactic theory and the projection problem. *Linguistic Inquiry, 10,* 533–581.

Baker, L. (1982). An evaluation of the role of metacognitive deficits in learning disabilities. *Topics in Learning and Learning Disabilities, 2,* 27–36.

Baker, L., & Brown, A. (1980). *Metacognitive skills and reading* (Tech. Rep. No. 188). Urbana, IL: University of Illinois, Center for the Study of Reading.

Bakker, D.J. (1992). Neuropsychological classification and treatment of dyslexia. *Journal of Learning Disabilities, 25,* 102–109.

Baldwin, L.S., & Henry, M.K. (1985). Reading and language arts: A design for integrated instruction. In C.S. Simon (Ed.), *Communication skills and classroom success: Therapy methodologies for language-learning disabled students.* San Diego: College-Hill Press.

Bandura, A. (1969). *Principles of learning modification.* New York: Holt, Rinehart & Winston, Inc.

Barrett, M., Zachman, L., & Huisingh, R. (1989). *Assessing semantic skills through everyday themes.* Moline, IL: Linguisystems.

Barrie-Blackley, S., Musselwhite, C.R., & Rogister, S.H. (1978). *Clinical oral language sampling: A handbook for students and clinicians.* Danville, IL: Interstate Printers and Publishers.

Barsch, R.H. (1968). *Enriching perception and cognition* (Vol. 2). Seattle: Special Child Publications.

Bartel, N.R., Grill, J.J., & Bartel, H.W. (1973). The syntagmatic-pardigmatic shift in learning disabled and normal children. *Journal of Learning Disabilities, 6,* 518–523.

Bartlett, F.C. (1932). *Remembering: A study in experimental and social psychology.* Cambridge, England: Cambridge University Press.

Bashir, A. (1973). *Error behavior and the reading process: Some germinal thoughts.* Cambridge, MA: Harvard University School of Education.

Bashir, A.S., Kuban, K., Kleinman, S.N., & Scavuzzo, A. (1983). Issues in language disorders: Considerations of cause, maintenance, and change. In J. Miller, D.E. Yoder, & R. Schiefelbusch (Eds.), *Contemporary issues in language intervention.* Rockville, MD: The American Speech-Language-Hearing Association.

Bassett, R.E., Whittington, N., & Staton-Spicer, A. (1978). The basics in speaking and listening for high school graduates: What should be assessed? *Communication Education, 27,* 300–307.

Bates, E. (1976). Pragmatics and sociolinguistics in child language. In D.M. Morehead & A.E. Morehead (Eds.), *Normal and deficient child language.* Baltimore: University Park Press.

Bates, E., & MacWhinney, B. (1987). Competition, variation and language learning. In B. MacWhinney (Ed.), *Mechanisms of language acquisition.* Hillsdale, NJ: Lawrence Erlbaum Associates.

Bauer, R.H. (1977). Memory processes in children with learning disabilities: Evidence of deficient rehearsal. *Journal of Experimental Child Psychology, 23,* 415–430.

Bauer, R.H. (1979). Memory, acquisition and category clustering in learning disabled children. *Journal of Experimental Child Psychology, 27,* 365–383.

Bauer, R.H. (1988). Toward a megatheory of learning disabilities. *Journal of Learning Disabilities, 21,* 230–232.

Benninck, C.D. (1982). Individual differences in cognitive style, working memory and semantic integration. *Journal of Research in Personality, 16,* 267–280.

Berko, J. (1958). The child's learning of English morphology. *Word, 14,* 150–177.

Berlin, L., Blank, M., & Rose, S.A. (1980). Language of instruction: The hidden complexities. *Topics in Language Disorders, 1,* 47–58.

Bernard-Opitz, V. (1982). Pragmatic analysis of the communication of an autistic child. *Journal of Speech and Hearing Disorders, 47,* 99–108.

Bernstein, D., & Tiegerman, B. (1989). *Language and communication disorders in children* (2nd ed.). Columbus, OH: Charles E. Merrill.

Berry, M.F. (1980). *Teaching linguistically handicapped children.* Englewood Cliffs, NJ: Prentice Hall, Inc.

Berry, M.F., & Eisenson, J. (1956). *Speech disorders: Principles and practices of therapy.* New York: Appleton-Century-Crofts, Inc.

Best, D.L., & Ornstein, P.A. (1986). Children's generation and communication of mnemonic organization strategies. *Developmental Psychology, 22,* 845–853.

Bever, T.G., Lackner, J., & Kirk, R. (1969). The underlying structures of sentences are the primary units of immediate speech processing. *Perception and Psychophysics, 5,* 225–234.

Bigler, E.D. (1987). Neuropathology of acquired cerebral trauma. *Journal of Learning Disabilities, 20,* 458–473.

Bjorklund, D.F., & Zeman, B.R. (1982). Children's organization and metamemory awareness in their recall of familiar information. *Child Development, 53,* 779–810.

Blachman, B.A. (1989). Phonological awareness and word recognition: Assessment and intervention. In A.G. Kamhi & H.W. Catts (Eds.), *Reading disabilities: A developmental perspective.* Boston: College-Hill Press.

Black, J.B. (1984). The architecture of the mind [Review of *The architecture of cognition*]. *Contemporary Psychology, 29,* 853–854.

Blagden, C., & McConnell, N. (1985). *Interpersonal language skill assessment.* Moline, IL: Linguisystems.

Blalock, G., & Dixon, N. (1982). Improving prospects for the college-bound learning disabled. *Topics in Learning and Learning Disabilities, 2,* 69–78.

Blanchowicz, C. (1986). Making connections: Alternatives to the vocabulary notebook. *Journal of Reading, 29,* 643–649.

Blank, M., & Marquis, M.A. (1987). *Directing discourse.* Tucson, AZ: Communication Skill Builders.

Blank, M., & Franklin, E. (1980). Dialogue with preschoolers: A cognitively-based system of assessment. *Applied Psycholinguistics, 1,* 127–150.

Blank, M., Rose, S.A., & Berlin, L.J. (1978). *The language of learning: The preschool years.* New York: Grune & Stratton.

Blank, M., & White, S.J. (1986). Questions: A powerful form of classroom exchange. *Topics in Language Disorders, 6,* 1–12.

Blashfield, R.K. (1993). Taxonomic models of possible relevance to the classification of learning disabilities. In G.R. Lyon, D.B. Gray, J.F. Kavanagh, & N. Krasnegor (Eds.), *Better understanding learning disabilities: New views from research and their implications for education and public policies.* Baltimore: Paul H. Brookes Publishing Co.

Blodgett, E., & Cooper, E. (1987). *Analysis of language of learning: The practical test of metalinguistics.* Moline, IL: Linguisystems.

Bloom, C.P. (1988). The roles of schemata in memory for text. *Discourse Processes, 11,* 305–318.

Bloom, L. (1970). *Language development: Form and function in emerging grammars.* Cambridge, MA: The M.I.T. Press.

Bloom, L., & Lahey, M. (1978). *Language development and language disorders.* New York: John Wiley & Sons.

Bloom, L., Lightbown, P., & Hood, L. (1975). Structure and variation in child language. *Monographs of the Society for Research in Child Development, 40*(Serial No. 160).

Bloome, D., & Knott, G. (1985). Teacher-student discourse. In N. Ripich & F.M. Spinelli (Eds.), *School discourse problems.* San Diego: College Hill Press.

Board of Trustees of the Council for Learning Disabilities. (1986). Measurement and training of perceptual and perceptual-motor functions (position statement). *Learning Disability Quarterly, 9,* 247.

Boder, E. (1971). Developmental dyslexia: Prevailing diagnostic concepts and a new diagnostic approach. In H.R. Myklebust (Ed.), *Progress in Learning Disabilities* (Vol. II). New York: Grune & Stratton.

Boehm, A. (1971). *Boehm Test of Basic Concepts.* New York: The Psychological Corporation.

Bohannon, J., & Hirsh-Pasek, K. (1984). Do children say as they are told? A new perspective on motherese. In L. Feagens, C. Garvey, & R. Golinkoff (Eds.), *The origins and growth of communication.* Norwood, NJ: Ablex Publ. Corp.

Bohannon, J., & Warren-Leubecker, A. (1989). Theoretical approaches to language acquisition. In J. Berko Gleason (Ed.), *The development of language* (2nd ed.). Columbus, OH: Charles E. Merrill.

Borden, G., Gerber, A., & Milsark, G. (1983). Production and perception of the /r/-/l/ contrast in Korean adults learning English. *Language Learning, 38,* 499–526.

Borkowski, J.G., Estrada, M.T., Milstead, M., & Hale, C.A. (1989). General problem-solving skills: Relations between metacognition and strategic processing. *Learning Disabilities Quarterly, 12,* 57–70.

Borkowski, J.G., Johnston, M.B., & Reid, M.K. (1987). Metacognition, motivation, and controlled performance. In S.J. Ceci (Ed.), *Handbook of cognitive, social, and neuropsychological aspects of learning disabilities* (Vol. 2). Hillsdale, NJ: Lawrence Erlbaum Associates.

Borkowski, J.G., Milstead, M., & Hale, C. (1988). Components of children's metamemory: Implications for strategy generalization. In F.E. Weinert & M. Perlmutter (Eds.), *Memory development: Universal changes and individual differences.* Hillsdale, NJ: Lawrence Erlbaum Associates.

Borkowski, J.G., Weyhing, R.S., & Carr, M. (1988). Effects of attributional retraining on strategy-based reading comprehension in learning disabled students. *Journal of Educational Psychology, 80,* 46–53.

Bos, C.S., & Filip, D. (1982). Comprehension monitoring skills in learning disabled and average students. *Topics in Learning and Learning Disabilities, 2,* 79–86.

Bow, J.N. (1988). A comparison of intellectually superior male reading achievers and underachievers from a neuropsychological perspective. *Journal of Learning Disabilities, 21,* 118–123.

Bower, G.H., & Cirilo, R.K. (1985). Cognitive psychology and text processing. In T.A. van Dijk (Ed.), *Handbook of discourse analysis. Vol. 1: Disciplines of discourse.* London: Academic Press.

Bowerman, M. (1973). Structural relationships in child utterances: Syntactic or semantic? In T.E. Moore (Ed.), *Cognitive development and the acquisition of language.* New York: Academic Press.

Bowerman, M. (1974). Development of concepts underlying language. In R.L. Schiefelbusch & L.L. Lloyd (Eds.), *Language perspectives—acquisition, retardation, and intervention.* Baltimore: University Park Press.

Bowerman, M. (1979). The acquisition of complex sentences. In P. Fletcher & M. Garman (Eds.), *Language acquisition: Studies in first language development.* Cambridge, England: Cambridge University Press.

Bradley, L. (1983). The organization of visual, phonological and motor strategies in learning to read and spell. In U. Kirk (Ed.), *Neuropsychology of language, reading, and spelling.* New York: Academic Press.

Bradley, L., & Bryant, P.E. (1978). Difficulties in auditory organization as a possible cause of reading backwardness. *Nature, 271,* 746–747.

Bradley, L., & Bryant, P.E. (1983). Categorizing sounds and learning to read: A causal connection. *Nature, 301,* 419–421.

Bradley, L., & Bryant, P.E. (1985). *Rhyme and reason in reading and spelling.* IARLD Monograph No. 1. Ann Arbor: University of Michigan Press.

Brady, S., Mann, V., & Schmidt, R. (1987). Errors in short-term memory for good and poor readers. *Memory and Cognition, 15,* 444–453.

Brady, S., Shankweiler, D., & Mann, V. (1983). Speech perception and memory coding in relation to reading ability. *Journal of Experimental Child Psychology, 35,* 345–367.

Braine, M.D.S. (1971). On two types of models of the internalization of grammars. In D. Slobin (Ed.), *The ontogenesis of grammar.* New York: Academic Press.

Brainerd, C.J., Kingman, J., & Howe, M.L. (1986). Long-term memory development and learning disability: Storage and retrieval loci of disabled/nondisabled differences. In S.J. Ceci (Ed.), *Handbook of cognitive, social, and neuropsychological aspects of learning disabilities.* Hillsdale, NJ: Lawrence Erlbaum Associates.

Bransford, J.D., & Franks, J.J. (1971). The abstraction of linguistic ideas. *Cognitive Psychology, 2,* 331–350.

Bransford, J.D., & Johnson, M.K. (1972). Contextual prerequisites for understanding: Some investigations of comprehension and recall. *Journal of Verbal Learning and Verbal Behavior, 11,* 717–726.

Bricker, W.A., & Bricker, D.D. (1974). An early language training strategy. In R.L. Schiefelbusch & L.L. Lloyd (Eds.), *Language perspectives: Acquisition, retardation and intervention.* Baltimore: University Park Press.

Bridwell-Bowles, L. (1987). Writing with computers: Implications from research for the language impaired. *Topics in Language Disorders, 7,* 78–85.

Briggs, M.H., & Chan, S. (1987). *Leadership development curriculum.* Unpublished manuscript, UAP Center for Child Development and Developmental Disorders. Children's Hospital, Los Angeles.

Brinton, B., & Fujiki, M. (1982). A comparison of request-response sequences in the discourse of normal and language-disordered children. *Journal of Speech and Hearing Disorders, 47,* 57–62.

Brinton, B., Fujiki, M., & Sonnenberg, E.A. (1988). Responses to requests for clarification by linguistically normal and language-impaired children in conversation. *Journal of Speech and Hearing Research, 53,* 383–391.

Brinton, B., Fujiki, M., Winkler, E., & Loeb, D.F. (1986). Responses to requests for clarification in linguistically normal and language-impaired children. *Journal of Speech and Hearing Disorders, 51,* 370–377.

Broadbent, D.E. (1958). *Perception and communication.* New York: Pergamon Press.

Brookshire, R.H. (1974). Differences in responding to auditory verbal material by adult aphasics. *Acta Symbolica, 5,* 1–18.

Brown, A.L. (1975). The development of memory: Knowing, knowing about knowing, and knowing how to know. In H.W. Reese (Ed.), *Advances in child development and behavior* (Vol. 10). New York: Academic Press.

Brown, A.L. (1979). Theories of memory and the problems of development: Activity, growth and knowledge. In L.S. Cermak & F.I. Craik (Eds.), *Levels of processing in human memory.* Hillsdale, NJ: Lawrence Erlbaum Associates.

Brown, A.L. (1980). Metacognitive development and reading. In R.J. Spiro, B.C. Bruce, & W.F. Brewster (Eds.), *Theoretical issues in reading comprehension.* Hillsdale, NJ: Lawrence Erlbaum Associates.

Brown, A.L., Bransford, J.D., Ferrara, R.A., & Campione, J.C. (1983). Learning, remembering, and understanding. In P.H. Mussen (Ed.), *Handbook of child psychology.* New York: John Wiley & Sons.

Brown, A.L., & Palinscar, A.S. (1982). Inducing strategic learning from texts by means of informed self-control training. *Topics in Learning and Learning Disabilities, 2,* 1–18.

Brown, E.K. (1974). *Cognitive mechanisms of children exhibiting learning disabilities.* Paper presented at the International Symposium on Learning Disabilities, Miami Beach. (ERIC Document Reproduction Service No. ED 097 406)

Brown, G., Anderson, A., Shillcock, R., & Yule, G. (1984). *Teaching talk: Strategies for production and assessment.* Cambridge, England: Cambridge University Press.

Brown, H.D. (1971). Children's comprehension of relativized English sentences. *Child Development, 42,* 1923–1936.

Brown, R. (1957). Linguistic determinism and the parts of speech. *Journal of Abnormal and Social Psychology, 55,* 1–5.

Brown, R. (1973). *A first language: The early stages.* Cambridge, MA: Harvard University Press.

Brown, R., & Hanlon, C. (1970). Derivational complexity and the order of acquisition in child speech. In J. Hayes (Ed.), *Cognition and the development of language.* New York: John Wiley & Sons.

Bruck, M. (1986). Social and emotional adjustments of learning disabled children: A review of the issues. In S.J. Ceci (Ed.), *Handbook of cognitive, social and neuropsychological aspects of learning disabilities.* Hillsdale, NJ: Lawrence Erlbaum Associates.

Bruck, M., & Hebert, M. (1982). Correlates of learning disabled children's peer interaction patterns. *Learning Disability Quarterly, 5,* 353–362.

Bruner, J.S. (1964). The course of cognitive growth. *American Psychologist, 19,* 1–15.

Bruner, J.S. (1975). From communication to language. *Cognition, 3,* 255–287.

Bryan, T., Bay, M., & Donahue, M. (1988). Implications of the learning disabilities definition for the regular education initiative. *Journal of Learning Disabilities, 21,* 23–28.

Bryan, T., Donahue, M., & Pearl, R. (1981). Learning disabled children's peer interactions during a small group problem solving task. *Learning Disability Quarterly, 4,* 13–22.

Bryan, T.H., & Bryan, J.H. (1978). Social interaction of learning disabled children. *Learning Disability Quarterly, 1,* 33–38.

Bryden, M.P. (1982). *Laterality: Functional asymmetry in the intact brain.* New York: Academic Press.

Bryen, D.N. (1981). Language and language problems. In A. Gerber & D.N. Bryen, *Language and learning disabilities.* Baltimore: University Park Press. (Reprinted in Gerber, A., & Bryen, D.N. [1981]. *A speech-language pathologist's guide to language and learning disabilities.* Phoenix: RCL Publications.)

Bryen, D.N., & Gerber, A. (1981). Assessing language and its use. In A. Gerber & D.N. Bryen, *Language and learning disabilities* (pp. 115–158). Baltimore: University Park Press.

Bunce, B.H. (1989). Using a barrier game format to improve children's referential skills. *Journal of Speech and Hearing Disorders, 54,* 33–43.

Bunce, B.H. (1990). Bilingual/bicultural children and education. In L. McCormick & R.L. Schiefelbusch (Eds.), *Early language intervention: An introduction* (2nd ed.). Columbus, OH: Charles E. Merrill.

Bunce, B.H. (1991). Referential communication skills: Guidelines for therapy. *Language, Speech, and Hearing Services in Schools, 22,* 296–301.

Burke, D., Worthley, J., & Martin, J. (1988). I'll never forget what's-her-name: Aging and the tip of the tongue experience in everyday life. In M.M. Gruneberg, P.E. Morris, & R.N. Sykes (Eds.), *Practical aspects of memory: Current research and issues.* New York: John Wiley & Sons.

Bush, W.J. (1976). Psycholinguistic remediation in the schools. In P.L. Newcomer & D.D. Hammill (Eds.). *Psycholinguistics in the schools.* Columbus, OH: Charles E. Merrill Publ. Co.

Bush, W.J., & Giles, M.T. (1969). *Aids to psycholinguistic teaching.* Columbus, OH: Charles E. Merrill Publ. Co.

Butler, K.G. (1984). The language of the schools. *Asha, 26,* 31–35.

Butler, K.G. (1988). *The language of instruction.* Paper presented at the annual convention of the American Speech/Language/Hearing Association, Boston.

Buttrill, J., Niizawa, J., Biemer, C., Takahashi, C., & Hearn, S. (1989). Serving the language learning adolescent: A strategies-based model. *Language Speech and Hearing Services in Schools, 20,* 185–203.

Byrne, B. (1981). Deficient syntactic control in poor readers: Is a weak phonetic memory code responsible? *Applied Psycholinguistics, 3,* 201–212.

Calfee, R., Lindamood, P., & Lindamood, C. (1973). Acoustic-phonetic skills and reading—kindergarten through twelfth grade. *Journal of Educational Psychology, 64,* 293–298.

Calfee, R., & Sutter-Baldwin, L. (1982). Oral language assessment through formal discussion. *Topics in Language Disorders, 2,* 45–55.

Calvert, M.B., & Murray, S.L. (1985). Environmental communication profile: An assessment procedure. In C.S. Simon (Ed.), *Communication skills and classroom success: Assessment of language-learning disabled children.* San Diego: College Hill Press.

Cambourne, B.L., & Rousch, P.D. (1982). How do learning disabled children read? *Topics in Learning and Learning Disabilities, 2,* 59–68.

Campbell, S., & Whitaker, H. (1986). Cortical maturation and developmental neurolinguistics. In J.E. Obrzut & G.W. Hynd (Eds.), *Child neuropsychology: Theory and research* (Vol. I). Orlando, FL: Academic Press.

Campbell, T.F., & McNeil, M.R. (1985). Effects of presentation rate and divided attention on auditory comprehension in children with an acquired language disorder. *Journal of Speech and Hearing Research 28,* 513–520.

Canale, M. (1983). On some dimensions of language proficiency. In J.W. Oller (Ed.), *Issues in language testing research.* Rowley, MA: Newbury House.

Cantwell, D.P., & Baker, L. (1991). Association between attention deficit–hyperactivity disorder and learning disorders. *Journal of Learning Disabilities, 24,* 88–95.

Caplan, B., & Kinsbourne, M. (1982). Cognitive style and dichotic asymmetries of disabled readers. *Cortex, 18,* 357–366.

Carbo, M., Dunn, R., & Dunn, K. (1986), *Teaching children to read through their individual reading styles.* Reston, VA: Reston Publishing Co.

Carey, S. (1978). The child as word learner. In M. Halle, J. Bresnan, & G.A. Miller (Eds.), *Linguistic theory and psychological reality.* Cambridge, MA: The MIT Press.

Carey, S. (1982). Semantic development: The state of the art. In E. Wannner & L.R. Gleitman (Eds.), *Language acquisition: The state of the art.* Cambridge, England: Cambridge University Press.

Carlberg, C., & Kavale, K. (1980). The efficacy of special versus regular classroom placement for exceptional children: A meta-analysis. *Journal of Special Education, 14,* 295–309.

Carnine, D., & Woodward, J. (1988). Paradigms lost: Learning disabilities and the new ghost in the old machine. *Journal of Learning Disabilities, 21,* 233–236.

Carroll, J.B. (1961). Fundamental considerations in testing for English proficiency of foreign students. In *Testing the English proficiency of foreign students.* Washington, DC: Center for Applied Linguistics.

Carrow, E. (1973). *Test of Auditory Comprehension of Language.* Hingham, MA: Teaching Resources Corp.

Carrow-Woolfolk, E., & Lynch, J.I. (1982). *An integrative approach to language disorders in children.* New York: Grune & Stratton.

Cartelli, L.M. (1978). Paradigmatic language training for learning disabled children. *Journal of Learning Disabilities, 11,* 313–318.

Carver, C.S., & Scheier, M.F. (1981). *Attention and self-regulation: A control-theory approach to human behavior.* New York: Springer-Verlag.

Catts, H.W. (1986). Speech production/phonological deficits in reading-disordered children. *Journal of Learning Disabilities, 19,* 504–508.

Catts, H.W. (1989). Phonological processing deficits and reading disabilities. In A.G. Kamhi & H.W. Catts (Eds.), *Reading disabilities: A developmental language perspective.* Boston: College Hill Press.

Cazden, C.B. (1988). *Classroom discourse: The language of teaching and learning.* Portsmouth, NH: Heinemann.

Ceci, S.J. (1982). Extracting meaning from stimuli: Automatic and purposive processing of the language-based learning disabled. *Topics in Learning and Learning Disabilities, 2,* 46–53.

Ceci, S.J. (1984). A developmental study of learning disabilities and memory. *Journal of Experimental Child Psychology, 38,* 352–371.

Ceci, S.J., & Baker, J.G. (1987). How shall we conceptualize the language problems of learning disabled children? In S.J. Ceci (Ed.), *Handbook of cognitive, social and neuropsychological aspects of learning disabilities.* Hillsdale, NJ: Lawrence Erlbaum Associates.

Ceci, S.J., & Baker, J.G. (1989). On learning . . . more or less: A knowledge x process x context view of learning disabilities. *Journal of Learning Disabilities, 22,* 90–99.

Ceci, S.J., Ringstrom, M., & Lea, S.E.G. (1981). Do language-learning disabled children have impaired memories? In search of underlying process. *Journal of Learning Disabilities, 14,* 159–162.

Cermak, L.S., & Moliotis, P. (1987). Information processing deficits in children with learning disabilities. In H.L. Swanson (Ed.), *Advances in learning and behavioral disabilities: Memory and learning disabilities.* Hillsdale, NJ: Lawrence Erlbaum Associates.

Chall, J.S. (1989). *From language to reading and reading to language.* Paper presented at the American Speech-Language-Hearing Association's National Forum on Schools—Partnership in Education: Toward a Literate America, Washington, D.C.

Chaney, C. (1990). Evaluating the whole language approach to language arts: The pros and cons. *Language, Speech, and Hearing Services in Schools, 21,* 244–249.

Chapman, K.L., & Terrell, B.Y. (1988). Verb-alizing: Facilitating action word usage in young language-impaired children. *Topics in Language Disorders, 8,* 1–11.

Chappell, G.E. (1980). Oral language performance of upper elementary school students obtained via story reformulation. *Language Speech and Hearing Services in Schools, 11,* 236–251.

Chappell, G.E. (1985). Description and assessment of language disabilities in junior high school students. In C.S. Simon (Ed.), *Communication skills and classroom success: Assessment of language-learning disabled students.* San Diego: College Hill Press.

Cherry, C. (1953). Some experiments on the recognition of speech with one and with two ears. *Journal of the Acoustical Society of America,, 25,* 975–979.

Cherry, R., & Kruger, B. (1983). Selective abilities of learning disabled and normal children. *Journal of Learning Disabilities, 16,* 202–205.

Chomsky, C. (1976). After decoding: What? *Language Arts, 53,* 288–296.

Chomsky, N. (1957). *Syntactic structures.* The Hague: Mouton.

Chomsky, N. (1959). A review of Skinner's "verbal behavior." *Language, 35,* 26–58.

Chomsky, N. (1965). *Aspects of the theory of syntax*. Cambridge, MA: The MIT Press.

Chomsky, N. (1968). *Language and mind*. New York: Harcourt, Brace & World Inc.

Chomsky, N. (1975). *Reflections on language*. New York: Pantheon.

Chomsky, N. (1980). Language without cognition. In M. Piattelli-Palmarini (Ed.), *Language and learning: The debate between Jean Piaget and Noam Chomsky*. Cambridge, MA: Harvard University Press.

Chomsky, N. (1981). *Lectures on government and binding*. Dordrecht, Holland: Foris.

Christensen, S.S., & Luckett, C.H. (1990). Getting into the classroom and making it work! *Language, Speech, and Hearing Services in Schools, 21,* 110–113.

Cirilo, R.K. (1981). Referential coherence and text structure in story comprehension. *Journal of Verbal Learning and Verbal Behavior, 20,* 358–366.

Clark, E.V. (1983). Meanings and concepts. In P.H. Mussen (Ed.), *Handbook of child psychology* (4th ed.). New York: John Wiley & Sons.

Clark, H.H., & Clark, E.V. (1968). Semantic distinctions and memory for complex sentences. *Quarterly Journal of Experimental Psychology, 20,* 129–139.

Clark, H.H., & Clark, E.V. (1977). *Psychology and language: An introduction to psycholinguistics*. New York: Harcourt Brace Jovanovich.

Clements, S.D. (1973). Minimal brain dysfunction in children. In S.G. Sapir & A.C. Nitzburg (Eds.), *Children with learning problems*. New York: Brunner/Mazel.

Cohen, C.K., & Schiller, J.S. (1981). Group training of auditory processing skills. In A. Gerber & D.N. Bryen, *Language and learning disabilities* (pp. 295–304). Baltimore: University Park Press.

Collins, J.T., & Hagen, J.W. (1979). A constructivist account of development of perception, attention and memory. In G.A. Hale & M. Lewis (Eds.), *Attention and cognitive development*. New York: Plenum Press.

Connell, P. (1986). Teaching subjecthood to language-disordered children. *Journal of Speech and Hearing Research, 29,* 481–492.

Connell, P.J. (1988). Induction, generalization, and deduction: Models for defining language generalization. *Language Speech and Hearing Services in the Schools, 19,* 282–291.

Conrad, R. (1972). Speech and reading. In J.F. Kavanaugh & I. Mattingly (Eds.), *Language by ear and by eye*. Cambridge, MA: The MIT Press.

Cooley, E.J., & Ayers, R.R. (1988). Self-concept and success-failure attributions of nonhandicapped students and students with learning disabilities. *Journal of Learning Disabilities, 21,* 174–178.

Cooney, J.B., & Swanson, H.L. (1987). Memory and learning disabilities: An overview. In H.L. Swanson (Ed.), *Advances in learning and behavioral disabilities: Memory and learning disabilities*. Greenwich, CT: JAI Press.

Copeland, A.P.A., & Reiner, E.M. (1984). The selective attention of learning disabled children: Three studies. *Journal of Abnormal Psychology, 12,* 455–470.

Copeland, A.P.A., & Wisniewski, N.M. (1981). Learning disability and hyperactivity: Deficits in selective attention. *Journal of Experimental Child Psychology, 32,* 88-101.

Corsale, K., & Ornstein, P.A. (1980). Developmental changes in children's use of semantic information in recall. *Journal of Experimental Child Psychology, 30,* 231–245.

Corsaro, W.A. (1981). The development of social cognition in preschool children: Implications for language learning. *Topics in Language Disorders, 2,* 22–95.

Costello, J.M. (1983). Generalization across settings: Language intervention with children. In J. Miller, D.E. Yoder, & R. Schiefelbusch (Eds.), *Contemporary issues in language intervention*. ASHA Reports 12. Rockville, MD: The American Speech-Language-Hearing Association.

Cotugno, A.J. (1987). Cognitive control functioning in hyperactive and nonhyperactive learning disabled children. *Journal of Learning Disabilities, 20,* 563–567.

Cowan, N. (1984). On short and long auditory stores. *Psychological Bulletin, 96,* 341–370.

Craik, F.I., & Levy, B.A. (1976). The concept of primary memory. In W.K. Estes (Ed.), *Handbook of learning and cognitive processes: Vol. 4. Attention and memory*. Hillsdale, NJ: Lawrence Erlbaum Associates.

Craik, F.I., & Lockhart, R.S. (1972). Levels of processing: A framework for memory research. *Journal of Verbal Learning and Verbal Behavior, 11,* 671–684.

Craik, F.I., & Tulving, E. (1975). Depth of processing and the retention of words in episodic memory. *Journal of Experimental Psychology: General, 104,* 268–294.

Crain, S., & McKee, C. (1985). *The acquisition of structural constraints on anaphora*. Paper presented at the Boston University Conference on Language Development, Boston.

Crain, S., & McKee, C. (1987). *Cross linguistic analysis of coreference relations*. Paper presented at the Boston University Conference on Language Development, Boston.

Crain, S., & Nakayama, M. (1987). Structure-dependence in grammar formation. *Language, 63,* 522–543.

Crais, E.R. (1990). World knowledge to word knowledge. *Topics in Language Disorders, 10,* 45–62.

Crais, E.R., & Chapman, R.S. (1987). Story recall and inferencing skills in language/learning disabled and nondisabled children. *Journal of Speech and Hearing Disorders, 52,* 50–55.

Creaghead, N.A., & Tattershall, S.S. (1985). Observation and assessment of classroom pragmatic skills. In C.S. Simon (Ed.), *Communication skills and classroom success: Assessment of language-learning disabled students*. San Diego: College Hill Press.

Cross, T.G. (1978). Mothers' speech and its association with rate of linguistic development in young children. In N. Waterson & C. Snow (Eds.), *The development of communication*. New York: John Wiley & Sons.

Cross, T.G. (1981). Parental speech as primary linguistic data: Some complexities in the study of the effect of the input in language acquisition. In P.S. Dale & D. Ingram (Eds.), *Child language: An international perspective*. Baltimore: University Park Press.

Cruikshank, W. (1955). *Psychology of exceptional children and youth*. Englewood Cliffs, NJ: Prentice-Hall.

Crystal, D. (1979). *Working with LARSP*. New York: Elsevier.

Crystal, D. (1982). *Profiling linguistic disability*. London: Edward Arnold.

Crystal, D. (1987). Toward a 'bucket' theory of language disability: Taking account of interaction between linguistic levels. *Clinical Linguistics and Phonetics, 1,* 7–22.

Crystal, D., Fletcher, P., & Garman, M. (1976). *The grammatical analysis of language disability*. London: Edward Arnold.

Culatta, B., Page, J., & Ellis, J. (1983). Story telling as a communicative performance screening tool. *Language Speech and Hearing Services in Schools, 14,* 66–74.

Cummins, J.P. (1983). Language proficiency and academic achievement. In J.W. Oller (Ed.), *Issues in language testing research*. Rowley, MA: Newbury House.

Cummins, J.P. (1984). *Bilingualism and special education: Issues in assessment and pedagogy*. San Diego: College Hill Press.

Curtiss, S. (1981). Dissociation between language and cognition: Cases and implications. *Journal of Autism and Developmental Disorders, 11,* 15–30.

Czudner, G., & Rourke, B.P. (1972). Age differences in visual reaction time of "brain-damaged" and normal children under regular and irregular preparatory interval conditions. *Journal of Experimental Child Psychology, 13,* 516–526.

Dalby, J.T., & Gibson, D. (1981). Functional cerebral lateralization in subtypes of disabled readers. *Brain and Language, 14,* 34–48.

Dale, P.S., & Cole, K.N. (1991). What's normal? Specific language impairment in an individual differences perspective. *Language, Speech, and Hearing Services in Schools, 22,* 80–83.

Damico, J. (1980). Pragmatic versus morphological/syntactic criteria for language referrals. *Language, Speech and Hearing Services in Schools, 11,* 85–94.

Damico, J.S. (1985a). Clinical discourse analysis: A functional language assessment technique. In C.S. Simon (Ed.), *Communication skills and classroom success: Assessment of language-learning disabled students*. San Diego: College Hill Press.

Damico, J.S. (1985b). *The effectiveness of direct observation as a language assessment technique*. Unpublished doctoral dissertation, University of New Mexico, Albuquerque.

Damico, J.S. (1987). Addressing language concerns in the schools: The SLP as consultant. *Journal of Childhood Communication Disorders, 11,* 17–40.

Damico, J.S. (1988). The lack of efficacy in language therapy: A case study. *Language, Speech and Hearing Services in Schools, 19,* 51–67.

Damico, J.S. (1990). Prescriptionism as a motivating mechanism: An ethnographic study in the public schools. *Journal of Childhood Communication Disorders, 13,* 85–92.

Damico, J.S. (1991). Descriptive assessment of communicative ability in limited English proficient students. In E.V. Hamayan & J.S. Damico (Eds.), *Limiting bias in the assessment of bilingual students*. Austin, TX: PRO-ED.

Damico, J.S., & Oller, J.W. (1985). *Spotting language problems*. San Diego: Los Amigos Research Associates.

Daneman, M., & Carpenter, P.A. (1983). Individual differences in integrating information between and within sentences. *Journal of Experimental Psychology: Learning, Memory and Cognition, 9,* 561–584.

Danielewicz, J.M. (1984). The interaction between text and context: A study of how adults and children use spoken and written language in four contexts. In A.D. Pellegrini & T.D. Yawkey (Eds.), *The development of oral and written language in social context*. Norwood, NJ: Ablex.

Das, J.P., & Varnhagen, C.K. (1986). Neuropsychological functioning and cognitive processing. In J.E. Obrzut & G.W. Hynd (Eds.), *Child neuropsychology: Vol. 1. Theory and research*. Orlando, FL: Academic Press.

Davidson, R.E. (1976). The role of metaphor and analogy in learning. In J.R. Levin & V.L. Allen (Eds.), *Cognitive learning in children: Theories and strategies*. New York: Academic Press.

Day, P. (1985). *Means for enhancing efficiency of interdisciplinary team decision making. (ERIC Document Reproduction Service No. ED 266 621)* Paper presented at CAID, St. Augustine, FL.

de Beaugrande, R. (1985). Text linguistics in discourse studies. In T.A. van Dijk (Ed.), *Handbook of discourse analysis, Vol. 1: Disciplines of discourses*. London: Academic Press.

Deese, J. (1965). *The structure of associations in language and thought*. Baltimore: Johns Hopkins University Press.

de Hirsch, K. (1981). Unready children. In A. Gerber & D.N. Bryen, *Language and learning disabilities* (pp. 61–74). Baltimore: University Park Press.

de Hirsch, K., Jansky, J., & Langsford, W. (1965). *Predicting reading failure*. New York: Harper & Row.

DeMarie-Dreblow, D., & Miller, P. (1988). The development of children's strategies for selective attention: Evidence for a transitional period. *Child Development, 59,* 1504–1513.

Denckla, M.B. (1972). Clinical syndromes in learning disabilities: A case for "splitting" and "lumping." *Journal of Learning Disabilities, 5,* 26–33.

Denckla, M.B., & Rudel, R.G. (1976a). Naming of object drawings by dyslexic and other learning disabled children. *Brain and Language, 3,* 1–15.

Denckla, M.B., & Rudel, R.G. (1976b). Rapid "automatized" naming (RAN): Dyslexia differentiated from other learning disabilities. *Neuropsychologia, 14,* 471–479.

Denckla, M.B., Rudel, R.G., & Broman, M. (1980). The development of spatial orientation skill in normal, learning disabled and neurologically impaired children. In D. Caplan (Ed.), *Biological studies of mental processes*. Cambridge, MA: The MIT Press.

Dennis, M. (1983). The developmental dyslexic brain and the written language skills of children with one hemisphere. In U. Kirk (Ed.), *Neuropsychology of language, reading, and spelling*. New York: Academic Press.

Dennis, M., & Kohn, B. (1975). Comprehension of syntax in infantile hemiplegia after cerebral hemidecortication: Left hemisphere superiority. *Brain and Language, 2,* 472–482.

DeRenzi, E., & Vignolo, L.A. (1962). The Token Test: A sensitive test to detect receptive disturbances in aphasics. *Brain, 85,* 665–678.

Derwing, B.L., & Baker, W.J. (1979). Recent research on the acquisition of English morphology. In P. Fletcher & M. Garman (Eds.), *Language acquisition: Studies in first language development*. Cambridge, England: Cambridge University Press.

Despain, A.D., & Simon, C.S. (1987). Alternative to failure: A junior high school language development-based curriculum. *Journal of Childhood Communication Disorders, 11,* 139–179.

DiSimoni, F. (1978). *The Token Test for Children*. Hingham, MA: Teaching Resources.

Doehring, D.G. (1985). Reading disability subtypes: Interaction of reading and nonreading deficits. In B.P. Rourke (Ed.), *Neuropsychology of learning disabilities*. New York: The Guilford Press.

Doehring, D.G., Trites, R.L., Patel, P.G., & Fiedorowicz, C.A.M. (1981). *Reading disabilities: The interaction of reading, language and neuropsychological deficits*. New York: Academic Press.

Dollaghan, C.A. (1987). Comprehension monitoring in normal and language-impaired children. *Topics in Language Disorders, 7,* 45–60.

Dollaghan, C.A., & Kaston, N. (1986). A comprehension monitoring program for language-impaired children. *Journal of Speech and Hearing Disorders, 51,* 264–271.

Donahue, M. (1981). Requesting strategies of learning disabled children. *Applied Psycholinguistics, 2,* 213–234.

Donahue, M. (1984). Learning disabled children's comprehension and production of syntactic devices for marking given versus new information. *Applied Psycholinguistics, 5,* 101–116.

Donahue, M. (1985). Communicative style in learning disabled children: Some implications for classroom discourse. In D.N. Ripich & F.M. Spinelli (Eds.), *School discourse problems*. San Diego: College Hill Press.

Donahue, M. (1986). Linguistic and communicative development in learning disabled children. In S.J. Ceci (Ed.), *Handbook of cognitive, social and neuropsychological aspects of learning disabilities*. Hillsdale, NJ: Lawrence Erlbaum Associates.

Donahue, M., & Bryan T. (1983). Conversational skills and modelling in learning disabled boys. *Applied Psycholinguistics, 4,* 251–278.

Donahue, M., Pearl, R., & Bryan, T. (1982). Learning disabled children's syntactic proficiency on a communicative task. *Journal of Speech and Hearing Disorders, 47,* 397–402.

Dooling, D., & Lackman, R. (1971). Effects of comprehension on retention of prose. *Journal of Experimental Psychology, 88,* 216–222.

Dore, J. (1979). Conversation and preschool language development. In P. Fletcher & M. Garman (Eds.), *Language acquisition*. Cambridge: Cambridge University Press.

Doris, J.L. (1993). Some historical notes on the definition and prevalence of learning disabilities. In G.R. Lyon, D.B. Gray, J.F. Kavanagh, & N. Krasnegor (Eds.), *Better understanding learning disabilities: New views from research and their implications for education and public policies*. Baltimore: Paul H. Brookes Publishing Co.

Douglas, V.I. (1983). Attentional and cognitive problems. In M. Rutter (Ed.), *Developmental neuropsychiatry*. New York: Guilford Press.

Douglas, V.I., & Peters, K.G. (1979). Toward a clearer definition of the attentional deficits of hyperactive children. In G.A. Hale & M. Lewis (Eds.), *Attention and cognitive development*. New York: Plenum Press.

Duane, D.D. (1989). Commentary on dyslexia and neurodevelopmental pathology. *Journal of Learning Disabilities, 22,* 219–220.

Duchan, J.F., & Katz, J. (1983). Language and auditory processing: Top-down plus bottom-up. In E.Z. Lasky & J. Katz (Eds.), *Central auditory processing disorders*. Baltimore: University Park Press.

Dudley-Marling, C.C. (1985). The pragmatic skills of learning disabled children. *Journal of Learning Disabilities, 18,* 193–199.

Dudley-Marling, C.C., & Rhodes, L.K. (1987). Pragmatics and literacy. *Language, Speech and Hearing Services in Schools, 18*, 41–52.

Duffy, F., Denckla, M., Bartels, S., & Sandini, G. (1980). Dyslexia: Regional differences in brain electrical activity by topographic mapping. *Annals of Neurology, 7*, 412–420.

Duncan, J.C., & Perozzi, J.A. (1987). Concurrent validity of a pragmatic protocol. *Language Speech and Hearing Services in Schools, 18*, 80–85.

Dunn, L.M. (1965) *Peabody Picture Vocabulary Test*. Minneapolis: American Guidance Service.

Dunn, L.M., & Dunn, L.M. (1981). *Peabody Picture Vocabulary Test—Revised*. Circle Pines, MN: American Guidance Service.

Durkin, K. (1986). Introduction. In K. Durkin (Ed.), *Language development in the school years*. Cambridge, MA: Brookline Books.

Durkin, K., Crowther, R., & Shire, B. (1986). Children's processing of polysemous vocabulary in the school years. In K. Durkin (Ed.), *Language development in the school years*. Cambridge, MA: Brookline Books.

Dykman, R.A. & Dykman, P.T. (1991). Attention deficit disorders and specific reading disability: Separate but often overlapping disorders. *Journal of Learning Disabilities, 24*, 96–103.

Edwards, D., & Mercer, N. (1989). Reconstructing context: The conventionalization of classroom knowledge. *Discourse Processes, 12*, 91–104.

Egeland, B. (1974). Training impulsive children in the use of more efficient scanning techniques. *Child Development, 45*, 165–171.

Ehri, L. (1979). Linguistic insight: Threshold of reading acquisition. In T. Waller & G. Mackinnon (Eds.), *Reading research*. New York: Academic Press.

Ehri, L.C. (1989). The development of spelling knowledge and its role in reading acquisition and reading disability. *Journal of Learning Disabilities, 22*, 356–365.

Ehrlich, S. (1979). Semantic memory: A free elements system. In C.R. Puff (Ed.), *Memory organization and structure*. New York: Academic Press.

Eibling, H.H., Jackson, C.L., & Perrone, V. (Eds). (1977). *Two centuries of progress: United States history*. River Forest, IL: Laidlaw Brothers.

Eimas, P., Siqueland, E., Jusczyk, P., & Vigorito, K. (1971). Speech perception in infants. *Science, 303*, 259–260.

Eisenson, J. (1968). Developmental aphasia: A speculative view with therapeutic implications. *Journal of Speech and Hearing Disorders, 33*, 3–13.

Elliott, L.L., & Busse, L.A. (1987). Auditory processing by learning disabled young adults. In D.J. Johnson & J.W. Blalock (Eds.), *Adults with learning disabilities*. Orlando, FL: Grune & Stratton.

Elliott, L.L., & Hammer, M.A. (1988). Longitudinal changes in auditory discrimination in normal children and children with language-learning problems. *Journal of Speech and Hearing Disorders, 53*, 467–474.

Elliott, L.L., Hammer, M.A., & Scholl, M.E. (1989). Fine-grained auditory discrimination in normal children and children with language-learning problems. *Journal of Speech and Hearing Research, 32*, 112–119.

Englert, C.S., Raphael, T.E., Anderson, L.M., Gregg, S.L., & Anthony, H.M. (1989). Exposition: Reading, writing and the metacognitive knowledge of learning disabled students. *Learning Disabilities Research, 5*, 5–24.

Epstein, M.A., Shaywitz, S.E., Shaywitz, B.A., & Woolston, J.L. (1991). The boundaries of attention deficit disorder. *Journal of Learning Disabilities, 24*, 78–86.

Ervin-Tripp, S. (1970). Discourse agreement: How children answer questions. In J.R. Hayes (Ed.), *Cognition and the development of language*. New York: John Wiley & Sons.

Esterly, D.L., & Griffin, J.C. (1987). Preschool programs for children with learning disabilities. *Journal of Learning Disabilities, 20*, 571–573.

Estes, W.K. (1976). Introduction to Volume 4. In W.K. Estes (Ed.), *Handbook of learning and cognitive processes: Vol. 4. Attention and memory* (p. 14). Hillsdale, NJ: Lawrence Erlbaum Associates.

Eysenck, M.W. (1982). *Attention and arousal*. New York: Springer-Verlag.

Feagans, L., & Appelbaum, M.I. (1986). Validation of language subtypes in learning disabled children. *Journal of Educational Psychology, 78*, 358–364.

Feagans, L., & Short, E.J. (1984). Developmental differences in the comprehension and production of narratives by reading disabled and normally achieving children. *Child Development, 55*, 1727–1736.

Feinberg, C.L. (1981). The pre-academic language classroom. In A. Gerber & D.N. Bryen, *Language and learning disabilities* (pp. 249–268). Baltimore: University Park Press.

Feldman, H., Goldin-Meadow, S., & Gleitman, L.R. (1978). Beyond Herodotus: The creation of language by linguistically deprived deaf children. In A. Lock (Ed.), *Action, symbol and gesture: The emergence of language*. New York: Academic Press.

Felton, R.H., & Wood, F.B. (1989). Cognitive deficits in reading disability and attention disorder. *Journal of Learning Disabilities, 22*, 3–13.

Ferguson, C. (1977). Baby talk as a simplified register. In C. Snow & C. Ferguson (Eds.), *Talking to children: Language input and acquisition*. London: Cambridge University Press.

Ferraro, A. (1985). Pragmatics. In T.A. van Dijk (Ed.), *Handbook of discourse analysis, Vol. 2: Dimensions of discourse*. London: Academic Press.

Feuerstein, R. (1980). *Instrumental enrichment: An intervention program for cognitive modifiability*. Baltimore: University Park Press.

Fey, M.E. (1986). *Language intervention with young children*. San Diego: College Hill Press.

Fey, M.E. (1988). Generalization issues facing language interventionists: An introduction. *Language, Speech and Hearing Services in the Schools, 19*, 272–281.

Fey, M.E., Warr-Leeper, G., Webber, S.A., & Disher, L.M. (1988). Repairing children's repairs: Evaluation and facilitation of children's clarification requests and responses. *Topics in Language Disorders, 8*, 63–84.

Fillmore, C. (1968). The case for case. In E. Bach & T. Harms (Eds.), *Universals in linguistic theory*. New York: Holt, Rinehart & Winston.

Fillmore, C.J. (1985). Linguistics as a tool for discourse analysis. In T.A. van Dijk (Ed.), *Handbook of discourse analysis, Vol. 1: Disciplines of discourse*. London: Academic Press.

Fisk, A.D., & Schneider, E. (1984). Memory as a function of attention, level of processing and automatization. *Journal of Experimental Psychology, 10*, 181–197.

Fisk, J.L., & Rourke, B.P. (1983). Neuropsychological subtyping of learning disabled children: History, methods, implications. *Journal of Learning Disabilities, 16*, 529–531.

Flavell, J.H. (1977). *Cognitive development*. Englewood Cliffs, NJ: Prentice Hall, Inc.

Flavell, J.H. (1985). *Cognitive development* (2nd ed.). Englewood Cliffs, NJ: Prentice Hall, Inc.

Flavell, J.H., Beach, D.R., & Chinsky, J.M. (1966). Spontaneous verbal rehearsal in a memory task as a function of age. *Child Development, 37*, 238–299.

Flavell, J.H., Friederichs, A.G., & Hoyt, J.D. (1970). Developmental changes in memorization processes. *Cognitive Psychology, 1*, 324–340.

Flavell, J.H., & Wellman, H.M. (1977). Metamemory. In R.V. Kail & J.W. Hagen (Eds.), *Perspectives on the development of memory and cognition*. Hillsdale, NJ: Lawrence Erlbaum Associates.

Fletcher, J.M. (1985). External validation of learning disability subtypes. In B.P. Rourke (Ed.), *Neuropsychology of learning disabilities*. New York: The Guilford Press.

Fletcher, J.M., Francis, D.J., Rourke, B.P., Shaywitz, S.E., & Shaywitz, B.S. (1993). Classification of learning disabilities: Relationships with other disorders. In G.R. Lyon, D.B. Gray, J.F. Kavanagh, & N. Krasnegor (Eds.), *Better understanding learning disabilities: New views from research and their implications for education and public policies*. Baltimore: Paul H. Brookes Publishing Co.

Fletcher, J.M., Morris, R.D., & Francis, D.J. (1991). Methodological issues in the classification of attention-related disorders. *Journal of Learning Disabilities, 24*, 72–77.

Fletcher, J.M., & Satz, P. (1985). Cluster analysis and the search for learning disability subtypes. In B.P. Rourke (Ed.), *Neuropsychology of learning disabilities*. New York: Guilford Press.

Fletcher, J.M., Satz, P., & Scholes, R. (1981). Developmental changes in the linguistic performance correlates of reading achievement. *Brain and Language, 13*, 78–90.

Fodor, J.A., & Bever, T.G. (1965). The psychological reality of linguistic segments. *Journal of Verbal Learning and Verbal Behavior, 4*, 414–420.

Fodor, J.A., Bever, T.G., & Garrett, M.F. (1974). *The psychology of language*. New York: McGraw-Hill Book Co.

Forrest-Pressley, D.L., & Waller, T.G. (1984). Knowledge and monitoring abilities of poor readers. *Topics in Learning and Learning Disabilities, 3*, 73–80.

Foss, D.J., & Hakes, D.T. (1978). *Psycholinguistics: An introduction to the psychology of language*. Englewood Cliffs, NJ: Prentice Hall, Inc.

Foster, C.R., Giddan, J.J., & Stark, J. (1972). *ACLC: Assessment of Children's Language Comprehension*. Palo Alto, CA: Consulting Psychologists Press.

Fowler, A., Gelman, R., & Gleitman, L.R. (1980). *A comparison of normal and retarded language equated on MLU*. Paper presented at the Boston University Conference on Language Development, Boston.

Fox, B., & Routh, D.K. (1975). Analyzing spoken language into words, syllables, and phonemes: A developmental study. *Journal of Psycholinguistic Research, 4*, 331–342.

Fox, B., & Routh, D.K. (1976). Phonemic analysis and synthesis as word-attack skills. *Journal of Educational Psychology, 68*, 70–74.

Fox, B., & Routh, D.K. (1984). Phonemic analysis and synthesis as word attack skills: Revisited. *Journal of Educational Psychology, 76*, 1059–1064.

Freedle, R., & Hale, G. (1979). Acquisition of new comprehension schemata for expository prose by transfer of a narrative schema. In R. Freedle (Ed.), *New directions in discourse processing* (Vol. II). Norwood, NJ: Ablex Publ. Corp.

Fried, I., Tanguay, P.E., Boder, E. Doubleday, C., & Greensite, M. (1981). Developmental dyslexia: Electrophysiologic evidence of clinical subgroups. *Brain and Language, 12*, 14–22.

Friendly, M. (1979). Methods for finding graphic representations of associative memory structures. In C.R. Puff (Ed.), *Memory organization and structure*. New York: Academic Press.

Frostig, M., Lefever, D.W., & Whittlesey, J.R.B. (1964). *Marianne Frostig Test of Visual Perception*. Palo Alto, CA: Consulting Psychologists Press.

Fuchs, L.S., & Maxwell, L. (1988). Interactive effects of reading mode, production format and structural importance of text among LD pupils. *Learning Disability Quarterly, 11*, 97–105.

Fuller, P.W. (1978). Attention and the EEG alpha rhythm in learning disabled children. *Journal of Learning Disabilities, 11*, 303–312.

Furrow, D., Nelson, K., & Benedict, H. (1979). Mothers' speech to children and syntactic development: Some simple relations. *Journal of Child Language, 6*, 423–442.

Gajar, A.H. (1989). A computer analysis of written language variables and a comparison of compositions written by university students with and without learning disabilities. *Journal of Learning Disabilities, 22*, 125–130.

Galaburda, A.M. (1988). *Ordinary and extraordinary brain development: "Nature and nurture" and dyslexia*. Paper presented at the meeting of the Orton Dyslexia Society, Tampa, FL.

Galaburda, A.M. (1989). Learning disability: Biological, societal or both? A response to Gerald Coles. *Journal of Learning Disabilities, 22*, 278–282.

Galaburda, A.M., Sherman, G.F., Rosen, G.D., Aboitz, F., & Geshwind, N. (1985). Developmental dyslexia: Four consecutive patients with cortical anomalies. *Annals of Neurology, 18*, 222–233.

Gallagher, T., & Darnton, B.A. (1978). Conversational aspects of the speech of language-impaired children: Revision behaviors. *Journal of Speech and Hearing Research, 21*, 118–133.

Gallagher, T.M. (1983). Pre-assessment: A procedure for accommodating language use variability. In T.M. Gallagher & C.A. Prutting (Eds.), *Pragmatic assessment and intervention issues in language*. San Diego: College Hill Press.

Gardner, H. (1983). *Frames of mind: The theory of multiple intelligences*. New York: Basic Books, Inc.

Garner, R., & Reis, R. (1981). Monitoring and resolving comprehension obstacles: An investigation of spontaneous text lookbacks among upper grade good and poor comprehenders. *Reading Research Quarterly, 16*, 569–582.

Garnett, K. (1986). Telling tales: Narratives and learning disabled children. *Topics in Language Disorders, 6*, 44–56.

Garnham, A., Oakhill, J., & Johnson-Laird, P.N. (1982). Referential continuity and the coherence of discourse. *Cognition, 11*, 29–46.

Gavilek, J.R., & Palinscar, A.S. (1988). Contextualism as an alternative worldview of learning disabilities: A response to Swanson's "Toward a metatheory of learning disabilities." *Journal of Learning Disabilities, 21*, 278–281.

Gelzheiser, L.M. (1984). Generalization from categorical memory tasks to prose by learning disabled adolescents. *Journal of Educational Psychology, 76*, 1128–1138.

Gerber, A. (1981). Remediation of language processing problems of the school-age child. In A. Gerber & D.N. Bryen, *Language and learning disabilities* (pp. 159–215). Baltimore: University Park Press.

Gerber, A., & Bryen, D.N. (1981). *Language and learning disabilities*. Baltimore: University Park Press.

Gerber, A., Goehl, H., & Heuer, R. (1988). *Temple University Short Syntax Inventory—Revised*. East Aurora, NY: Slosson Educational Publications.

Gerber, A., & Mastriano, B. (1991). *Preschool language intervention: A reasoned approach*. Phoenix: ECL Publications.

Gerber, A.J. (1970). A pilot program in the training of Black elementary school children in functional bi-dialectalism. *Journal of the Pennsylvania Speech and Hearing Association, 3*, 30–39.

Gerber, M.M. (1986). Generalization of spelling strategies by LD students as a result of contingent imitation/modeling and mastery criteria. *Journal of Learning Disabilities, 19*, 530–537.

Gerber, M.M., & Hall, R.J. (1987). Information processing approaches to studying spelling deficiencies. *Journal of Learning Disabilities, 20*, 34–42.

German, D. (1982). Word-finding substitutions in children with learning disabilities. *Language Speech and Hearing Services in Schools, 13*, 223–230.

German, D.J. (1986). *Test of Word Finding (TWF)*. Allen, TX: DLM Teaching Resources.

German, D.J. (1987). Spontaneous language profiles of children with word finding problems. *Language Speech and Hearing Services in Schools, 18*, 217–230.

German, D.J., & Simon, E. (1991). Analysis of children's word-finding skills in discourse. *Journal of Speech and Hearing Research, 34*, 309–316.

Gibson, E., & Rader, N. (1979). The perceiver as performer. In G.A. Hale & M. Lewis (Eds.), *Attention and cognitive development*. New York: Plenum Press.

Gibson, E.J. (1969). *Principles of perceptual learning and development*. New York: Appleton-Century-Crofts.

Gibson, E.J., & Levin, H. (1975). *The psychology of reading*. Cambridge, MA: The MIT Press.

Gillet, J.W., & Temple, C.(1986). *Understanding reading problems: Assessment and instruction*. Boston: Little, Brown and Co.

Glass, A.L., & Perna, J. (1986). The role of syntax in reading disability. *Journal of Learning Disabilities, 19*, 354–359.

Glazer, S.M. (1989). Oral language and literacy development. In D.S. Strickland & L.M. Morrow (Eds.), *Emerging literacy: Young children learn to read and write*. Newark, DE: International Reading Association.

Gleitman, H. (1986). *Psychology* (2nd ed.). New York: Norton & Co.

Gleitman, L.R., Landau, B., & Wanner, E. (1988). Where learning begins: Initial representations for language learning. In F. Newmeyer (Ed.), *The Cambridge linguistic survey*. New York: Cambridge University Press.

Gleitman, L.R., Newport, E.L., & Gleitman, H. (1984). The current status of the motherese hypothesis. *Journal of Child Language, 11,* 43–79.

Gleitman, L.R., & Wanner, E. (1982). Language acquisition: The state of the state of the art. In E. Wanner & L.R. Gleitman (Eds.), *Language acquisition: The state of the art*. Cambridge, England: Cambridge University Press.

Glosser, G., & Koppell, S. (1987). Emotional-behavioral patterns in children with learning disabilities: Lateralized hemispheric differences. *Journal of Learning Disabilities, 20,* 365–368.

Goehl, H. (1983). *Auditory processing: Controversy and challenge*. Miniseminar, Pennsylvania Speech and Hearing Association Convention, Pittsburgh, PA.

Goldman, R., Fristoe, M., & Woodcock, R. (1970). *Goldman-Fristoe-Wooodcock Test of Auditory Discrimination*. Circle Pines, MN: Guidance Service Inc.

Goldstein, D., & Cohen, W.D. (1987). Affect and cognition in learning disabilities. In S.J. Ceci (Ed.), *Handbook of cognitive, social, neuropsychological aspects of learning disabilities* (Vol. 2). Hillsdale, NJ: Lawrence Erlbaum Associates.

Goldstein, K. (1942). *Aftereffects of brain injuries in war*. New York: Grune & Stratton.

Golinkoff, R., Hirsh-Pasek, K., Cauley, K., & Gordon, L. (1987). The eyes have it: Lexical and syntactic comprehension in a new paradigm. *Journal of Child Language, 14,* 23–45.

Goodman, K. (1986). *What's whole about whole language?* Portsmouth, NH: Heinemann.

Goodman, K., & Goodman, Y. (1979). Learning to read is natural. In L.B. Resnick & P.B. Weaver (Eds.), *Theory and practice in early reading*. Hillsdale, NJ: Lawrence Erlbaum Associates.

Gordon, C.J., & Braun, C. (1985). Metacognitive processes: Reading and writing narrative discourse. In D.L. Forrest-Pressley, G.E. MacKinnon, & T.G. Waller (Eds.), *Metacognition, cognition, and human performance* (Vol. II). Orlando, FL: Academic Press.

Gordon, H.W. (1983). The learning disabled are cognitively right. *Topics in Learning and Learning Disabilities, 3,* 29–39.

Graham, S. (1990). The role of production factors in learning disabled students' compositions. *Journal of Educational Psychology, 82,* 781–791.

Graham, S., & Harris, K.R. (1987). Improving composition skills of inefficient learners with self-instructional strategy training. *Topics in Language Disorders, 7,* 68–77.

Graves, D.H. (1987). *Writing: Teachers and children at work*. Portsmouth, NH: Heinemann.

Graves, D.H. (1991). *Build a literate classroom*. Portsmouth, NH: Heinemann.

Graves, D.H., & Hansen, J. (1983). The author's chair. *Language Arts, 60,* 176–183.

Gray, B.B., & Ryan, B.P. (1973). *A language program for the nonlanguage child*. Champaign, IL: Research Press.

Gray, B.B., & Ryan, B.P. (1975). *Monterey language program*. Palo Alto, CA: Monterey Learning Systems.

Green, J.L., & Harker, J.O. (Eds.). (1988). *Multiple perspective analyses of classroom discourse*. Norwood, NJ: Ablex Publ. Corp.

Green, J.L., Weade, R., & Graham, K. (1988). Lesson construction and student participation: A sociolinguistic analysis. In J.L. Green & J.D. Harker (Eds.), *Multiple perspective analyses of classroom discourse*. Norwood, NJ: Ablex Publ. Corp.

Greenberg, K.L. (1987). Defining, teaching, and testing basic writing competence. *Topics in Language Disorders, 7,* 31–41.

Greenfield, P.M., & Smith, J.H. (1976). *The structure of communication in early language development*. New York: Academic Press.

Grice, H.P. (1975). Logic and conversation. In P. Cole & H.L. Morgan (Eds.), *Syntax and semantics, Vol. 3: Speech acts*. New York: Academic Press.

Griffin, K., & Hannah, L. (1960). A study of the results of an extremely short instructional unit in listening. *Journal of Communication, 10,* 135–139.

Grimshaw, J. (1986). *Linguistic mistakes: The role of negative evidence in language learning*. Paper presented at the Boston University Conference on Language Development, Boston.

Griswold, P.C., Gelzheiser, L.M., & Sheperd, M.J. (1987). Does a production deficiency hypothesis account for vocabulary learning among adolescents with learning disabilities? *Journal of Learning Disabilities, 20,* 620–626.

Gruenewald, L.J., & Pollak, S.A. (1975). Analyzing language interaction in academics. *Journal of Learning Disabilities, 8,* 11–17.

Gruenewald, L.J., & Pollak, S.A. (1990). *Language interaction in curriculum and instruction*. Austin, TX: PRO-ED.

Grunwell, P. (1986). Aspects of phonological development in later childhood. In K. Durkin (Ed.), *Language development in the school years*. Cambridge, MA: Brookline Books.

Guess, D., Keogh, W., & Sailor, W. (1978). Generalization of language behavior: Measurement and training tactics. In R.L. Schiefelbusch (Ed.), *Bases of language intervention* (pp. 373–395). Baltimore: University Park Press.

Guess, D., Sailor, W., & Baer, D.M. (1974). To teach language to retarded children. In R.L. Schiefelbusch & L.L. Lloyd (Eds.), *Language perspectives: Acquisition, retardation, and intervention*. Baltimore: University Park Press.

Gulich, E., & Quasthoff, U.M. (1985). Narrative analysis. In T.A. van Dijk (Ed.), *Handbook of discourse analysis, Vol. 2: Dimensions of discourse*. London: Academic Press.

Guttentag, R.E. (1984). The mental effort requirement of cumulative rehearsal: A developmental study. *Journal of Experimental Child Research, 37,* 92–106.

Guyer, B.L., & Friedman, M.P. (1975). Hemispheric processing and cognitive styles in learning disabled and normal children. *Child Development, 46,* 658–668.

Hagen, J.W., Barclay, C.R., & Newman, R.S. (1982). Metacognition, self-knowledge and learning disabilities: Some thoughts on knowing and doing. *Topics in Learning and Learning Disabilities, 2,* 19–26.

Hagen, J.W., & Hale, G.H. (1973). The development of attention in children. In A.D. Pick (Ed.), *Minnesota symposium on child psychology* (Vol. 7). Minneapolis: University of Minnesota Press.

Hagen, J.W., & Kail, R.V. (1975). The role of attention in perceptual and cognitive development. In W.M. Cruikshank & D.P. Hallahan (Eds.), *Perceptual and learning disabilities in children: II. Research and theory.* Syracuse, NY: Syracuse University Press.

Hahn, E. (1961). Indications for direct, nondirect and indirect methods in speech correction. *Journal of Speech and Hearing Disorders, 26,* 230–237.

Hakes, D., Evans, J., & Brannon, L. (1976). Understanding sentences with relative clauses. *Memory and Cognition, 4,* 283–290.

Hale, G.A. (1979). Development of children's attention to stimulus components. In G.A. Hale & M. Lewis (Eds.), *Attention and cognitive development.* New York: Plenum Press.

Hall, M. (1976). *Teaching reading as a language experience.* Columbus, OH: Charles E. Merrill.

Hallahan, D.P., Gajar, A.H., Cohen, S.B., & Tarver, S.G. (1978). Selective attention and locus of control in learning disabled and normal children. *Journal of Learning Disabilities, 11,* 231–236.

Hallahan, D.P., & Kauffman, J. (1976). *Introduction to learning disabilities: A psycho-behavioral approach.* Englewood Cliffs, NJ: Prentice Hall.

Hallahan, D.P., Keller, C.E., McKinney, J.D., Lloyd, J.W., & Bryan, T. (1988). Examining the research base of the regular education initiative: Efficacy studies and the Adaptive Learning Environment Model. *Journal of Learning Disabilities, 21,* 29–35.

Hallahan, D.P., Tarver, S.G., Kaufman, J.M., & Graybeal, N.L. (1978). A comparison of the effects of reinforcement and response cost on the selective attention of learning disabled children. *Journal of Learning Disabilities, 11,* 430–438.

Halliday, M.A.K. (1975). *Learning how to mean: Explorations in the development of language.* New York: Elsevier.

Halliday, M.A.K. (1985). Dimensions of discourse analysis: Grammar. In T.A. van Dijk (Ed.), *Handbook of discourse analysis: Vol. 2. Dimensions of discourse.* London: Academic Press.

Halliday, M.A.K., & Hasan, R. (1976). *Cohesion in English.* London: Longman.

Hamburger, H., & Crain, S. (1982). Relative acquisition. In S. Kuczaj (Ed.), *Language development* (Vol. 2). Hillsdale, NJ: Lawrence Erlbaum Associates.

Hammill, D.D. (1985). *Detroit Test of Learning Aptitude—2.* Austin, TX: PRO-ED.

Hammill, D.D. (1990a). A brief history of learning disabilities. In P. Myers & D. Hammill (Eds.), *Learning disabilities: Basic concepts, assessment practices, and instructional strategies* (4th ed.), Austin, TX: PRO-ED.

Hammill, D.D. (1990b). On defining learning disabilities: An emerging consensus. *Journal of Learning Disabilities, 23,* 74–84.

Hammill, D.D., Brown, V.L., Larsen, S.C., & Wiederholt, J.L. (1980). *Test of Adolescent Language.* Allen, TX: DLM.

Hammill, D.D., & Larsen, S.C. (1988). *Test of Written Language—2.* Austin, TX: PRO-ED.

Hammill, D.D., Leigh, J.E., McNutt, G., & Larsen, S.C. (1981). A new definition of learning disabilities. *Journal of Learning Disabilities, 4,* 336–342. (Reprinted from *Learning Disability Quarterly, 4,* 336–342, 1981.)

Hansen, J., & Pearson, P.D. (1983). An instructional study: Improving the inferential comprehension of good and poor fourth-grade readers. *Journal of Educational Psychology, 75,* 821–829.

Hardy, B.W., McIntyre, C.W., Brown, A.S., & North, A.J. (1989). Visual and auditory coding confusability in students with and without learning disabilities. *Journal of Learning Disabilities, 22,* 646–651.

Harris, G.P. (1979). *Classification skills in normally achieving and learning disabled seven- and nine-year old boys.* Unpublished doctoral dissertation, Northwestern University, Chicago.

Harste, J.C., & Burke, C.L. (1980). Examining instructional assumptions: The child as informant. *Theory into Practice, 19,* 170–176.

Hart, B., & Rogers-Warren, A. (1978). A milieu approach to teaching language. In R.L. Schiefelbusch (Ed.), *Language intervention strategies* (pp. 193–235). Baltimore: University Park Press.

Hartlage, L.C., & Telzrow, C.F. (1983). The neuropsychological basis of educational intervention. *Journal of Learning Disabilities, 16,* 521–527.

Haslam, R.H., Dalby, J.T., Johns, R.D., & Rademaker, A.W. (1981). Cerebral asymmetry in developmental dyslexia. *Archives of Neurology, 38,* 679–682.

Haslett, B.J. (1983). Children's strategies for maintaining cohesion in their written and oral stories. *Communication Education, 32,* 91–104.

Haslett, B.J. (1987). *Communication: Strategic action in context.* Hillsdale, NJ: Lawrence Erlbaum Associates.

Haviland, S.E., & Clark, H.H. (1974). What's new? Acquiring new information as a process in comprehension. *Journal of Verbal Learning and Verbal Behavior, 13,* 512–521.

Haynes, W.O., Haynes, M.D., & Strickland-Helms, D.F. (1989). Alpha hemispheric asymmetry in children with learning disabilities and normally achieving children during story comprehension and rehearsal prior to narrative production. *Journal of Learning Disabilities, 22,* 391–396.

Heath, S.B. (1983). *Ways with words: Language, life and work in communities and classrooms.* Cambridge, England: Cambridge University Press.

Heath, S.B. (1986a). Sociocultural contexts of language development. In Bilingual Education Office: *Beyond language: Social and cultural factors in schooling language minority students.* Los Angeles: Evaluation, Dissemination, and Assessment Center.

Heath, S.B. (1986b). Taking a cross-cultural look at narratives. *Topics in Language Disorders, 7,* 84–94.

Heavey, C.L., Adelman, H.S., Nelson, P., & Smith, D.C. (1989). Learning problems, anger, perceived control and misbehavior. *Journal of Learning Disabilities, 22,* 46–50.

Hedberg, N.L., & Stoel-Gammon, C. (1986). Narrative analysis: Clinical procedures. *Topics in Language Disorders, 7,* 58–69.

Helfgott, J.A. (1976). Phonemic segmentation and blending skills of kindergarten children: Implications for beginning reading acquisition. *Contemporary Educational Psychology, 1,* 157–169.

Henker, B., & Whalen, C.K. (1989). Hyperactivity and attention deficits. *American Psychologist, 44,* 216–223.

Heyman, R.D. (1986). Formulating topics in the classroom. *Discourse Processes, 9,* 37–55.

Hier, D.B., LeMay, M., Rosenberger, P.B., & Perlo, V.P. (1978). Developmental dyslexia: Evidence for a subgroup with a reversal of cerebral asymmetry. *Archives of Neurology, 35,* 90–92.

Hirsh-Pasek, K., Golinkoff, R., Braidi, S., & McNally, L. (1986). *"Daddy throw": On the existence of implicit negative evidence for subcategorization errors.* Paper presented at the Boston University Conference on Language Development, Boston.

Hirst, W. (1986). The psychology of attention. In J.E. LeDoux & W. Hirst (Eds.), *Mind and brain: Dialogues in cognitive neuroscience.* Cambridge, England: Cambridge University Press.

Hiscock, M. (1983). Do learning disabled children lack functional hemispheric lateralization? *Topics in Learning and Learning Disabilities, 3,* 14–28.

Hiscock, M., & Kinsbourne, M. (1987). Specialization of the cerebral hemispheres: Implications for learning. *Journal of Learning Disabilities, 20,* 130–143.

Hoffman, J.E., Houck, M.R., MacMillan, F.W. III, Simons, R.F., & Oatman, L.C. (1985). Event-related potentials elicited by automatic targets: A dual-task analysis. *Journal of Experimental Psychology: Human Perception and Performance, 11,* 50–61.

Hoffman, L.P. (1990). The development of literacy in a school-based program. *Topics in Language Disorders, 10,* 81–92.

Hoffman, P.R. (1990). Spelling, phonology, and the speech-language pathologist: A whole language perspective. *Language, Speech, and Hearing Services in the Schools, 21,* 238–243.

Holcomb, W.R., Hardesty, R.A., Adams, N.A., & Ponder, H.M. (1987). WISC-R types of learning disabilities: A profile analysis with cross validation. *Journal of Learning Disabilities, 20,* 369–373.

Holmes, B.C. (1985). The effects of strategy and sequenced materials on the inferential comprehension of disabled readers. *Journal of Learning Disabilities, 18,* 542–546.

Hornby, P. (1971). Surface structure and topic-comment distinction: A developmental study. *Child Development, 42,* 1975–1988.

Hornstein, N., & Lightfoot, D. (Eds.). (1981). *Explanation in linguistics: The logical problem of language acquisition.* New York: Longman.

Horowitz, E.C. (1981). Popularity, decentering ability and role-taking skills in learning disabled and normal children. *Learning Disability Quarterly, 4,* 23–30.

Horton, D.L., & Mills, C.B. (1984). Human learning and memory. *Annual Review of Psychology, 35,* 361–394.

Hoskins, B. (1983). Semantics. In C. Wren (Ed.), *Language learning disabilities.* Rockville, MD: Aspen Systems Corp.

Hoskins, B. (1990). Language and literacy: Participating in the conversation. *Topics in Language Disorders, 10,* 46–62.

Houck, C.K., & Billingsley, B.S. (1989). Written expression of students with and without learning disabilities: Differences across the grades. *Journal of Learning Disabilities, 22,* 561–572.

Howell, M.J., & Manis, F.R. (1986). Developmental and reader ability differences in semantic processing efficiency. *Journal of Educational Psychology, 78,* 124–129.

Hresko, W.P., Rosenberg, S., & Buchanan, L. (1978). *Use of the Carrow Test of Auditory Comprehension with learning disabled children.* Paper presented at the Annual Meeting of the Council for Exceptional Children, Kansas City, KS.

Hubbell, R.D. (1981). *Children's language disorders.* Englewood Cliffs, NJ: Prentice-Hall.

Hughes, M., & Sussman, H.M. (1983). An assessment of cerebral dominance in language disordered children via a time-sharing paradigm. *Brain and Language, 19,* 48–64.

Hull, G. (1987). Current views of error and editing. *Topics in Language Disorders, 7,* 55–65.

Hunt, E., Lunneborg, C., & Lewis, J. (1975). What does it mean to be high verbal? *Cognitive Psychology, 7,* 194–227.

Hyams, N. (1983). *The acquisition of parameterized grammar.* Unpublished doctoral dissertation, City University of New York.

Hyams, N. (1986). *Language acquisition and the theory of parameters.* Dordrecht, Holland: Foris.

Hymes, D. (1971). Competence and performance in linguistic theory. In R. Huxley & D. Ingram (Eds.), *Language acquisition: Models and methods.* New York: Academic Press.

Hynd, G.W. (1992). Neurological aspects of dyslexia: Comment on the Balance Model. *Journal of Learning Disabilities, 25,* 110–112.

Hynd, G.W., Hynd, C.R., Sullivan, H.G., & Kingsbury, T.B. (1987). Regional cerebral blood flow (rCBF) in developmental dyslexia: Activation during reading in a surface and deep dyslexic. *Journal of Learning Disabilities, 20,* 294–300.

Hynd, G.W., & Obrzut, J.E. (1981). Development of reciprocal hemispheric inhibition in normal and learning disabled children. *The Journal of General Psychology, 104,* 203–212.

Hynd, G.W., & Semrud-Clikeman, M. (1989). Dyslexia and neurodevelopmental pathology: Relationships to cognition, intelligence, and reading acquisition. *Journal of Learning Disabilities, 22,* 204–216.

Idol-Maestas, L. (1980). Oral language responses of children with reading difficulties. *Journal of Speech Education, 14,* 386–404.

Iglesias, A. (1985). Cultural conflict in the classroom: The communicatively different child. In D.N. Ripich & F.M. Spinelli (Eds.), *School discourse problems.* San Diego: College Hill Press.

Iglesias, A., Pena, E., & Quinn, R. (1991). *Classroom collaboration: A process not a product.* Paper presented at Annual Convention of the American Speech-Language-Hearing Association, Atlanta.

Individuals with Disabilities Education Act of 1990 (PL 101-476). (October 30, 1990). Title 20, U.S.C. 1400 et seq: *U.S. Statutes at Large, 104,* 1103–1151.

Ingram, D. (1976). *Phonological disability in children.* London: Edward Arnold.

Ingram, D. (1979). Phonological patterns in the speech of young children. In P. Fletcher & M. Garman (Eds.), *Language acquisition: Studies in first language development.* Cambridge, England: Cambridge University Press.

Isaacson, S. (1985). Assessing written language skills. In C.S. Simon (Ed.), *Communication skills and classroom success: Assessment of language-learning disabled students.* San Diego: College Hill Press.

Israel, L. (1984). Word knowledge and word retrieval: Phonological and semantic strategies. In G.P. Wallach & K.G. Butler (Eds.), *Language learning disabilities in school-age children.* Baltimore: Williams & Wilkins.

Jacoby, L.L., & Craik, F.I. (1979). Effects of elaboration of processing at encoding and retrieval: Trace distinctiveness and recovery of initial context. In L.S. Cermak & F.I. Craik (Eds.), *Levels of processing in human memory.* Hillsdale, NJ: Lawrence Erlbaum Associates.

James, C.T. (1972). Theme and imagery in the recall of active and passive sentences. *Journal of Verbal Learning and Verbal Behavior, 11,* 205–211.

James, W. (1890). *The principles of psychology* (Vol. 1). New York: Holt.

Jansky, J., & de Hirsch, K. (1972). *Preventing reading failure.* New York: Harper & Row.

Jarvella, R.J., & Herman, S.J. (1972). Clause structure of sentences and speech processing. *Perception and Psychophysics, 11,* 381–382.

Jenkins, J.R., & Heliotis, J.G. (1981). Reading comprehension instruction: Findings from behavioral and cognitive psychology. *Topics in Language Disorders, 1,* 25–42.

Jimenez, J.E., & Rumeau, M.A. (1989). Writing disorders and their relationship to reading-writing methods: A longitudinal study. *Journal of Learning Disabilities, 22,* 195–199.

Johnson, D.J., & Blalock, J.W. (1987). Summary of problems and needs. In D.J. Johnson & J.W. Blalock (Eds.), *Adults with learning disabilities.* Orlando, FL: Grune & Stratton.

Johnson, D.J., & Myklebust, H.R. (1967). *Learning disabilities: Educational principles and practices.* New York: Grune & Stratton.

Johnson, M.K., & Hasher, L. (1987). Human learning and memory. *Annual Review of Psychology, 38,* 631–668.

Johnston, J.R. (1982). Narratives: A new look at communication problems in older language-disordered children. *Language Speech and Hearing Services in Schools, 13,* 144–155.

Johnston, J.R. (1988). Generalization: The nature of change. *Language Speech and Hearing Services in Schools, 19,* 314–329.

Johnston, J.R. (1991). The continuing relevance of cause: A reply to Leonard's "Specific language impairment as a clinical category." *Language, Speech, and Hearing Services in Schools, 22,* 75–79.

Johnston, J.R., & Schery, T.K. (1976). The use of grammatical morphemes by children with communication disorders. In D.M. Morehead & A.E. Morehead (Eds.), *Normal and deficient child language.* Baltimore: University Park Press.

Johnston, W.A., & Dark, V.J. (1986). Selective attention. *Annual Review of Psychology, 37,* 43–75.

Jorgensen, C., Barrett, M., Huisingh, R., & Zachman, L. (1981). *The Word Test.* Moline, IL: Linguisystems.

Joshko, M., & Rourke, B.P. (1985). Neuropsychological subtypes of learning disabled children who exhibit the ACID pattern on the WISC, 65. In B.P. Rourke (Ed.), *Neuropsychology of learning disabilities.* New York: Guilford Press.

Kagan, J. (1983). Retrieval difficulty in reading disability. *Topics in Learning and Learning Disabilities, 3,* 75–83.

Kagan, S. (1985). Dimensions of cooperative classroom structures. In R. Slavin, S. Sharan, S. Kagan, R.H. Lazarowitz, C. Webb, & R. Schmuck (Eds.), *Learning to cooperate, cooperating to learn*. New York: Plenum Press.

Kail, R., & Leonard, L.B. (1986). Sources of word-finding problems in language-impaired children. In S.J. Ceci (Ed.), *Handbook of cognitive, social and neuropsychological aspects of learning disabilities*. Hillsdale, NJ: Lawrence Erlbaum Associates.

Kail, R., & Strauss, M.S. (1984). Development of human memory: An historical overview. In R. Kail & N.E. Spear (Eds.), *Comparative perspectives on the development of memory*. Hillsdale, NJ: Lawrence Erlbaum Associates.

Kamhi, A.G. (1988). A reconceptualization of generalization and generalization problems. *Language, Speech and Hearing Services in Schools, 19*, 304–313.

Kamhi, A.G. (1989). Causes and consequences of reading disabilities. In A.G. Kamhi & H.W. Catts (Eds.), *Reading disabilities: A developmental language perspective*. Boston: College-Hill Press.

Kamhi, A.G., & Catts, H.G. (1986). Toward an understanding of developmental language and reading disorders. *Journal of Speech and Hearing Disorders, 51*, 337–347.

Kamhi, A.G., & Catts, H.W. (1989). *Reading disabilities: A developmental language perspective*. Boston: College-Hill Press.

Kamhi, A.G., Catts, H.W., Mauer, D., Apel, K., & Gentry, B.F. (1988). Phonological and spatial processing abilities in language- and reading-impaired children. *Journal of Learning Disabilities, 53*, 316–327.

Kamhi, A.G., & Johnston, J.R. (1982). Towards an understanding of retarded children's linguistic deficiencies. *Journal of Speech and Hearing Research, 25*, 435–445.

Kamhi, A.G., & Koenig, L.A. (1985). Metalinguistic awareness in normal and language-disordered children. *Language Speech and Hearing Services in Schools, 16*, 199–210.

Katz, B., Baker, G., & Macnamara, J. (1974). What's in a name? On the child's acquisition of proper and common nouns. *Child Development, 45*, 169–273.

Katz, J. (1972). *Semantic theory*. New York: Harper & Row.

Katz, J. (1977). The staggered spondaic word test. In R.W. Keith (Ed.), *Central auditory dysfunction*. New York: Grune & Stratton.

Kauffman, J.M., Gerber, M.M., & Semmel, M.I. (1988). Arguable assumptions underlying the regular education initiative. *Journal of Learning Disabilities, 21*, 6–11.

Kauffman, J.M., & Hallahan, D.P. (1976). *Teaching children with learning disabilities*. Columbus, OH: Charles E. Merrill.

Kaufman, A., & Kaufman, N. (1983). *Kaufman Assessment Battery for Children*. Circle Pines, MN: American Guidance Service.

Kaufman, D.K. (1987). *"Who's him?": Evidence for principle B in children's grammar*. Paper presented at the Boston University Conference on Language Development, Boston.

Kaufman, D.K. (1988). *Grammatical and cognitive interactions in the study of children's knowledge of binding theory and reference relations*. Doctoral dissertation, Temple University, Philadelphia.

Kavale, K.A. (1981). Functions of the Illinois Test of Psycholinguistic Abilities (ITPA): Are they trainable? *Exceptional Children, 47*, 496–510.

Kavale, K.A. (1982). A comparison of learning disabled and normal children on the Boehm Test of Basic Concepts. *Journal of Learning Disabilities, 15*, 160–161.

Kavale, K.A. (1988). Epistemological relativity in learning disabilities. *Journal of Learning Disabilities, 21*, 215–218.

Kavale, K.A. (1993). A science and theory in learning disabilities. In G.R. Lyon, D.B. Gray, J.F. Kavanagh, & N. Krasnegor (Eds.), *Better understanding learning disabilities: New views from research and their implications for education and public policies*. Baltimore: Paul H. Brookes Publishing Co.

Kavale, K.A., & Forness, S.R. (1985). *The science of learning disabilities*. San Diego: College Hill Press.

Kavale, K.A., & Mattson, P.D. (1983). "One jumped off the balance beam": meta-analysis of perceptual-motor training. *Journal of Learning Disabilities, 16*, 165–173.

Kawakami, A.J., & Hu-Pei-Au, K. (1986). Encouraging reading and language development in cultural minority children. *Topics in Language Disorders, 6*, 71–80.

Keeley, S., Shemberg, K., & Carbonell, J. (1976). Operant clinical intervention: Behavior management or beyond? *Behavior Therapy, 7*, 292–305.

Kemper, S. (1989). Synthesis/commentary: Factoring individual differences into the teachability of language. In M.L. Rice & R.L. Schiefelbusch (Eds.), *The teachability of language* (pp. 227–236). Baltimore: Paul H. Brookes Publishing Co.

Kempson, R.M. (1977). *Semantic theory*. Cambridge, MA: Cambridge University Press.

Kent, L.R., Klein, D., Falk, A., & Guenthe, H. (1972). A language acquisition program for the retarded. In J.E. McLean, D.E. Yoder, & R.L. Schiefelbusch (Eds.), *Language intervention with the retarded*. Baltimore: University Park Press.

Keogh, B.K. (1988). Improving services for problem learners: Rethinking and restructuring. *Journal of Learning Disabilities, 21*, 19–22.

Keogh, B.K. (1993). Linking purpose and practice: Social/political and developmental perspectives on classification. In G.R. Lyon, D.B. Gray, J.F. Kavanagh, & N. Krasnegor (Eds.), *Better understanding learning disabilities: New views from research and their implications for education and public policies*. Baltimore: Paul H. Brookes Publishing Co.

Keogh, B.K., & Becker, L. (1973). Early detection of learning problems: Questions, cautions, and guidelines. *Exceptional Children, 4,* 501–503.

Keogh, B.K., & Donlon, G.M. (1972). Field dependence: Impulsivity and learning disabilities. *Journal of Learning Disabilities, 5,* 331–336.

Keogh, B.K., Tchir, C., & Windeguth-Behn, A. (1974). Teachers' perception of educationally high risk children. *Journal of Learning Disabilities, 7,* 43–50.

Kephart, N.C. (1960). *The slow learner in the classroom.* Columbus, OH: Charles E. Merrill.

Kershner, J.R. (1983). Laterality and learning disabilities: Cerebral dominance as a cognitive process. *Topics in Learning and Learning Disabilities, 3,* 66–74.

Kershner, J.R., & Stringer, R.W. (1991). Effects of reading and writing on cerebral laterality in good readers and children with dyslexia. *Journal of Learning Disabilities, 24,* 560–567.

King, R.R., Jones, C., & Lasky, E. (1982). In retrospect: A fifteen-year follow-up report of speech-language disordered children. *Language, Speech, and Hearing Services in Schools, 13,* 24–32.

Kinsbourne, M. (1970). The cerebral basis of lateral asymmetries in attention. *Acta Psychologica, 33,* 193–201.

Kinsbourne, M. (1983). Models of learning disability. *Topics in Learning and Learning Disabilities, 3,* 1–13.

Kinsbourne, M., & Caplan, P.J. (1979). *Children's learning and attention problems.* Boston: Little, Brown.

Kinsbourne, M., & Hiscock, M. (1981). Cerebral lateralization and cognitive development: Conceptual and methodological issues. In G.W. Hynd & J.E. Obrzut (Eds.), *Neuropsychological assessment and the school-age child: Issues and procedures.* New York: Grune & Stratton, Inc.

Kinsbourne, M., & McMurray, J. (1975). The effects of cerebral dominance on time sharing between speaking and tapping by preschool children. *Child Development, 46,* 240–242.

Kintsch, W. (1977). On comprehending stories. In M.A. Just & P.A. Carpenter (Eds.), *Cognitive processes in comprehension.* Hillsdale, NJ: Lawrence Erlbaum Associates.

Kintsch, W. (1982). Discourse processing: Comprehension and recall of text. In A. Flammer & W. Kintsch (Eds.), *Memory for text.* Amsterdam: North-Holland Publ. Co.

Kintsch, W. (1988). The role of knowledge in discourse comprehension: A construction-integration model. *Psychological Review, 95,* 163–182.

Kintsch, W., & van Dijk, T.A. (1978). Toward a model of text comprehension and production. *Psychological Review, 85,* 363–394.

Kirchner, D.M., & Skarakis-Doyle, E. (1983). Developmental language disorders: A theoretical perspective. In T.M. Gallagher & C.A. Prutting (Eds.), *Pragmatic assessment and intervention issues in language.* San Diego: College Hill Press.

Kirk, S.A., & Kirk, W.D. (1975) *Psycholinguistic learning disabilities: Diagnosis and remediation.* Urbana, IL: University of Illinois Press.

Kirk, S.A., McCarthy, J.J., & Kirk, W.D. (1968). *Illinois Test of Psycholinguistic Abilities* (rev. ed.). Urbana, IL: University of Illinois Press.

Klahr, D., & Wallace, J.G. (1976). *Cognitive development: An information-processing view.* Hillsdale, NJ: Lawrence Erlbaum Associates.

Klees, M., & LeBrun, A. (1972). Analysis of the figurative and operative processes of thought of 40 dyslexic children. *Journal of Learning Disabilities, 5,* 390.

Klein, M.D., & Harris, K.C. (1986). Classroom communication functions of four learning-handicapped students. *Language, Speech, and Hearing Services in School, 17,* 318–328.

Klein-Konigsberg, H. (1984). Semantic integration and language learning disabilities: From research to assessment and intervention. In G.P. Wallach & K.G. Butler (Eds.), *Language learning disabilities in school-age children.* Baltimore: Williams & Wilkins.

Klekan-Aker, J.S. (1985). Syntactic abilities in normal and language deficient middle school children. *Topics in Language Disorders, 5,* 46–54.

Kolligian, K., & Sternberg, R.J. (1987). Intelligence, information processing, and specific learning disabilities: A triarchic synthesis. *Journal of Learning Disabilities, 20,* 8–17.

Koorland, M.A. (1986). Applied behavior analysis and the correction of learning disabilities. In J.F. Torgeson & B.Y.L. Wong (Eds.), *Psychological and educational perspectives on learning disabilities.* Orlando, FL: Academic Press.

Koriat, A., & Melkman, R. (1987). Depth of processing and memory organization. *Psychological Research, 49,* 183–188.

Kulhavy, R.W., Schwartz, N.H., & Peterson, S. (1986). Working memory: The encoding process. In G.D. Phye & T. Andre (Eds.), *Cognitive classroom learning: Understanding, thinking and problem solving.* Orlando, FL: Academic Press.

LaBerge, D. (1976). Perceptual learning and attention. In K.W. Estes (Ed.), *Handbook of learning and cognitive processes, Vol 4: Attention and memory.* Hillsdale, NJ: Lawrence Erlbaum Associates.

LaBerge, D., Petersen, R.J., & Norden, M.J. (1977). Exploring the limits of cueing. In S. Dornic (Ed.), *Attention and performance VI.* Hillsdale, NJ: Lawrence Erlbaum Associates.

LaBerge, D., & Samuels, S.J. (1974). Toward a theory of automatic information processing in reading. *Cognitive Psychology, 6,* 293–323.

Labov, W. (1972). *Language in the inner city*. Philadelphia: University of Pennsylvania Press.

LaBuda, M.C., & DeFries, J.C. (1988). Cognitive abilities in children with reading disabilities and controls: A follow-up study. *Journal of Learning Disabilities, 21,* 562–566.

Laesch, K.B., & van Kleeck, A. (1987). The cloze test as an alternative measure of language proficiency of children considered for exit from bilingual programs. *Language Learning, 37,* 171–189.

Laffey, D.G., & Laffey, J.L. (1986). Vocabulary teaching: An investment in literacy. *Journal of Reading, 29,* 650–652.

Landau, B., & Gleitman, L.R. (1985). *Language and experience*. Cambridge, MA: Harvard University Press.

Lange, G. (1978). Organization-related processes in children's recall. In P.A. Ornstein (Ed.), *Memory development in children*. Hillsdale, NJ: Lawrence Erlbaum Associates.

Languis, M.L., & Wittrock, M.C. (1986). Integrating neuropsychological and cognitive research: A perspective for bridging brain-behavior relationship. In J.E. Obrzut & G.W. Hynd (Eds.), *Child neuropsychology: Vol. 1. Theory and research*. Orlando, FL: Academic Press.

LaPointe, L.L. (1983). Aphasia intervention with adults: Historical, present and future approaches. In J. Miller, D. Yoder, & R. Schiefelbusch (Eds.), *Contemporary issues in language intervention*. Rockville, MD: The American Speech-Language-Hearing Association.

Larsen, S.C., Rogers, D., & Sowell, V. (1976). The use of selected perceptual tests in differentiating between normal and learning disabled children. *Journal of Learning Disabilities, 9,* 85–90.

Larson, V.L., & McKinley, N.L. (1987). *Communication assessment and intervention strategies for adolescents*. Eau Claire, WI: Thinking Publications.

Lasky, E.Z. (1983). Parameters affecting auditory processing. In E. Lasky & J. Katz (Eds.), *Central auditory processing disorders*. Baltimore: University Park Press.

Lasky, E.Z. (1985). Comprehension and processing of information in clinic and classroom. In C.S. Simon (Ed.), *Communication skills and classroom success: Therapy methodologies for the language-learning disabled student*. San Diego: College Hill Press.

Lasky, E.Z., & Chapandy, A.M. (1976). Factors affecting language comprehension. *Language Speech and Hearing Services in Schools, 7,* 159–169.

Lasky, E.Z., Weidner, W.E., & Johnson, J.P. (1976). Influence of linguistic complexity, rate of presentation and interphrase pause time on auditory-verbal comprehension of adult aphasic patients. *Brain and Language, 3,* 395–396.

Lassman, F.M. (1980). The examination of speech, language, and hearing in the NINCDS Collaborative Perinatal Project. In P.J. LaBenz & E.S. LaBenz (Eds.), *Early correlates of speech, language, and hearing*. Littleton, MA: PSG Publ. Co.

Laughton, J., & Hasenstab, M.S. (1986). *The language learning process*. Rockville, MD: Aspen Publishers.

Lee, D.M., & Allen, R.V. (1961). *Learning to read through experience* (2nd ed.). New York: Appleton-Century-Crofts.

Lee, L.L. (1974). *Developmental Sentence Analysis*. Evanston, IL: Northwestern University Press.

Lenchner, O., Gerber, M.M., & Routh, D.K. (1990). Phonological awareness tasks as predictors of decoding ability: Beyond segmentation. *Journal of Learning Disabilities, 23,* 240–247.

Lenneberg, E.H. (1964). *New directions in the study of language*. Cambridge, MA: The MIT Press.

Lenz, B.K., & Hughes, C.A. (1990). A word identification strategy for adolescents with learning disabilities. *Journal of Learning Disabilities, 23,* 149–159.

Leonard, L.B. (1976). *Meaning in child language; Issues in the study of early semantic development*. New York: Grune & Stratton.

Leonard, L.B. (1978). Cognitive factors in early linguistic development. In R.L. Schiefelbusch (Ed.), *Bases of language intervention* (pp. 67–96). Baltimore: University Park Press.

Leonard, L.B. (1991). Specific language impairment as a clinical category. *Language, Speech, and Hearing Services in Schools, 22,* 66–68.

Leonard, L.B., Nippold, N.A., Kail, R., & Hale, C.A. (1983). Picture naming in language-impaired children. *Journal of Speech and Hearing Research, 26,* 609–615.

Lerner, J. (1985). *Learning disabilities: Theories, diagnosis and teaching strategies*. Boston: Houghton Mifflin Co.

Lerner, J.W. (1971). *Children with learning disabilities*. Boston: Houghton Mifflin.

Levi, G., Capozzi, F., Fabrizi, A., & Sechi, S. (1982). Language disorders and prognosis for reading disabilities in developmental age. *Perceptual and Motor Skills, 54,* 1119–1122.

Levi, G., Musatti, L., Piredda, M.L., & Sechi, E. (1984). Cognitive and linguistic strategies in children with reading disabilities in an oral story-telling task. *Journal of Learning Disabilities, 17,* 406–410.

Levin, J.R. (1976). What have we learned about maximizing what children learn? In J.R. Levin & V.L. Allen (Eds.), *Cognitive learning in children: Theories and strategies*. New York: Academic Press.

Levin, J.R., & Allen, V.L. (1976). *Cognitive learning in children: Theories and strategies*. New York: Academic Press.

Levine, M.D., Hooper, S., Montgomery, J., Reed, M., Sandler, A., Swartz, C., & Watson, T. (1993). Learning disabilities: An interactive developmental paradigm. In G.R. Lyon, D.B. Gray, J.F. Kavanagh, & N. Krasnegor (Eds.), *Better understanding learning disabilities: New views from research and their implications for education and public policies*. Baltimore: Paul H. Brookes Publishing Co.

Lewis, A. (1980). The early identification of children with learning difficulties. *Journal of Learning Disabilities, 13,* 51–57.

Lewis, B.A. (1990). Familial phonological disorders: Four pedigrees. *Journal of Speech and Hearing Disorders, 55,* 160–170.

Lewis, B.A., Ekelman, B.L., & Aram, D.M. (1989). A familial study of severe familial phonological disorders. *Journal of Speech and Hearing Research, 32,* 713–724.

Liben, L.S. (1977). Memory from a cognitive-developmental perspective. In W.F. Overton & J.M. Gallagher (Eds.), *Knowledge and development: Vol. 1. Advances in research and theory.* New York: Plenum Press.

Liberman, A.M., Cooper, F.S., Shankweiler, D.P., & Studdert-Kennedy, M. (1967). Perception of the speech code. *Psychological Review, 74,* 431–461.

Liberman, I.Y. (1987). Language and literacy: The obligations of the schools of education. In *Intimacy with language: A forgotten basic in teacher education.* Baltimore: The Orton Dyslexia Society.

Liberman, I.Y., Mann, V.A., Shankweiler, D., & Werfelman, M. (1982). Children's memory for recurring linguistic and nonlinguistic material in relation to reading ability. *Cortex, 18,* 367–375.

Liberman, I.Y., & Shankweiler, D. (1979). Speech, the alphabet, and teaching to read. In L. Resnick & P. Weaver (Eds.), *Theory and practice of early reading.* Hillsdale, NJ: Lawrence Erlbaum Associates.

Liles, B.Z. (1985). Cohesion in the narratives of normal and language disordered children. *Journal of Speech and Hearing Research, 28,* 123–133.

Liles, B.Z. (1987). Episode organization and cohesive conjunctions in narratives of children with and without language disorders. *Journal of Speech and Hearing Research, 30,* 185–196.

Liles, B.Z., Cooker, H.S., Kass, M., & Carey, B.J. (1976). Effects of pause time on auditory comprehension of language disordered children. *Journal of Communication Disorders, 11,* 365–379.

Limber, T. (1976). Unraveling competence, performance and pragmatics in the speech of young children. *Journal of Child Language, 3,* 309–318.

Lipsky, D.K., & Gartner, A. (1989). The current situation. In D.K. Lipsky & A. Gartner (Eds.), *Beyond separate education: Quality education for all* (pp. 3–24). Baltimore: Paul H. Brookes Publishing Co.

Loban, W.D. (1963). *The language of elementary school children.* Champaign, IL: National Council of Teachers of English.

Loban, W.D. (1976). *Language development: K–12.* Urbana, IL: National Council of Teachers of English.

Locke, J. (1983). *Phonological acquisition and change.* New York: Academic Press.

Loftus, G.R., & Loftus, E.F. (1976). *Human memory: The processing of information.* Hillsdale, NJ: Lawrence Erlbaum Associates.

Loper, A.B. (1982). Metacognitive training to correct academic deficiency. *Topics in Learning and Learning Disabilities, 2,* 61–68.

Loper, A.B., & Hallahan, D.P. (1982). A consideration of the role of generalization in cognitive training. *Topics in Learning and Learning Disabilities, 2,* 62–67.

Lorsbach, T.C., & Gray, J.W. (1986). Item identification speed and memory span performance in learning disabled children. *Contemporary Educational Psychology, 11,* 68–78.

Lovaas, O.I. (1968). A program for the establishment of speech in psychotic children. In H.N. Sloane & B.D. MacAulay (Eds.), *Operant procedures in remedial speech and language training.* Boston: Houghton Mifflin Co.

Lovitt, T.C. (1975a). Characteristics of ABA: General recommendations and methodological limitations. *Journal of Learning Disabilities, 8,* 432–443.

Lovitt, T.C. (1975b). Applied behavioral analysis and learning disabilities. Part II: Specific research recommendations and suggestions for practitioners. *Journal of Learning Disabilities, 8,* 504–518.

Lovrinic, J.H. (1983). *Auditory processing: Controversy and challenge.* Miniseminar, Pennsylvania. Speech and Hearing Association Convention.

Lufi, D., & Cohen, A. (1988). Differential diagnosis of learning disability versus emotional disturbance using the WISC-R. *Journal of Learning Disabilities, 21,* 515–517.

Lund, K.A., Foster, G.E, & McCall-Perez, F.C. (1978). The effectiveness of psycholinguistic training: A re-evaluation. *Exceptional Children, 44,* 310–319.

Luria, A.R. (1980). *Higher cortical functions in man* (2nd ed.). New York: Basic Books.

Luria, A.R. (1981). *Language and cognition.* New York: John Wiley & Sons.

Lust, B. (Ed.). (1986). *Studies in the acquisition of anaphora: Vol. 1. Defining the constraints.* Dordrecht, Holland: D. Reidel.

Lust, B. (Ed.). (1987). *Studies in the acquisition of anaphora: Vol. 2. Applying the constraints.* Dordrect, Holland: D. Reidel.

Lyon, G.R. (1985a). Educational validation studies of learning disability subtypes. In B.P. Rourke (Ed.), *Neuropsychology of learning disabilities.* New York: The Guilford Press.

Lyon, G.R. (1985b). Identification and remediation of learning disability subtypes: Preliminary findings. *Learning Disabilities Focus, 1,* 21–35.

Lyon, G.R., Stewart, N., & Freedman, D. (1982). Neuropsychological characteristics of empirically derived subgroups of learning disabled readers. *Journal of Clinical Neuropsychology, 4,* 343–365.

Lyon, G.R., & Watson, B. (1981). Empirically derived subgroups of learning disabled readers: Diagnostic characteristics. *Journal of Learning Disabilities, 14,* 251–256.

MacCorquodale, K. (1969). B.F. Skinner's verbal behavior: A retrospective appreciation. *Journal of Experimental Analysis of Behavior, 12,* 831–841.

MacDonald, J.D., & Blott, J.P. (1974). Environmental language intervention: The rationale for a diagnostic and training strategy through rules, context and generalization. *Journal of Speech and Hearing Disorders, 39,* 244–256.

MacKay, D.G. (1973). Aspects of the theory of comprehension, memory, and attention. *Quarterly Journal of Experimental Psychology, 25,* 22–40.

Macken, M. (1980). Aspects of the acquisition of stop systems: A cross-linguistic perspective. In G.H. Yeni-Komshian, F. Kavanaugh, & C.A. Ferguson (Eds.), *Child phonology: Vol. 1. Production.* New York: Academic Press.

Maclean, M., Bryant, P., & Bradley, L. (1987). Rhymes, nursery rhymes, and reading in early childhood. *Merrill-Palmer Quarterly, 33,* 255–281.

MacMillan, D.L. (1993). Classification and definition in mental retardation—Similarities and differences with the field of learning disabilities. In G.R. Lyon, D.B. Gray, J.F. Kavanagh, & N. Krasnegor (Eds.), *Better understanding learning disabilities: New views from research and their implications for education and public policies.* Baltimore: Paul H. Brookes Publishing Co.

MacWhinney, B. (1987). The competition model. In B. MacWhinney (Ed.), *Mechanisms of language acquisition.* Hillsdale, NJ: Lawrence Erlbaum Associates.

MacWhinney, B. (1989). Competition and teachability. In M.L. Rice & R.L. Schiefelbusch (Eds.), *The teachability of language* (pp. 63–104). Baltimore: Paul H. Brookes Publishing Co.

Maheady, L., & Sainato, D.M. (1986). Learning disabled students' perceptions of social events. In S.J. Ceci (Ed.), *Handbook of cognitive, social and neuropsychological aspects of learning disabilities.* Hillsdale, NJ: Lawrence Erlbaum Associates.

Mandler, J.M. (1979). Categorical and schematic organization in memory. In C.R. Puff (Ed.), *Memory organization and structure.* New York: Academic Press.

Mandler, J.M. (1984). *Stories, scripts, and scenes: Aspects of schema theory.* Hillsdale, NJ: Lawrence Erlbaum Associates.

Mandler, J.M., & Johnson, N.S. (1977). Remembrance of things parsed: Story structure and recall. *Cognitive Psychology, 9,* 111–151.

Mann, L., & Sabatino, D. (1985). *Foundations of cognitive process in remedial and special education.* Rockville, MD: Aspen Systems Corp.

Mann, V.A. (1984). Longitudinal prediction and prevention of early reading difficulty. *Annals of Dyslexia, 34,* 117–135.

Mann, V.A., & Brady, S. (1988). Reading disability: The role of language deficiencies. *Journal of Consulting and Clinical Psychology, 56,* 811–816.

Manning, G., & Manning, M. (Eds.). (1989). *Whole language: Beliefs and practices, K–8.* Washington, DC: National Education Association.

Maratsos, M. (1986). *On the roles of input and tabulation.* Paper presented at the Boston University Conference on Language Development, Boston.

Marcel, T. (1980). Phonological awareness and phonological representation: Investigation of a specific spelling problem. In U. Frith (Ed.), *Cognitive processes in spelling.* London: Academic Press.

Margalit, M. (1989). Academic competence and social adjustment of boys with learning disabilities and boys with behavior disorders. *Journal of Learning Disabilities, 22,* 41–45.

Markman, E. (1979). Realizing that you don't understand: Elementary school children's awareness of inconsistencies. *Child Development, 50,* 643–655.

Martin, E.W. (1993). Learning disabilities and public policy: Myths and outcomes. In G.R. Lyon, D.B. Gray, J.P. Kavanagh, & N. Krasnegor (Eds.), *Better understanding learning disabilities: New views from research and their implications for education and public policies.* Baltimore: Paul H. Brookes Publishing Co.

Martin, L.J. (1986). Assessing current theories of cerebral organization. In S.J. Ceci (Ed.), *Handbook of cognitive, social and neuropsychological aspects of learning disabilities* (Vol. 1). Hillsdale, NJ: Lawrence Erlbaum Associates.

Martin, R.C., Jerger, S., & Breedin, S. (1987). Syntactic processing of auditory and visual sentences in a learning disabled child: Relations to short term memory. *Developmental Neuropsychology, 3,* 129–152.

Masland, R.L. (1975). Neurological bases and correlates of language disabilities: Diagnostic implications. *Acta Symbolica, VI* (Part 2), 1–34.

Massaro, D.W. (1976). Auditory information processing. In W. K.W. Estes (Ed.), *Handbook of learning and cognitive processes: Vol. 4. Attention and memory.* Hillsdale, NJ: Lawrence Erlbaum Associates.

Matkin, N.D., & Hook, P.E. (1983). A multidisciplinary approach to central auditory evaluation. In E.Z. Lasky & J. Katz (Eds.), *Central auditory processing disorders.* Baltimore: University Park Press.

Matlin, M.W. (1989). *Cognition* (2nd ed.). Orlando, FL: Holt, Rinehart and Winston, Inc.

Mattingly, I.G. (1972). Reading, the linguistic process and linguistic awareness. In J.F. Kavanaugh & I.G. Mattingly (Eds.), *Language by ear and by eye.* Cambridge, MA: The MIT Press.

Mattis, S., French, J.H., & Rapin, I. (1975). Dyslexia in children: Three independent neuropsychological syndromes. *Developmental Medicine and Child Neurology, 17,* 150–163.

Mazzie, C.A. (1987). An experimental investigation of the determinants of implicitness in spoken and written discourse. *Discourse Processes, 19,* 31–42.

McBride, J.E., & Levy, K. (1981). The early academic classroom for children with communication disorders. In A. Gerber & D.N. Bryen (Eds.), *Language and learning disabilities* (pp. 269–294). Baltimore: University Park Press.

McCarthy, B. (1980). *The 4mat system*. Oak Harbor, IL: Excel Inc.

McCarthy, D. (1972). *McCarthy Scales of Children's Abilities*. San Antonio, TX: The Psychological Corporation.

McCord, J.S., & Haynes, W.O. (1988). Discourse errors in students with learning disabilities and their normally achieving peers: Molar versus molecular views. *Journal of Learning Disabilities, 21,* 237–243.

McCue, P.M., Shelly, C., & Goldstein, G. (1986). Intellectual, academic and neuropsychological performance levels in learning disabled adults. *Journal of Learning Disabilities, 19,* 233–236.

McCutchen, D. (1987). Children's discourse skill: Form and modality requirements of schooled writing. *Discourse Processes, 10,* 267–286.

McDonald, E.T. (1964). *Articulation testing and treatment: A sensory-motor approach*. Pittsburgh: Stanwix House.

McGregor, K.K., & Leonard, L.B. (1989). Facilitating word-finding skills of language-impaired children. *Journal of Speech and Hearing Disorders, 54,* 141–147.

McKinney, J.D. (1989). Longitudinal research on the behavioral characteristics of children with learning disabilities. *Journal of Learning Disabilities, 22,* 141–150.

McKinney, J.D., & Hocutt, A.M. (1988). The need for policy analysis in evaluating the regular education initiative. *Journal of Learning Disabilities, 21,* 12–18.

McKinney, J.M. (1985). The search for subtypes of specific learning disability. *Annual Progress in Child Psychiatry and Child Development, 18,* 542–555.

McKinney, J.M., Short, E.J., & Feagans, L. (1985). Academic consequences of perceptual-linguistic subtypes of learning disabled children. *Learning Disabilities Research, 1,* 6–17.

McLean, J.E. (1983). Historical perspectives on the content of child language programs. In J. Miller, D.E. Yoder, & R.L. Schiefelbusch (Eds.), *Contemporary issues in language intervention*. Rockville, MD: The American Speech-Language-Hearing Association.

McLeod, J. (1965). *Some psychological and psycholinguistic aspects of severe reading disability in children*. Unpublished doctoral dissertation, University of Queensland, Australia.

McLeod, J. (1976). A reaction to psycholinguistics in the schools. In P.L. Newcomber & D.D. Hammill (Eds.), *Psycholinguistics in the schools*. Columbus, OH: Charles E. Merrill.

McNeill, D. (1966). A study of word association. *Journal of Verbal Learning and Verbal Behavior, 5,* 548–557.

McNeill, D. (1970). *The acquisition of language*. New York: Harper & Row.

Mehan, H. (1979). *Learning lesson: Social organization in the classroom*. Cambridge, MA: Harvard University Press.

Meichenbaum, D. (1980). Cognitive behavior modification with exceptional children: A promise yet unfulfilled. *Exceptional Education Quarterly, 1,* 83–88.

Meichenbaum, D.H., & Goodman, J. (1971). Training impulsive children to talk to themselves: A means of developing self-control. *Journal of Abnormal Psychology, 77,* 115–126.

Meline, T.J., & Brackin, S.R. (1987). Language-impaired children's awareness of inadequate messages. *Journal of Speech and Hearing Disorders, 52,* 263–270.

Menyuk, P. (1969). *Sentences children use*. Cambridge: The MIT Press.

Menyuk, P. (1988). *Language development: Knowledge and use*. Glenview, IL: Scott, Foresman and Co.

Menyuk, P., & Menn, L. (1979). Early strategies for the perception of words and sounds. In P. Fletcher & M. Garman (Eds.), *Language acquisition: Studies in first language development*. Cambridge, England: Cambridge University Press.

Merritt, D.D., & Liles, B.Z. (1987). Story grammar ability in children with and without language disorder: Story generation, story retelling, and story comprehension. *Journal of Speech and Hearing Research, 30,* 539–551.

Meyer, B.J. (1975). *The organization of prose and its effects on memory*. Amsterdam: Elsevier North-Holland Publishers.

Meyer, B.J. (1977). The structure of prose: Effects on learning and memory and implications for educational practice. In R.C. Anderson & R.J. Spiro (Eds.), *Schooling and the acquisition of knowledge*. Hillsdale, NJ: Lawrence Erlbaum Associates.

Miller, G.A. (1978). Practical and lexical knowledge. In E. Rosch & B.B. Lloyd (Eds.), *Cognition and categorization*. Hillsdale, NJ: Lawrence Erlbaum Associates.

Miller, G.E., Giovenco, A., & Rentiers, K.A. (1987). Fostering comprehension monitoring in below average readers through self-instruction training. *Journal of Reading Behavior, 19,* 379–394.

Miller, J. (1981). *Assessing language production in children*. Baltimore: University Park Press.

Miller, J., & Chapman, R. (1983). *SALT: Systematic analysis of language transcripts. User's manual*. Madison: University of Wisconsin.

Miller, J.F., & Yoder, D.E. (1972). A syntax teaching program. In J.E. McLean, D.E. Yoder, & R.L. Schiefelbusch (Eds.), *Language intervention with the retarded*. Baltimore: University Park Press.

Miller, J.F., & Yoder, D.E. (1974). An ontogenetic language teaching strategy for retarded children. In R.L. Schiefelbusch & L.L. Lloyd (Eds.), *Language perspectives—acquisition, retardation, and intervention*. Baltimore: University Park Press.

Miller, L. (1984). Problem solving and language disorders. In G.P. Wallach & K.G. Butler (Eds.), *Language learning disabilities in school-age children*. Baltimore: Williams & Wilkins.

Miller, L. (1989). Classroom-based language intervention. *Language Speech and Hearing Services in Schools, 20,* 153–169.

Miller, L. (1990). The roles of language and learning in the development of literacy. *Topics in Language Disorders, 10,* 1–24.

Miller, P.H., & Weiss, M.G. (1981). Children's attention allocation, understanding of attention and performance on the incidental learning task. *Child Development, 52,* 1183–1190.

Minskoff, E.H. (1976), Research on the efficacy of remediating psycholinguistic disabilities: Critique and recommendations. In P.L. Newcomer & D.D. Hammill (Eds.), *Psycholinguistics in the schools.* Columbus, OH: Charles E. Merrill Co.

Moffett, J. (1968). *Teaching the universe of discourse.* Boston: Houghton Mifflin Co.

Mokros, H.B., Poznanski, E.O., & Merrick, W.A. (1989). Depression and learning disabilities in children: A test of an hypothesis. *Journal of Learning Disabilities, 22,* 230–233.

Molfese, D.L., & Molfese, V.J. (1986). Psychophysiological indices of early cognitive processes and their relationship to language. In J.E. Obrzut & G.W. Hynd (Eds.), *Child neuropsychology: Theory and research* (Vol. 1). Orlando, FL: Academic Press.

Montague, M., Maddux, C.D., & Dereshiwsky, M.I. (1990). Story grammar and comprehension and production of narrative prose by students with learning disabilities. *Journal of Learning Disabilities, 23,* 190–197.

Moore, T., & Harris, A. (1978). Language and thought in Piagetian theory. In L. Siegel & C. Brainerd (Eds.), *Alternatives to Piaget.* New York: Academic Press.

Moran, M. (1981a). *A comparison of formal features of oral language of learning disabled, low achieving, and achieving secondary students* (Res. Rep. No. 35). Lawrence, KS: University of Kansas, Institute for Research in Learning Disabilities.

Moran, M. (1981b). *A comparison of formal features of written language of learning disabled, low achieving, and achieving secondary students* (Res. Rep. No. 34). Lawrence, KS: University of Kansas, Institute for Research in Learning Disabilities.

Moran, M.R. (1987). Individualized objectives for writing instruction. *Topics in Language Disorders, 7,* 42–54.

Moran, M.R. (1988). Reading and writing disorders in the learning disabled student. In N.J. Lass, L.V. McReynolds, J.L. Northern, & D.E. Yoder (Eds.), *Handbook of speech-language pathology and audiology.* Philadelphia: Brian C. Decker, Publishers.

Moran, M.R., & Byrne, M.C. (1977). Mastery of verb tense markers by normal and learning-disabled children. *Journal of Speech and Hearing Research, 20,* 529–542.

Morehead, D., & Ingram, D. (1973). Development of base syntax in normal and linguistically deviant children. *Journal of Speech and Hearing Research, 16,* 330–352.

Morice, R., & Slaghuis, W. (1985). Language performance and reading ability at 8 years of age. *Applied Psycholinguistics, 6,* 141–160.

Morine-Dershimer, G. (1988). Three approaches to sociolinguistic analysis: Introduction. In J.L. Green & J.O. Harker (Eds.), *Multiple perspective analysis of classroom discourse.* Norwood, NJ: Ablex.

Morris, R. (1993). Issues in empirical and clinical identification of learning disabilities. In G.R. Lyon, D.B. Gray, J.F. Kavanagh, & N. Krasnegor (Eds.), *Better understanding learning disabilities: New views from research and their implications for education and public policies.* Baltimore: Paul H. Brookes Publishing Co.

Morris, R., Blashfield, R., & Satz, P. (1986). Developmental classification of reading-disabled children. *Journal of Clinical and Experimental Neuropsychology, 8,* 371–392.

Morrison, F.J., Giordano, B., & Nagy, J. (1977). Reading disability: An information processing analysis. *Science, 196,* 77–79.

Muma, J.R. (1978). *Muma Assessment Program.* Lubbock, TX: Natural Child Publications.

Murray, S.L., Feinstein, C.B., & Blouin, A.G. (1985). The Token Test for Children: Diagnostic patterns and programming implications. In C.S. Simon (Ed.), *Communication skills and classroom success: Assessment of language-learning disabled students.* San Diego: College Hill Press.

Myers, N.A., & Perlmutter, M. (1978). Memory in the years from two to five. In P.A. Ornstein (Ed.), *Memory development in children.* Hillsdale, NJ: Lawrence Erlbaum Associates.

Myers, P.I., & Hammill, D.D. (1976). *Methods for learning disorders* (2nd ed.). New York: John Wiley & Sons.

Myers, P.I., & Hammill, D.D. (1990). *Learning disabilities: Basic concepts, assessment practices, and instructional strategies* (4th ed.). Austin, TX: PRO-ED.

Myklebust, H. (1954). *Auditory disorders in children: A manual for differential diagnostics.* New York: Grune & Stratton.

Myklebust, H. (1965). *Development and disorders of written language: Vol. 1: Picture story language test.* New York: Grune & Stratton.

Myklebust, H. (1971). *The Pupil Rating Scale.* New York: Grune & Stratton.

Naigles, L., Golinkoff, R., & Hirsh-Pasek, K. (1989). *Comprehension of the passive by two year olds.* Paper presented at the Boston University Conference on Language Development, Boston.

National Joint Committee on Learning Disabilities. (1988). Letter to NJCLD member organizations. Baltimore: NJCLD.

National Joint Committee on Learning Disabilities. (1991). Providing appropriate education for students with learning disabilities in regular education classrooms. *Asha, 33,* 15–17.

Naus, M.J., & Halasz, F.G. (1979). Developmental perspectives on cognitive processing and semantic memory structure. In L.S. Cermak & F.I.M. Craik (Eds.), *Levels of processing in human memory.* Hillsdale, NJ: Lawrence Erlbaum Associates.

Naus, M.J., Ornstein, P.A., & Hoving, K.L. (1978). Developmental implications of multistore and depth-of-processing models of memory. In P.A. Ornstein (Ed.), *Memory development in children*. Hillsdale, NJ: Lawrence Erlbaum Associates.

Naylor, H. (1980). Reading disability and lateral asymmetry: An information processing analysis. *Psychological Bulletin, 87,* 531–545.

Neisser, U. (1979). The control of information pickup in selective looking. In A. Pick (Ed.), *Perception and its development: A tribute to Eleanor J. Gibson*. Hillsdale, NJ: Lawrence Erlbaum Associates.

Nelson, C.M., & Polsgrove, L. (1984). Behavior analysis in special education: White rabbit or white elephant? *Remedial and Special Education (RASE), 5,* 6–17.

Nelson, K. (1977). The syntagmatic-paradigmatic shift revisited: A review of research and theory. *Psychological Bulletin, 84,* 93–116.

Nelson, N.W. (1981). An eclectic model of language intervention for disorders of listening, speaking, reading and writing. *Topics in Language Disorders, 1,* 1–24.

Nelson, N.W. (1984). Beyond information processing: The language of teachers and textbooks. In G.P. Wallach & K.G. Butler (Eds.), *Language learning disabilities in school-age children*. Baltimore: Williams & Wilkins.

Nelson, N.W. (1985). Teacher talk and child listening—fostering a better match. In C.S. Simon (Ed.), *Communication skills and classroom success: Assessment of language-learning disabled students*. San Diego: College Hill Press.

Nelson, N.W. (1986a). Individual processing in classroom settings. *Topics in Language Disorders, 6,* 13–27.

Nelson, N.W. (1986b). What is meant by meaning (and how can it be taught)? *Topics in Language Disorders, 6,* 1–14.

Nelson, N.W. (1988a). Reading and writing. In M. Nippold (Ed.), *Later language development: Ages nine through nineteen*. Boston: College Hill Press.

Nelson, N.W. (1988b). *Planning individualized speech and language intervention programs*. Tucson, AZ: Communication Skill Builders.

Nelson, N.W. (1989). Curriculum-based language assessment and intervention. *Language Speech and Hearing Services in Schools, 20,* 170–184.

Newcomer, P.L., Barenbaum, E.M.E., & Nodine, B.F. (1988). Comparison of story production of LD, normal-achieving and low-achieving children under two modes of production. *Learning Disability Quarterly, 11,* 82–96.

Newcomer, P.L., & Hammill, D.D. (1976). *Psycholinguistics in the schools*. Columbus, OH: Charles E. Merrill Co.

Newcomer, P.L., & Hammill, D.D. (1977). *Test of Linguistic Development*. Austin, TX: PRO-ED.

Newman, J.E., Lovett, M.W., & Dennis, M. (1986). The use of discourse analysis in neurolinguistics: Some findings from the narratives of hemidecorticate adolescents. *Topics in Language Disorders, 7,* 31–44.

Newport, E.L., Gleitman, L.R., & Gleitman, H. (1977). Mother, I'd rather do it myself: Some effects and non-effects of maternal speech style. In C. Snow & C. Ferguson (Eds.), *Talking to children: Language input and acquisition*. Cambridge, MA: Cambridge University Press.

Nichols, E.G., Inglis, J., Lawson, J.S., & MacKay, I. (1988). A cross-validation study of patterns of cognitive ability in children with learning difficulties, as described by factorially defined WISC–R verbal and performance IQs. *Journal of Learning Disabilities, 21,* 504–508.

Nippold, M.A. (1985). Comprehension of figurative language in youth. *Topics in Language Disorders, 5,* 1–20.

Nippold, M.A. (1988a). Figurative Language. In M.A. Nippold (Ed.), *Later language development: Ages nine through nineteen*. Boston: College Hill Press.

Nippold, M.A. (1988b). The literate lexicon. In M.A. Nippold (Ed.), *Later language development: Ages nine through nineteen*. Boston: College Hill Press.

Nippold, M.A. (1991). Evaluating and enhancing idiom comprehension in language-disordered students. *Language, Speech, and Hearing Services in Schools, 22,* 100–106.

Nippold, M.A., & Fey, S.H. (1983). Metaphoric understanding in preadolescents having history of language acquisition difficulties. *Language, Speech and Hearing Services in Schools, 14,* 171–180.

Nippold, M.A., & Martin, S.T. (1989). Idiom interpretation in isolation versus context: A developmental study with adolescents. *Journal of Speech and Hearing Research, 32,* 59–66.

Nix, D., & Schwarz, M. (1979). Toward a phenomenology of reading comprehension. In R.O. Freedle (Ed.), *New directions in discourse processing*. Norwood, NJ: Ablex Publ. Co.

Norman, D. (1972). The role of memory in the understanding of language. In J.F. Kavanaugh & I.G. Mattingly (Eds.), *Language by ear and by eye*. Cambridge, MA: The M.I.T. Press.

Norris, J.A. (1989). Providing language remediation in the classroom: An integrated language-to-reading intervention method. *Language, Speech and Hearing Services in Schools, 20,* 205–218.

Norris, J.A., & Bruning, R.H. (1988). Cohesion in the narratives of good and poor readers. *Journal of Speech and Hearing Disorders, 53,* 416–424.

Norris, J.A., & Damico, J. (1990). Whole language in theory and practice: Implications for language intervention. *Language, Speech, and Hearing Services in Schools, 21,* 212–220.

Norris, J.A., & Hoffman, P.R. (1990). Language intervention within naturalistic environments. *Language, Speech, and Hearing Services in Schools, 21,* 72–84.

O'Boyle, M.W. (1986). Hemispheric laterality as a basis for learning: What we know and don't know. In G.D. Phye & T. Andre (Eds.), *Cognitive classroom learning*. Orlando, FL: Academic Press.

O'Brien, B.J. (1987). Antecedent search process and the structure of text. *Journal of Experimental Psychology: Learning, Memory and Cognition, 13*, 178–190.

Obrzut, J.E. (1989). Dyslexia and neurodevelopmental pathology: Is the neurodiagnostic technology ahead of the psycho-educational technology? *Journal of Learning Disabilities, 22*, 217–218.

Obrzut, J.E., & Boliek, C.A. (1986). Lateralization characteristics in learning disabled children. *Journal of Learning Disabilities, 19*, 308–314.

Obrzut, J.E., & Hynd, G.W (1983). The neurobiological and neurophysiological foundations of learning disabilities. *Journal of Learning Disabilities, 16*, 515–520.

Obrzut, J.E., & Hynd, G.W. (1986). Child neuropsychology: An introduction to theory and research. In J.E. Obrzut & G.W. Hynd (Eds.), *Child neuropsychology: Vol. 1. Theory and research*. Orlando, FL: Academic Press.

Obrzut, J.E., Hynd, G.W., & Boliek, C.A. (1986). Lateral asymmetries in learning disabled children: A review. In S.J. Ceci (Ed.), *Handbook of cognitive, social and neuropsychological aspects of learning disabilities* (Vol. 1). Hillsdale, NJ: Lawrence Erlbaum Associates.

Obrzut, J.E., Hynd, G.W., Obrzut, A., & Leitgeb, J.L. (1980). Time-sharing and dichotic listening asymmetry in normal and learning disabled children. *Brain and Language, 11*, 181–194.

Obrzut, J.E., Hynd, G.W., Obrzut, A., & Pirozzolo, F.J. (1981). Effect of directed attention on cerebral asymmetries in normal and learning disabled children. *Developmental Psychology, 17*, 118–125.

Obrzut, J.E., Obrzut, A., Bryden, M.P., & Bartels, S.G. (1985). Information processing and speech lateralization in LD children. *Brain and Language, 25*, 87–101.

Ochs, E. (1977). Planned and unplanned discourse. In T. Givon (Ed.), *Syntax and semantics: Discourse and syntax*. New York: Academic Press.

Oleron, P. (1977). *Language and mental development*. Hillsdale, NJ: Lawrence Erlbaum Associates.

Oller, J.W., Jr. (1979). *Language test at school*. London: Longman.

Oller, J.W., Jr. (1983). A consensus for the eighties? In J.W. Oller (Ed.), *Issues in language testing research*. Rowley, MA: Newberry House.

Olson, D. (1977a). From utterance to text: The bias of language in speech and writing. *Harvard Educational Review, 47*, 257–281.

Olson, D.R. (1977b). The language of instruction: On the literate bias of schooling. In R.C. Anderson & R.J. Spiro (Eds.), *Schooling and the acquisition of knowledge*. Hillsdale, NJ: Lawrence Erlbaum Associates.

Olson, D. (1982). The language of schooling. *Topics in Language Disorders, 2*, 1–12.

Olson, G.M. (1973). Developmental changes in memory and the acquisition of language. In T.E. Moore (Ed.), *Cognitive development and the acquisition of language*. New York: Academic Press.

Olson, R., Wise, B., Conners, F., Rack, J., & Fuller D. (1989). Specific deficits in component reading and language skills: Genetic and environmental influences. *Journal of Learning Disabilities, 22*, 339–348.

Ornstein, P.A. (1978). Introduction: The study of children's memory. In P.A. Ornstein (Ed.), *Memory development in children*. Hillsdale, NJ: Lawrence Erlbaum Associates.

Ornstein, P.A., Baker-Ward, L., & Naus, M.J. (1988). The development of mnemonic skill. In F.E. Weinert & M. Perlmutter (Eds.), *Memory development: Universal changes and individual differences*. Hillsdale, NJ: Lawrence Erlbaum Associates.

Ornstein, P.A., & Corsale, K. (1979). Organizational factors in children's memory. In C.R. Puff (Ed.), *Memory organization and structure*. New York: Academic Press.

Ornstein, P.A., & Naus, M.J. (1978). Rehearsal processes in children's memory. In P.A. Ornstein (Ed.), *Memory development in children*. Hillsdale, NJ: Lawrence Erlbaum Associates.

Ornstein, P.A., Naus, M.J., & Stone, B.P. (1977). Rehearsal training and developmental differences in memory. *Developmental Psychology, 13*, 15–24.

Ortiz, A.A. (1988). Evaluating educational contexts in which language minority children are served. *Bilingual Special Education Newsletter, 7*, 1–4.

Orton, S.T (1937). *Reading, writing and speech problems in children*. New York: Norton Publ. Co.

Osgood, C.E., & Sebeok, T.A. (Eds.). (1954). Psycholinguistics: A survey of theory and research problems. *Journal of Abnormal and Social Psychology, 52* (Suppl.).

Owens, R.E. Jr. (1984). *Language development: An introduction*. Columbus, OH: Charles E. Merrill.

Ozols, E.J., & Rourke, B.P. (1988). Characteristics of young learning disabled children classified according to patterns of academic achievement: Auditory-perceptual and visual-perceptual abilities. *Journal of Clinical Child Psychology, 17*, 44–52.

Page, J.L., & Stewart, S.R. (1985). Story grammar skills in school-age children. *Topics in Language Disorders, 5*, 16–30.

Palinscar, A.S. (1989). *Roles of the speech-language pathologist in disadvantaged children's pursuit of literacy*. Paper presented at the American Speech-Language-Hearing Association's National Forum on Schools—Partnership in Education: Toward a Literate America, Washington, DC.

Palinscar, A.S., & Brown, A.L. (1984). Reciprocal teaching of comprehension fostering and comprehension monitoring activities. *Cognition and Instruction, 1,* 117—175.

Palinscar, A.S, & Brown, A.L. (1986). Interactive teaching to promote independent learning from text. *Reading Teacher, 39,* 771–777.

Palinscar, A.S., & Brown, D.A. (1987). Enhancing instructional time through attention to metacognition. *Journal of Learning Disabilities, 20,* 66–75.

Pany, D., Jenkins, J.R., & Schreck, J. (1982). Vocabulary instruction: Effects on word knowledge and reading comprehension. *Learning Disability Quarterly, 5,* 202–215.

Parasuraman, R. (1984). The psychobiology of sustained attention. In J.S. Warm (Ed.), *Sustained attention in human performance.* New York: John Wiley & Sons.

Paris, S., & Oka, E.R. (1989). Strategies for comprehending text and coping with reading difficulties. *Learning Disability Quarterly, 12,* 32–42.

Paris, S.G. (1978). The development of inference and transformation as memory operations. In P.A. Ornstein (Ed.), *Memory development in children.* Hillsdale, NJ: Lawrence Erlbaum Associates.

Paris, S.G., & Jacobs, J.E. (1984). The benefits of informed instruction for children's reading awareness and comprehension skills. *Child Development, 55,* 2083–2093.

Parish, R. (1989). *Young children at risk: Language development and intervention.* Paper presented at the American Speech-Language-Hearing Association's National Forum on Schools—Partnership in Education: Toward a Literate America, Washington, DC.

Parker, G.M. (1990). *Team players and team work.* San Francisco: Jossey-Bass.

Parker, T.B., Freston, C.W., & Drew, C.J. (1975). Comparison of verbal performance of normal and learning disabled children as a function of input organization. *Journal of Learning Disabilities, 8,* 386–392.

Parkins, R.A., Roberts, R.J., Reinarz, S.J., & Varney, N.R. (1987). *CT asymmetries in adult developmental dyslexics.* Paper presented at the annual meeting of the International Neuropsychological Society, Washington, DC.

Parnell, M.M., Amerman, J.D., & Harting, R.D. (1986). Responses of language-disordered children to Wh-questions. *Language Speech and Hearing Services in Schools, 17,* 95–106.

Pascual-Leone, J., & Smith, J. (1969). The encoding and decoding of symbols by children: A new experimental paradigm and a neo-Piagetian model. *Journal of Experimental Child Psychology, 8,* 328–355.

Pea, R. (1982). Origins of verbal logic: Spontaneous denials by two- and three-year-olds. *Journal of Child Language, 9,* 597–626.

Pearl, R. (1987). Social cognitive factors in learning disabled children's social problems. In S.J. Ceci (Ed.), *Handbook of cognitive, social and neuropsychological aspects of learning disabilities.* Hillsdale, NJ: Lawrence Erlbaum Associates.

Pearson, P.D., & Spiro, R.J. (1980). Toward a theory of reading comprehension instruction. *Topics in Language Disorders, 1,* 71–88.

Peck, C.A. (1989). Assessment of social communicative competence. *Seminars in Speech and Language, 10,* 1–15.

Pehrsson, R.S., & Robinson, H.A. (1985). *The semantic organizer approach to writing and reading instruction.* Rockville, MD: Aspen Systems Corp.

Pelham, W.E. (1986). The effects of psychostimulant drugs on learning and academic achievement in children with attention disorders and learning disabilities. In J.K. Torgeson & B.Y.L. Wong (Eds.), *Psychological and educational perspectives on learning disabilities.* Orlando, FL: Academic Press.

Pellegrino, J.W., & Goldman, S.R. (1987). Information processing and elementary mathematics. *Journal of Learning Disabilities, 20,* 23–32.

Perera, K. (1984). *Children's writing and reading: Analyzing classroom language.* New York: Basil Blackwell, Inc.

Perfetti, C.A. (1979). Levels of language and levels of process. In L.S. Craik & F.I. Cermak (Eds.), *Levels of processing in human memory.* Hillsdale, NJ: Lawrence Erlbaum Associates.

Perfetti, C.A. (1985). *Reading ability.* New York: Oxford University Press.

Perfetti, C.A. (1987). Language, speech, and print: Some asymmetries in the acquisition of literacy. In R. Horowitz & S.J. Samuels (Eds.), *Comprehending oral and written language.* San Diego: Academic Press.

Perfetti, C.A., & Lesgold, A.M. (1977). Discourse comprehension and sources of individual differences. In M.A. Just & P.A. Carpenter (Eds.), *Cognitive processes in comprehension.* Hillsdale, NJ: Lawrence Erlbaum Associates.

Perfetti, C.A., & McCutchen, D. (1982). Speech processes in reading. *Speech and Language: Advances in Basic Research and Practice, 7,* 237–269.

Perkins, W.H.W. (1971). *Speech pathology: An applied behavioral science.* St. Louis: The C.V. Mosby Co.

Perlmutter, L. (1986). Personality variables and peer relations of children and adolescents with learning disabilities. In S.J. Ceci (Ed.), *Handbook of cognitive, social and neuropsychological aspects of learning disabilities.* Hillsdale, NJ: Lawrence Erlbaum Associates.

Perlmutter, M. (1984). Continuities and discontinuities in early human memory paradigms, processes and performance. In R. Kail & N.E. Spear (Eds.), *Comparative perspectives on the development of memory.* Hillsdale, NJ: Lawrence Erlbaum Associates.

Perlmutter, M. (1988). Research on memory and its development: Past, present, and future. In F.E. Weinert & M. Perlmutter (Eds.), *Memory development: Universal changes and individual differences.* Hillsdale, NJ: Lawrence Erlbaum Associates.

Peterson, C., & McCabe, A. (1983). *Developmental psycholinguistics: Three ways of looking at a child's narrative.* New

York: Plenum Press.

Petry, S. (1977). Word association and the development of lexical memory. *Cognition, 5,* 57–71.

Pflaum, S.W., & Pascarella, E.T. (1980). Interactive effects of prior reading achievement and training in context on the reading of learning disabled children. *Reading Research Quarterly, 16,* 138–158.

Phelps-Gunn, T., & Phelps-Terasaki, D. (1982). *Written language instruction.* Rockville, MD: Aspen Systems Corp.

Phelps-Terasaki, D., Phelps-Gunn, T., & Stetson, E.G. (1983). *Remediation and instruction in language.* Rockville, MD: Aspen Publications.

Piaget, J. (1962). *Plays, dreams, and imitation in childhood.* New York: W.W. Norton & Co.

Piaget, J. (1980). About the fixed nucleus and innateness. In M. Piattelli-Palmarini (Ed.), *Language and learning: The debate between Jean Piaget and Noam Chomsky.* Cambridge, MA: Harvard University Press.

Piaget, J., & Inhelder, B. (1973). *Memory and intelligence.* New York: Basic Books.

Pinker, S. (1985). *Visual cognition.* Cambridge, MA: The MIT Press.

Pirozzolo, F.J., Dunn, K., & Zetusky, W. (1983). Physiological approaches to subtypes of developmental reading disability. *Topics in Learning and Learning Disabilities, 3,* 40–47.

Pirozzolo, F.J., & Hansch, E.C. (1982). The neurobiology of developmental reading disorders. In R.N. Malatesha & P.G. Aaron (Eds.), *Neuropsychological and neurolinguistic aspects of reading disorders.* New York: Academic Press.

Pirozzolo, F.J., & Papanicolaou, A.C. (1986). Plasticity and recovery of the central nervous system. In J.E. Obrzut & G.W. Hynd (Eds.), *Child neuropsychology: Theory and research* (Vol. 1). Orlando, FL: Academic Press.

Pirozzolo, F.J., & Rayner, K. (1979). Cerebral organization and reading disability. *Neuropsychologia, 17,* 485–489.

Pisoni, D.B., & Sawusch, J.R. (1975). Some stages of processing in speech perception. In A. Cohen & S. Nootenboom (Eds.), *Structure and process in speech perception.* Heidelberg: Springer-Verlag.

Pomerance, A. (1991). *The student-tutor orientation: A collaborative whole-language tutor training that includes students.* Adult Basic Education Fall Workshop, Commonwealth of Pennsylvania, Radnor, PA.

Poplin, M.S. (1988a). The reductionist fallacy in learning disabilities: Replicating the past by reducing the present. *Journal of Learning Disabilities, 21,* 389–400.

Poplin, M.S. (1988b). Holistic/constructivist principles of the teaching/learning process: Implications for the field of learning disabilities. *Journal of Learning Disabilities, 21,* 401–416.

Porch, B.E. (1979). *Porch Index of Communicative Ability in Children.* Palo Alto: Consulting Psychologists Press.

Posner, M. (1973). *Cognition: An introduction.* Glenview, IL: Scott, Foresman & Co.

Posner, M., & Boies, S.J. (1971). Components of attention. *Psychological Review, 78,* 391–408.

Pratt, A.C., & Brady, S. (1988). Relation of phonological awareness to reading disability in children and adults. *Journal of Educational Psychology, 80,* 319–323.

Pressley, M., Borkowski, J.G., & O'Sullivan, J.T. (1984). Memory strategy instruction is made of this: Metamemory and durable strategy use. *Educational Psychologist, 19,* 94–107.

Pressley, M., Borkowski, J.G., & O'Sullivan, J. (1985). Children's metamemory and the teaching of memory strategies. In D.L. Forrest-Pressley, G.E. MacKinnon, & T.G. Waller (Eds.), *Metacognition, cognition, and human performance* (Vol. I). Orlando, FL: Academic Press.

Pressley, M., Forrest-Pressley, D., & Elliot-Faust, D.J. (1988). What is strategy instructional enrichment and how to study it: Illustrations from research on children's prose memory and comprehension. In F.E. Weinert & M. Perlmutter (Eds.), *Memory development: Universal changes and individual differences.* Hillsdale, NJ: Lawrence Erlbaum Associates.

Pressley, M., Johnson, C.J., & Symons, S. (1987). Elaborating to learn and learning to elaborate. *Journal of Learning Disabilities, 20,* 76–91.

Pressley, M., & Levin, J.R. (1987). Elaborative learning strategies for the inefficient learner. In S.J. Ceci (Ed.), *Handbook of cognitive, social and neuropsychological aspects of learning disabilities.* Hillsdale, NJ: Lawrence Erlbaum Associates.

Pressley, M., McDaniel, M.A., Turnure, J.E., Wood, B., & Ahmad, M. (1987). Generation of precision of elaboration: Effects on intentional and incidental learning. *Journal of Experimental Psychology: Learning, Memory and Cognition, 13,* 291–300.

Prince, E.F. (1981). Toward a taxonomy of given/new information. In P. Cole (Ed.), *Radical pragmatics.* New York: Academic Press.

Prutting, C.A. (1982). Pragmatic and social competence. *Journal of Speech and Hearing Disorders, 4,* 123–134.

Prutting, C.A., & Kirchner, D.M. (1983). Applied pragmatics. In T.M. Gallagher & C.A. Prutting (Eds.), *Pragmatic assessment and intervention issues in language.* San Diego: College Hill Press.

Prutting, C.A., & Kirchner, D.M. (1987). A clinical appraisal of the pragmatic aspects of language. *Journal of Speech and Hearing Disorders, 52,* 105–119.

Pullis, M., & Smith, D.C. (1981). Social cognitive development of learning disabled children: Implications of Piaget's theory for research and intervention. *Topics in Learning and Learning Disabilities, 1,* 43–56.

Rabinowitz, M., & Chi, M.T.H. (1987). An interactive model of strategic processing. In S.J. Ceci (Ed.), *Handbook of cognitive, social and neuropsychological aspects of learning disabilities.* Hillsdale, NJ: Lawrence Erlbaum Associates.

Read, C. (1978). Children's awareness of language with emphasis on sound systems. In A. Sinclair, R. Jarvella, & W. Levelt (Eds.), *The child's conception of language.* New York: Springer-Verlag.

Rees, N.S. (1973). Auditory processing factors in language disorders: The view from Procrustes' bed. *Journal of Speech and Hearing Disorders, 38,* 304–315.

Rees, N.S. (1978a). I don't understand what you mean by comprehension. *Journal of Speech and Hearing Disorders, 43,* 208–219.

Rees, N.S. (1978b). Pragmatics of language: Application to normal and disordered language development. In R.L. Schiefelbusch (Ed.), *Bases of language intervention* (pp. 191–268). Baltimore: University Park Press.

Rees, N.S. (1981). Saying more than we know: Is auditory processing disorder a meaningful concept? In R.W. Keith (Ed.), *Central auditory and language disorders in children.* Boston: College Hill Press.

Rees, N.S. (1983). Language intervention with children. In J. Miller, D.E. Yoder, & R.L. Schiefelbusch (Eds.), *Contemporary issues in language intervention.* Rockville, MD: The American Speech-Language-Hearing Association.

Reeves, W.H. (1980). Auditory learning disabilities and emotional disturbance: Diagnostic differences. *Journal of Learning Disabilities, 13,* 199–202.

Reid, D.K., & Hresko, W.P. (1981). *A cognitive approach to learning disabilities.* New York: McGraw-Hill Book Co.

Restle, F. (1974). Critique of pure memory. In R.L. Solso (Ed.), *Theories in cognitive psychology: The Loyola symposium.* Hillsdale, NJ: Lawrence Erlbaum Associates.

Reynolds, M.C., & Wang, M.C. (1983). Restructuring "special" school programs: A position paper. *Policy Studies Review, 2,* 189–212.

Rice, M.L., Sell, M.A., & Hadley, P.A. (1990). The Social Interactive Coding System (SICS): An on-line, clinically relevant descriptive tool. *Language Speech and Hearing Services in Schools, 21,* 2–14.

Richard, G.J., & Hanner, M.A. (1987). *Language Processing Test.* Moline, IL: Linguisystems.

Richards, G.P., Samuels, S.J., Turnure, J.E., & Ysseldyke, J.E. (1990). Sustained and selective attention in children with learning disabilities. *Journal of Learning Disabilities, 23,* 129–136.

Riedlinger-Ryan, K.J., & Shewan, C.M. (1984). Comparison of auditory language comprehension skills in learning-disabled and academically-achieving adolescents. *Language Speech and Hearing Services in Schools, 15,* 127–136.

Ring, B.C. (1976). Effects of input organization on auditory short-term memory. *Journal of Learning Disabilities, 9,* 59–63.

Ripich, D.N., & Griffith, P.L. (1988). Narrative abilities of children with learning disabilities and nondisabled children: Story structure, cohesion and propositions. *Journal of Learning Disabilities, 21,* 165–173.

Ripich, D.N., & Spinelli, F.M. (1985). *School discourse problems.* San Diego: College Hill Press.

Risley, T., & Wolf, M. (1968). Establishing functional speech in echolalic children. In H.N. Sloane & B.D. MacAulay (Eds.), *Operant procedures in remedial speech and language training.* New York: Houghton Mifflin Co.

Rosch, E. (1978). Principles of categorization. In E. Rosch & B.B. Lloyd (Eds.), *Cognition and categorization.* Hillsdale, NJ: Lawrence Erlbaum Associates.

Rosen, G.D., Sherman, G.F., & Galaburda, A.M. (1986). Biological interactions in dyslexia. In J.E. Obrzut & G.W. Hynd (Eds.), *Child neuropsychology* (Vol. 1). Orlando, FL: Academic Press, Inc.

Rosenberger, P.B., & Hier, D.B. (1980). Cerebral asymmetry and verbal intellectual deficits. *Annals of Neurobiology, 8,* 300–304.

Ross, A.O. (1976). *Psychological aspects of learning disabilities & reading disorders.* New York: McGraw-Hill Book Co.

Roth, F.P. (1986). Oral narrative abilities of learning disabled students. *Topics in Language Disorders, 7,* 21–30.

Roth, F.P. (1987) *Discourse abilities of learning disabled children: Patterns and intervention strategies.* Workshop presented at the Language Learning Disabilities Conference, Emerson College, Boston.

Roth, F.P., & Spekman, N.J. (1984). Assessing the pragmatic abilities of children. Parts 1 and 2. *Journal of Speech and Hearing disorders, 49,* 2–17.

Roth, F.P., & Spekman, N.J. (1986). Narrative discourse: Spontaneously generated stories of learning disabled and normally achieving students. *Journal of Speech and Hearing Disorders, 51,* 8–23.

Roth, F.P., & Spekman, N.J. (1989a) Higher-order language processes and reading disabilities. In A.G. Kamhi & H.W. Catts (Eds.), *Reading disabilities: A developmental perspective.* Boston: College Hill Press.

Roth, F.P., & Spekman, N.J. (1989b). The oral syntactic proficiency of learning disabled students: A spontaneous story sampling analysis. *Journal of Speech and Hearing Research, 32,* 67–77.

Rourke, B.P. (1983). Reading and spelling disabilities: A developmental neuropsychological perspective. In U. Kirk (Ed.), *Neuropsychology of language, reading and spelling.* New York: Academic Press.

Rourke, B.P. (1985). Overview of learning disability subtypes. In B.P. Rourke (Ed.), *Neuropsychology of learning disabilities.* New York: The Guilford Press.

Rourke, B.P., & Czudner, G. (1972). Age differences in auditory reaction time of "brain-damaged" and normal children under regular and irregular preparatory interval conditions. *Journal of Experimental Clinical Psychology, 14,* 372–378.

Rourke, B.P., & Finlayson, M.A.J. (1978). Neuropsychological significance of variations in patterns of academic performance: Verbal and visual-spatial abilities. *Journal of Abnormal Child Psychology, 6,* 121–133.

Rourke, B.P., & Fisk, J.L. (1981). Socio-emotional disturbances of learning disabled children: The role of central processing deficits. *Bulletin of the Orton Society, 31,* 77–88.

Rourke, B.P., Fisk, J.L., & Strang, J.D. (1986). *Neuropsychological assessment of children: A treatment-oriented approach.* New York: The Guilford Press.

Rowe, M.B. (1987). Wait time: Slowing down may be a way of speeding up. *American Education, 11,* 81–97.

Rubin, A. (1980). A theoretical taxonomy of the differences between oral and written language. In R.J. Spiro, B.C. Bruce, & W.F. Brewer (Eds.), *Theoretical issues in reading comprehension.* Hillsdale, NJ: Lawrence Erlbaum Associates.

Rubin, D.L. (1987). Divergence and convergence between oral and written communication. *Topics in Language Disorders, 7,* 1–18.

Rubin, H., & Liberman, I. (1983). Exploring the oral and written language errors made by language disabled children. *Annals of Dyslexia, 33, 111–120.*

Rudel, R.G. (1988). Disorders of attention. In R.G. Rudel, J.M. Holmes, & J.R. Pardel (Eds.), *Assessment of developmental learning disorders.* New York: Basic Books.

Rueckl, J.G., & Oden, G.C. (1986). The integration of contextual and featural information during word identification. *Journal of Memory and Language, 25,* 445–460.

Rumelhart, D.E. (1977a). *Introduction to human information processing.* New York: John Wiley & Sons.

Rumelhart, D.E. (1977b). Understanding and summarizing brief stories. In D. LaBerge & S.J. Samuels (Eds.), *Basic processes in reading: Perception and comprehension.* Hillsdale, NJ: Lawrence Erlbaum Associates.

Rumelhart, D.E., & McClelland, J.L. (1982). An interactive activation model of context effects in letter perception: Part 2. The contextual enhancement effect and some tests and extensions of the model. *Psychological Review, 89,* 60–94.

Russell, L.H. (1981). Legal and philosophical considerations in service delivery. In A. Gerber & D.N. Bryen, *Language and learning disabilities* (pp. 219–247). Baltimore: University Park Press.

Rutter, M. (1984). Issues and prospects in developmental neuropsychiatry. In M. Rutter (Ed.), *Developmental neuropsychiatry.* Edinburgh: Churchill Livingston.

Rutter, M., Chadwick, O., & Schaffer, D. (1983). Head injury. In M. Rutter (Ed.), *Developmental neuropsychiatry.* New York: Guilford Press.

Ryan, E. (1980). Metalinguistic development and reading. In F.B. Murray (Ed.), *Language awareness and reading.* Newark, DE: International Reading Association.

Ryan, E.B., Short, E., & Weed, K.A. (1986). The role of cognitive strategy training in improving the academic performance of learning disabled children. *Journal of Speech and Hearing Disorders, 19,* 521–529.

Sabatino, D.A., Miller, P.F., & Schmidt, W. (1981). Can intelligence be modified through cognitive training? *Journal of Special Education, 2,* 125–144.

Sachs, J., & Truswell, L. (1978). Comprehension of two-word instructions by children in the one-word stage. *Journal of Child Language, 5,* 17–24.

Sailor, W., Anderson, J.L., Halveson, A.T., Doering, K., Filler, J., & Goetz, L. (1989). *The comprehensive local school: Regular education for all students with disabilities.* Baltimore: Paul H. Brookes Publishing Co.

Samuels, S.J. (1987a). Factors that influence listening and reading comprehension. In R. Horowitz & S.J. Samuels (Eds.), *Comprehending oral and written language.* San Diego: Academic Press.

Samuels, S.J. (1987b). Information processing abilities and reading. *Journal of Learning Disabilities, 20,* 18–22.

Sanders, M. (1979). *Clinical assessment of learning problems.* Boston: Allyn & Bacon Inc.

Sanders, N.M. (1973). Classroom questions: What kinds? In G.D. Spache & E.B. Spache (Eds.), *Reading in the elementary schools* (3rd ed.). Boston: Allyn & Bacon.

Sandman, C.A., & Wilhardt, L. (1988). Performance of nondisabled adults and adults with learning disabilities on a computerized multiphasic cognitive memory battery. *Journal of Learning Disabilities, 21,* 179–185.

Santos, O.B. (1989). Language skills and cognitive processes related to poor reading comprehension performance. *Journal of Learning Disabilities, 22,* 131–133.

Satz, P. (1977). Laterality tests: An inferential problem. *Cortex, 13,* 208–212.

Satz, P., & Morris, R. (1981). Learning disability subtypes: A review. In F.J. Pirozzolo & M.C. Wittrock (Eds.), *Neuropsychological and cognitive processes in reading.* New York: Academic Press.

Satz, P., Rardin, D., & Ross, J.R. (1971). An evaluation of a theory of specific dyslexia. *Child Development, 42,* 2002–2021.

Savage-Rumbaugh, S. (1987). Communication, symbolic communication and language: A reply to Seidenberg and Petitto. *Journal of Experimental Psychology: General, 116,* 1–5.

Savage-Rumbaugh, S., MacDonald, K., Sevcik, R.A., Hopkins, W.D.W., & Rupert, E. (1986). Spontaneous symbol acquisition and communicative use by pygmy chimpanzees (*Panpaniscus*). *Journal of Experimental Psychology: General, 115,* 211–235.

Sawyer, D.J. (1985). Language problems observed in poor readers. In C.S. Simon (Ed.), *Communication skills and classroom success.* San Diego: College Hill Press.

Schacter, D.L., & Graf, P. (1986). Effects of elaborative processing on implicit and explicit memory for new associations. *Journal of Experimental Psychology: Learning, Memory, and Cognition, 12,* 432–444.

Schank, R., & Abelson, R. (1977). *Scripts, plans, goals, and understanding.* Hillsdale, NJ: Lawrence Erlbaum Associates.

Schlesinger, I.M. (1971). Relational concepts underlying language. In R.L. Schiefelbusch & L.L. Lloyd (Eds.), *Language perspectives: Acquisition, retardation, and intervention*. Baltimore: University Park Press.

Schneider, W. (1985). Developmental trends in the metamemory-memory behavior relationship: An integrative review. In D.L. Forrest-Pressley, G.H., MacKinnon, & T.G. Waller (Eds.), *Metacognition, cognition, and human performance* (Vol. I), Orlando, FL: Academic Press.

Schory, M.E. (1990). Whole language and the speech-language pathologist. *Language, Speech, and Hearing Services in Schools, 21,* 206–211.

Schuele, M., & van Kleeck, A. (1987). Precursors to literacy: Assessment and intervention. *Topics in Language Disorders, 7,* 32–44.

Schumaker, J.B., & Deshler, D.D. (1984). Setting demand variables: A major factor in program planning for the LD adolescent. *Topics in Language Disorders, 4,* 22–40.

Schumaker, J.B., Deshler, D.D., Alley, G.R., Warner, M.M., & Denton, P.H. (1982). Multipass: A learning strategy for improving reading comprehension. *Learning Disabilities Quarterly, 5,* 295–304.

Schumaker, J.B., Deshler, D.D., & Ellis, E.S. (1986). Intervention issues related to the education of LD adolescents. In J.K. Torgeson & B.Y.L. Wong (Eds.), *Psychological and educational perspectives on learning disabilities*. Orlando, FL: Academic Press.

Schunk, D.H. (1986). Verbalization and children's self-regulating behavior. *Contemporary Educational Psychology, 11,* 347–369.

Schwabe, A.M., Olswang, L.B., & Kriegsmann, E. (1986). Requests for information: Linguistic, cognitive, pragmatic, and environmental variables. *Language, Speech and Hearing Services in Schools, 17,* 38–55.

Schworm, R.W., & Birnbaum, R. (1989). Symptom expression is hyperactive children. *Journal of Learning Disabilities, 22,* 35–40.

Scinto, L.F.M. (1986). *Written language and psychological development*. Orlando, FL: Academic Press.

Scott, C.M. (1988a). A perspective on the evaluation of school children's narratives. *Language, Speech and Hearing Services in Schools, 19,* 67–79.

Scott, C.M. (1988b). Spoken and written syntax. In M.A. Nippold (Ed.), *Later language development: Ages nine through nineteen*. Boston: College Hill Press.

Scott, C.M. (1989). Problem writers: Nature, assessment, and intervention. In A.G. Kamhi & H.V. Catts (Eds.), *Reading disabilities: A developmental perspective*. Boston: College Hill Press.

Seidenberg, M.S., & Petitto, L.A. (1979). Signing behavior in apes: A critical review. *Cognition, 2,* 177–215.

Seidenberg, M.S., & Petitto, L.A. (1987). Communication, symbolic communication and language: Comment on Savage-Rumbaugh, McDonald, Sevcik, Hopkins and Rupert. (1986). *Journal of Experimental Psychology: General, 116,* 279–287.

Seidenberg, P.L. (1988). Cognitive and academic instructional intervention for learning disabled adolescents. *Topics in Language Disorders, 8,* 58–71.

Seidenberg, P.L., & Bernstein, D.K. (1986). The comprehension of similes and metaphors by learning-disabled and nonlearning-disabled children. *Language Speech and Hearing Services in Schools, 17,* 219–230.

Semel, E.M., & Wiig, E.H. (1975). Comprehension of syntactic structures and critical verbal elements by children with learning disabilities. *Journal of Learning Disabilities, 8,* 53–58.

Semel, E.M., & Wiig, E.H. (1980). *Clinical evaluation of language functions*. Columbus, OH: Charles E. Merrill.

Senf, G.M. (1972). *An information integration theory and its application to normal reading acquisition and reading disability*. Presentation to the Leadership Training Institute in Learning Disabilities, Tucson, AZ (ERIC Document Reproduction Service No. ED127584).

Seymour, P.H.K., & Porpodas, C.D. (1980). Lexical and non-lexical processing of spelling in dyslexia. In U. Frith (Ed.), *Cognitive processes in spelling*. London: Academic Press.

Shaffer, D., O'Connor, P.A., Shafer, S., & Prupis, S. (1984). Neurological "soft signs": their origins and significance for behaviors. In M. Rutter (Ed.), *Developmental neuropsychiatry*. Edinburgh: Churchill Livingstone.

Shankweiler, D., & Liberman, I.Y. (1972). Misreading: A search for causes. In J.F. Kavanaugh & I.G. Mattingly (Eds.), *Language by ear and by eye: The relationship between speech and reading*. Cambridge, MA: The M.I.T. Press.

Shapiro, K.L., Ogden, N., & Lind-Blad, F. (1990). Temporal processing in dyslexia. *Journal of Learning Disabilities, 23,* 99–107.

Sharan, S. (1980). Cooperative learning in small groups: Recent methods and effects on achievement, attitudes, and ethnic relations. *Review of Educational Research, 50,* 241–272.

Share, D.L., Jorm, A.F.A, MacLean, R., & Matthews, R. (1984). Sources of individual differences in reading acquisition. *Journal of Educational Psychology, 76,* 1309–1324.

Shatz, M. (1982). On mechanisms of language acquisition: Can features of the communicative environment account for development? In E. Wanner & L.R. Gleitman (Eds.), *Language acquisition: The state of the art*. Cambridge, England: Cambridge University Press.

Shatz, M., Hoff-Ginsberg, E., & Maciver, D. (1989). Induction and the acquisition of English auxiliaries: The effect of differentially enriched input. *Journal of Child Language, 16,* 121–140.

Shaughnessy, M.P. (1977). *Errors and expectations: A guide for the teacher of basic writing*. New York: Oxford University Press.

Shaywitz, S.E., Escobar, M.D., Shaywitz, B.A., Fletcher, J.M., & Makuch, R. (1992). Evidence that dyslexia may represent the lower tail of a normal distribution of reading disability. *New England Journal of Medicine, 326,* 145–151.

Shaywitz, S.E., & Shaywitz, B.A. (1988). Attention deficit disorder: Current perspectives. In J.F. Kavanaugh & T.J. Truss, Jr. (Eds.), *Learning disabilities: Proceedings of the National Conference*. Parkton, MA: York Press.

Shaywitz, S.E., & Shaywitz, B.A. (1991). Introduction to the special series on attention deficit disorders. *Journal of Learning Disabilities, 24,* 68–71.

Sherman, J.C., & Lust, B. (1988). *Children are in control*. Paper presented at the Boston University Conference on Language Development, Boston.

Shiffrin, R.M., & Schneider, W. (1984). Automatic and controlled processing revisited. *Psychological Review, 91,* 269–276.

Shilo, V. (1979). *Memory processing in learning disabled children*. Unpublished doctoral dissertation, Graduate School and University Center, City University of New York.

Shilo, V. (1981). *Word associations in learning disabled children*. Unpublished master's thesis, Emerson College, Boston.

Shinn-Streiker, T. (1986). Patterns of cognitive style in normal and handicapped children. *Journal of Learning Disabilities, 19,* 572–576.

Short, E.J., & Ryan, E.B. (1984). Metacognitive differences between skilled and less skilled readers: Remediating deficits through story grammar and attributional training. *Journal of Educational Psychology, 76,* 225–235.

Shulman, B. (1985). *Test of Pragmatic Skills*. Tucson, AZ: Communication Skill Builders.

Shuy, R.W. (1981). A holistic view of language. *Research in the Teaching of English, 15,* 101–111.

Shuy, R.W. (1988). Identifying dimensions of classroom language. In J.L. Green & J.O. Harker (Eds.), *Multiple perspective analyses of classroom discourse*. Norwood, NJ: Ablex Publ. Corp.

Siegel, L.S., & Linder, B.A. (1984). Short-term memory processes in children with reading and arithmetic learning disabilities. *Developmental Psychology, 20,* 200–207.

Siegel, L.S., & Ryan, E.B. (1984). Reading disability as a language disorder. *Remedial and Special Education (RASE), 5,* 28–33.

Siegel, L.S., & Ryan, E.B. (1988). Development of grammatical-sensitivity, phonological, and short-term memory skills in normally achieving and learning disabled children. *Developmental Psychology, 24,* 28–37.

Silliman, E.R. (1984). Interactional competencies in the instructional context: The role of teaching discourse in learning. In G.P. Wallach & K.G. Butler (Eds.), *Language learning disabilities in school-age children*. Baltimore: Williams & Wilkins.

Silliman, E.R., & Lamanna, M.L. (1986). Interactional dynamics of turn disruption: Group and individual effects. *Topics in Language Disorders, 6,* 28–43.

Silva, P.A., McGee, R., & Williams, S.M. (1983). Developmental language delay from three to seven years and its significance for low intelligence and reading difficulties at age seven. *Developmental Medicine and Child Neurology, 25,* 783–793.

Silver, L.B. (1981). The relationship between learning disabilities, hyperactivity, distractibility and behavior problems. A clinical analysis. *Journal of the American Academy of Child Psychiatry, 20,* 385–397.

Silver, L.B. (1987). The "magic cure": A review of current controversial approaches for treating learning disabilities. *Journal of Learning Disabilities, 20,* 498–504.

Silverstein, S. (1974). *Where the sidewalk ends*. New York: Harper & Row.

Simon, C.S. (1979). *Communicative competence: A functional-pragmatic approach to language therapy*. Tucson, AZ: Communication Skill Builders.

Simon, C.S. (1980). *Suggested strategies for a functional-pragmatic approach to language therapy*. Tucson, AZ: Communication Skill Builders.

Simon, C.S. (1984). Functional-pragmatic evaluation of communication skills in school-aged children. *Language, Speech and Hearing Services in Schools, 15,* 83–98.

Simon, C.S. (1985). The language-learning disabled student: Description and therapy implications. In C.S. Simon (Ed.), *Communication skills and classroom success: Therapy methodologies for language-learning disabled students*. San Diego: College-Hill Press.

Simon, C.S. (1986). *Evaluating communicative competence: A functional-pragmatic procedure*. Tucson, AZ: Communication Skill Builders.

Simon, C.S. (1987). Out of the broom closet and into the classroom: The emerging SLP. *Journal of Childhood Communication Disorders, 11,* 41–66.

Simon, C.S. (1989). *Classroom Communication Screening Procedure for Early Adolescents: A handbook for assessment and intervention*. Tempe, AZ: Communi-Cog Publications.

Simon, H.A. (1972). On the development of the processor. In S. Farnham-Diggory (Ed.), *Information processing in children*. New York: Academic Press.

Sinatra, R. (1989). Verbal/visual processing for males disabled in print acquisition. *Journal of Learning Disabilities, 20,* 69–71.

Sinclair, J.M. (1985). On the integration of linguistic description. In T.A. van Dijk (Ed.), *Handbook of discourse analysis, Vol. 2: Dimensions of discourses*. London: Academic Press.

Sinclair, R.L., & Ghory, W.J. (1987). Becoming marginal. In H.T. Trueba (Ed.), *Success or failure: Learning and the language minority student*. Cambridge, MA: Newbury House.

Sinclair-de Zwart, H. (1973). Language acquisition and cognitive development. In T.E. Moore (Ed.), *Cognitive development and the acquisition of language*. New York: Academic Press.

Sipes, S., & Engle, R.W. (1986). Echoic memory processes in good and poor readers. *Journal of Experimental Psychology: Learning, Memory and Cognition, 12*, 402–412.

Skinner, B.F. (1957). *Verbal behavior*. New York: Appleton-Century-Crofts.

Slavin, R.E. (1983). *Cooperative learning*. New York: Longman.

Slavin, R.E. (1985). An introduction to cooperative learning. In R. Slavin, S. Sharan, S. Kagan, R.H. Lazarowitz, C. Webb, & R. Schmuck (Eds.), *Learning to cooperate, cooperating to learn*. New York: Plenum Press.

Slobin, D.I. (1982). Universal and particular in the acquisition of language. In E. Wanner & L.R. Gleitman (Eds.), *Language acquisition: The state of the art*. Cambridge, England: Cambridge University Press.

Smith, F. (1973). *Psycholinguistics and reading*. New York: Holt, Rinehart & Winston, Inc.

Smith, F. (1982). *Writing and the writer*. New York: Holt, Rinehart & Winston, Inc.

Snider, V.E. (1989). Reading comprehension performance of adolescents with learning disabilities. *Learning Disability Quarterly, 12*, 87–96.

Snow, C., & Ferguson, C. (1977). *Talking to children: Language input and acquisition*. Cambridge, England: Cambridge University Press.

Snow, C., Midkiff-Borunda, S., Small, A., & Proctor, A. (1984). Therapy as social interaction: Analyzing the contexts for language remediation. *Topics in Language Disorders, 4*, 72–85.

Snow, C.E. (1981). Social interaction and language acquisition. In P.S. Dale & D. Ingram (Eds.), *Child language: An international perspective*. Baltimore: University Park Press.

Snyder, L.S., & Downey, D.M. (1991). The language-reading relationship in normal and reading-disabled children. *Journal of Speech and Hearing Research, 34*, 129–140.

Solso, R.L. (1974). Memory and the efficacy of cues or "yes, I know!" vs. "why didn't I think of that?" In R.L. Solso (Ed.), *Theories of cognitive psychology: The Loyola symposium*. Hillsdale, NJ: Lawrence Erlbaum Associates.

Spear, L.C., & Sternberg, R.J. (1986). An information-processing framework for understanding reading disability. In S.J. Ceci (Ed.), *Handbook of cognitive, social, and neuropsychological aspects of learning disabilities*. Hillsdale, NJ: Lawrence Erlbaum Associates.

Speece, D.L. (1993). Broadening the scope of classification research: Conceptual and ecological perspectives. In G.R. Lyon, D.B. Gray, J.F. Kavanagh, & N. Krasnegor (Eds.), *Better understanding learning disabilities: New views from research and their implications for education and public policies*. Baltimore: Paul H. Brookes Publishing Co.

Spekman, N.J. (1981). Dyadic verbal communication abilities of learning disabled and normally achieving fourth- and fifth-grade boys. *Learning Disability Quarterly, 4*, 139–151.

Spiro, R.J. (1980). Constructive processes in prose comprehension and recall. In R.J. Spiro, B.D. Bruce, & W.F. Brewer (Eds.), *Theoretical issues in reading comprehension*. Hillsdale, NJ: Lawrence Erlbaum Associates.

Spreen, O., & Haaf, R.G. (1986). Empirically derived learning disability subtypes: A replication attempt and longitudinal patterns over 15 years. *Journal of Learning Disabilities, 19*, 170–180.

Sroufe, L.A., Sonies, B.C., West, W.D., & Wright, F.S (1973). Anticipatory heart rate deceleration and reaction time in children with and without referral for learning disabilities. *Child Development, 44*, 267–273.

Staats, A.W., & Staats, C.K. (1966). *Complex human behavior*. New York: Holt, Rinehart, and Winston.

Stainback, S., & Stainback, W. (1989). Integration of students with mild and moderate handicaps. In D.K. Lipsky & A. Gartner (Eds.), *Beyond separate education: Quality education for all* (pp. 41–52). Baltimore: Paul H. Brookes Publishing Co.

Stankov, L. (1983). Attention and intelligence. *Journal of Educational Psychology, 75*, 471–490.

Stanovich, K.E. (1984). The interactive-compensatory model of reading: A confluence of developmental, experimental, and educational psychology. *RASE (Remedial and Special Education), 5*, 11–19.

Stanovich, K.E. (1986). Matthew effects in reading: Some consequences of individual differences in the acquisition of literacy. *Reading Research Quarterly, 21*, 360–407.

Stanovich, K.E. (1988). Explaining the differences between the dyslexic and the garden variety poor reader: The phonological-core variable-difference model. *Journal of Learning Disabilities, 21*, 590–604.

Stanovich, K.E. (1993). The construct validity of discrepancy definitions of reading disability. In G.R. Lyon, D.B. Gray, J.F. Kavanagh, & N. Krasnegor (Eds.), *Better understanding learning disabilities: New views from research and their implications for education and public policies*. Baltimore: Paul H. Brookes Publishing Co.

Stark, R.E., Bernstein, L.E., Condino, R., Bender, M., Tallal, P., & Catts, H. (1984). Four year follow-up study of language impaired children. *Annals of Dyslexia, 34*, 49–68.

Stein, C.L., Cairns, H.S., & Zurif, E.B. (1984). Sentence comprehension limitations related to syntactic deficits in reading disabled children. *Applied Psycholinguistics, 5*, 305–322.

Stein, N., & Glenn, C. (1979). An analysis of story comprehension in elementary school children. In R.O. Freedle (Ed.), *New directions in discourse processing* (Vol. II). Norwood, NJ: Ablex Publ. Corp.

Stein, P.A., & Hoover, J.H. (1989). Manifest anxiety in children with learning disabilities. *Journal of Learning Disabilities, 22,* 66–71.

Stellern, J. Collins, J., & Bayne, M. (1987). A dual-task investigation of language-spatial lateralization. *Journal of Learning Disabilities, 20,* 551–556.

Stellern, J. Collins, J., Cassairt, A., & Gutierrez, R. (1986). Interference asymmetry involving concurrent tasks performed by Native American Indian students. *Developmental Neuropsychology, 2,* 241–255.

Sternberg, R.J., & Wagner, R.K. (1982). Automatization failure in learning disabilities. *Topics in Learning and Learning Disabilities, 2,* 1–11.

Stevens, R.J. (1988). Effects of strategy training on the identification of the main ideas of expository passages. *Journal of Educational Psychology, 80,* 21–26.

Stewart, S.R. (1985). Development of written language proficiency: Methods for teaching text structure. In C.S. Simon (Ed.), *Communication skills and classroom success: Therapy methodologies for language-learning disabled students.* San Diego: College Hill Press.

Stewig, J. (1990). *Read to write: Using children's literature as a springboard for teaching writing* (3rd ed.). Katonah, NY: R.C. Owen.

Stickler, K.R. (1987). *Guide to analysis of language transcripts.* Eau Claire, WI: Thinking Publications.

Strand, K.E. (1982). *The development of idiom comprehension in language disordered children.* Paper presented at the Symposium on Research in Child Language Disorders, Madison, WI.

Strauss, A., & Lehtinen, L. (1947). *Psychopathology and education of the brain-injured child.* New York: Grune & Stratton.

Striffler, N., & Willig, S. (1981). *The communication screen; A preschool speech-language screening tool.* Tucson, AZ; Communication Skill Builders.

Strominger, A.Z., & Bashir, A.S. (1977). *A nine-year follow-up of language-disordered children.* Paper presented at the Annual Convention of the American Speech-Language-Hearing Association, Chicago.

Studdert-Kennedy, M. (1989). *A developmental approach to the role of speech perception in child language development.* Paper presented at a Symposium on Central Auditory Perception in Language Processing, Temple University, Philadelphia.

Studdert-Kennedy, M., Liberman, A.M., Harris, K.S., & Cooper, F.S. (1970). Motor theory in speech perception: A reply to Lane's critical review. *Psychological Review, 77,* 234–249.

Suiter, M.L., & Potter, R.E. (1978). The effects of paradigmatic organization on recall. *Journal of Learning Disabilities, 11,* 247–250.

Sulzby, E., Teale, W.H., & Kamberlis, G. (1989). Emergent writing in the classroom: Home and school connections. In D.S. Strickland & L.M. Morrow (Eds.), *Emergent literacy: Young children learn to read and write.* Newark, DE: International Reading Association.

Swanson, H.L. (1982). Strategies and constraints—a commentary. *Topics in Learning and Learning Disabilities, 2,* 79–81.

Swanson, H.L. (1983). A study of nonstrategic linguistic coding in visual recall of learning disabled readers. *Journal of Learning Disabilities, 16,* 209–216.

Swanson, H.L. (1984a). Effect of cognitive effort on learning disabled and nondisabled readers' recall. *Journal of Learning Disabilities, 17,* 67–74.

Swanson, H.L. (1984b). Semantic and visual memory codes in learning disabled readers. *Journal of Experimental Child Psychology, 37,* 124–140.

Swanson, H.L. (1985). Assessing learning disabled children's intellectual performance: An information processing perspective. In K. Gadow (Ed.), *Advances in learning and behavior disabilities* (Vol. 4). Greenwich, CT: JAI Press.

Swanson, H.L. (1986). Learning disabled readers' verbal coding difficulties: A problem of storage or retrieval? *Learning Disabilities Research, 1,* 73–82.

Swanson, H.L. (1987). Information processing theory and learning disabilities: A commentary and future perspective. *Journal of Learning Disabilities, 20,* 155–166.

Swanson, H.L. (1988a). Memory subtypes in learning disabled readers. *Learning Disability Quarterly, 11,* 342–357.

Swanson, H.L. (1988b). Toward a metatheory of learning disabilities. *Journal of Learning Disabilities, 21,* 196–209.

Swanson, H.L. (1989). Strategy instruction: Overview of principles and procedures for effective use. *Learning Disability Quarterly, 12,* 3–15.

Swanson, H.L. (1993). Learning disabilities from the perspective of cognitive psychology. In G.R. Lyon, D.B. Gray, J.F. Kavanagh, & N. Krasnegor (Eds.). *Better understanding learning disabilities: New views from research and their implications for education and public policies.* Baltimore: Paul H. Brookes Publishing Co.

Swanson, H.L., Cochran, K.F., & Ewers, C.A. (1990). Can learning disabilities be determined from working memory performance? *Journal of Learning Disabilities, 23,* 59–68.

Swanson, H.L., & Obrzut, J.E. (1985). Learning disabled readers' recall as a function of distinctive encoding, hemispheric processing and selective attention. *Journal of Learning Disabilities, 18,* 409–418.

Swanson, H.L., & Rathgeber, A.J. (1986). The effects of organizational dimensions on learning disabled readers' recall. *Journal of Educational Research, 79,* 155–162.

Tallal, P., & Piercy, M. (1973). Developmental aphasia: Impaired rate of nonverbal processing as a function of sensory modality. *Neuropsychologia, 11*, 389–398.

Tallal, P., & Piercy, M. (1974). Developmental aphasia: Rate of auditory processing and selective impairment of consonant perception. *Neuropsychologia, 12*, 83–93.

Tallal, P., & Piercy, M. (1978). Defects of auditory perception in children with developmental dysphasia. In M.A. Wyke (Ed.), *Developmental dysphasia*. New York: Academic Press.

Tallal, P., Stark, R., Kallman, C., & Mellits, D. (1981). A reexamination of some nonverbal perceptual abilities of language-impaired and normal children as a function of age and sensory modality. *Journal of Speech and Hearing Research, 24*, 351–357.

Tannen, D. (1979). What's in a frame? Surface evidence for underlying expectations. In R.O. Freedle (Ed.), *New directions in discourse processings* (Vol. II). Norwood, NJ: Ablex Publ. Corp.

Tannen, D. (1982). Oral and literate strategies in spoken and written discourse. *Language, 58*, 1–20.

Tarver, S.G., Hallahan, D.P., Kaufman, J.M., & Ball, D.W. (1976). Verbal rehearsal and selective attention in children with learning disabilities: A developmental lag. *Journal of Experimental Child Psychology, 22*, 375–385.

Tattersall, S., & Creaghead, N. (1985). A comparison of communication at home and school. In D.N. Ripich & F.M. Spinelli (Eds.), *School discourse problems*. San Diego: College Hill Press.

Teale, W.H., & Sulzby, E. (1986). Introduction: Emergent literacy as a perspective for examining how young children become writers and readers. In W.H. Teale & E. Sulzby (Eds.), *Emergent literacy*. Norwood, NJ: Ablex.

Teale, W.H., & Sulzby, E. (1989). Emergent literacy: New perspectives. In D.S. Strickland & L.M. Morrow (Eds.), *Emerging literacy: Young children learn to read and write*. Newark, DE: International Reading Association.

Tenenberg, M. (1988). Diagramming question cycle sequences. In J.L. Green & J.O. Harker (Eds.), *Multiple perspective analyses of classroom discourse*. Norwood, NJ: Ablex Publ. Co.

Terrell, B.Y. (1985). Learning the rules of the game: Discourse skills in early childhood. In D.N. Ripich & F.M. Spinelli (Eds.), *School discourse problems*. San Diego: College Hill Press.

Tharp, R.G., & Gallimore, R. (1988). *Rousing minds to life: Teaching, learning and schooling in social context*. Cambridge, England: Cambridge University Press.

Thomas, C. Englert, C.S., & Morsinck, C. (1984). Modifying the classroom program in language. In C.V. Morsinck (Ed.), *Teaching special needs students in regular classrooms*. Boston: Little, Brown.

Thorndyke, P.W. (1977). Cognitive structures in comprehension and memory of narrative discourse. *Cognitive Psychology, 9*, 77–110.

Tomblin, J.B. (1984). Specific abilities approach: An evaluation and an alternative method. In W.H. Perkins (Ed.), *Language handicaps in children*. New York: Thieme-Stratton, Inc.

Tomblin, J.B. (1989). Familial concentration of developmental language impairment. *Journal of Speech and Hearing Disorders, 54*, 287–295.

Tomblin, J.B. (1991). Examining the cause of specific language impairment. *Language, Speech, and Hearing Services in Schools, 22*, 69–74.

Torgeson, J.K. (1977). Memorization processes in reading disabled children. *Journal of Educational Psychology, 69*, 571–578.

Torgeson, J.K. (1979). Factors related to poor performance on rote memory tasks in reading disabled children. *Learning Disabilities Quarterly, 2*, 17–23.

Torgeson, J.K. (1982). The learning disabled child as an inactive learner: Educational implications. *Topics in Learning and Learning Disabilities, 2*, 45–52.

Torgeson, J.K. (1986). Learning disabilities theory: Its current state and future prospects. *Journal of Learning Disabilities, 19*, 399–407.

Torgeson, J.K. (1988a). Applied research and metatheory in the context of contemporary cognitive theory. *Journal of Learning Disabilities, 21*, 271–274.

Torgeson, J.K. (1988b). Studies of learning disabled children who perform poorly on memory span tasks. *Journal of Learning Disabilities, 21*, 605–612.

Torgeson, J.K. (1993). Variations on theory in learning disabilities. In G.R. Lyon, D.B. Gray, J.F. Kavanagh, & N. Krasnegor (Eds.), *Better understanding learning disabilities: New views from research and their implications for education and public policies*. Baltimore: Paul H. Brookes Publishing Co.

Torgeson, J.K., & Greenstein, J.J. (1982). Why do some learning disabled children have poor memories? Does it make a difference? *Topics in Learning and Learning Disabilities, 2*, 54–61.

Torgeson, J.K., & Houck, G. (1980). Processing deficiencies in learning disabled children who perform poorly on the digit span task. *Journal of Educational Psychology, 72*, 141–160.

Tough, J. (1981). *Talk for teaching and learning*. Portsmouth, NH: Heinemann.

Treiman, R., & Baron, J. (1983). Individual differences in spelling: The Phoenician-Chinese distinction. *Topics in Learning and Learning Disabilities, 3*, 33–40.

Treisman, A.M. (1960). Contextual cues in selective listening. *Quarterly Journal of Experimental Psychology, 12*, 242–248.

Treisman, A.M. (1986). Features and objects in visual processing. *Scientific American, 255*, 114b–125.

Treisman, A.M., & Gelade, G. (1980). A feature-integration theory of attention. *Cognitive Psychology, 12,* 97–136.

Treisman, A.M., & Souther, J. (1985). Search asymmetry: A diagnostic for preattentive processing of separable features. *Journal of Experimental Psychology: General, 114,* 285–310.

Truesdale, S.P. (1990). Whole-body listening: Developing active auditory skills. *Language, Speech, and Hearing Services in Schools, 21,* 183–184.

Tucker, J.A. (1985). Curriculum-based assessment: An introduction. *Exceptional Children, 52,* 199–204.

Tulving, E. (1972). Episodic and semantic memory. In E. Tulving & W. Donaldson (Eds.), *Organization of memory.* New York: Academic Press.

Tulving, E. (1985). How many memory systems are there? *American Psychologist, 40,* 385–398.

Tulving, E. (1986). What kind of hypothesis is the distinction between episodic and semantic memory? *Journal of Experimental Psychology: Learning, Memory, and Cognition, 12,* 307–311.

Tulving, E., Mandler, G., & Baumel, R. (1964). Interaction of two sources of information in tachistoscopic word recognition. *Canadian Journal of Psychology, 18,* 62–71.

Tulving, E., & Thomson, D.M. (1973). Encoding specificity and retrieval processes. *Psychological Review, 80,* 352–373.

Tunmer, W.E., & Cole, P.G. (1985). Learning to read: A metalinguistic act. In C.S. Simon (Ed.), *Communication skills and classroom success: Therapy methodologies for language-learning disabled students.* San Diego: College Hill Press.

Turnure, J., Buium, N., & Thurlow, M. (1976). The effectiveness of interrogatives for promoting verbal elaboration productivity in young children. *Child Development, 47,* 851–855.

Updike, J. (1986). *Roger's version.* New York: Alfred A. Knopf.

van der Wissel, A. (1988). Hampered production of words as a characteristic of school failure. *Journal of Learning Disabilities, 21,* 517–518.

van Dijk, T.A. (1977). Semantic macro-structures and knowledge frames in discourse comprehension. In M.A. Just & P.A. Carpenter (Eds.), *Cognitive processes in comprehension.* Hillsdale, NJ: Lawrence Erlbaum Associates.

van Dijk, T.A. (1985). Semantic discourse analysis. In T.A. van Dijk (Ed.), *Handbook of discourse analysis, Vol. 2: Dimensions of discourse.* London: Academic Press.

van Dijk, T.A. (1987). Episodic models in discourse processing. In R. Horowitz & S.J. Samuels (Eds.), *Comprehending oral and written language.* San Diego: Academic Press, Inc.

van Dijk, T.A., & Kintsch, W. (1983). *Strategies of discourse comprehension.* New York: Academic Press.

Van Dongen, R., & Westby, C.E (1986). Building the narrative mode of thought through children's literature. *Topics in Language Disorders, 7,* 70–83.

Van Kleeck, A. (1984a). Assessment and intervention: Does "meta" matter? In G.P. Wallach & K.G. Butler (Eds.), *Language learning disabilities in school-age children.* Baltimore: Williams & Wilkins.

Van Kleeck, A. (1984b). Metalinguistic skills: Cutting across spoken and written language and problem-solving abilities. In G.P. Wallach & K.G. Butler (Eds.), *Language learning disabilities in school-age children.* Baltimore: Williams & Wilkins.

Van Kleeck, A. (1990). Emergent literacy: Learning about print before learning to read. *Topics in Language Disorders, 10,* 25–45.

Van Kleeck, A., & Richardson, A. (1988). Language delay in the child. In N.J. Lass, L.V. McReynolds, J.R. Northern, & D.E. Yoder (Eds.), *Handbook of speech-language pathology and audiology.* Philadelphia: Brian C. Decker Inc.

Van Kleeck, A., & Schuele, C.M. (1987). Precursors to literacy: Normal development. *Topics in Language Disorders, 7,* 13–31.

Van Riper, C. (1954). *Speech correction: Principles and methods* (3rd ed.). Englewood Cliffs, NJ: Prentice-Hall, Inc.

Vellutino, F. (1977). Alternative conceptualizations of dyslexia: Evidence in support of a verbal deficit hypothesis. *Harvard Educational Review, 47,* 334–354.

Vellutino, F. (1979). *Dyslexia: Theory and research.* Cambridge, MA: The M.I.T. Press.

Vellutino, F.R., & Scanlon, D.M. (1985). Verbal memory in poor and normal readers: Developmental differences in the use of linguistic codes. In D.B. Gray & J.F. Kavanaugh (Eds.), *Biobehavioral measures of dyslexia.* Parkton, MD: York Press.

Vellutino, F.R., & Scanlon, D.M. (1987). Linguistic coding and metalinguistic awareness: Their relationship to verbal memory and code acquisition in poor and normal readers. In D.B. Yaden & S. Templeton (Eds.), *Metalinguistic awareness and beginning literacy.* Portsmouth, NH: Heinemann.

Vetter, D.K. (1982). Language disorders and schooling. *Topics in Language Disorders, 2,* 13–19.

Vogel, S.A. (1975). *Syntactic abilities in normal and dyslexic children.* Baltimore: University Park Press.

Vygotsky, L. (1962). *Thought and language.* Cambridge, MA: The M.I.T. Press.

Wallach, G.P. (1977). *Reading disabilities and language.* Paper presented at the Northeast Conference of the American Speech and Hearing Association, Boston.

Wallach, G.P. (1984). Later language learning: Syntactic structures and strategies. In G.P. Wallach & K.G. Butler (Eds.), *Language learning disabilities in school-age children.* Baltimore: Williams & Wilkins.

Wallach, G.P. (1990). Magic buries Celtics: Looking for broader interpretations of language learning and literacy. *Topics in Language Disorders, 10,* 63–80.

Wallach, G.P., & Goldsmith, S.C. (1975). *Sentence processing in normal and learning disabled children: A look at auditory–*

verbal and visual–verbal channels. Paper presented at the American Speech-Language-Hearing Association Convention, Washington, DC.

Wallach, G.P., & Miller, L. (1988). *Language intervention and academic success*. Boston: College Hill Publications.

Wang, M.C. (1989). Adaptive instruction: An alternative for accommodating student diversity through the curriculum. In D.K. Lipsky & A. Gartner (Eds.), *Beyond separate education: Quality education for all* (pp. 99–119). Baltimore: Paul H. Brookes Publishing Co.

Wang, M.C., & Baker, E.T. (1985–1986). Mainstreaming programs: Design features and effects. *Journal of Special Education, 19*, 503–521.

Wang, M.C., & Birch, J.W. (1984). Effective special education in regular classes. *Exceptional Children, 50*, 391–398.

Wang, M.C., & Reynolds, M.C. (1985). Avoiding the "Catch 22" in special education reform. *Exceptional Children, 51*, 497–502.

Wanner, E., & Gleitman, L.R. (1982). *Language acquisition: The state of the art*. Cambridge, England: Cambridge University Press.

Warren, S.F. (1988). A behavioral approach to language generalization. *Language, Speech and Hearing Services in the Schools, 19*, 292–303.

Warren, S.F., & Kaiser, A.P. (1986). Incidental language teaching: A critical review. *Journal of Speech and Hearing Disorders, 51*, 291–299.

Waryas, C.L., & Stremel-Campbell, K. (1978). Grammatical training for the language-delayed child. In R. Schiefelbusch (Ed.), *Language intervention strategies* (pp. 145–192.) Baltimore: University Park Press.

Weaver, P.A., & Dickinson, D.K. (1982). Scratching below the surface structure: Exploring the usefulness of story grammar. *Discourse Processes, 5*, 225–243.

Webb, N.M. (1985). Student interaction and learning in small groups: A research summary. In R. Slavin, S. Sharan, S. Kagan, R.H. Lazarowitz, C. Webb, & R. Schmuck (Eds.), *Learning to cooperate, cooperating to learn*. New York: Plenum Press.

Wechsler, D. (1949). *Wechsler Intelligence Scale For Children*. New York: The Psychological Corporation.

Wechsler, D. (1955). *Manual for the Wechsler Adult Intelligence Scale*. New York: The Psychological Corporation.

Wechsler, D. (1974). *Wechsler Intelligence Scale for Children–Revised*. New York: The Psychological Corporation.

Weidner, W.E., & Lasky, E.Z. (1976). The interaction of rate and complexity of stimulus on the performance of adult aphasic subjects. *Brain and Language, 3*, 34–40.

Weiner, C.A., & Creighton, J.M. (1987). Documenting and facilitating "school readiness language" in the kindergarten classroom. *Journal of Childhood Communication Disorders, 11*, 125–137.

Weisberg, R.W. (1980). *Memory, thought, and behavior*. New York: Oxford University Press.

Wellman, H.M. (1988). The early development of memory strategies. In F.E. Weinert & M. Perlmutter (Eds.), *Memory development: Universal changes and individual differences*. Hillsdale, NJ: Lawrence Erlbaum Associates.

Werner, H., & Strauss, A.A. (1941). Pathology of the figure-background relationship in the child. *Journal of Abnormal Social Psychology, 36*, 236–248.

Westby, C.E. (1985). Learning to talk—talking to learn: Oral-literate language differences. In C.S. Simon (Ed.), *Communication skills and classroom success: Therapy methodologies for language-learning disabled students*. San Diego: College Hill Press.

Westby, C.E. (1987). *Cultural differences in child socialization: Implications for assessment and intervention*. Paper presented at Temple University, Philadelphia, PA.

Westby, C.E. (1989). Assessing and remediating text comprehension problems. In A.G Kamhi & H.W. Catts (Eds.), *Reading disabilities: A developmental language perspective*. Boston: College Hill Press.

Westby, C.E. (1990). The role of the speech-language pathologist in whole language. *Language, Speech, and Hearing Services in Schools, 21*, 228–237.

Westby, C.E., & Rouse, G.R (1985). Culture in education and the instruction of language learning disabled children. *Topics in Language Disorders, 5*, 15–28.

Westby, C.E., Van Dongen, R., & Maggart, Z. (1989). Assessing narrative competence. *Seminars in Speech and Language, 10*, 63–76.

Wexler, K. (1982). A principle theory for language acquisition. In E. Wanner & L.R. Gleitman (Eds.), *Language acquisition: The state of the art*. Cambridge, England: Cambridge University Press.

Wexler, K., & Chien, Y.C. (1985). *The development of lexical anaphors and pronouns*. Paper presented at the Boston University Conference on Language Development, Boston.

Wexler, K., & Culicover, P. (1980). *Formal principles of language acquisition*. Cambridge, MA: The MIT Press.

White, E.J. (1979). *Dysnomia in the adolescent dyslexic and the developmentally delayed adolescent*. Unpublished doctoral dissertation, Boston University.

Whittlesey, B.W.A., & Brooks, L.B. (1988). Critical influence of particular experiences in the perception of letters, words and phrases. *Memory and Cognition, 16*, 387–399.

Wiederholt, J.L. (1985). *Formal reading inventory*. Austin, TX: PRO-ED.

Wiens, W.J. (1983). Metacognition and the passive learner. *Journal of Learning Disabilities, 16*, 144–149.

Wiig, E.H. (1984). Language disabilities in adolescents: A question of cognitive strategies. *Topics in Language Disorders, 4,* 41–58.

Wiig, E. (1989). *Steps in language competence: Developing metalinguistic strategies.* San Antonio: The Psychological Corporation.

Wiig, E.H., & Becker-Caplan, L. (1984). Linguistic retrieval strategies and word-finding difficulties among children with language disabilities. *Topics in Language Disorders, 4,* 1–18.

Wiig, E.H., Florence, D.P., Kutner, S.M., Sherman, B., & Semel, E.M. (1977). Perception and interpretation of explicit negations by learning disabled children and adolescents. *Perceptual and Motor Skills, 44,* 1251–1257.

Wiig, E.H., Lapointe, C.M., & Semel, E.M. (1977). Relationship among language processing and production abilities of learning disabled adolescents. *Journal of Learning Disabilities, 10,* 292–299.

Wiig, E.H., & Roach, M.A. (1975). Immediate recall of semantically varied "sentences" by learning disabled adolescents. *Perceptual and Motor Skills, 40,* 119–145.

Wiig, E.H., & Secord, W. (1988). *Test of Language Competence—Expanded edition.* San Antonio, TX: The Psychological Corporation.

Wiig, E.H., & Semel, E.M. (1973). Comprehension of linguistic concepts requiring logical operations by learning disabled children. *Journal of Speech and Hearing Research, 16,* 627–636.

Wiig, E.H., & Semel, E.M. (1974). Development of comprehension of logico-grammatical sentences by grade-school children. *Perceptual and Motor Skills, 38,* 171–176.

Wiig, E.H., & Semel, E.M. (1975). Productive language abilities in learning disabled adolescents. *Journal of Learning Disabilities, 8,* 578–586.

Wiig, E.H., & Semel, E.M. (1976). *Language disabilities in children and adolescents.* Columbus, OH: Charles E. Merrill.

Wiig, E.H., & Semel, E.M. (1984). *Language assessment and intervention for the learning disabled.* Columbus, OH: Charles E. Merrill.

Wiig, E.H., Semel, E.M., & Abele, E. (1981). Perception and interpretation of ambiguous sentences by learning disabled twelve-year-olds. *Learning Disabilities Quarterly, 4,* 3–12.

Wiig, E.H., Semel, E.M., & Nystrom, L.A. (1982). Comparison of rapid naming abilities in learning disabled and academically achieving eight-year olds. *Language Speech and Hearing Services in Schools, 13,* 11–23.

Wilkinson, L.C., & Milosky, L.M. (1987). School-age children's metapragmatic knowledge of requests and responses in the classroom. *Topics in Language Disorders, 7,* 61–70.

Will, M. (1986). *Educating students with learning problems—A shared responsibility: A report to the Secretary.* Washington, DC: U.S. Department of Education, Office of Special and Rehabilitative Services.

Will, M. (1989). Foreword. In W. Sailor, J.L. Anderson, A.T. Halvorsen, K. Doering, J. Filler, & L. Goetz, *The comprehensive local school: Regular education for all students with disabilities* (pp. vi–viii). Baltimore: Paul H. Brookes Publishing Co.

Willeford, J.A. (1985). Assessment of central auditory disorders in children. In M.L. Pinheiro & F.E. Musiek (Eds.), *Assessment of central auditory dysfunction: Foundations and clinical correlates.* Baltimore: Williams & Wilkins.

Williams, M.D., & Hollan, J.D. (1982). The process of retrieval from very long-term memory. *Cognitive Science, 5,* 87–119.

Willis, W.G., & Widerstrom, A.H. (1986). Structure and function in prenatal and postnatal neuropsychological development: A dynamic interaction. In J.E. Obrzut & G.W. Hynd (Eds.), *Child neuropsychology: Vol. 1. Theory and research.* Orlando, FL: Academic Press.

Wing, C.S. (1990). A preliminary investigation of generalization to untrained words following two treatments of children's word-finding problems. *Language, Speech, and Hearing Services in Schools, 21,* 151–156.

Wingfield, A., & Byrnes, D.L. (1981). *The psychology of human memory.* New York: Academic Press.

Winograd, T. (1977). A framework for understanding discourse. In M.A. Just & P.A. Carpenter (Eds.), *Cognitive processes in comprehension.* Hillsdale, NJ: Lawrence Erlbaum Associates.

Witelson, S.F. (1976). Abnormal right hemisphere specialization in developmental dyslexia. In R.M. Knights & D.J. Bakker (Eds.), *The neuropsychology of learning disorders: Theoretical approaches.* Baltimore: University Park Press.

Wolf, M. (1982). The word-retrieval process and reading in children and aphasics. In K. Nelson (Ed.), *Children's language* (Vol. 3). Hillsdale, NJ: Lawrence Erlbaum Associates.

Wolf, M. (1984). Naming, reading, and the dyslexias: A longitudinal overview. *Annals of Dyslexia, 34,* 87–115.

Wong, B.Y.L. (1980). Activating the inactive learner: Use of questions/prompts to enhance comprehension and retention of implied information in learning disabled children. *Learning Disability Quarterly, 3,* 29–37.

Wong, B.Y.L. (1982). Understanding learning disabled students' reading problems: Contributions from cognitive psychology. *Topics in Learning and Learning Disabilities, 1,* 43–50.

Wong, B.Y.L. (1985a). Metacognition and learning disabilities. In D.L. Forrest-Pressley, G.E. McKinnon, & T.G. Waller (Eds.), *Metacognition, cognition, and human performance.* Orlando, FL: Academic Press.

Wong, B.Y.L. (1985b). Self-questioning instructional research. *Review of Educational Research, 55,* 227–268.

Wong, B.Y.L. (1986). Problems and issues in the definition of learning disabilities. In J.K. Torgeson & B.Y.L. Wong (Eds.), *Psychological and educational perspectives on learning disabilities.* Orlando, FL: Academic Press, Inc.

Wong, B.Y.L. (1987). How do the effects of metacognitive research impact on the learning disabled individual? *Learning Disabilities Quarterly, 10,* 189–195.

Wong, B.Y.L., & Jones, W. (1982). Increasing metacomprehension in learning disabled and normally achieving students through self-questioning training. *Learning Disabilities Quarterly, 5,* 228–246.

Wong, B.Y.L., & Wilson, M. (1984). Investigating awareness of and teaching passage organization in learning disabled children. *Journal of Learning Disabilities, 17,* 477–482.

Wong, B.Y.L., Wong, R., & Foth, D. (1977). Recall and clustering of verbal materials among normal and poor readers. *Bulletin of the Psychonomic Society, 10,* 375–376.

Woodcock, R. (1973). *Woodcock Reading Mastery Tests.* Circle Pines, MI: American Guidance Service.

Woodcock, R.W., & Johnson, M.B. (1977). *Woodcock-Johnson Psychoeducational Battery.* Hingham, MA: Teaching Resources Corporation.

Woodcock, R., & Johnson, M.B. (1978). *Woodcock-Johnson Psycho-educational Battery: Part 1. Test of cognitive ability.* Hingham, MA: Teaching Resources.

Woody-Ramsey, J., & Miller, P.H. (1988). The facilitation of selective attention in preschoolers. *Child Development, 59,* 1497–1503.

Worden, P., Malmgren, I., & Gabourie, P. (1982). Memory for stories in learning disabled adults. *Journal of Learning Disabilities, 15,* 145–152.

Worden, P.E. (1986). Prose comprehension and recall in disabled learners. In S.J. Ceci (Ed.), *Handbook of cognitive, social and neuropsychological aspects of learning disabilities.* Hillsdale, NJ: Lawrence Erlbaum Associates.

Worden, P.E. (1987). The four M's—Memory strategies, metastrategies, monitoring, and motivation. In S.J. Ceci (Ed.), *Handbook of cognitive, social, and neuropsychological aspects of learning disabilities.* Hillsdale, NJ: Lawrence Erlbaum Associates.

Worden, P.E., & Nakamura, G.V. (1983). Story comprehension and recall in learning disabled vs. normal college students. *Journal of Educational Psychology, 74,* 633–641.

Wren, C.T. (1983). *Language learning disabilities: Diagnosis and remediation.* Rockville, MD: Aspen Systems Corporation.

Yoshinaga-Itano, C., & Downey, D.M. (1986). A hearing-impaired child's acquisition of schemata: something's missing. *Topics in Language Disorders, 7,* 45–57.

Yussen, S.R. (1985). The role of metacognition in contemporary theories of cognitive development. In D.L. Forrest-Pressley, G.E. MacKinnon, & T.G. Waller (Eds.), *Metacognition, cognition, and human performance* (Vol. I). Orlando, FL: Academic Press.

Zachman, L. Barrett, M., Huisingh, R., & Jorgensen, C. (1984). *Test of Problem Solving.* Moline, IL: Linguisystems.

Zigmond, N. (1993). Learning disabilities from an educational perspective. In G.R. Lyon, D.B. Gray, J.F. Kavanagh, & N. Krasnegor (Eds.), *Better understanding learning disabilities: New views from research and their implications for education and public policies.* Baltimore: Paul H. Brookes Publishing Co.

Index

Page numbers followed by f, n, or t indicate figures, footnotes, or tables, respectively.